Imaging in Nephrology

Antonio Granata • Michele Bertolotto
Editors

Imaging in Nephrology

Springer

Editors
Antonio Granata
Department of Nephrology and Dialysis
"Cannizzaro" Emergency Hospital
Catania
Italy

Michele Bertolotto
Department of Radiology
Cattinara Hospital, University of Trieste
Trieste, Italy

ISBN 978-3-030-60792-0 ISBN 978-3-030-60794-4 (eBook)
https://doi.org/10.1007/978-3-030-60794-4

This Springer imprint is published by the registered company Springer Nature Switzerland AG
The registered company address is: Gewerbestrasse 11, 6330 Cham, Switzerland

Thank you

To our wives, Grazia and Rosaria, partners for life, who have always been aware of our passion for medical practice.

To our beloved children, Salvo, Noemi and Sara, secretly wishing them to be able to write even more intriguing pages in their work and life.

Antonio Granata
Michele Bertolotto

Foreword

Since the very beginning of our specialty, we as nephrologists have had trouble looking for a reliable tool not only to show us the functional and anatomical conditions of the kidneys but to also be an easily repeatable exam that would not compromise the patient's well-being.

Serum creatinine can only inform us when filtration function has already been substantially reduced while urinalysis and urinary albumin excretion, though highly informative on some qualitative aspects of the renal conditions, do not completely intercept all types of renal function imbalance (especially on tubular function) and inform us even less on the anatomical kidney changes. On the other hand, renal biopsy, though highly informative on the structural alterations of renal parenchyma, is a not an easily repeatable exam.

In this scenario, the nephrology community has enthusiastically welcomed ultrasound (US) techniques since their first development. Many nephrologists have started to dedicate more and more of their working time to the US techniques, which have undergone incredible technological improvements since their initial discovery.

Nowadays, the application of US techniques in nephrology has increasingly extended to fields of highly sophisticated diagnostics and new interventional therapies, hence requiring highly specialized medical skills, including more and more complex knowledge and experience for the nephrologists and radiologists who are involved in this field.

Presently, Antonio Granata and Michele Bertolotto are the perfect examples of top medical professionals in this field, presenting themselves as ideal candidates for sharing their top level experience with all the medical doctors interested in this exciting field of modern medicine.

Antonio and Michele coauthored this impressive book, where the reader will find everything required for an easy and complete understanding of the several US techniques and countless ways to apply them on the field.

Besides being a precise and detailed description of the presented US techniques, this volume is heavily enriched with high-resolution images to help and fascinate the reader even more.

I enthusiastically accepted to write a short presentation of this book, which I sincerely believe represents a great and useful piece of scientific work. I firmly believe this volume will be highly appreciated by the scientific community and will fascinate any reader who decides to read it. Happy reading!

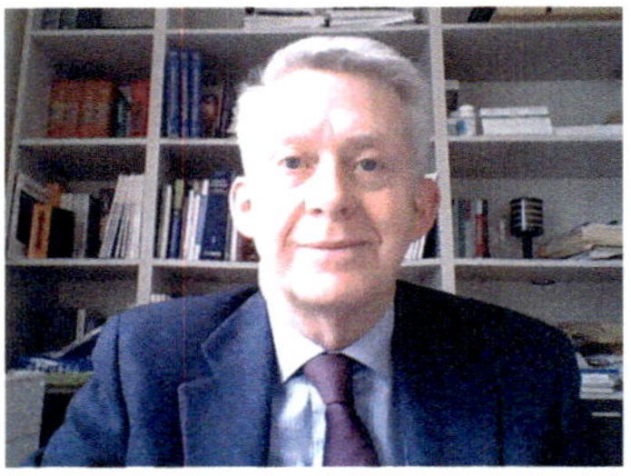

Piergiorgio Messa
President of Italian Society of Nephrology,
Chief of Nephrology, Dialysis and
Renal Transplant Unit
"Policlinico" Hospital -
University of Milan
Milan, Italy

Foreword

Modern ultrasound has, to date, acquired a crucial role among the several imaging modalities available, particularly for the evaluation of nephrological diseases.

This imaging modality is recognized as an effective tool in the clinical management of all kidney diseases, and when I was asked to present this innovative and very well-written book, I was sincerely honored.

Antonio Granata and Michele Bertolotto are internationally renowned leaders in their clinical, diagnostic, and operational setting. They have acquired an outstanding expertise as demonstrated by numerous and remarkable contributions to the literature, as well as by lecturing in international and national congresses, teaching courses, and by their society roles. I have had the privilege to work with both of them for many years and by the beginning I appreciated their preparation, seriousness, and scientific integrity.

The book provides a comprehensive and wide-ranging guide to current and emerging applications of nephrological ultrasonography with the main aim of helping the reader to learn how, when, and why to use properly ultrasound techniques in various clinical settings, including, for example: complications following renal transplantation, arteriovenous fistulas, renal artery stenosis, non-stenotic renal artery pathology, renal vein pathology, aortic disease, and acute renal failure. The most recent US techniques such as US elastography, contrast-enhanced ultrasonography, and color Doppler imaging are explained, starting by limitations and showing how to do the proper and tailored examinations.

I was one of the first in literature to use the term of multiparametric Ultrasound and especially in this fields, this approach is fundamental to achieve the best results for clinical and research purposes. This volume is superbly and abundantly illustrated by photographs and ultrasound images, all realized with state-of-the-art and high-end equipment. These well-chosen illustrations strongly enhance the didactic and educational value of this book.

Therefore, for the above reasons, I am strongly convinced that this book will be very useful for all medical doctors interested in the use of ultrasound techniques in nephrology and will be especially for nephrologists seeking to incorporate ultrasonography into their practice.

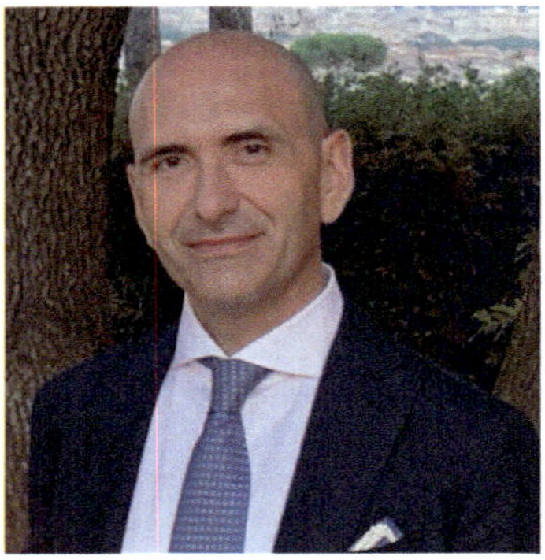

Vito Cantisani
Ass. Prof. of Radiology,
Chairman of Ultrasound Unit
Policlinico Umberto I,
Univ. Sapienza, Roma
Vice-Dean of Medicine and Dentistry,
Univ. Sapienza,
President of Italian Society of Ultrasound
in Medicine and Biology
Rome, Italy

Contents

About the Editors

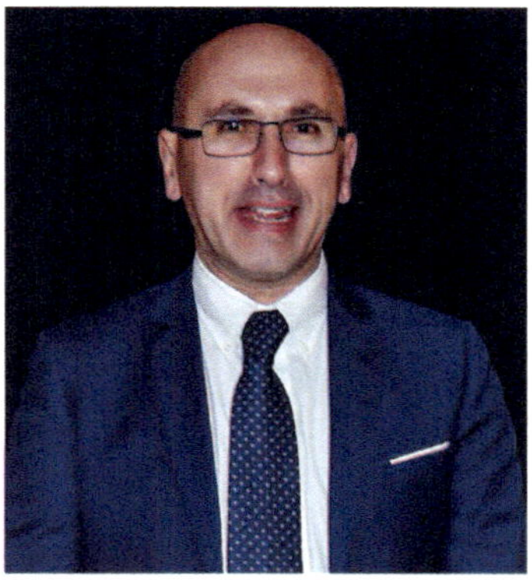

Antonio Granata is an Italian specialist in Nephrology and Internal Medicine. He headed the Nephrology and Dialysis Department in Agrigento Hospital from 2011 to 2019. Since 2019 he has been heading the Department of Nephrology and Dialysis of the "Cannizzaro" Emergency Hospital in Catania. His main fields of interest range from clinical nephrology to rare kidney diseases, from ultrasound diagnostics to interventional nephrology. He is a member of the Board of Directors of the Italian Society of Ultrasound in Medicine and Biology (SIUMB) and of the Italian Society of Nephrology (SIN). He is a member of the European Society of Nephrology, Dialysis and Transplantation (ERA-EDTA). Speaker at several national and international conferences, he authored several articles, book chapters, and books such as "Italian Manual of Central Venous Catheterization" and "Doppler Ultrasound in Daily Nephrological Clinical Practice." Antonio Granata is heading the SIUMB Advanced School of Ultrasound in Nephrology and Vascular Access in Catania. He is Adjunct Professor in Nephrology at Trieste University Medical School.

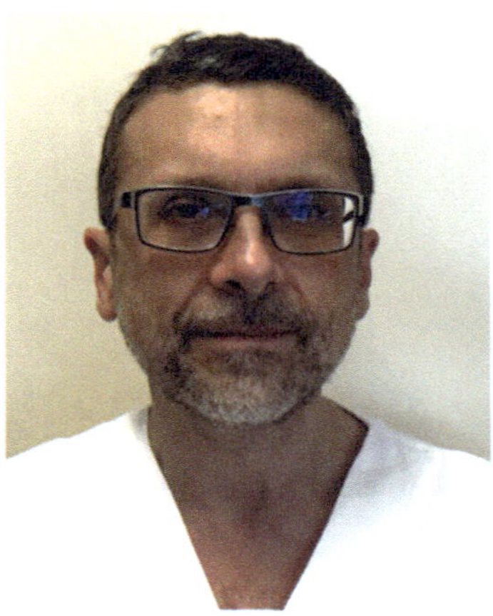

Michele Bertolotto was born in Genoa, Italy. After training in medical biophysics, he graduated in medicine and completed a Residency in Radiology at the University of Genoa. He serves as associate professor in the Department of Radiology at the University of Trieste, Italy. He is chief of ultrasound since 2010, and he is currently head of the II level University of Trieste Master in Urologic, Andrologic and Nephrologic Ultrasound.

He devotes the majority of his time to clinical practice as senior consultant in genitourinary radiology. His research activity concerns several fields of diagnostic imaging, with contributions mainly focused on abdominal and genitourinary radiology, dealing with the use of color Doppler modes and CEUS.

Prof. Bertolotto had several commitments in the European Society of Radiology and in the European Society of Urogenital Radiology (ESUR). He is currently serving as ESUR President-elect. Invited speaker in more than 400 meetings, his research activity is documented by more than 200 full papers, 85 book chapters, and 3 books.

Part I

General Principles

Doppler Signal and Doppler Waveform Analysis

1

Luca Aiani and Alberto Martegani

1.1 Doppler Effect in Ultrasound

B-mode ultrasonography is used to determine the "morphology" of anatomical structures and organs; Doppler methods have the potential to offer "functional" information through blood circulation analysis.

Color Doppler, power Doppler, and spectral analysis provide a noninvasive, real-time imaging of these hemodynamic phenomena.

1.1.1 Doppler Effect

The Doppler effects the change in frequency of a wave for an observer/receiver moving relative to its source: the frequency increases if the sound-emitting object moves towards the observer, and decreases if the sound-emitting object moves away from the observer [1–4].

When a sound wave is emitted by a sinusoidal source (pure-tone source), its speed (c), frequency (f), and wavelength (λ) are connected by the equation

$$c = f \cdot \lambda$$

Notice that the velocity of the waves is a fixed property of the medium.

If the source is fixed, a series of concentric waves are seen. The waves spread all around from the source in all directions, on the same wavelength (Fig. 1.1a).

If the source moves at a certain speed, in a specific direction, the distance between two consecutive peaks of waves is shortened on the direction towards the source is moving and increases on the opposite direction (Fig. 1.1b). As the propagation speed is fixed, also the wave frequency changes but in the opposite way.

Focusing on the case of a fixed source, and on reflected waves emitted by an obstacle moving relative to the source, we can observe a change in the frequency of the reflective wave towards the incident one. This frequency shift is proportional to the relative speed and it is defined as Doppler shift.

It is named after the Austrian physicist Christian Doppler, who proposed it in 1842 in Prague.

In mathematical terms

$$\Delta F = \frac{2\,\mathrm{Fi} \cdot v \cdot \cos\theta}{c}.$$

where

L. Aiani (✉) · A. Martegani
Department of Radiology, Valduce Hospital,
Como, Italy

A. Granata, M. Bertolotto (eds.), *Imaging in Nephrology*,
https://doi.org/10.1007/978-3-030-60794-4_1

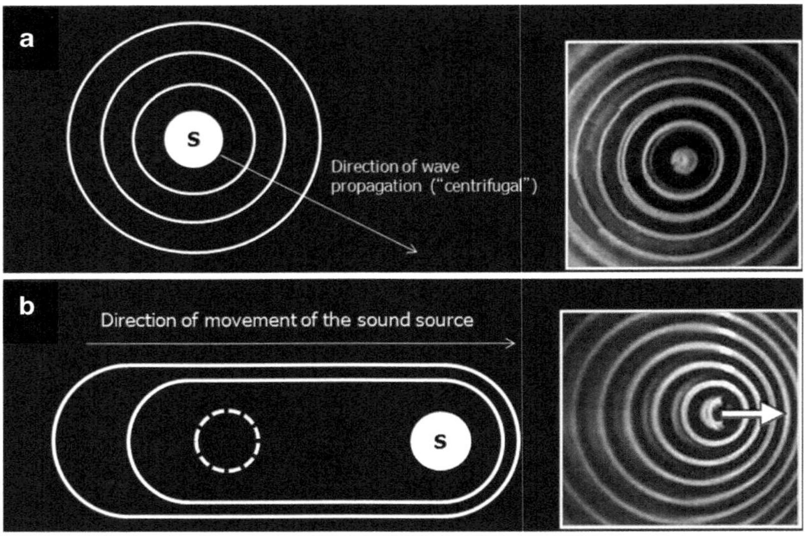

Fig. 1.1 (**a**) When the sound source (S) is fixed, the waves maintain a constant phase difference. (**b**) The figure shows a moving sound source (S): the shorter wavelength of the forward-emitted waves and the longer wavelength of the backward-going ones

- ΔF = frequency shift between the incident and the reflective wave
- Fi = original emission frequency of ultrasonic Doppler probe
- v = velocity of reflecting medium
- c = speed of the wave within the medium; for human tissues it is estimated to be 1540 m/s
- cos θ = cosine of the angle between the original wave and the direction of the moving reflector. This angle is referred to as angle of insonation or Doppler angle.

1.1.2 Doppler Effect: From Theory to Clinical Applications

Concerning hemodynamic flow characteristics, red cells at the center of the vessel move faster than those at the vessel wall.

Sample volume Doppler analysis includes several different frequencies called Doppler spectrum.

The spectrum is made of different frequencies with their characteristics (e.g., direction).

Spectral analysis is generally made with real-time fast Fourier transform (FFT) which is a standard system analysis tool for viewing the spectral content of a signal or sequence (the vertical axis represents frequencies and the horizontal axis represents time).

The number of red blood cells moving with a specific velocity (Doppler amplitude) can be represented by different gradations of gray corresponding to different frequencies.

The laminar flow spectrum is characterized by a maximum concentration of frequencies ("narrow band of frequencies") in systolic phase as all the red blood cells are accelerated in the same way from the center to the periphery.

During diastolic phase, the velocity decreases more at the vessel wall than at the center producing a shift that grows progressively and determines a spectrum with a large band of frequencies.

Doppler waveform in the laminar flow is characterized by a narrow and large spectrum in systolic and diastolic phase, respectively, by a systolic window and by a regular profile.

Turbulent and chaotic flow shows irregularity profile of the spectrum ("broadening").

Considering the flow direction, the machine can represent the spectral frequency over/under the baseline depending on its direction towards the transducer (Fig. 1.2).

The "Doppler signal" contains various information relating the blood flow:

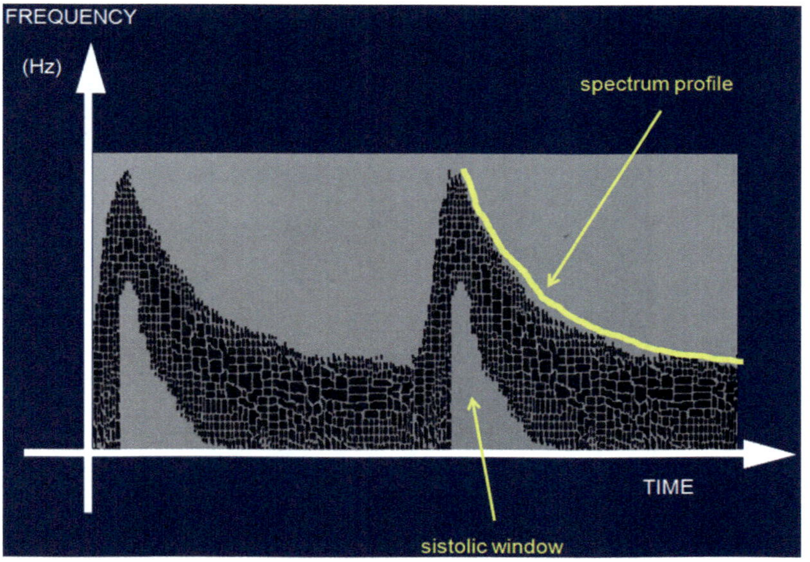

Fig. 1.2 Diagram shows a normal arterial spectrum obtained with Doppler US. The arterial flow is pulsed and moves towards the transducer. Doppler signal amplitude (red blood cell flow velocity) is represented with a gray tone in the spectrum. The spectrum profile (yellow line) is regular and the acoustic window is well defined (laminar flow indicators)

- Velocity of the flow (correlated to ΔF)
- Direction of the flow
- Number of red blood cells contained within the sample volume (correlated to the amplitude or intensity of the Doppler signal)

Red blood cells are easily estimated through power Doppler (PD) technology which correlates the flow phenomena to a chromatic code that is not influenced by flow velocity or insonation angle.

For that reason, PD technology is more sensitive in identifying a slow flow, although it is more susceptible to artifacts due to the vessel walls and anatomical structures around the vessel. These artifacts can severely compromise the information quality.

Once we have defined the flow characteristics measured by the machinery, it is important to "set up" the ultrasound machine appropriately, considering all the parameters (e.g., PRF, gain, color box dimension, Fi, and cos θ) [5–10].

The use of high transmission frequency (Fi) is convenient but it is important to remember that high frequency means high spatial resolution but limited depth of penetration. This is an inevitable compromise. Therefore medical ultrasound devices use sound waves in the range of 1.5–5 MHz for studying deep abdominal vessels (aorta, renal, and parenchymal arteries) whereas higher frequencies (5–10 MHz) are used for superficial vessels.

Considering the insonation angle, Doppler frequency is proportional to its cosine, so when θ is 90° (cos 90° = 0) and the ultrasound beam is perpendicular to the direction of blood flow, it cannot be used to measure velocity. Doppler shift will be greatest when the angle of incidence is 0° degrees (cos 0° = 1) when the ultrasound beam lines up perfectly parallel with blood flow (Fig. 1.3).

Therefore, the optimal angle of incidence is obtained through oblique scans (30°–60°), this also because the backscattering effect in B-mode imaging is maximum for 90° angles.

Assuming the velocity measurements as a function of the insonation angle: angles closed to 0° ensure an accurate flow velocity evaluation.

Conversely, with angles more than 60° the measurement is unreliable as it can result in more than 20% error (Fig. 1.4).

It follows that 10° variation of the insonation angle results in a reliable evaluation (<10% error) of the flow velocity with a transducer under 30° oriented.

The same variation of the insonation angle, considering scanning angles over 60°, results in more than 30% error [11].

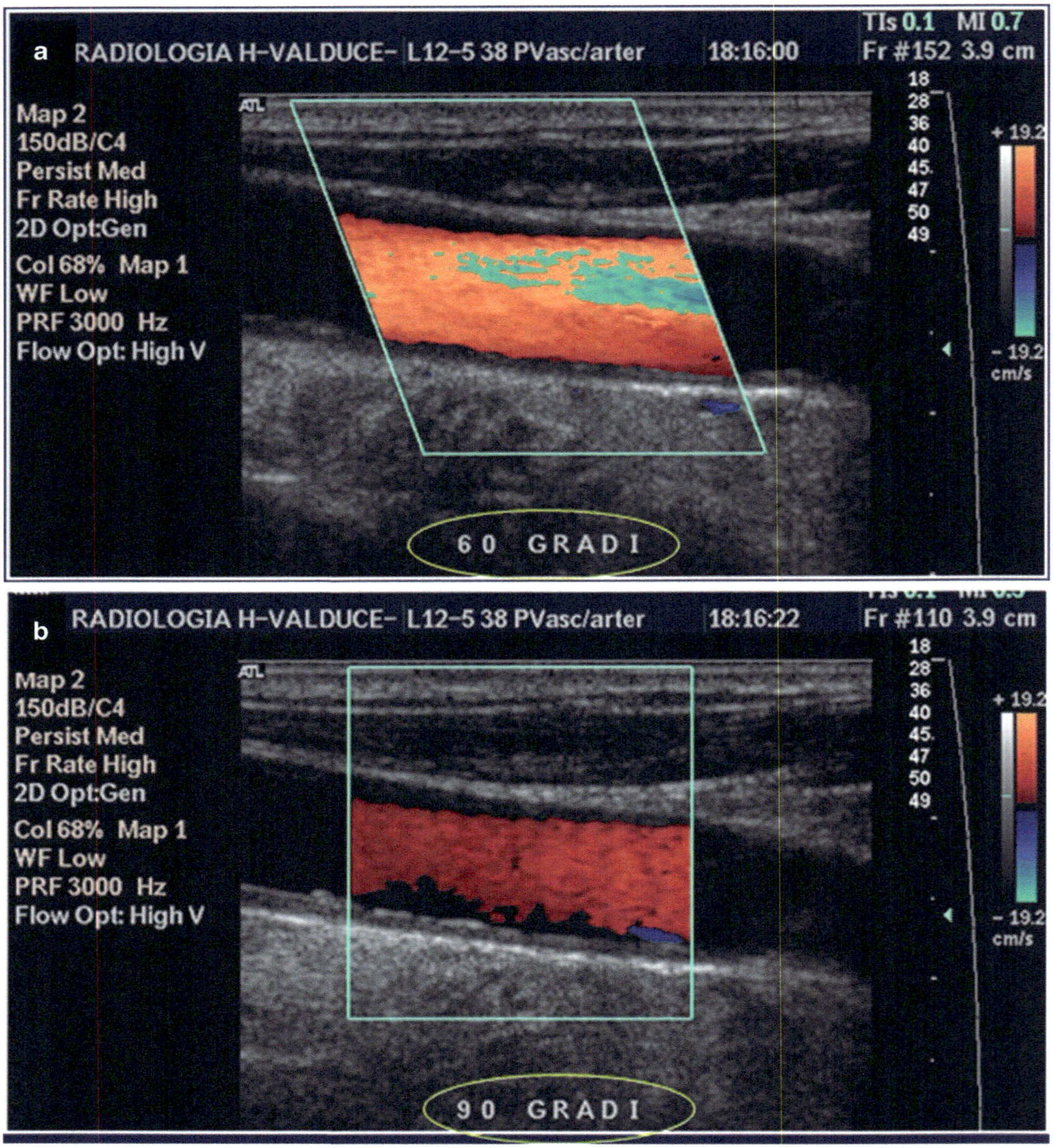

Fig. 1.3 Different color Doppler maps at different insonation angles (common carotid artery). (**a**) To 60° incidence angle to the vascular carotid axis ensures a good signal. (**b**) Considering the same regulation parameters settled for that specific vascular district, the Doppler signal is less efficient with near to 90° incidence angle to the vascular axis

Proper selection of insonation angle for studying abdomen with convex or microconvex transducer requires appropriate anatomic windows for optimal scans.

This aspect is highly operator dependent as it is related to specialist's skills and experience. Small transducer or phase-arrayed transducer (e.g., cardiological device) can be easily managed thanks to their small size.

For superficial structure analysis with linear array, the insonation angle is improved with steering technology. Through this technique, the

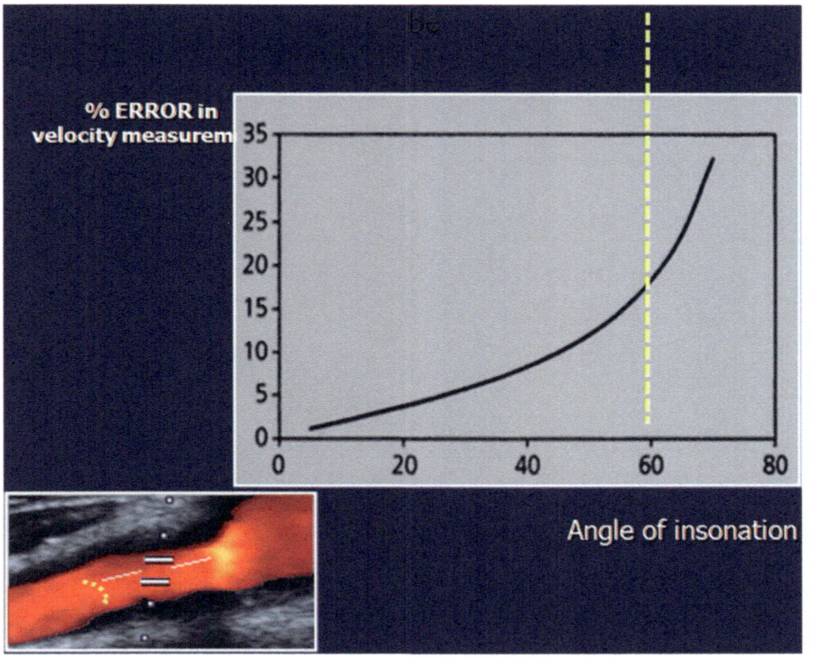

Fig. 1.4 Correlation diagram to percentage error in velocity measurements as a function of the angle of insonation. Angles which measure more than 60° show a rapid change of the slope value. The variation coefficient of the blood flow velocity is very high for angles between 70° and 80°, whereas the variation is minimum for angles between 40° and 50°. For that reason, over 60° the measurement is unreliable. Angles under 60° or better under 30° (if technically feasible) are preferable to measuring velocity

angle of the beam with respect to the transducer can be changed. Steering technology enables to increase the insonation angle up to 25°–30° more than those obtained manually (Fig. 1.5).

Assuming that insonation angle (θ), ΔF, Fi, and propagation velocity are known, it is possible to calculate the blood flow velocity (v) which is the real unknown quantity of Doppler equation.

In everyday practice to perform a good Doppler examination, the operator will make many changes in the parameters and will try different probe positions to optimize the image.

Power and gain: Color flow uses higher intensity power than B-mode. Attention should be paid to safety indices. Power and gain should be set to obtain good signal for flow and to minimize the signals from surrounding tissue.

Frequency selection: Many scanner/transducer combinations permit changes of frequency. High frequencies give better sensitivity to low flow and have better spatial resolution. Low frequencies have better penetration and are less susceptible to aliasing at high velocities.

Pulse repetition frequency (PRF): Low pulse repetition frequencies should be used to examine low velocities but aliasing may occur if high velocities are encountered.

Region of interest (box color): Because more pulses are needed to look at flow than for the B-mode image, reducing the width and maximum depth of the color flow area under investigation will usually improve frame rate (FR) and may allow a higher color scan line density with improved spatial resolution.

Focus: The focus should be at the level of the area of interest. This can make a significant difference to the appearance and accuracy of the image.

1.2 Doppler Ultrasound Technology Systems

According to their ultrasound emission mode, Doppler equipment can be classified into continuous-wave Doppler (continuous-wave Doppler—CW) or pulsed-wave Doppler (pulsed-wave Doppler—PW). During the last decades the PW ultrasound has undergone a considerable technological improvement which has allowed to switch from duplex scanner into color Doppler

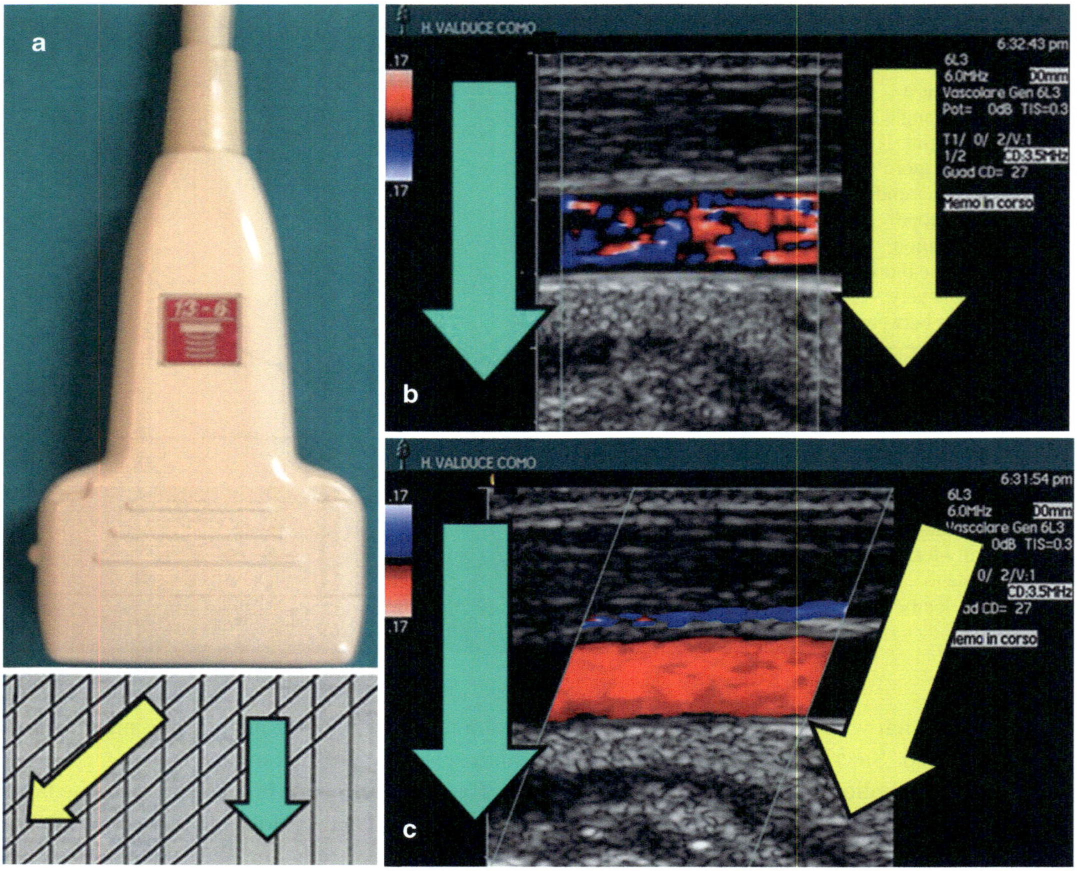

Fig. 1.5 A linear prober generates two separated acoustic beams for B-mode and Doppler imaging; with Doppler the beam is possibly steered at preselected angles (**a**). The system displays simultaneously B-mode and color Doppler imaging (**b**, **c**); considering the same regulation parameters settled steering technology improves the blood flow information (**c**)

and power Doppler. These most up-to-date equipment allow an anatomical imaging of the vascular or parenchymal (morphological data) flows and to obtain at the same time a spectral display of the flow speed (functional information) [12–14].

1.2.1 Continuous-Wave Doppler (CW)

In CW technology, i.e., simple and low-cost technology, the transducer employs two piezoelectric crystals, one for transmitting and the other for a nonstop receiving placed nearby.

This instrument allows to measure the flow direction and speed without limits of sampling: very fast flows, such as those that are generated in the case of tight aortic valvular stenosis, can be properly evaluated. For its feature CW recognizes an elective use in cardiology.

This technology shows a very high sensitivity enabling to detect the presence of extremely slow flows and limited flow rates. The main criticality of these devices is their inefficacy to focus the depth of the flow signals and to sum up the ones coming from all vessels included in the US beam even if localized at different depths (Fig. 1.6a).

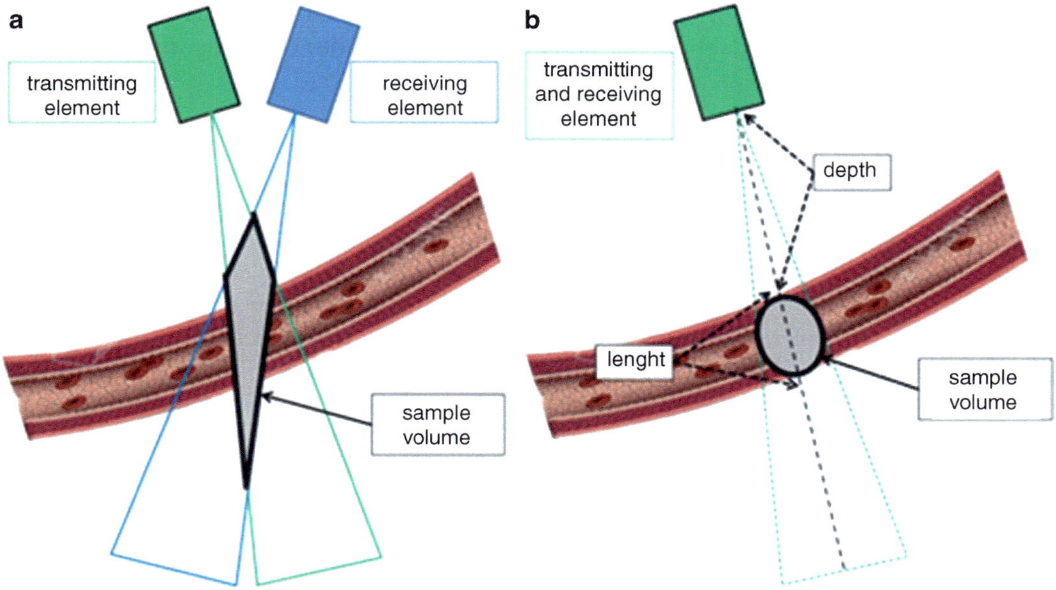

Fig. 1.6 Test volume with continuous (**a**) and pulsed (**b**) Doppler technology. In continuous Doppler system transmitting and receiving elements are separated and the sample volume is determined by the overlap of the two ultrasound beams. In pulsed Doppler system the same transducer element is used for transmitting and receiving. Depth and length of the sample volume are controlled by the operator

1.2.2 Pulsed-Wave Doppler (PW)

In this type of ultrasound technology the transducer transmits and receives the pulse by employing the same piezoelectric crystal. Ultrasound is emitted in short pulses intervaled by corresponding short pauses; in this period of time the piezoelectric crystal waits for listening to the reflected way. As ultrasound speed propagation in organic tissues is well known, it is possible to change the depth of specific regions and to select the measurement interval by modifying the time gap between emission and reception impulse.

In this way it is possible to select a real sample volume according to the desired dimensions and depth: e.g., it is possible to functionally typify a specific vessel positioned at a certain depth by excluding the above and below vascular structures (Fig. 1.6b).

The depth of the sampling volume (h_v) is given by the relation

$$h_v = \frac{c \cdot \tau}{2}.$$

where c is the sound wave propagation speed in tissues and τ the interval between direct wave emission and reception of the reflected one.

This ultrasound technology does not allow to simultaneously display the vessel morphology forcing to proceed almost "blindfold."

1.2.3 Duplex Scanner

The problem is worked out by the duplex scanner systems that can be considered as an evolution of the pulsed-wave systems. These ultrasound machines allow to obtain a double scan. It is possible to display a B-mode image of the vessel and to obtain simultaneously a Doppler sampling of a specific sample volume by employing the same transducer.

The introduction of duplex scanner systems has revolutionized the use of ultrasound in vascular diagnostics, offering a repeatable and noninvasive method that allows to simultaneously assess the vessel morphology and the blood flow velocity speed as well.

Nevertheless the impossibility to display the whole frequency spectrum is still a limit in the use of this equipment; this is due to the so-called aliasing effect.

The capability to sample correctly an analogical signal, as the one coming from a reflected acoustic wave in a blood flow, depends on the pulse repetition frequency (PRF) selected, which corresponds to the frequency emission of pulse train.

The maximum Doppler frequency that can be measured correctly is half the PRF commonly called "Nyquist frequency."

The phenomenon has been known since a long time and can be exemplified as the effect of the apparent opposite rotation of the carriage wheels in old movies, where half the frequency change of the carriage spokes ("Nyquist frequency") is higher than the frequency of sampling (number of film frames per second—frame rate).

If the blood flow is very fast and/or the angle between the direction of the incident wave and speed is small, such as to produce a high Doppler frequency, a high PRF will have to be used. Nevertheless a high PRF can reduce the length of interval between the emission and reception of the pulse and consequently the depth of the sampling volume we intend to operate with. As a matter of fact the deeper the sampled vessel is, the lower the PRF must be to let the pulse train to go and return from the target. In conclusion fast and deep flows cannot be detected.

There is an additional restriction in the duplex scanner systems related to the different response of the system to the incidence angle of the acoustic wave when operating in Doppler mode or B-mode. As a matter of fact, the optimal angle of insonation in B-mode is 90°, while in Doppler mode is 0°. Consequently the optimal inclination of duplex equipment must be a compromise between 0° and 90°.

Usually an angle between 30° and 60° is used because these angles allow an accurate velocimetric sampling without compromising the B-mode display of the vascular structure.

1.2.4 Color Doppler (CD) and Power Doppler (PD) Technology

The CD is an extension and an enhancement of the duplex system thanks to the exploitation of the B-mode grayscale image on which a colorimetric dynamic image, representing flow rates, is superimposed [15–17]. In other words all flows present inside the sampled surface are evidenced; direction, speed, dispersion, and turbulence are specified. The flow direction is identified according to conventional color assignment: red for flow towards, and blue for flow away.

Velocity is mapped in chromatic red scale mainly red hues (from red to yellow for flow towards) and mainly blue hues (from blue to light blue for flows away).

Color display of vascular structures allows to assess average speed (but not the absolute one assessed by spectral analysis) in a given instant.

The simultaneous presence of different colors (velocity dispersion) allows to assess how particles inside a vessel can have different speed: laminar flows show a gradual speed dispersion from the center to the periphery of the vessel (Fig. 1.7a, b). In the presence of a significant stenosis, acceleration and flow turbulence are mapped with a mosaic of colors (aliasing) in which the dispersion speed is chaotic (Fig. 1.7c).

The physical and operating features of the machine and its limits are more or less similar to those of pulsed-wave Doppler and duplex which exploit the spectral analysis.

An important difference, however, consists of the fact that CD displays only the average speed of the different particles. From this point of view CD shows a lack of information compared to spectral analysis which displays also modal speed and peak systolic velocity (PSV) which is very important in hemodynamic stenosis quantification.

PD color mapping shows an imaging mode similar to CD; nevertheless its monochrome mapping represents Doppler signal power but not its frequency and direction [18, 19].

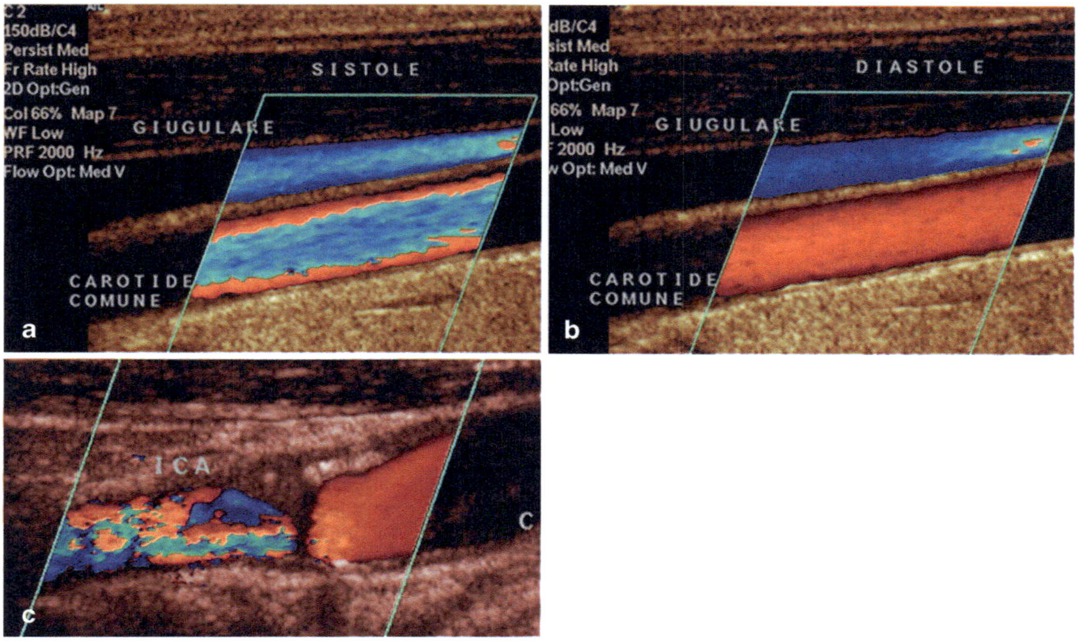

Fig. 1.7 Color Doppler imaging of the blood flow. (**a**, **b**) Laminar flow with a parabolic profile shows the highest velocities at the axial center of the vessel: velocities are lowest adjacent to the vessel wall. Different colors between systole and diastole are due to different flow velocities. (**c**) With a severe stenosis, the flow becomes turbulent and it is represented as a mosaic of colors ("aliasing"); the phenomenon is evident in the downstream segment of the stenosis

In summary the differences between CD and PD are related to the displaying mode of the two techniques. CD reproduces the average of the frequency shift which is directly proportional to the cosine of the insolation angle; PD reproduces a signal power which corresponds to the integral of the spectral curve.

The advantages of PD are related to its high sensitivity in representing flow phenomena, to the persistence of the chromatic resolution, to a better signal/noise ratio, and to a lack of the aliasing artifact. The disadvantages are related to its inability to represent the flow direction and its better sensitivity towards artifacts generated by movements of anatomical structures which can cause a significant decay of the image quality (Fig. 1.8).

1.3 Hemodynamic Principles

The blood is a viscous fluid with a liquid part and a corpuscular part. The flow of a fluid in a pipe of cross section occurs under certain conditions creating concentric layers sliding one over the other at a different speed which is maximum in the center of the vessel and minimum at its periphery [20, 21].

In these conditions the blood flow is called "laminar"; the cause of this particular configuration is owed to the internal friction of the fluid (viscosity) which shows a maximum level between the vessel wall and the fluid and a minimum level in the center of the vessel. This, therefore, determines a laminar flow with a parabolic scroll profile.

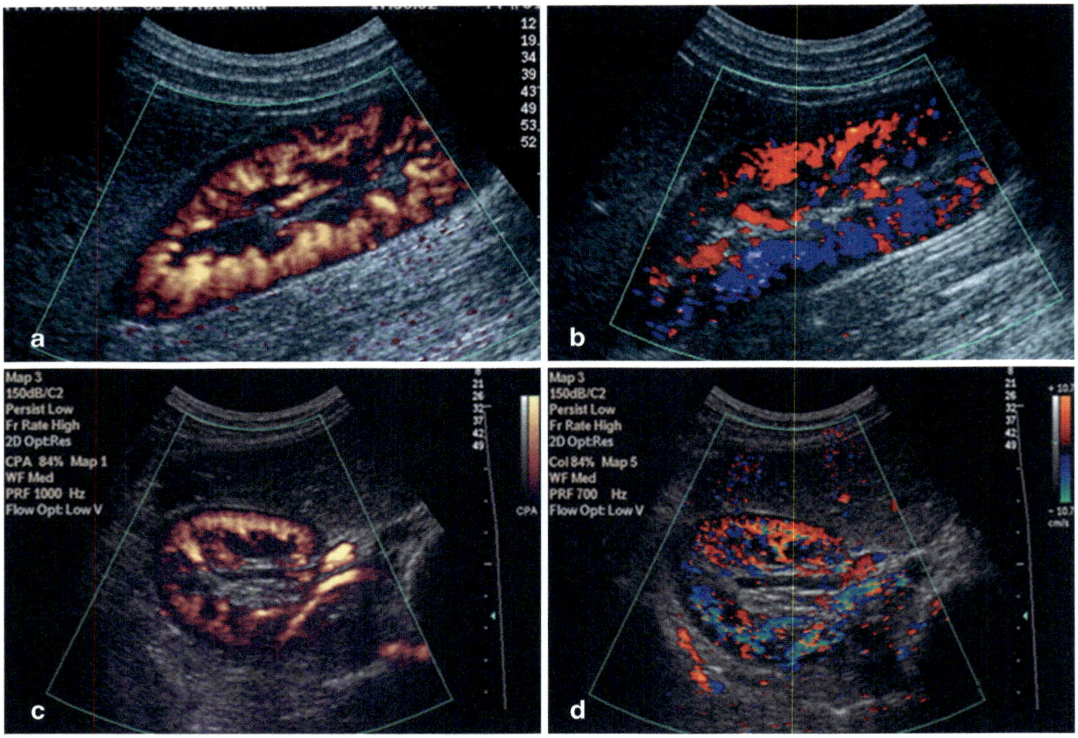

Fig. 1.8 Longitudinal and transverse scans of the kidney with power Doppler and color Doppler. Power Doppler (**a**) is more sensitive than color Doppler (**b**) in showing parenchymal flow of the cortical zone but it cannot represent the flow direction. Power Doppler (**c**) compared with color Doppler (**d**) shows a good signal-to-noise ratio without aliasing artifact in the transverse image of the kidney

Greater caliber vessels (such as the aorta) show during systole a more flat and uniform flow profile: i.e., when the diameter of a vessel tends to increase the parabolic flow profile tends to flatten (Fig. 1.9a).

Any alteration of the flow pipe geometry may cause a change of the flow speed profile; for example, this may occur in the presence of bending, expansion, or narrowing of the duct (Fig. 1.9b–d).

Under conditions of flow narrowing two main effects may be generated: the maximum speed cannot occur in the center of the duct and a turbulent flow can be originated. Flow conditions which turn a laminar flow into a turbulent flow are defined by the Reynolds number formula.

According to the theory the pressure increase determines a raise of the flow velocity up to a certain value beyond which the flow remains constant; in other words the speed of the fluid increases up to a certain limit beyond which turbulent movements are generated transforming the pressure in thermal energy (heat) rather than kinetic energy (speed).

At first this forms an "unstable" flow which progressively becomes "turbulent" [22–25].

The speed limit of a flow, in the presence of same pipe diameter, viscosity, and density, is provided by the formula expressed by the Reynolds number:

$$\mathrm{Re} = \frac{D \cdot V}{\delta \cdot \mu}.$$

where

- D is the pipe diameter.
- V is the velocity of the fluid.
- δ is the density of the fluid.
- μ is the viscosity of the fluid.

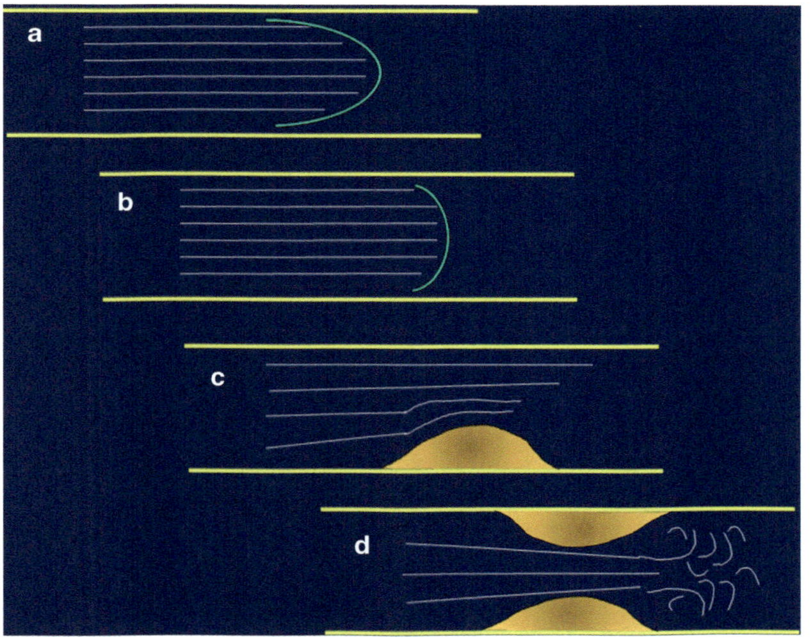

Fig. 1.9 Different velocity profiles of the blood flow associated to different vessel conditions. (**a**, **b**) Parabolic and flat profiles in laminar flow. Disturbed (**c**) and turbulent flow (**d**) in the presence of mild to severe stenosis, respectively

The critical threshold of transition from a laminar flow into a turbulent one corresponds to a value of Reynolds number which is equal to about 2000.

1.4 Doppler Signal Semeiotics

1.4.1 Interpretation of the Spectral Curve

The Doppler signals from a vascular structure are related to the speed of red blood cells. Flow speed changes in response to physiological or pathological causes can then be detected with this method. A simple qualitative assessment of the spectral curve of these signals allows to evaluate its main features (venous versus arterial) [26, 27].

1.4.1.1 The Arterial Flow

The arterial flow presents a typical "pulsed" flow reaching a maximum speed during systole (peak systolic velocity—PSV) and a minimum speed during diastole (end diastolic velocity—DV).

The arterial Doppler pattern of afferent vessels in organs with low resistance such as encephalon and parenchyma (kidney) presents all the times a pulsed but nonstop flow, to ensure a minimal blood supply even during the diastolic phase.

The Doppler curve is characterized by an initial period of fast flow velocity increase (systolic phase) corresponding to the contraction of the left ventricle. After the cardiac muscle relaxation, a sudden reduction but partial of the flow speed occurs; this is due to the low peripheral vascular resistance. Along the descending branch a further incisure (a small ascending branch) is noticeable due to kinetic phenomena induced by the closure of the semilunar aortic valves. Two peaks originate; the first one (early systolic peak—ESP) represents the extension of the ascending segment of the outflow tract and the second peak is less acute, lower, or higher than the early systolic peak. In the renal district, the presence of a higher late systolic peak is usually observed in young individuals with a low renal resistance and a good renal vascular compliance (Fig. 1.10).

During the diastolic phase the only propulsive force is provided by the relaxation of the aortic walls that, thanks to their elastic return, release the kinetic energy accumulated during the cardiac ejection; in this phase the tracking presents a reduction of the velocimetric values which nevertheless keep on remaining above the zero line.

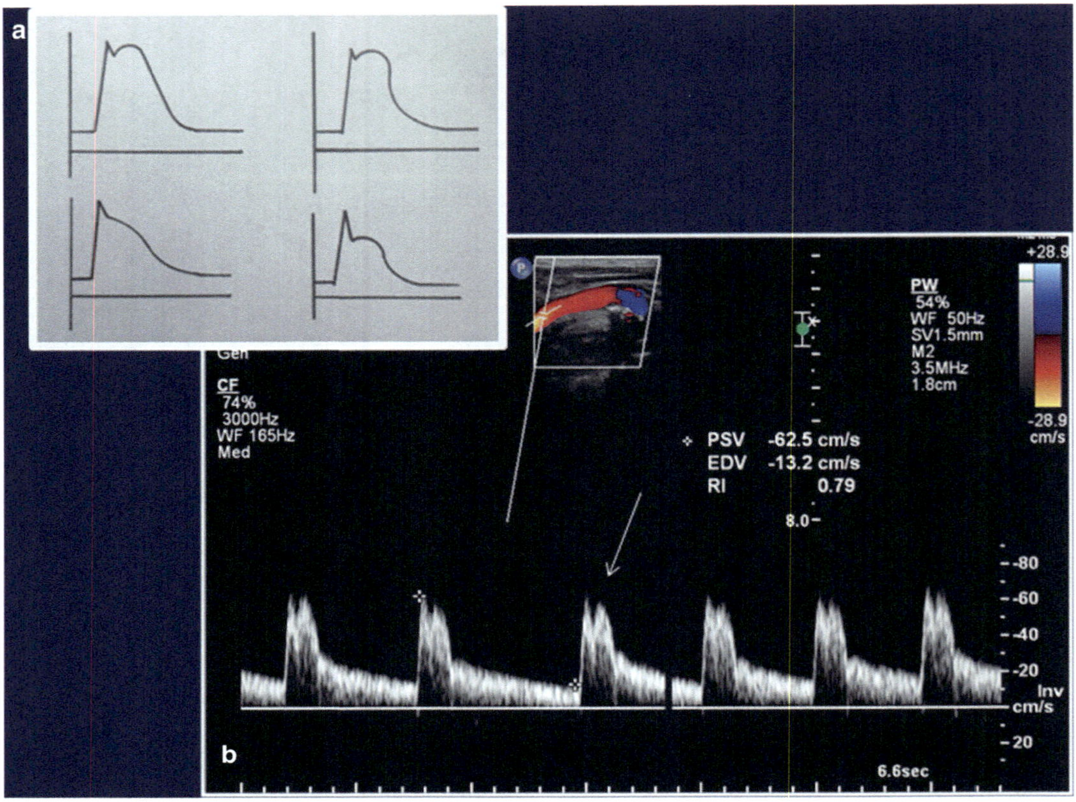

Fig. 1.10 (**a**) Different morphologies of the early systolic peak (ESP). (**b**) Doppler sonogram with dicrotic wave (white arrow)

The Doppler tracking of the arterial vessels afferent to high vascular resistance districts (upper or lower limbs) presents a pulsed appearance without a continuous flow. The initial period of the velocimetric complex is similar to that of low-resistivity vessels. A sudden and constant reduction of the flow velocity occurs in consequence of the cardiac muscle relaxation during the diastolic phase which in the presence of high peripheral resistance achieves the zero line and for a short period of time presents a flow-reverse wave called Windkessel effect.

The extent of this reversed flow also depends on the elasticity of the wall of the arteries (Fig. 1.11).

1.4.1.2 The Venous Flow

On the contrary, the veins present the so defined "continuous" flow with a modest velocity modulation usually affected by the cyclic cardiac activity, more evident in vessels closer to the heart and by respiration.

Such modulations, in the renal district, are more evident in the right renal vein due to its short length and for its position on the caval vein which is almost parallel to the axis of the vessel.

The loss of the regular "rhythm" of venous signals can be caused by the presence of a proximal obstruction close to the outflow.

An amplitude increase of the phasic oscillations indicates a proximal venous stasis with

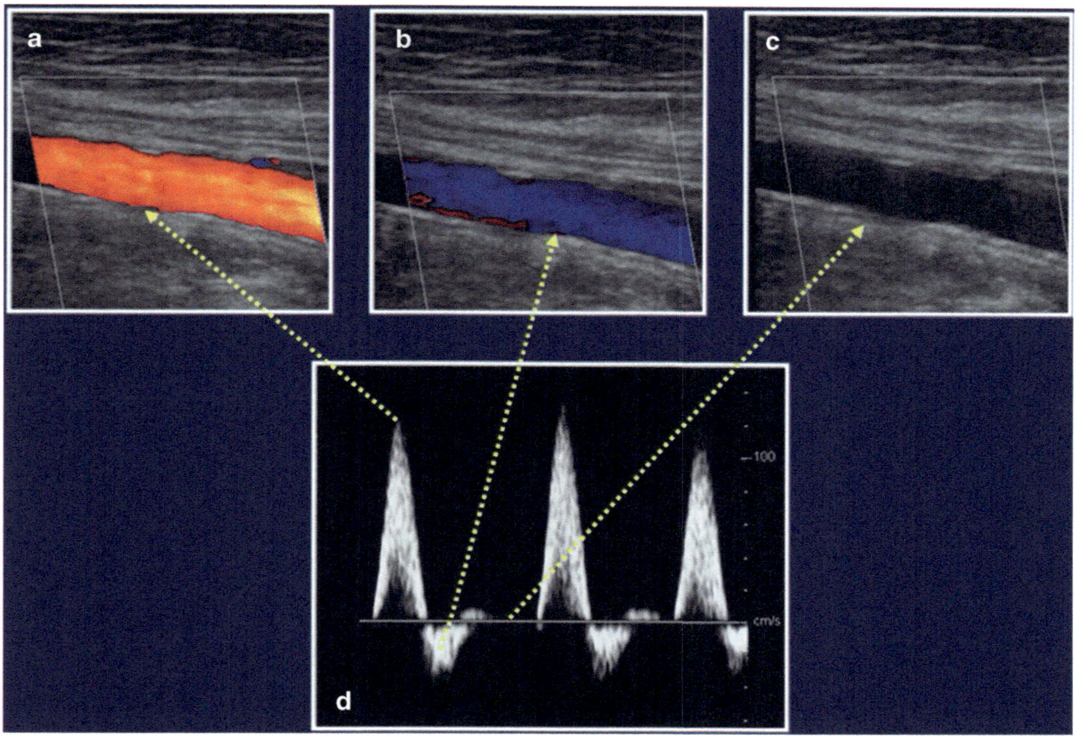

Fig. 1.11 High-resistive superficial femoral artery Doppler waveform. (**a**) Color flow image shows normal flow direction and high velocity of the femoral artery during systole. (**b**) Reverse flow in early diastolic flow (low velocity) based on the Windkessel effect in spectral analysis. (**c**) End diastolic flow is pulsed and unrecordable. (**d**) Spectral analysis shows blood flow velocity and direction

vasodilation of the venous system; in the right chronic heart failure a biphasic venous flow occurs (Fig. 1.12).

1.4.2 Parameters of the Spectral Curve

1.4.2.1 Quantitative Parameters

Quantitative parameters allow to express Doppler ultrasound curve related to local flow speed; the most commonly used parameters are peak systolic speed (PSV), end diastolic speed (DV), and average speed (AV).

After setting the insonation angle, the device assesses automatically the velocimetric parameters. The obtained velocimetric flow parameters provide a rough estimate of the actual speed. Considering the cosine function between speed and angles, the velocimetric estimate is reliable for angles below 60°.

Velocimetric values obtained with angles over 60° can be subjected to important errors and therefore cannot be accepted.

Main renal artery PSV values 100 ± 20 cm/s are considered as normal.

The average speed (AV), in young solitary kidney-transplanted patients, is higher. Moving towards the renal parenchyma a gradual reduction of the systolic peak speed can be observed; nevertheless both waveforms and systo-diastolic ratio remain unchanged. The possibility measures the flow rate both in normal and pathological vessels, in a noninvasive way, making this technique extremely interesting.

Flow rate can be calculated with ultrasound by measuring the diameter and/or the section vessel multiplied by AV.

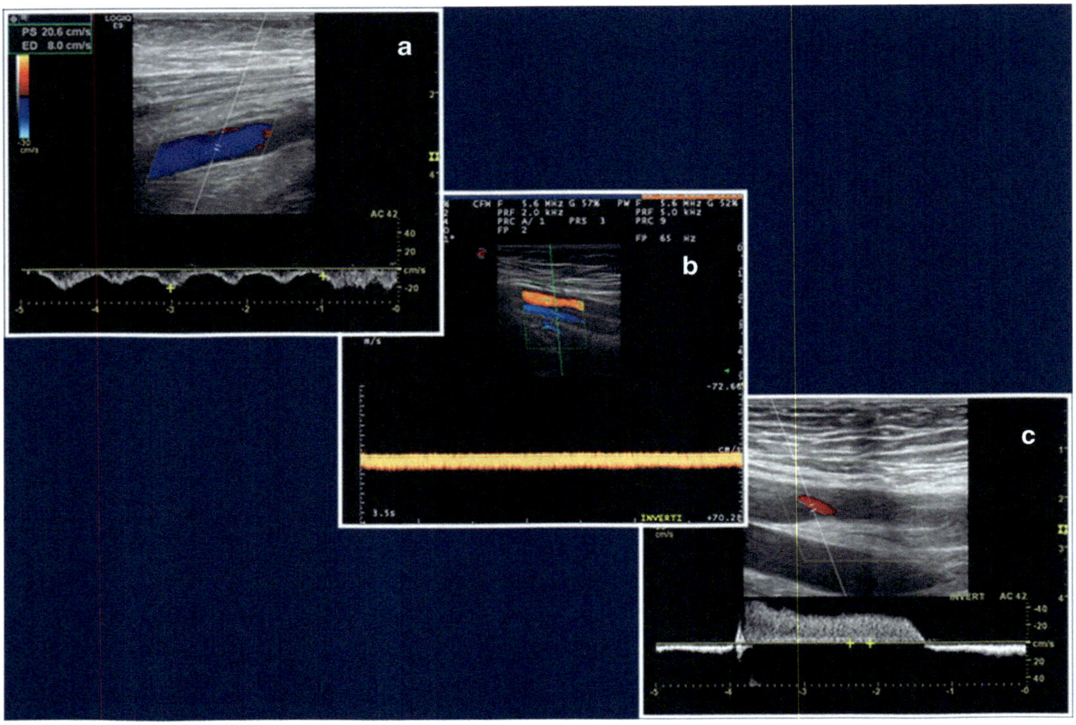

Fig. 1.12 Doppler waveform in venous system. (**a**) Venous flow velocity modulated by heart activity in a proximal cardiac vessel. (**b**) Continuous venous flow. (**c**) Reverse flow (venous reflux) with Valsalva maneuver

Nevertheless, rate flow measuring is affected by the complexity of the venous and arterial flow, by the incidence angle, as well as by the vessel caliber (and therefore by the vessel cross-sectional area) [28–30].

1.4.2.2 Semiquantitative Parameters

These parameters express the morphological features of the Doppler ultrasound curve and depend on the upstream and downstream flows [31–33]. The most commonly used parameters are the resistive index (RI), pulsatility index (PI), acceleration time (AT), acceleration index (AI), and velocimetric renal/aortic ratio (RAR) (Fig. 1.13).

Resistive index (***RI***) expresses the ratio which exists between difference of systolic and diastolic velocity with systolic velocity:

$$RI = \frac{PSV - DV}{PSV}.$$

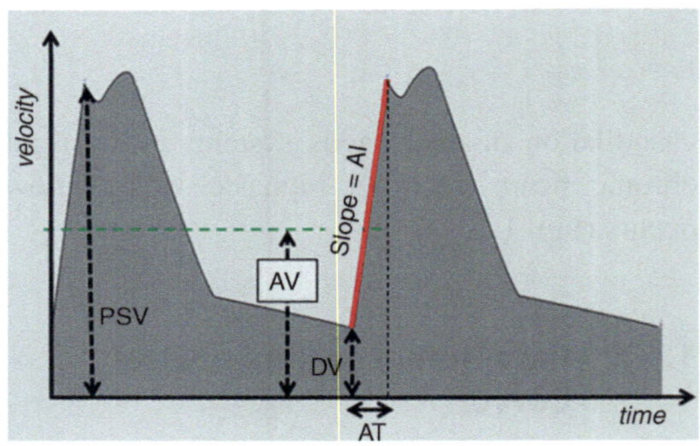

Fig. 1.13 Scheme of spectral Doppler. The vertical axis represents the frequency shift (velocity scale) and the horizontal axis represents time. The peak systolic velocity (PSV), the end diastolic velocity (DV), the average velocity (AV), the slope (acceleration index = AI), and the acceleration time (AT) are parameters commonly used in waveform quantification

Small impedance of organ and tissues determines a low resistance index; this condition is typical of carotid vessels and renal district (Fig. 1.14) [34–38].

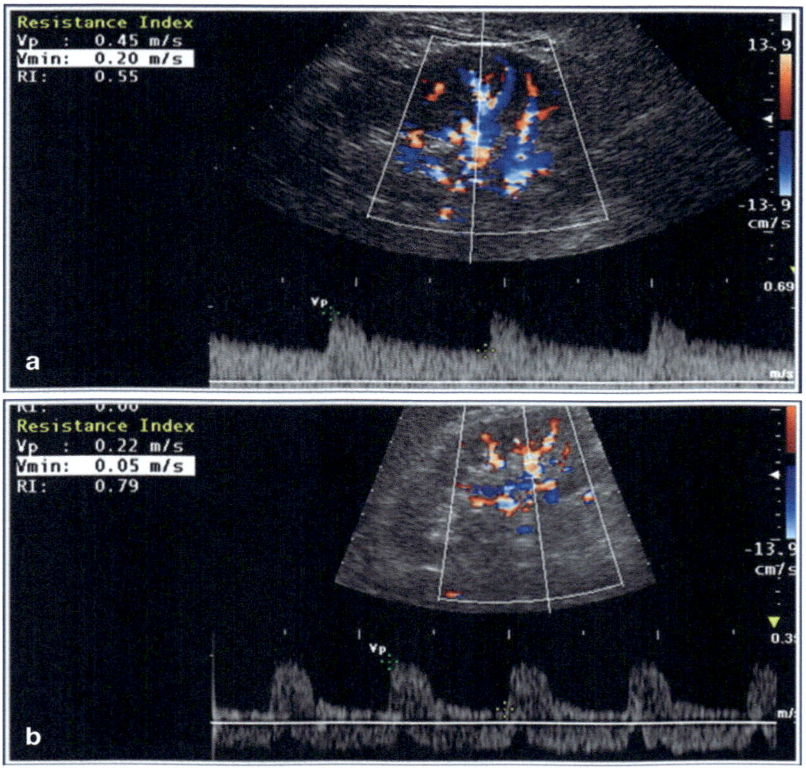

Fig. 1.14 Intrarenal arterial Doppler waveform. (**a**) Intraparenchymal renal Doppler in normal subject: the intrarenal resistive index (IR) is 0.55. (**b**) Intraparenchymal renal Doppler in a patient with renal disease: the intrarenal resistive index is significantly higher (IR = 0.79)

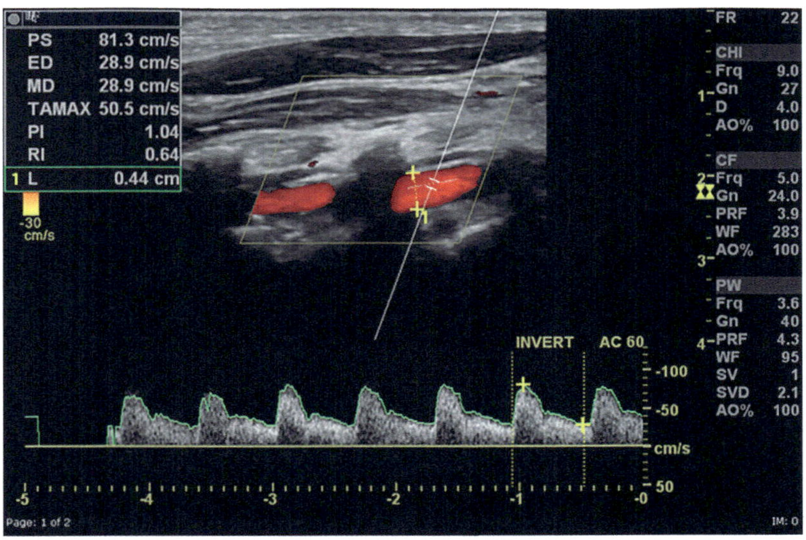

Fig. 1.15 Assessment of semiquantitative values for the arterial Doppler waveform of vertebral artery (automatic trace). Resistive index (RI) = 0.64. Pulsatility index (PI) = 1.04. Peak systolic velocity (PSV) = 81.3 cm/s. Diastolic velocity (DV) = 28.9 cm/s. Average velocity (TAMAX) = 50.5 cm/s

Pulsatility index (PI) expresses the ratio which exists between difference of systolic and diastolic velocity with average velocity:

$$\mathrm{PI} = \frac{\mathrm{PSV} - \mathrm{DV}}{\mathrm{AV}}.$$

Unlike RI, this index, since it includes the average speed as denominator, takes into consideration the way the velocimetric curve achieves the telediastolic speed during the diastole. For this reason two curves with the same RI could have a different PI (Fig. 1.15). To determine

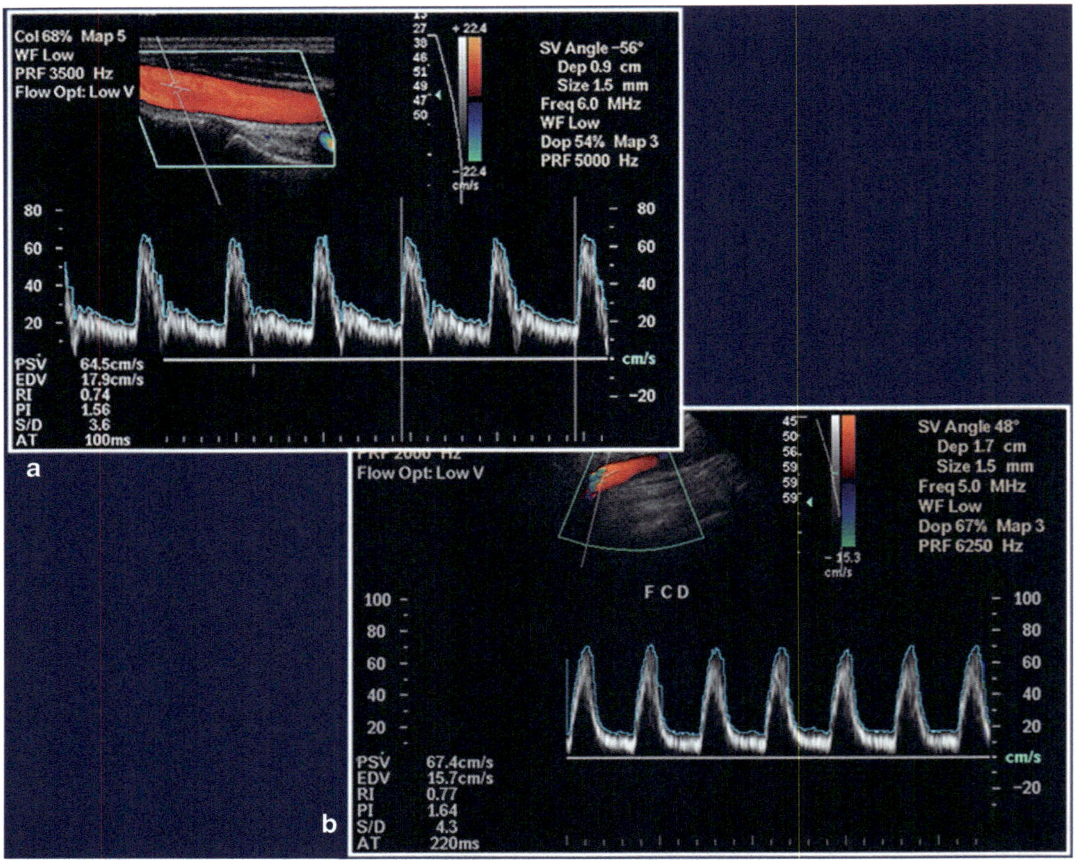

Fig. 1.16 Doppler waveform (automatic trace). (**a**) Normal Doppler waveform shows a rapid upstroke in systole which correlates to a normal acceleration time (AT = 100 ms). (**b**) Post-stenotic Doppler waveform is defined by a slope reduction of the ascendant branch with an increased acceleration time (AT = 220 ms)

PI it is necessary to calculate the average flow speed tracking automatically or manually the Doppler ultrasound curve.

Acceleration time (AT) takes into account the necessary time to achieve the maximum systolic speed expressed by the slope of the ascending branch of the ultrasound Doppler curve [32, 39]. Usually it does not have to exceed 70 ms (Fig. 1.16).

Since this index does not depend on angle it can be easily obtained. Nevertheless, this index can result erroneously normal in the presence of a post-stenotic curve since the real PSV value is unknown.

Acceleration index (AI) is a value which clearly indicates the slope of the ascending branch of the ultrasound Doppler curve allowing to suspect the existence of an upstream stenosis. By knowing the insonation angle and consequently the PSV value of that, AI can be calculated. This index is expressed in m/s^2; normal value is included in an interval of 8 ± 4 m/s^2. Patients with upstream stenosis of the sampled vessel show a lower acceleration index (AI) (Fig. 1.17).

Velocimetric renal/aortic ratio (RAR) expresses the ratio between the peak systolic velocity in renal artery (PSVRA) and in abdominal aorta.

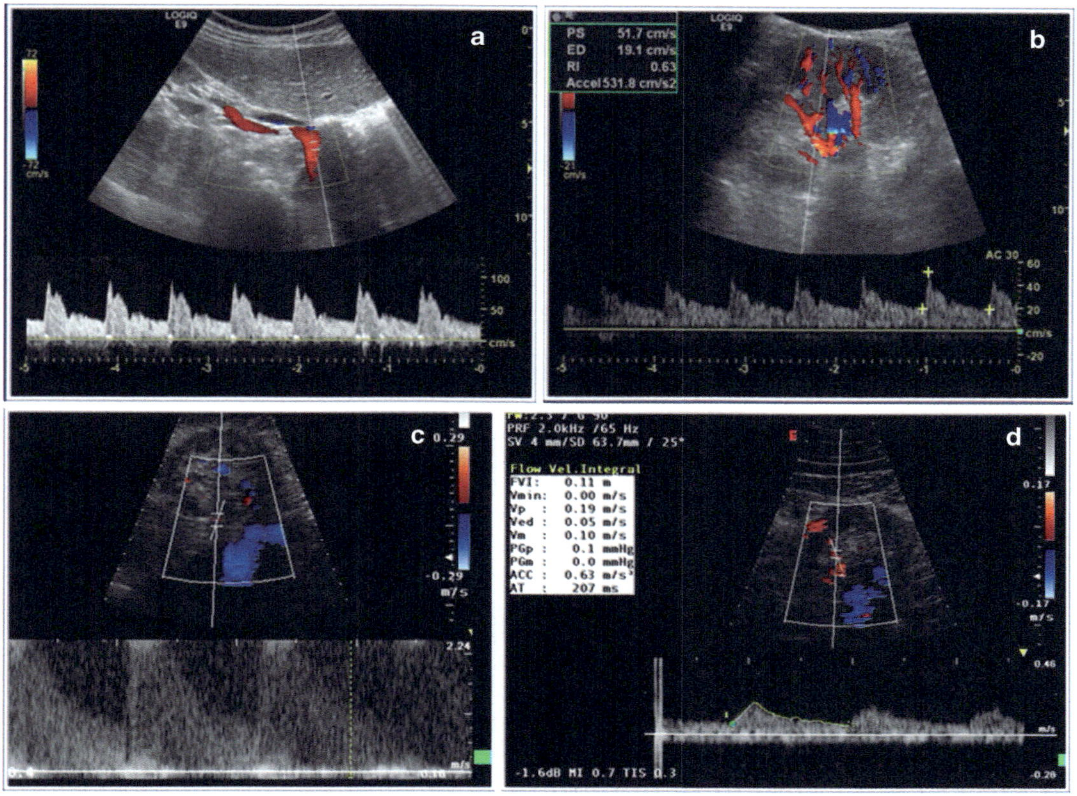

Fig. 1.17 Intrarenal and extrarenal Doppler waveform. (**a**) Normal waveform obtained from the main renal artery demonstrates a regular peak systolic velocity (PSV less than 1 m/s). (**b**) Doppler parenchymal wave is regularly modulated with normal form (PSV = 52 cm/s, RI = 0.63, and AI = 5.3 m/s^2). (**c**) Hemodynamically significant stenosis of the main renal artery shows a Doppler waveform with increased peak systolic velocity (PSV > 2.24 m/s), spectrum broadening, and reduction of the percentage systolic window. (**d**) Post-stenotic Doppler waveform (pulsus parvus et tardus waveform) shows an increased acceleration time (AT = 207 ms) and an acceleration index reduction (AI = 0.63 m/s^2)

1.4.3 Alterations of the Spectral Curve

1.4.3.1 Effects of Stenosis and Dilatations

When a stenosis of the vascular lumen occurs, hemodynamic effects related to the velocimetric curve depending on the dimensions and geometric features of the obstruction are noticeable. The main event which may happen in the presence of a stenosis is an increase of systolic speed peak.

Stenosis over 50% usually can originate a progressive increase of systolic and diastolic peak speed.

Velocimetric increase allows to maintain an acceptable flow up to 85% of the lumen.

Stenosis over 90% ("tight stenosis") can cause a very high systolic jet which can affect the vessel for a few centimeters after the stenosis region (Fig. 1.18).

Pre-occlusive stenosis, on the contrary, can cause a flow rate decrease and a relevant speed reduction distal to the lesion; this hemodynamic condition anticipates the occlusion of the vessel lumen. Furthermore, the presence of a stenosis causes a loss of the laminar flow regimes and consequently a vortex formation in the downstream area close to the lesion and close to the

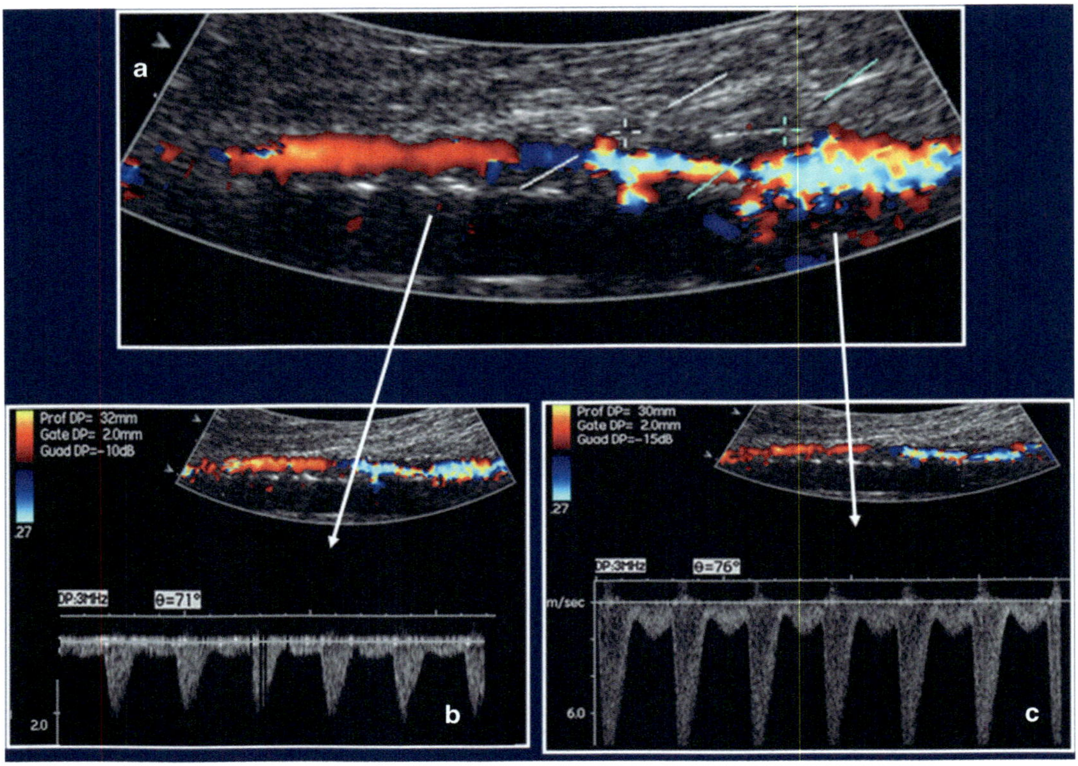

Fig. 1.18 Hemodynamically significant stenosis of the high-resistive superficial femoral artery. (**a**) Color Doppler of the stenosis shows a diameter and flow reduction and it leads to "aliasing" phenomenon. (**b**) The velocimetry is normal upstream of the stenosis (PSV = 1.2 mt/s). (**c**) Spectral Doppler waveform of the stenotic area; increased peak systolic velocity is seen (PSV = 6 m/s). The peak velocity "ratio" is more than 5

vessel walls; red blood cells move chaotically in all directions achieving very high speed.

This pattern determines the appearance of an irregular spectral profile (spectrum broadening), an ultrasound Doppler enlargement of spectrum track, and the disappearance of the systolic window (region below the curve) (Fig. 1.19) [40–42].

Distal to stenosis, it is observed, on the ultrasound Doppler tracking, a slope reduction both of the ascending branch (due to a decrease of the propulsive force) and of the descending branch (due to a peripheral compensatory vasodilatation); a "tardus and parvus" pulse appears (Fig. 1.20) [43–45].

In the proximal stenosis region, the velocimetric track is affected by the presence or absence of a collateral blood stream hemodynamically effective.

Due to lack of collateral blood stream the ultrasound Doppler curve appears as "slowed down"; that is, it shows a reduction in the systolic speed and the disappearance anterograde diastolic flow; pulsatility and resistance index tend to increase accordingly. In general, these phenomena are more evident close to the stenosis.

In the presence of an effective collateral blood stream such alterations can be barely detectable (Fig. 1.21). Unlike narrowing, in the presence of a vessel lumen dilatation (aneurysm) the ultra-

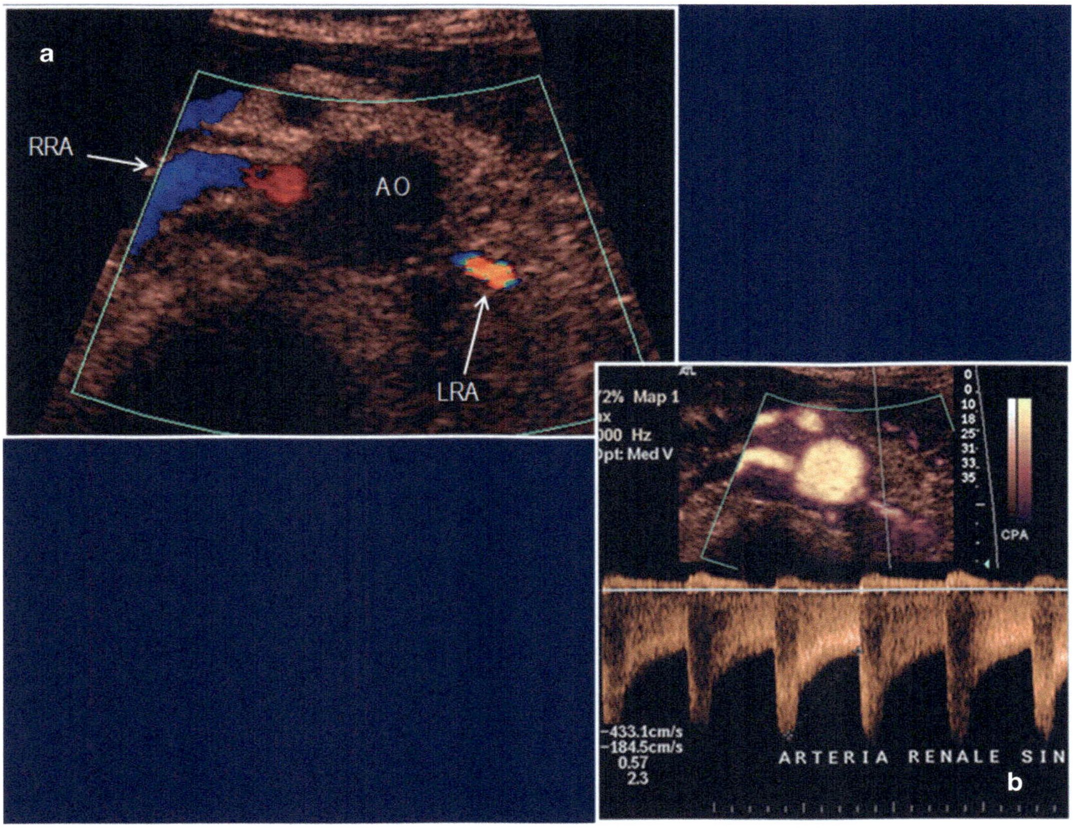

Fig. 1.19 Hemodynamically significant stenosis of the left renal artery. (**a**) Color Doppler image of the left renal arterial stenosis (LRA) shows aliasing in contrast to the normal chromatic code of the right renal artery (RRA). (**b**) Doppler analysis of the stenosis shows an increased peak systolic velocity (PSV = 433 cm/s), an increased diastolic velocity (DV = 184 cm/s), and no more systolic window

sound Doppler spectrum shows a reduction of systolic speed peak with slow vortex or swirling blood flow patterns, a "slowdown" of the axial flow, and an increase of the radial one. These modifications generate a variation of the wall vessel tension causing a progressive growth of aneurysm growth.

1.4.3.2 Alterations of Peripheral Blood Stream

Different situations (physiological or pathological) related to a vascularized tissue or organ may cause an increase or a reduction of the perfusion resistances with consequent changes of the relation between systolic and diastolic phase in the ultrasound Doppler spectrum.

Increase of perfusion resistance, in consequence of blood vessel pathologies or vascularized tissue pathology (nephropathy), causes a difficulty in perfusion with a reduction of peak systolic speed, especially diastolic: an increase of the resistance and pulsatility index is observed besides a speed reduction. Following a vascular and tubulointerstitial damage, in the renal district, caused by a critical stenosis of the main artery (chronic stenosis) a progressive increase of the intraparenchymal resistive index can be observed; this parenchymal vascular pattern

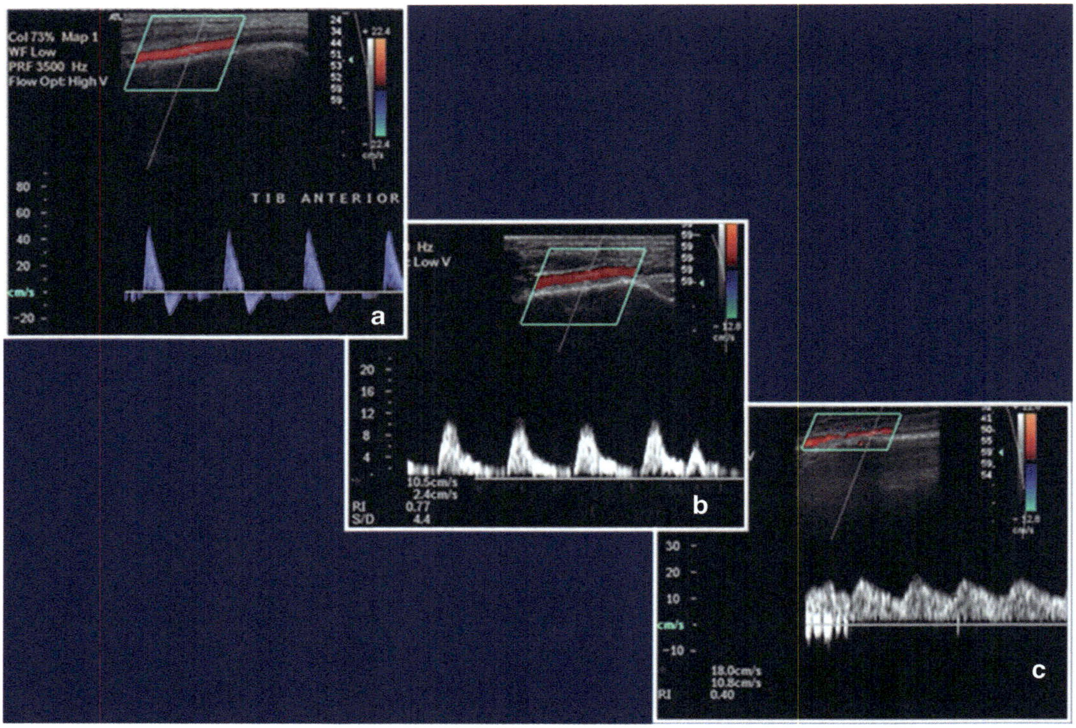

Fig. 1.20 Doppler waveform of peripheral arteries. (**a**) Spectral analysis without upstream stenosis (RI = 1). (**b**) Spectral Doppler waveform of a stenotic area shows an antegrade diastolic flow due to the reduction of the peripheral functional reserve (RI = 0.77). (**c**) Spectral Doppler waveform of a severe stenotic area shows an important antegrade diastolic flow due to a more severe peripheral functional reserve (RI = 0.40)

shows a chronic ischemia with a renal damage which reduces any successful possibility of revascularization.

Vascular resistance reduction determines a velocity increase of diastolic flow. This phenomenon can be secondary to a vasodilatation of a specific area or in the presence of fistulas (i.e., micro-arteriovenous fistulas of newly formed vessels due to neoplasia or in the presence of hemodialysis *macro*-arteriovenous *fistulas*): this induces a reduction of the resistive index and of the pulsatility index.

1.4.3.3 Arterial Wall Elasticity

Aging, hypertension, diabetes, atherosclerosis, or vascular prostheses (stent) determine a hardening of vessel walls causing a reduction of arterial wall elasticity. This condition determines an increase of vascular resistance and a velocimetric increase (not pathological); velocimetric curve shows an earlier dicrotic wave and an increase of the above index in the parenchymal tissues physiologically with a low resistance.

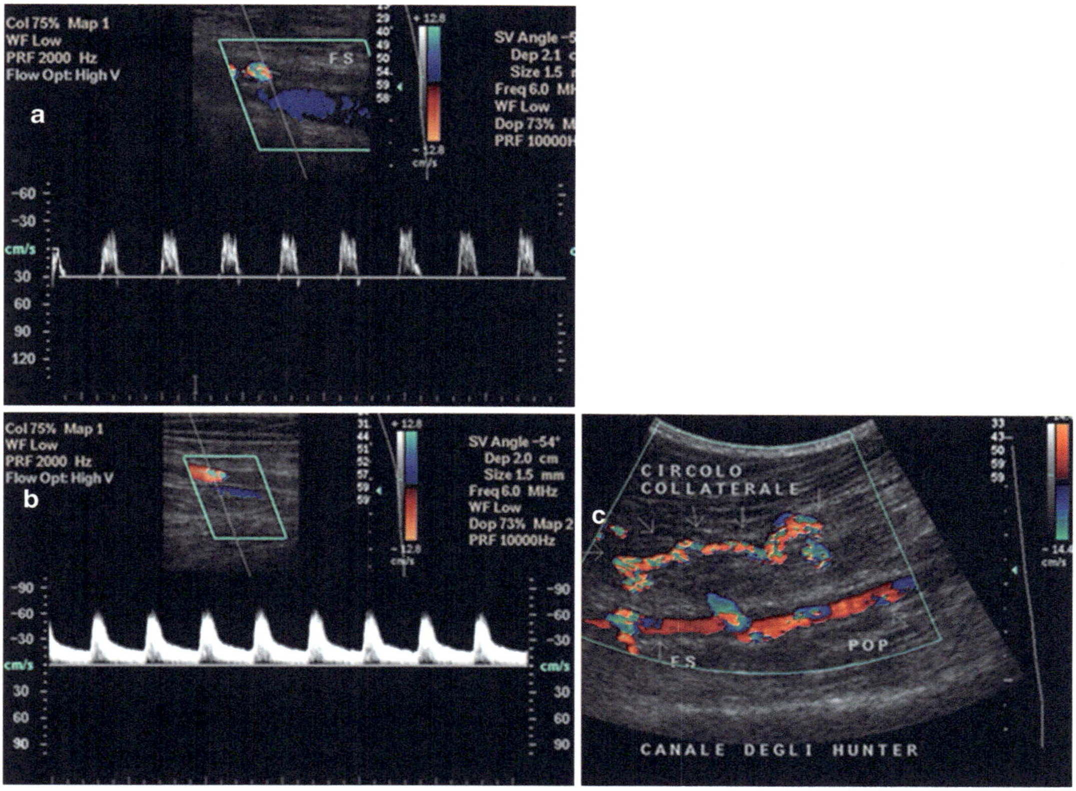

Fig. 1.21 Doppler spectral waveform analysis of a stenotic superficial femoral artery depending on the collateral circulation. (**a**) Without collateral circulation, the Doppler waveform shows a systolic morphology due to the absence of the diastolic flow. The velocity decreases (<30 cm/s) so the curve is defined to be "slowed down." (**b**) When the collateral flow is efficient, the Doppler curve upstream the stenosis demonstrates a reduction of the PSV (60 cm/s) and a partial component of the diastolic flow is seen. (**c**) Color Doppler image shows a hypertrophic collateral circulation (white arrows) with increased velocity over the femoral-popliteal axis

References

1. Taylor KJ, Holland S. Doppler US. Part 1. Basic principles, instrumentation and pitfalls. Radiology. 1990;174:297–307.
2. Kremkau FW. Doppler principles. Semin Roentgenol. 1992;17:6–16.
3. Kremkau FW. Diagnostic ultrasound. In: Principles and instruments. Part II: Doppler principles. 6th ed. St. Louis: Saunders, Elseviers; 2005. p. 157–248.
4. Burns PN. Principles of Doppler and color flow. Radiol Med. 1993;Suppl 1:S3–S16.
5. Kremkau FW. Principles and pitfalls of real-time color-flow imaging. In: Bernstein EF, editor. Vascular diagnosis. 4th ed. St. Louis: Mosby-Year Book; 1993.
6. Rabbia C, Matricardi L. "Eco-color-Doppler vascolare" III Edizione. Torino: Edizioni Minerva; 2006.
7. Taylor KJW. Clinical application of carotid Doppler ultrasound. In: Taylor KJW, Burns PN, Wells PNT, editors. Clinical applications of Doppler ultrasound. 8th ed. New York: Raven Press; 1988.
8. Winkler P, Hemke K, Mahl M. Major pitfalls in Doppler investigations. Part II Low flow velocities and colour Doppler applications. Pediatr Radiol. 1990;20:304–10.
9. Mitchel DJ. Color-Doppler imaging: principles, limitations and artifacts. Radiology. 1990;177:1–10.
10. Dauzat M, Laroche JF, De Bray JM, et al. Ultrasonographie vasculaire diagnostique. Theorie et pratique. Editions. Paris: Vigot; 1991.
11. Gill RW. Measurement of blood flow in ultrasound: accuracy and sources of error. Ultrasound Med Biol. 1995;11:625–41.

12. Boote EJ. Doppler ultrasound techniques: concept of blood flow detection and flow dynamics. Radiographics. 2003;23:1315–27.
13. Evans DH, McDicken WN, editors. Doppler ultrasound. Physics, instrumentation and signal processing. Chapter 4: Doppler systems: a general overview. Baffins Lane, Chichester (E): Wiley and Sons Ed; 2000. p. 43–70.
14. Hedrick WR, Hykes DI, Starchman DE. Doppler physics and instrumentation. In: Hedrick WR, Hykes DL, Starchman DE, editors. Ultrasound physics and instrumentation. 4th ed. St. Louis: Elsevier, Mosby; 2005. p. 205–19.
15. Remkau FW. Principles and instrumentation. In: Merritt CRB, editor. Doppler color imaging. New York: Churchill Livingstone; 1992.
16. Kremkau FW. Doppler color imaging. Principles and instrumentation. Clin Diagn Ultrasound. 1992;27:7–60.
17. Merrit CRB. Doppler color flow imaging. JCU. 1987;15:591–7.
18. Martinoli C, Pretolesi F, Crespi G, et al. Power Doppler sonography: clinical application. Eur J Radiol. 1998;27(S2):S133–40.
19. Rubin JM. Power Doppler. Section III: new imaging techniques. Technology. Eur Radiol. 1999;9:S318–22.
20. Berne RM, Levy MN, Physiology. 4th edn, 1998. Mosby Inc, Emodinamica. Ed. Italiana Casa editrice Ambrosiana 2000; pp. 422–437.
21. Milnor WR. Hemodynamics. Baltimore: Williams & Wilkins Ed; 1989. p. 1–408.
22. Batten JR, Neren RM. Model study of flow in curved and planar arterial bifurcations. Cardiovasc Res. 1982;16:178–86.
23. Ku DN, Giddens DP, Philips DJ, Strandness DE. Hemodynamics of the normal human carotid bifurcation: in vitro and in vivo studies. Ultrasound Med Biol. 1985;11:13–26.
24. Nichols WW, O'Rourke MF. McDonald's blood flow in arteries. 3rd edn. London: Edward Arnold Ed; 1990.
25. Middleton WD, Foley WD, Lawson TL. Flow reversal in normal carotid bifurcation: color doppler flow imaging analysis. Radiology. 1988;167:207–15.
26. Burns PN. The physical principles of Doppler and spectral analysis. J Clin Ultrasound. 1987;15:567–90.
27. Dauzat M. Notions théoriques et thechnologiques élémentaires. Bases de l'interpretation des signaux Doppler. In: Ultrasonographie vasculaire diagnostique. Vigot, Paris: Théorie et pratique. Ed; 1991. p. 3–35.
28. Meola M. Color-Doppler of renovascular diseases. G Ital Nefrol. 2007;24:425–45.
29. Holland CK, Clancy MJ, Taylor KJW. Volumetric flow estimation in vivo and in vitro using pulsed-Doppler ultrasound. Ultrasound Med Biol. 1996;22:591–603.
30. Burns PN. Measuring volume flow with Doppler ultrasound: an old nut. Ultrasound Obstet Gynecol. 1992;2:238–41.
31. Platt JF, Rubin JM, Ellis JH. Acute renal obstruction: evaluation with intrarenal duplex Doppler and conventional US. Radiology. 1993;186:685.
32. Handa N, Fukunaga R, Uehara A, et al. Echo Doppler velocimeter in the diagnosis of hypertensive patients: the renal artery Doppler technique. Ultrasound Med Biol. 1986;12:945–52.
33. Mostbeck GH, Kain R, Mallek R, et al. Duplex Doppler US in patients with medical renal disease. Histopathologic correlation. J Ultrasound Med. 1991;10:189–94.
34. Tublin ME, Bude RO, Platt JF. Review: the resistive index in renal Doppler sonography. Where do we stand? Am J Roentgenol. 2003;180:885–92.
35. Tedesco MA, Natale F, Mocerino R, et al. Renal resistive index and cardiovascular organ damage in a large population of 36 hypertensive patients. J Hum Hypertens. 2007;21:291–6.
36. Kim SH, Kim VH, Choi BI, et al. Duplex Doppler US in patients with medical renal disease: resistive index vs serum creatinine. Clin Radiol. 1992;45:85–7.
37. Napoli V, Bartolozzi C, et al. Duplex ultrasonographic study of the renal arteries before and after renal artery stenting. Eur Radiol. 2002;12(4):796.
38. Webb JAW. The role of ultrasonography in the diagnosis of intrinsic renal disease. Clin Radiol. 1994;49:589–91.
39. Stavros AT, Parker SH, Yakes WF, et al. Segmental stenosis of the renal artery: pattern recognition of tardus and parvus abnormalities with duplex sonography. Radiology. 1992;184:487–92.
40. House MK, Dowling RJ, King P, et al. Using Doppler sonography to reveal renal artery stenosis: an evaluation of the optimal imaging parameters. Am J Roentgenol. 1999;173:761–5.
41. Arbeille P, Bouin-Pineau MH, Herault S. Accuracy of the main Doppler methods for evaluating the degree of carotid stenoses (continuous wave, pulsed wave, and color Doppler). Ultrasound Med Biol. 1999;25:65–731.
42. Spencer MP, Reid JM. Quantification of carotid stenosis with continuous-wave (C-W) Doppler ultrasound. Stroke. 1979;10:326–30.
43. Grant EG, Benson CB, Moneta GL, et al. "Carotid artery stenosis: gray-scale and Doppler US diagnosis" Society of Radiologist in Ultrasound Consensus Conference. Radiology. 2003;229:340–6.
44. Favaretto E, Pili C, Amato A, et al. Analysis of agreement between Duplex ultrasound scanning and arteriography in patients with lower limb artery disease. J Cardiovasc Med. 2007;8:337–41.
45. Jorgensen JJ, Stranden E, Myhre HO, et al. Flow velocity patterns of the lower limb arteries investigated by a pulsed Doppler ultrasound flowmeter. A study in healthy control subjects. J Oslo City Hosp. 1984;34:109–14.

Grayscale Ultrasound Artifacts

2

Matilda Muça, Francesca Currò, Camilla Sachs, and Irene Campo

2.1 Introduction

The more frequent basic mode used in echography is the brightness mode (B-mode) and it provides a black-and-white two-dimensional image [1]. The B-mode imaging is created by converting the reflected waves in signals whose luminosity is modulated depending on the echo amplitude [2]. Often during the echographic exam acquisition artifacts may occur. To know the artifacts we should consider that the sound travels in straight lines, the registered echoes originate from reflectors placed along the transducer axis, the scattering strength of the imaged objects determinates the intensity of the returning echoes, and the distance is proportional to the round-trip travel time of 1540 ms [3]. Ultrasound artifacts seen in B-mode imaging can be subdivided into positive artifacts (increase in density and/or brightness, echoes reinforcement) and negative artifacts (decrease in density and/or brightness, echo absence, or shadows). There are also artifacts that determine the image deformation and those given from interaction of the beam phenomenon, grouping artifacts determined by equipment pre- and post-processing [2]. We can also divide the artifacts into those useful for diagnostic purposes (rear reinforcement, posterior acoustic shadowing, lateral acoustic shadows, comet-tail artifact, ring-down artifact, artifacts related to the velocity of propagation) and those that are sources of diagnostic errors (reverberation, mirror effect, refraction artifacts, partial-volume effect, and side lobe artifact) [3, 4]. In recent studies, the ultrasound artifacts seen in B-mode imaging are subdivided into those that are primarily related to structures and tissues with which the beam interacts and those that are primarily related to the beam properties and processing [4]. Basically a large part of ultrasound artifacts are the consequence of errors that arise from the ultrasound beam characteristics, velocity and attenuation errors, and presence of multiple echo paths [5].

M. Muça (✉)
Department of Radiology, Fuerth Hospital, University of Erlangen-Nürnberg, Erlangen, Germany

F. Currò
Department of Radiology, Maggiore Hospital, University of Trieste, Trieste, Italy

C. Sachs
Department of Radiology, Cattinara Hospital, University of Trieste, Trieste, Italy

I. Campo
Department of Radiology, Civile Hospital, Conegliano, Italy

2.2 Artifacts Related to Structures and Beam Interaction

2.2.1 Rear Reinforcement (Enhancement Artifact)

The increasing intensity of the echoes placed in the downstream area of a liquid collection creates this artifact which is pathognomonic of

A. Granata, M. Bertolotto (eds.), *Imaging in Nephrology*, https://doi.org/10.1007/978-3-030-60794-4_2

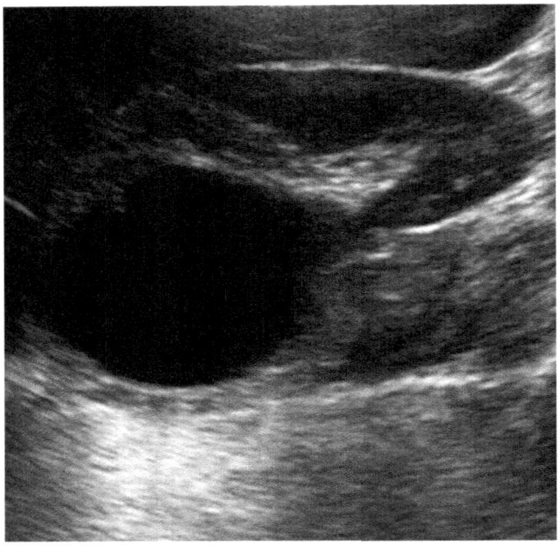

Fig. 2.1 Grayscale image demonstrating rear reinforcement with increasing intensity of the echoes placed in the downstream area of a liquid collection, in this case represented by a renal cyst. The beam does not undergo the normal attenuation phenomena. This artifact is pathognomonic of liquid collections

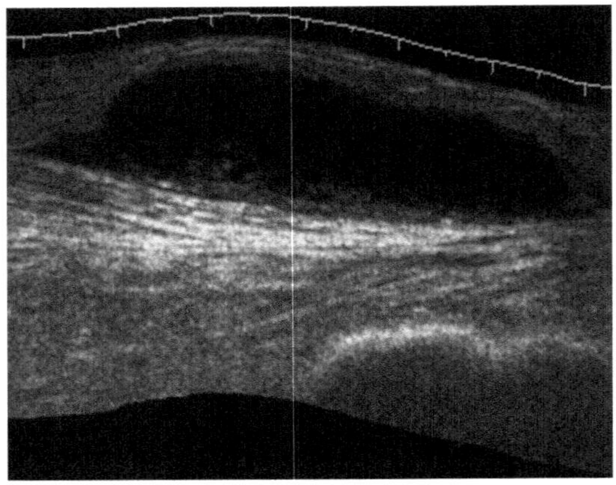

Fig. 2.2 Grayscale image demonstrating the acoustic enhancement artifact downstream of a hematoma in the rectus abdominis

liquid collections (Fig. 2.1) [2]. The beam amplitude deep into a liquid collection is increased because the ultrasound beam encounters a more weakly attenuating structure in its path than in the surrounding tissue [4]. The liquid collection structures attenuate less sound if compared with a solid structure so the strength of the sound pulse is higher after passing the liquid structure and this is shown as brightness deeply to a liquid structure [6]. The rear reinforcement is considered a positive artifact because it causes an increase in signal brightness and echoes reinforcement (Fig. 2.2). An ultrasonic beam which passes through a liquid structure is neither absorbed nor attenuated and does not produce echoes while in the sideways tissues the beam undergoes the normal attenuation phenomena. Therefore, downstream of the liquid collection, different intensity signals arrive and those passing through the liquid collection are more intense [2]. So echoes returning from tissues located deep into the liquid object will display significantly higher signals than the surrounding tissue, resulting in the enhancement artifact [4]. Given that the propagation velocity of the ultrasonic beam into liquids is lower than that in the surrounding parenchymal tissue, the signal travel time is higher and the posterior wall echoes are represented at greater distances than they really are. This phenomenon simulates a thickening of the posterior wall. The enhancement artifact is commonly encountered deep into fluid collections such as the urinary bladder, gallbladder, and cysts or even in case of a significant amount of ascitic fluid between the gallbladder and the transducer which generates a false thickening of the gallbladder wall [2, 4]. The small cysts may miss the rear reinforcement presenting echoes inside and shaded walls [2]. This artifact could be seen also in predominantly liquid lesions like abscesses or hemangioma (Figs. 2.3 and 2.4) and in solid lesions like metastasis (Figs. 2.5 and 2.6) or tumors (Figs. 2.7 and 2.8). The rear reinforcement, the absence of echoes within the liquid lesion, and the regular walls of the lesion are part of the triad of findings that classify a lesion as a cyst (Fig. 2.9).

2.2.2 Shadowing Artifacts

This artifact is caused by partial or complete attenuation of the ultrasound beam along its path due to absorption or reflection by an object or a tissue [4]. The rear shadow is a negative artifact because it determines signal decrease or disappearance. Limited or no energy arrives distally to

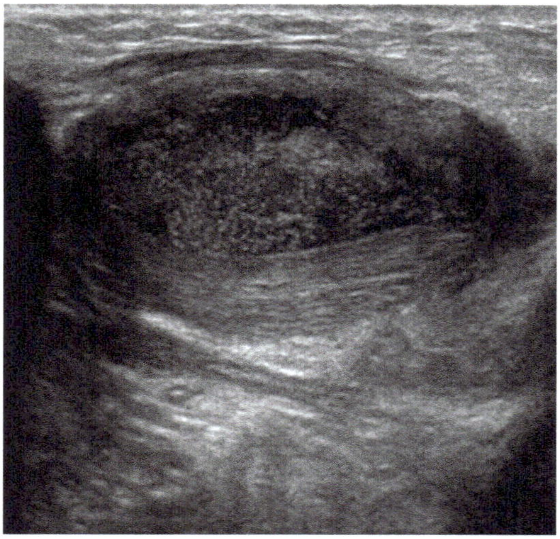

Fig. 2.3 Grayscale image demonstrating the rear reinforcement in one case of a submandibular gland abscess. This is to demonstrate that this artifact is present in any type of liquid collection

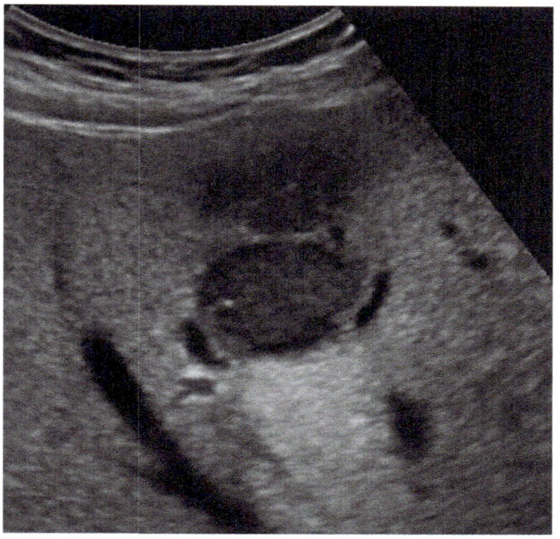

Fig. 2.5 Grayscale image showing the rear reinforcement that could be evident also distally to a solid nodule as in this case of hepatic metastases originated from a cancer of the tongue

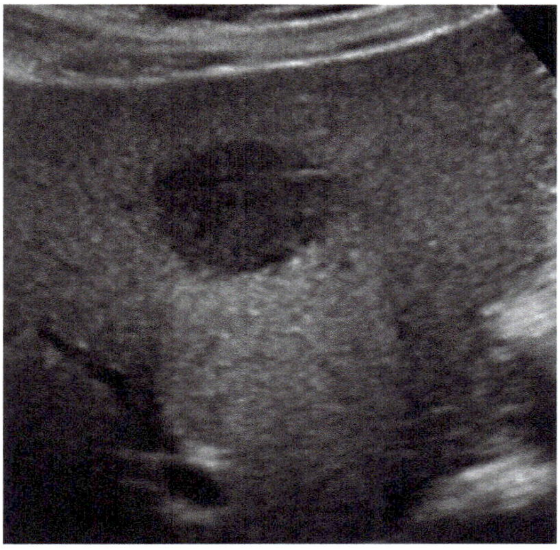

Fig. 2.4 The rear reinforcement is frequently observed in predominantly liquid formations like microcystic thyroid nodules or hepatic hemangiomas as in this case

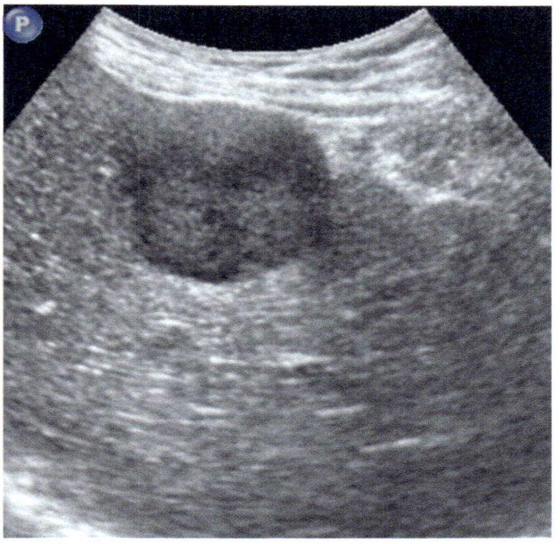

Fig. 2.6 Another grayscale image demonstrating the rear reinforcement in one case of hepatic metastasis originated from a cancer of the esophagus

an absorbent or reflective material and an area with weak or null echo signals is created. These areas are defined as rear shadows, acoustic shadows, or rear shadow cones and are classified as "clean" or "dirty" artifacts. The cleaned shadow cones have sharp margins, are echo free, and are determined primarily by absorption phenomena; typically shadow cones are observed deeply to large calcified structures that absorb the ultrasound beam (Figs. 2.10 and 2.11). The dirty shadow cones are determined mainly by reflection and reverberation phenomena; they have blurred margins, contain echoes inside, and are usually caused by air components that form an impenetrable barrier to sounds (Figs. 2.12 and 2.13) [2, 4]. The dense and rich-in-collagen

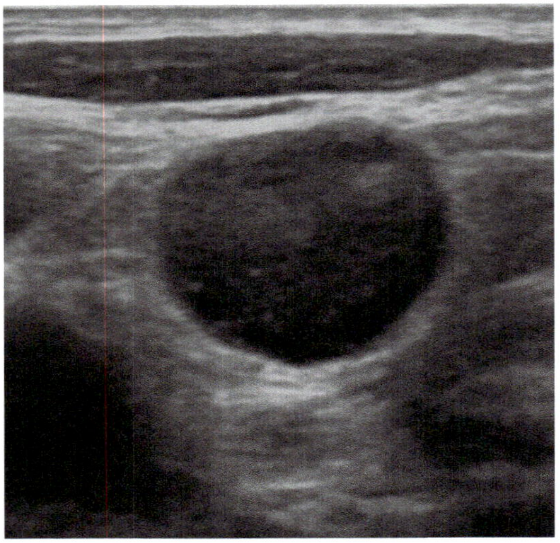

Fig. 2.7 A grayscale image demonstrating a modest rear reinforcement in one case of lateral-cervical lymphadenomegaly

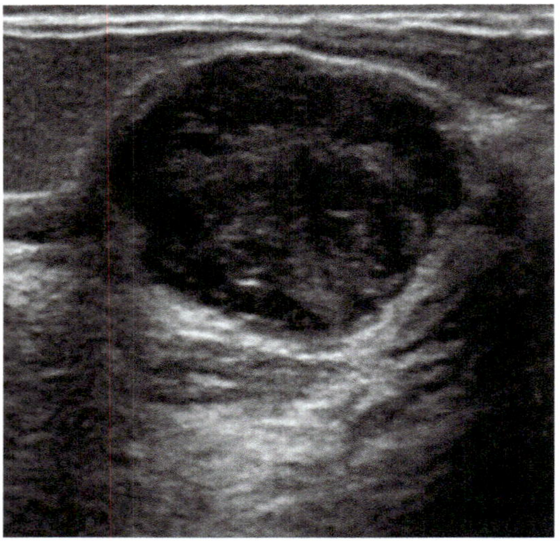

Fig. 2.8 A case of a breast phyllodes cancer with a fairly inhomogeneous echo structure and irregular edges where rear reinforcement is also seen

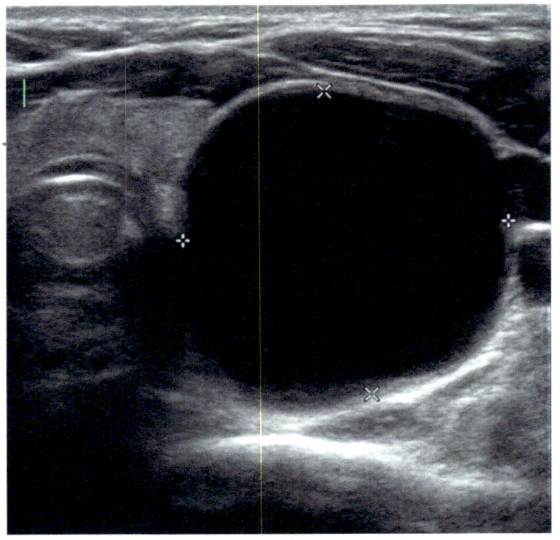

Fig. 2.9 Grayscale image demonstrating rear reinforcement of a thyroid cyst. The rear reinforcement together with the absence of echoes within the lesion and the regular walls of the lesion is so important that it is part of the triad of findings that classify a lesion as a cyst

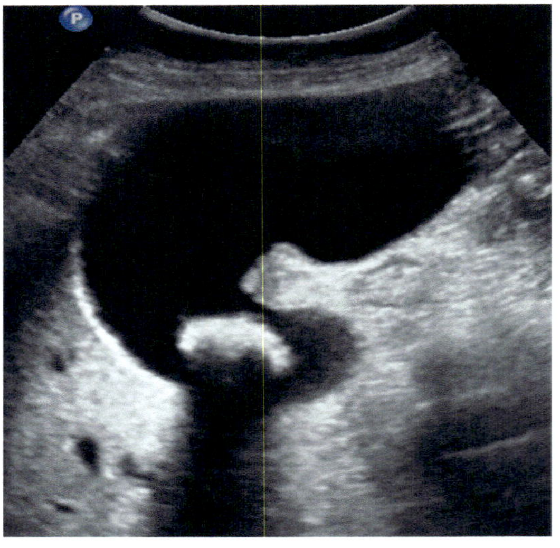

Fig. 2.10 Grayscale image demonstrating shadowing artifact. This artifact is due to the absence of echoes posteriorly to a structure because the structure reflects or absorbs much of the energy of the ultrasonic beam as in this case of gallbladder stone

parenchymal tissues determine shadows by absorption phenomena while calculations and calcifications by reflection and absorption phenomena. Generally calculations with more than 3 mm of diameter produce acoustic shadow, regardless of their chemical composition, whereas very small calculations, dimensionally comparable with the wavelength of the wave beam, are not detected because the shadow effect is masked by diffraction phenomena [2]. Caution should be taken when there is no complete view

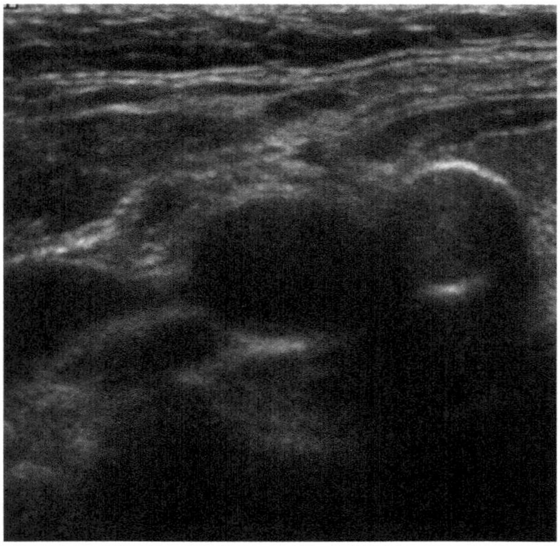

Fig. 2.11 Shadowing artifact in a grayscale image in which calcifications of the carotid artery wall are shown

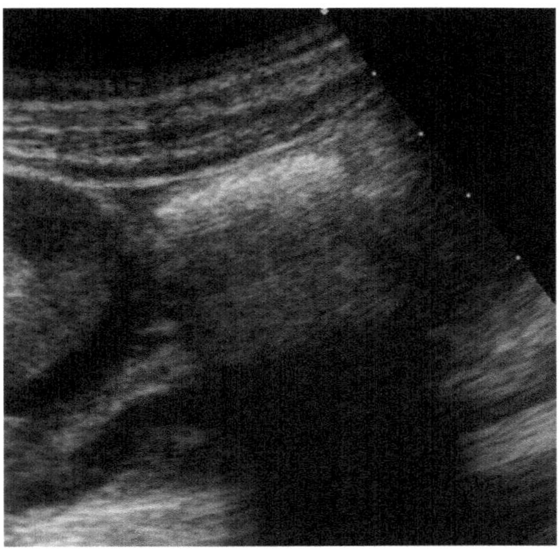

Fig. 2.12 It is necessary to differentiate the shadowing artifact produced from calculations from those produced from gas. Indeed those produced from gas are less marked than those produced from calcification and may present internal echoes (the "dirty" shadow) related to reverberations between the surface of the air bubble and the transducer as is shown in this grayscale image of an intestinal loop containing gas

of an organ because of the shadow artifact; in this situation lesions can be hidden in non-visible areas (Fig. 2.14). Scanning from a different transducer angle or an alternate window can resolve this issue [4, 7].

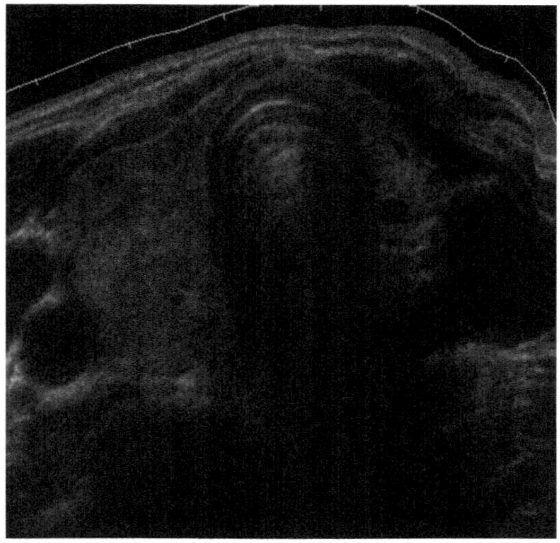

Fig. 2.13 Grayscale image showing a shadowing artifact in a filled-air structure (trachea)

2.2.3 Side Acoustic Shadows

The side acoustic shadows are the shadow cones observed at the side margins of a liquid collection. The ultrasonic beam that encounters a rounded liquid collection is partially reflected and partially refracted; refraction is greater for incidence angles larger than normal as it happens at the side margins of a liquid collection. As we said, the ultrasound beam travels at lower velocities in cystic formations than the surrounding tissue and the refracted beams converge toward the lower velocity tissue path. The refracted beams diverge when the incident beam encounters a lesion with regular and smooth wall which is crossed by the beam at higher velocity. Therefore the propagated beam over the side edges of the formation is attenuated and diverted and downstream of the reflection and refraction area the ultrasonic energy does not arrive. This appears on the display as an area without signals defined as side acoustic shadow (Fig. 2.15). In clinical practice the side acoustic shadows are seen basically at the lateral wall of the cysts (Figs. 2.16 and 2.17), but they may be present also in the existing interfaces between parenchymatous tissues with different acoustic impedance and velocity that the beam hits tangentially (Fig. 2.18). This artifact is seen for example

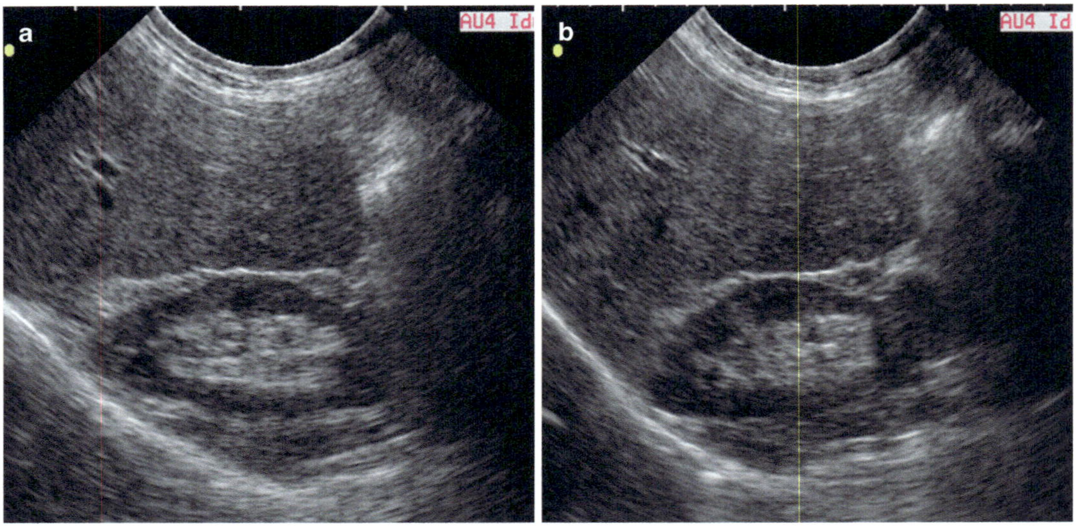

Fig. 2.14 Posteriorly to a structure that generates acoustic shadow can be hidden different pathologies. In this case the lower renal pole is hidden from gas contained in an intestinal loop (**a**) and after a deep breath and the probe reposition a lesion is shown at the lower renal pole (**b**)

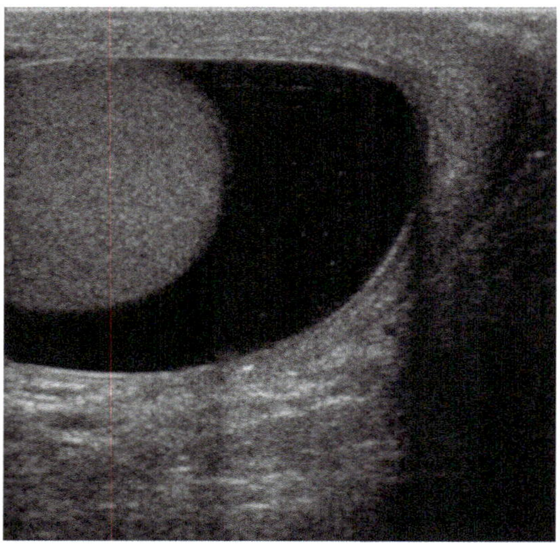

Fig. 2.15 Grayscale image demonstrating a side acoustic shadow artifact. It occurs while the ultrasound propagates with different velocity in round liquid structures than the surrounding tissues. An example of a side acoustic shadow artifact in a testicular varicocele

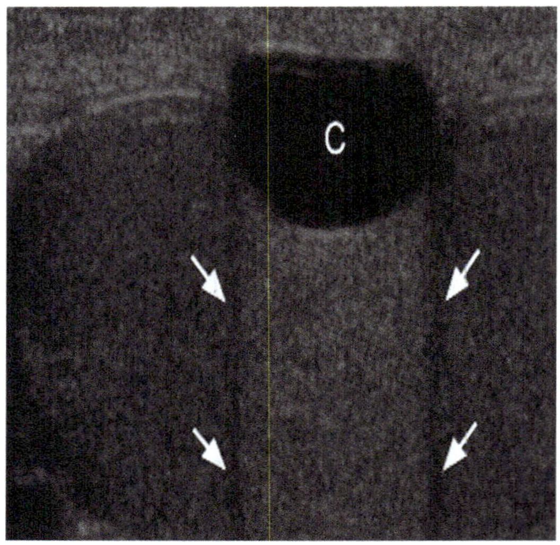

Fig. 2.16 A representation of the side acoustic shadow artifact (arrows) in a grayscale image of a cystic liver lesion (c)

between soft tissue and gallbladder, soft tissue and urinary bladder, liver and kidney, and muscle and fat [2].

2.2.4 Comet-Tail Artifact

The same tissue conditions that determine the posterior shadow, for example soft tissue—dense tissue or parenchymal tissue—gas interface, can

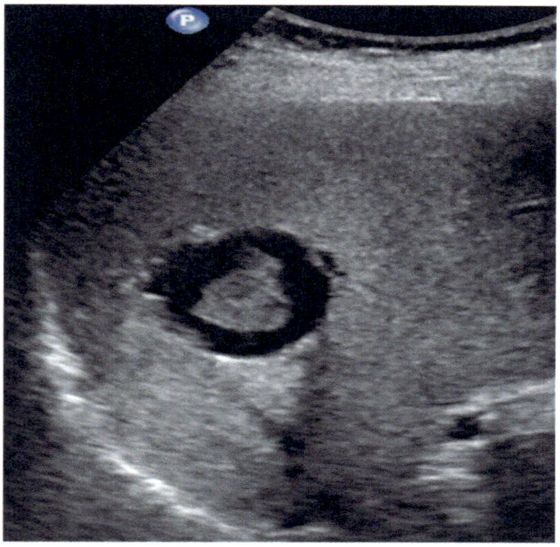

Fig. 2.17 Grayscale image showing a side acoustic shadow artifact in one subcapsular mixed liver lesion partly cystic (rear reinforcement artifact is also seen) and partly solid

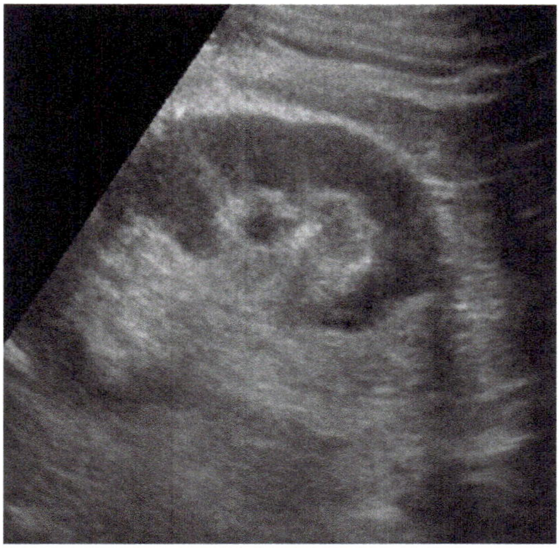

Fig. 2.18 Grayscale image demonstrating a side acoustic shadow artifact to the lower renal pole due to different acoustic impedance by the renal parenchyma and fat

simultaneously determine the onset of positive artifacts characterized by high signal brightness such as the comet-tail artifact and the ring-down artifact (Fig. 2.19) [2]. Multiple reverberations between the transducer and numerous closely spaced reflections cause the comet-tail artifact

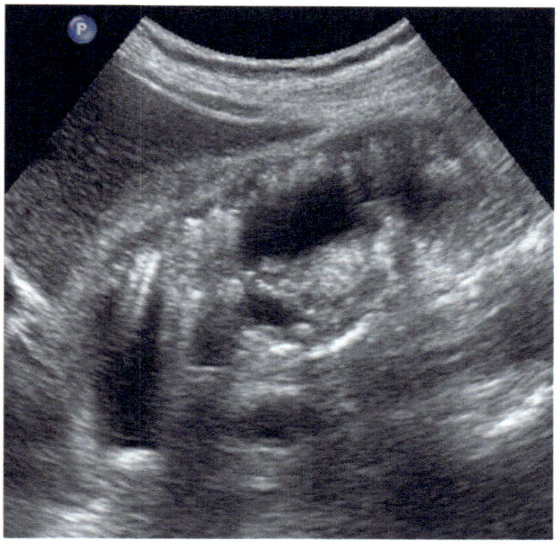

Fig. 2.19 Grayscale image demonstrating a comet-tail artifact. This artifact is projected distally to smaller structures with highly reflective anterior and posterior interfaces and is represented as a series of small echoes of triangular morphology as shown in this case in the stomach wall

[4]. It is shown as a series of dense echo stripes that originate from highly reflective interfaces like soft tissue-metal, soft tissue-mineral salts, and soft tissue-gas and are projected distally along the beam direction. They are formed by numerous small parallel echo bands disposed transversely to the beam direction which has generated them. These dense stripes are less wide if they are distant from the object that generated them. Unequal intervals can separate the bands which correspond to the distances between the reverberant elements [2].

In clinical practice this artifact can be determined by natural, pathological, or artificial gas-filled cavities, vessels and ducts, calculations, parenchymal and vessel wall calcifications (Fig. 2.20), metallic or plastic material catheters, clips, and intrauterine devices [2, 8]. Even cholesterol crystals or clusters of air microbubbles can cause the comet-tail artifact [4].

Lichtenstein et al. described a sensitivity of 92.5% and a specificity of 65.1% of the comet-tail artifact in diagnosing radiologic alveolar-interstitial syndrome of the lung parenchyma. In this case subpleural thickened interlobular septa

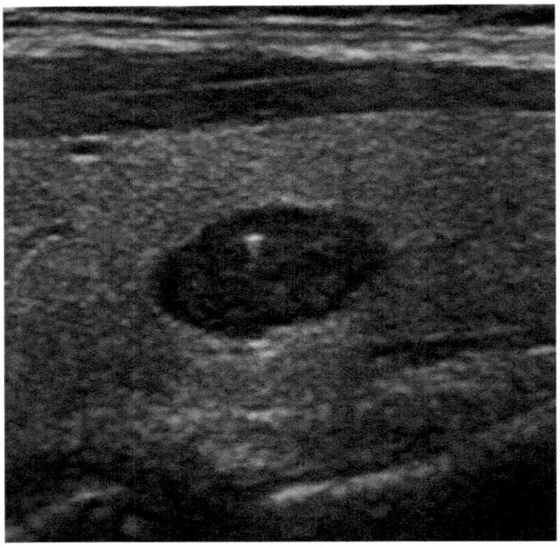

Fig. 2.20 Grayscale image demonstrating a comet-tail artifact usually observed in structures with crystal component, microcalcifications, clip, and metal needles. This is an example of comet-tail artifact in a colloid crystal of a hyperplastic thyroid nodule

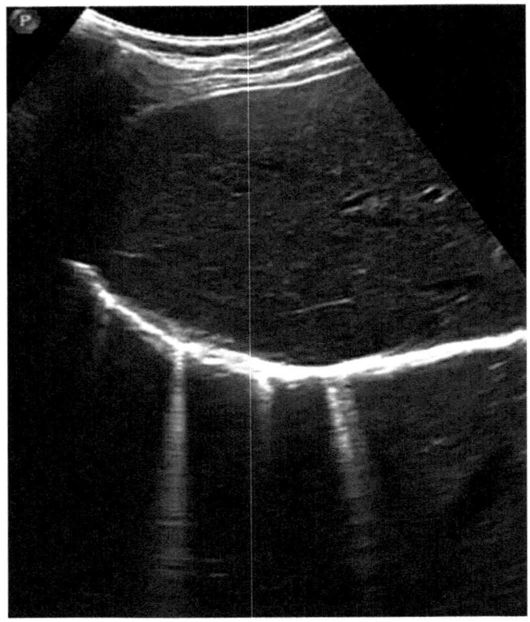

Fig. 2.21 Grayscale image in which a ring-down artifact is shown. This artifact originates from air microbubbles that resonate with the ultrasound beam. The ring-down artifact is represented by hyperechoic streaks or a continuous series of transverse parallel bands perpendicular to the beam direction. It arises distally to air bubbles

generate the artifact. Also in cases of acute pulmonary edema, chronic interstitial diseases, and ground-glass areas this artifact is present [9].

2.2.5 Ring-Down Artifact

It is formed upstream of a gas collection and appears as a continuous hyperechoic strip or a series of transverse parallel bands perpendicular to the beam direction (Fig. 2.21). The enclosed fluid between gas microbubbles generates this artifact. The ultrasound beam strikes the liquid contained in the microbubbles that enter in vibration and emit to the transducer a continuous reflected sound. The emitted signal is continuous, with gradually decreasing intensity and with periodic amplitude fluctuations. The bands of the ring-down artifact have two essential characteristics such as the periodicity that corresponds to the distance between the bands and the band thickness. These two parameters are constant for each ring-down artifact but change from a ring-down to another increasing or decreasing concordantly. The ring-down artifact is different from a comet-tail artifact which is rather a reverberation artifact and has both different appearance and formation mechanism, but they are both positive artifacts [2]. This artifact should be carefully evaluated and could be useful in patients with suspicion of bowel perforation (Fig. 2.22) or in case of surgical complications (Fig. 2.23).

2.2.6 Reverberation

Reverberation is caused by multiple reflections of the ultrasound beam between the transducer and a highly reflective interface [2]. Usually it is due to relevant differences in the acoustic impedance at the interface of two adjacent tissues [4]. When the ultrasonic wave beam meets an interface, an echo is formed and is recorded as part of the beam energy reflected back to the transducer while the remaining energy returns back to the subject tissue. This beam is then reflected a third time and returns back to the transducer to record a second echo. This phenomenon occurs until

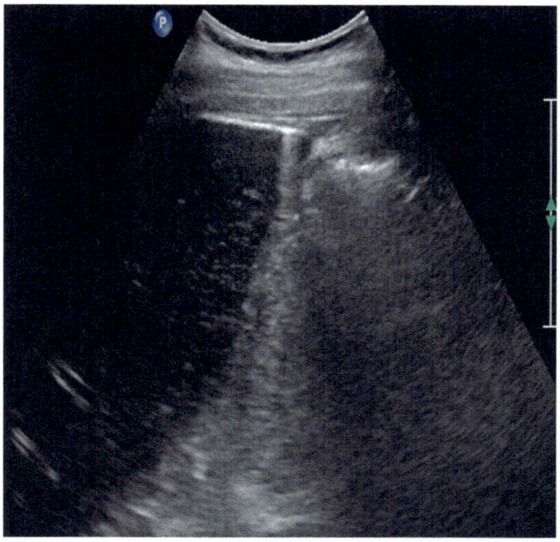

Fig. 2.22 Hyperechoic streak is shown between the liver and the anterior abdominal wall in this grayscale B-mode image. The patient was suffering from abdominal pain. The ring-down artifact in this case is due to the presence of air bubble between the liver and the anterior abdominal wall in a patient with abdominal perforation

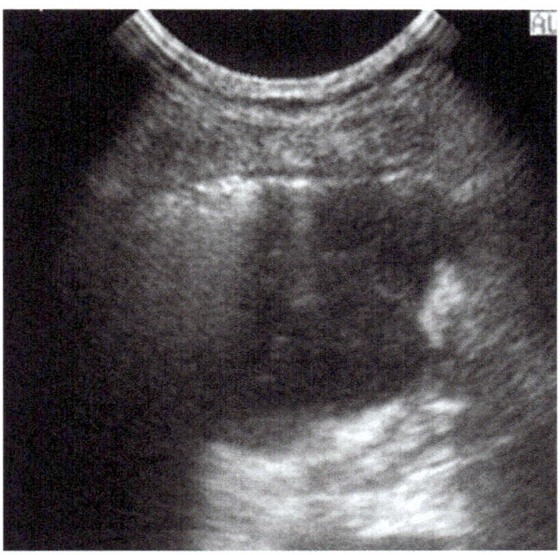

Fig. 2.23 Ultrasound grayscale image in a patient with fever after surgery where liquid collection and surface air bubbles in an abdominal abscess are shown

exhaustion of the energy for absorption [2]. This procedure repeated several times gives rise to multiple echoes [4]. As a result of these multiple reflections the transducer receives many returning pulses generated by the same beam and the

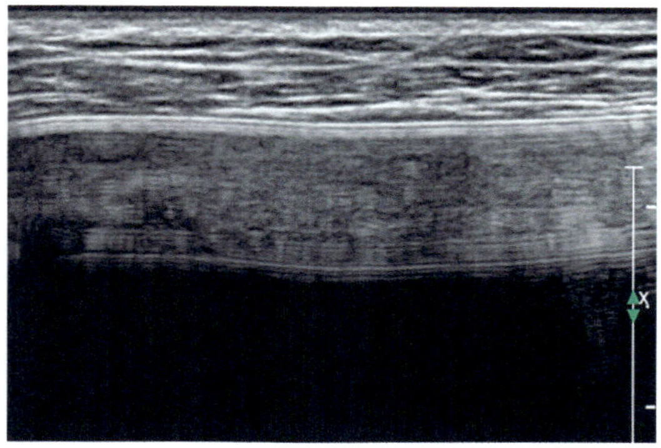

Fig. 2.24 Grayscale ultrasound image demonstrating the reverberation artifact from breast prosthesis. This artifact is seen when multiple reflections of the ultrasonic beam between the transducer and a highly reflective interface are generated

same interface; therefore the machine registers multiple echoes spaced from each other by progressively increasing times, shown on the display as increasing distances from the transducer (Fig. 2.24). Moreover, in addition to the real interface, we will have images of a second and third interface. The greater the intensity of the reflected signal the more evident the reverberation artifact. This is a very frequent phenomenon present in almost all ultrasound images and is usually projected as bright parallel lines at uniform intervals at progressively weaker intensity. This phenomenon occurs between different tissue interfaces, for example soft tissue-bone, bone-fluid, and fluid-gas. This artifact could be useful in identifying abnormal gas collections such as pneumobilia. However, reverberation often obscures the underlying structures and can mimic space-occupying masses (Fig. 2.25) [2, 4]. By selecting an imaging plane which does not include the highly reflective interface, the reverberation artifact can be avoided [4].

2.2.7 Rain Effect

The rain effect is due to multiple diffuse reflection types which occur between the transducer and the different layers of overlying soft tissues and a highly reflective interface typically represented by the proximal wall of a liquid collection.

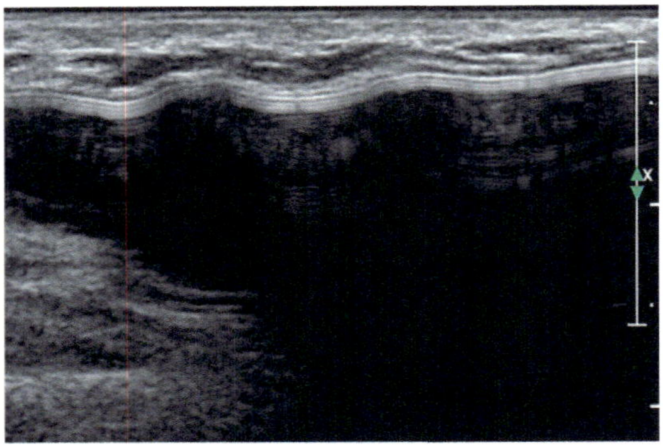

Fig. 2.25 Another case of reverberation artifact from breast prosthesis in a grayscale ultrasound image. Underlying structures can be obscured and the echoes of the artifact can mimic space-occupying diseases

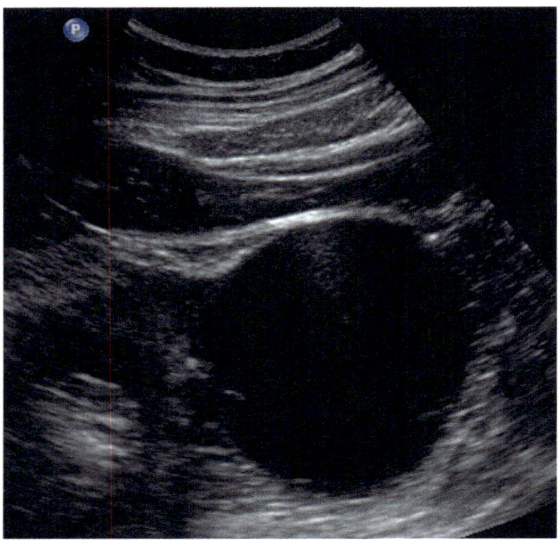

Fig. 2.26 Grayscale image showing a rain effect into a renal cystic lesion. This artifact is important for the differential diagnosis between a solid and a liquid element

The multiple diffuse reflection types have a low-to-medium brightness and are projected downstream a reflective interface to an area without echoes like a liquid collection. The rain effect is an important semeiological sign because it occurs only in the fluid-filled tissues (e.g., bladder, gallbladder, cysts, ascites) and it is often a differential diagnosis element between solid and liquid lesions (Fig. 2.26). Rain effect might mimic vegetating images or hide the presence of real pathologies [2].

2.2.8 Mirror Image Artifact

This is an artifact for which a normal or pathological object is placed between the transducer and a strong specular reflection interface [2]. Usually this artifact is caused by large reflective structures which redirect the beam in a different direction and when the echoes produced by the redirected sound reach the transducer; following the reverse path a displaced image will be generated [10]. When the beam invests the mass and reaches perpendicularly the specular interface, the time of flight for the ultrasound beam is prolonged. A second artifactual false image due to axial specular reflections and reverberations is created and this image is placed along the beam path downstream the interface [4]. On the other hand, when the beam is reflected by an obliquely disposed specular interface and thereafter invests the mass positioned upstream the interface, the machine does not reflect the real path of the beam and the false image is placed downstream the interface [2]. This phenomenon can generate a mirror image by registering the created echoes as equidistant by the object but on the opposite side of the reflector [4]. In clinical practice the mirror effect is often observed at the diaphragm (Fig. 2.27) and for example liver lesions can produce a second false image above the diaphragm (Fig. 2.28). The mirror effect can also occur at the posterior wall of the heart, the pleura, and the bowel. The duplication of the bladder image behind the sigma in the pelvic cavity produces a false mass effect (Fig. 2.29). By modifying the probe position and the patient posture, you can make sure that this is an artifact [2].

2.2.9 Lateral Displacement of the Image Artifact

It is caused by the beam refraction when it tangentially strikes the interface of a spherical or curve surface. If the so deviated beam encounters a different echogenicity element, compared to the tissue where it propagates after being deflected, the machine ignores the refraction and repro-

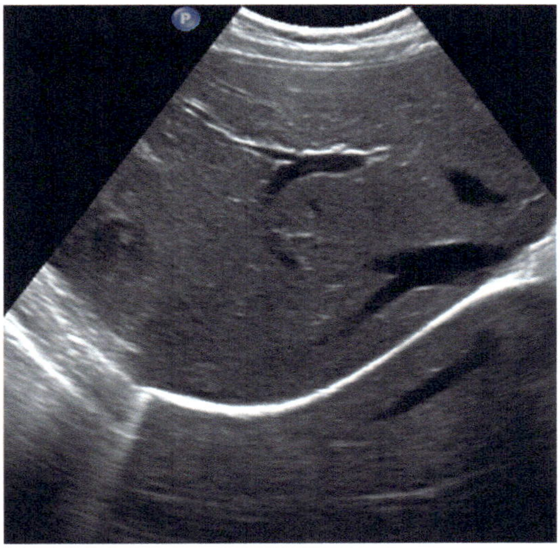

Fig. 2.27 Grayscale ultrasound image demonstrating the mirror effect at the level of the diaphragm. A normal or a pathological formation between the transducer and a highly reflective interface determines the formation of a second artifactual image

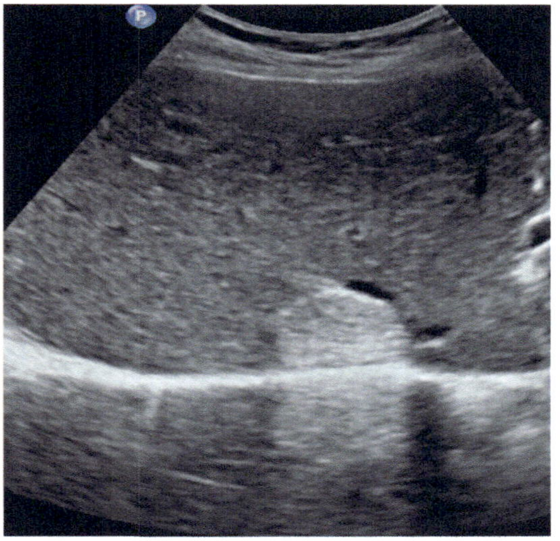

Fig. 2.28 A liver lesion that appears duplicated at the diaphragm in a grayscale ultrasound image due to the mirror effect

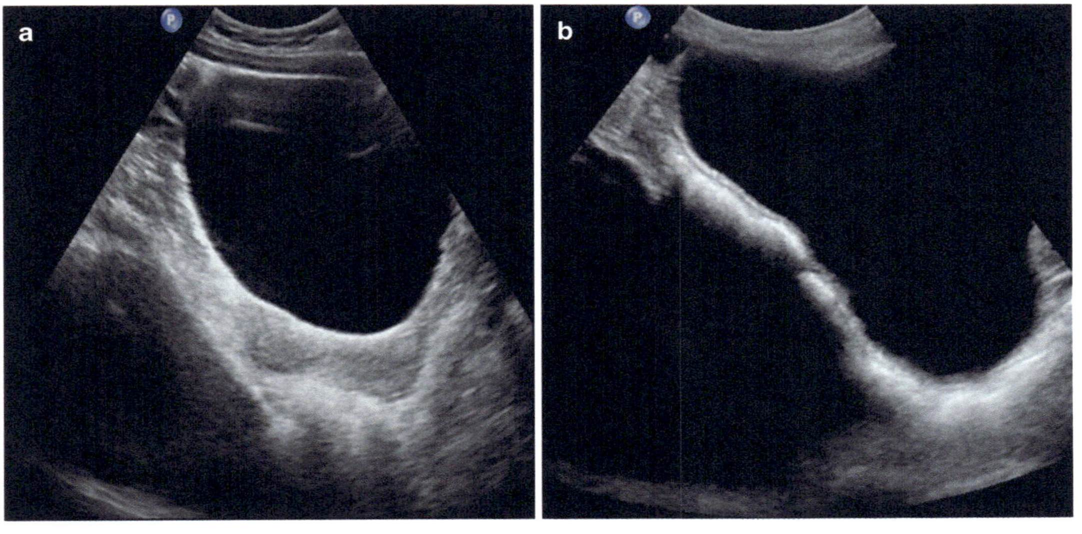

Fig. 2.29 Grayscale ultrasound image (**a**) demonstrating the mirror effect that creates a duplication of the image of the bladder which mimics a pelvic injury (**b**). This finding was not confirmed at the CT investigation

duces the image in the same direction that the beam had before being refracted. The reproduced image corresponds to the element that has determined it but is positioned laterally to the real location in the shadow caused by refraction. This artifact is comparable to what occurs in underwater images observed from the sea surface according to oblique lines of view compared to the water surface [2]. This artifact can be corrected by modifying the probe position.

2.2.10 Image Splitting or Refraction Artifact

It is an artifact caused by a twofold refraction of the beam which occurs when transverse scans in particular anatomical regions are performed; for example in suprapubic headquarters the beam undergoes a double refraction at the interfaces between the medial edges of the rectus abdominis, aponeurosis, and fat [2, 4]. When the sound passes obliquely through an interface between two media transmitting sound at different speeds the sound changes its direction and this depends on both the angle of the incident ultrasound beam and the difference in velocity between the two media [6]. Consequently a dual-lateral image shift is generated and any deeply placed object at the midline may appear duplicated (Fig. 2.30). Every object of dimensions less than 1 cm can be duplicated, whereas larger objects can be enlarged, distorted, or interrupted (Fig. 2.31) [2].

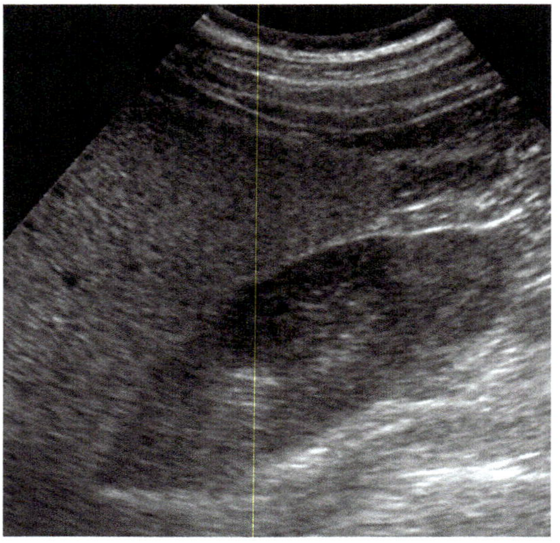

Fig. 2.31 At the level of the inferior pole of the kidney it is possible to recognize an alteration of the echogenicity that simulates a lesion because the refractions at the level of curved interfaces can partially duplicate the profile of the organs creating false images

2.2.11 Speed Error Artifact

The speed of sound in tissue is around 1540 m/s [11] and speed differences with which an ultrasonic beam is propagated in the parenchymatous tissues are modest. The propagation velocity in liquids is significantly lower (1480 m/s) and a cyst image will have the greatest diameter parallel to the beam axis [2]. A small round calculation will be crossed at higher velocity (almost threefold higher range of 3500–4600 m/s) [11] and will present the largest diameter perpendicular to the beam axis. When a considerable size organ like the diaphragm is reproduced by a beam that crossed partly a homogeneous tissue such as the liver and partly an inhomogeneous tissue (liver and liquid collection, liver and fat, etc.) the diaphragm appears as interrupted (Fig. 2.32). This is because the downstream portion of the inhomogeneous tissue is crossed with a lower velocity and will be reproduced further away from the transducer. So the additional time that the impulse has employed in crossing the liquid collection is translated by the probe in a greater distance. In skeletal muscle, a tissue poor of fat, the velocity of sound is greater than 1540 m/s and so the deeper objects will be dislocated and misrepresented as being shallower [4].

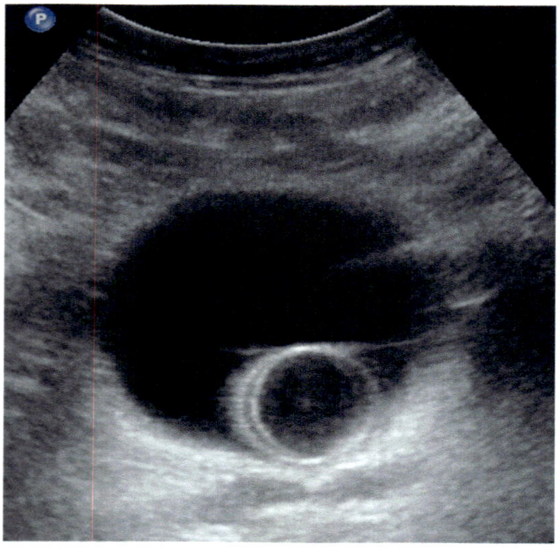

Fig. 2.30 Grayscale ultrasound image demonstrating the refraction artifact. The beam undergoes refraction when it affects tangentially on a curved interface and generates a distortion of the organ profile like in this case when the profile of a Foley catheter of the bladder is distorted

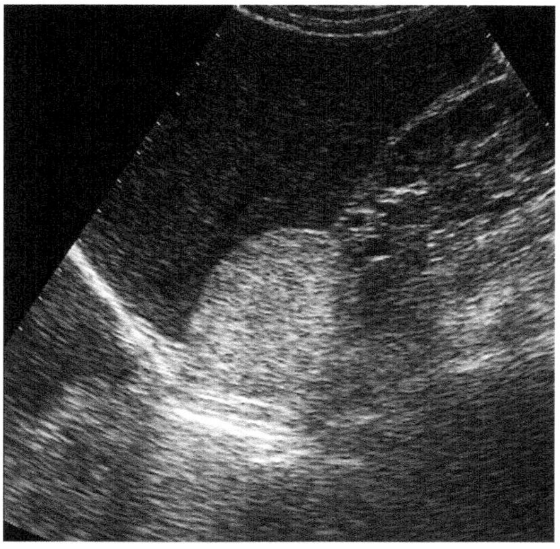

Fig. 2.32 Grayscale image showing a speed error artifact. The diaphragmatic profile abnormalities distal to a fluid-filled or adipose structure is shown

2.2.12 The Partial-Volume Effect (Artifacts Caused by the Layer Thickness)

It occurs when the layer we are investigating includes a fluid collection smaller than the layer thickness. We will observe that the image of the liquid collection contains echoes inside. The echo signals coming from tissues placed beside and laterally to the liquid collection are displayed in the monitor superimposed to the liquid collection therefore inside it. This effect may occur even if the liquid collection has equal or greater diameter than the layer thickness but the beam axis does not pass its center. In the layer thickness are then included a domed area of the fluid collection and a portion of the adjacent tissue and the echoes from this tissue are displayed on monitor overlapped to the liquid collection (Fig. 2.33). This artifact is dangerous when ultrasound-guided biopsies are performed because the needle tip can be positioned next to the biopsy region and not inside. For this reason a ductus which goes pricked should preferably be oriented perpendicularly to the layer [2].

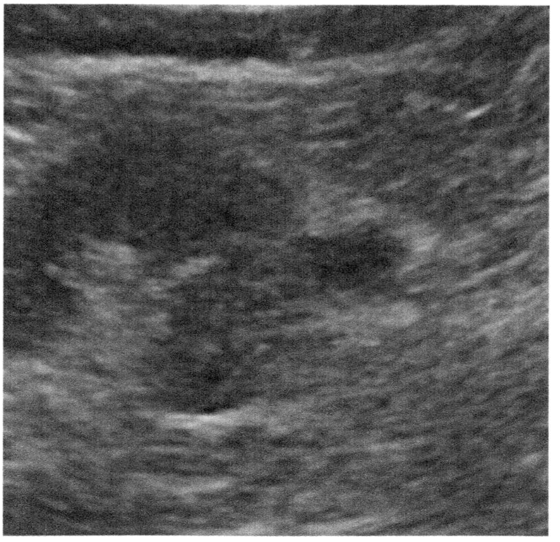

Fig. 2.33 Grayscale ultrasound image demonstrating a partial-volume effect. The ultrasound reproduces all the echoes coming from a tissue layer with the same thickness of the beam as in this case when a renal lesion is generated by the artifact and not confirmed with other exams

2.2.13 Side-Lobe Artifact

A rounded transducer emits an originally cylindrical main beam (*main lobe*) and multiple lateral beams with lower intensity (*side lobes*). When the main beam is directed into a liquid collection and strikes its distal wall simultaneously the lateral beams reach the lateral distal wall generating echoes within the echo-free image of the liquid formation. The liquid is anechoic but the artifact that depicts the echoes inside it is generated by side lobes affecting lateral and distal cavity walls (Figs. 2.34 and 2.35). The artifact can be observed in all liquid collections, for example into the gallbladder, simulating the presence of biliary sludge (Fig. 2.36). The flat surface of the true biliary sludge and the image shifting with the variation of patient decubitus position allow a correct diagnosis [2].

2.2.14 The Speckle Artifact

The speckle artifact results from interference patterns from echoes generated by closely spaced microstructure tissues that are too small to

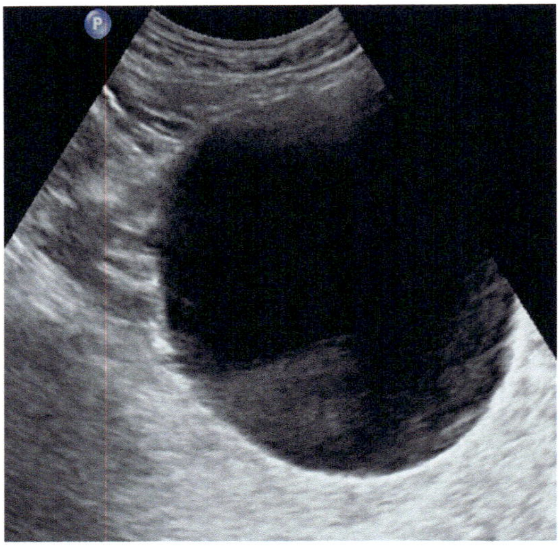

Fig. 2.34 Grayscale ultrasound image demonstrating a side-lobe artifact. In this case the side lobes are reflected from the bladder walls causing the appearance of echoes within the liquid. Differential diagnosis of urinary sediment must be considered

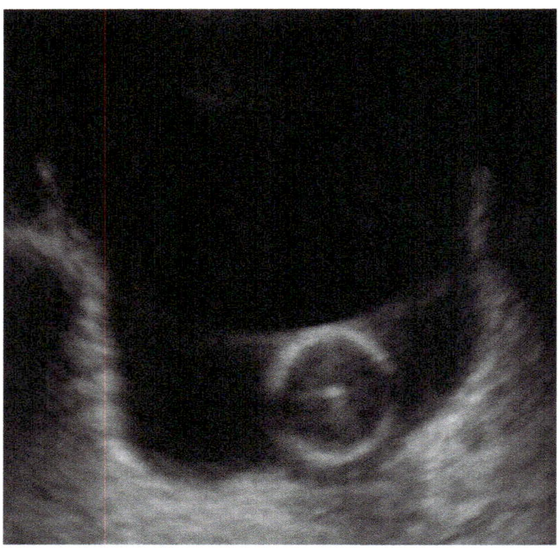

Fig. 2.35 Another case of a grayscale ultrasound image demonstrating a side-lobe artifact. In this case a similar image with urinary sediment is generated in a patient with a bladder catheter

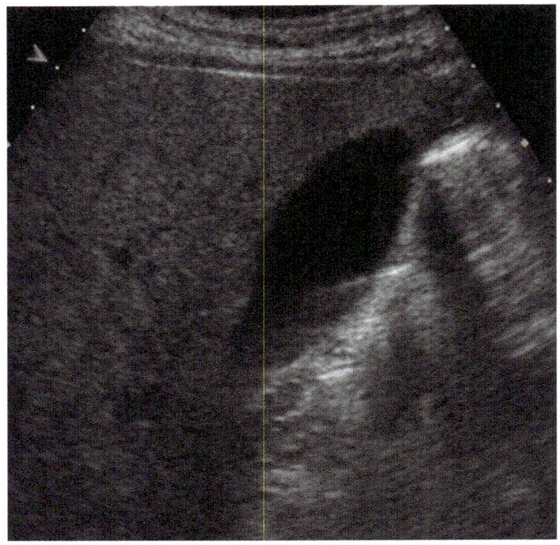

Fig. 2.36 Grayscale ultrasound image demonstrating a side-lobe artifact. In this case the side lobes are reflected from the gallbladder walls and an image of biliary sludge at the infundibula is generated

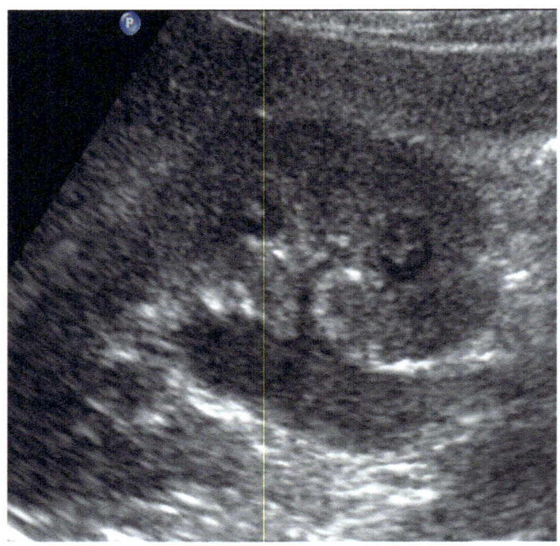

Fig. 2.37 Grayscale ultrasound image demonstrating a speckle artifact. Point sources give origin to a series of spherical waves like in this example of speckle artifact at the renal parenchyma

resolve. Punctiform sources give origin to a series of spherical waves and wavefront resulting from the interference of the waves produced by the individual elements (Fig. 2.37). It is a "structured" noise with a granular texture and it depends on the transducer characteristics and on the beam depth, frequency, and direction. Speckle is commonly seen even in homogeneous and solid tissues such as the liver and the kidneys which have granulated echo structure and their underlying microstructure is too small to be resolved by the transducer. Newer imaging techniques and the frequency and spatial compounding help minimize the speckle artifact [4].

2.3 Artifacts Related to Apparatus and to the Beam Properties and Processing

These artifacts also depend on the operator and are usually eliminated by resorting to the appropriate use of the apparatus or by choosing carefully the application parameters.

2.3.1 Range-Ambiguity Artifact

When all echoes are generated by the most recently transmitted pulse and another physical sonographic assumption fails, the range-ambiguity artifact is generated [2]. A high pulse frequency repetition records shallow objects accurately and the pulse repetition frequency is related to the field depth. When a distant echo returns to the crystal after a second pulse has been transmitted, deeper structures may be misregistered because the receiving timer inappropriately assigns its position relatively to that of the second pulse. The echo is subsequently positioned on the display nearer to the transducer than it really is. Clinically this artifact may result in projection of deeper solid or fluid structures in shallower tissues. The focal zone adjustment to assess deeper structures will help to better recognize this artifact and decreasing the pulse repetition frequency will minimize the artifact [4].

2.3.2 Artifacts from Incorrect Adjustment of Gain

This artifact is given by an incorrect adjustment of the overall (Fig. 2.38) or sectoral gain (Fig. 2.39) or by incorrect focusing (Fig. 2.40).

2.3.3 Artifacts Produced by the Ultrasound Malfunction

It is due to the rupture of the transducer elements (Fig. 2.41) or due to electrical interference (Fig. 2.42). This artifact often occurs even when there is an erroneous summary of the lines of view or malfunctioning of the video card:

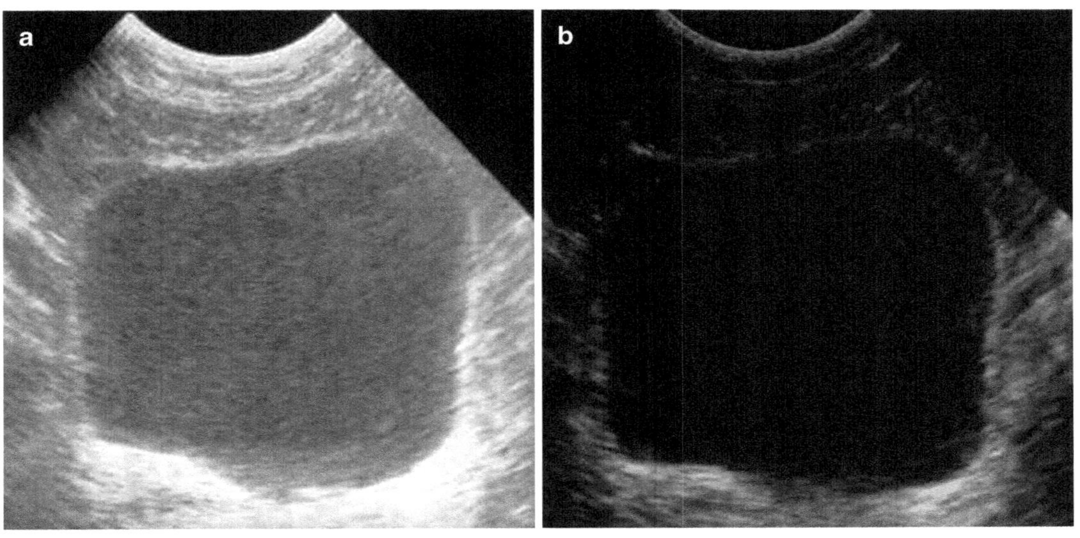

Fig. 2.38 Grayscale ultrasound image demonstrating an artifact generated by improper adjustment of the overall gain showing a very bright and poorly defined image of the bladder (**a**) that is corrected after the adjustment of the overall gain (**b**)

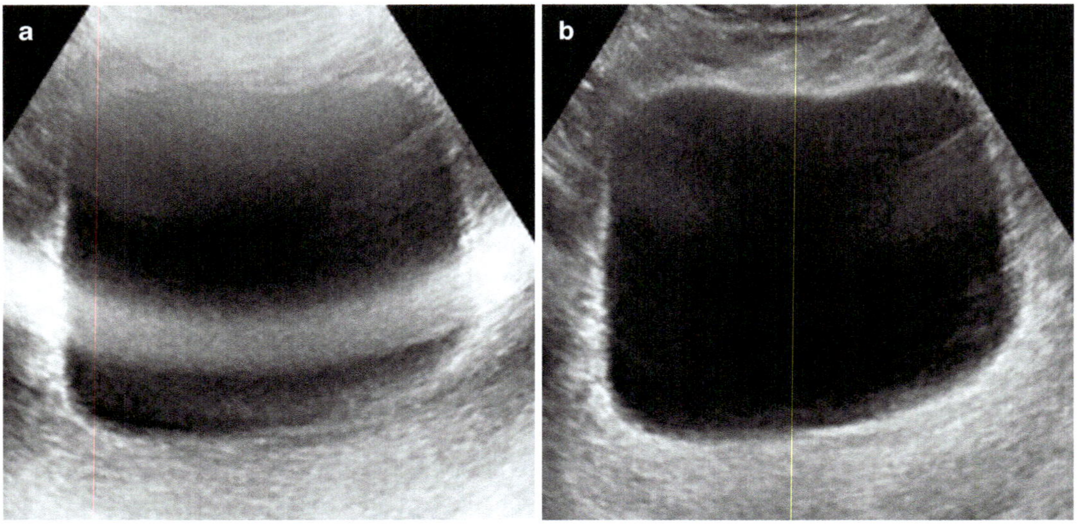

Fig. 2.39 Grayscale ultrasound image demonstrating an artifact generated by improper adjustment of the sectoral gain which generates a bright band at the bladder (**a**) that is eliminated after the adjustment of the sectoral gain (**b**)

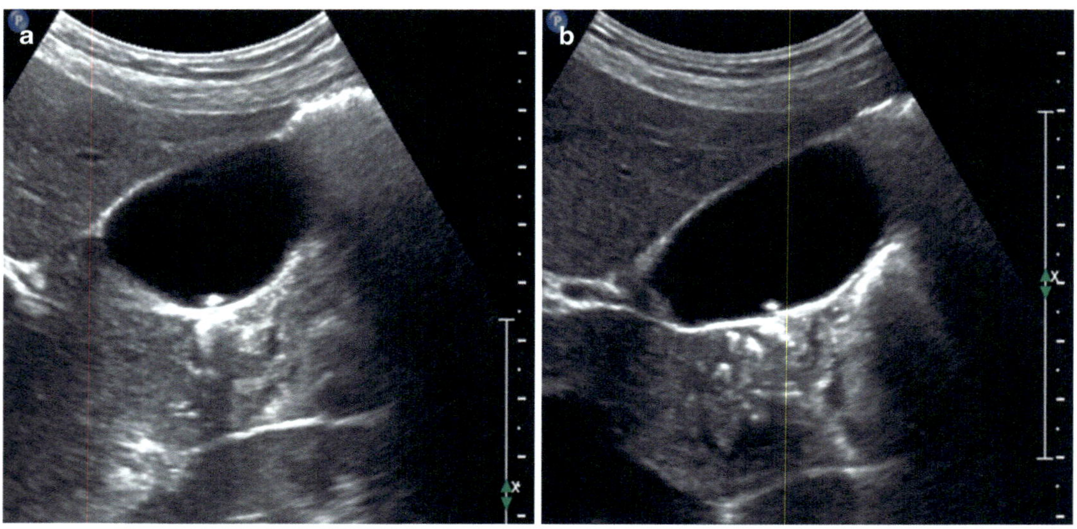

Fig. 2.40 Grayscale ultrasound image demonstrating an image alteration generated by incorrect focusing at the gallbladder (**a**) that is corrected after the adjustment of focusing (**b**)

- Rupture of the transducer elements
- Electrical interferences
- Erroneous summary of the lines of view
- Malfunctioning of the video card

2.3.4 Artifacts from Incorrect Image Processing

Erroneous summary of the lines of view (Fig. 2.43).

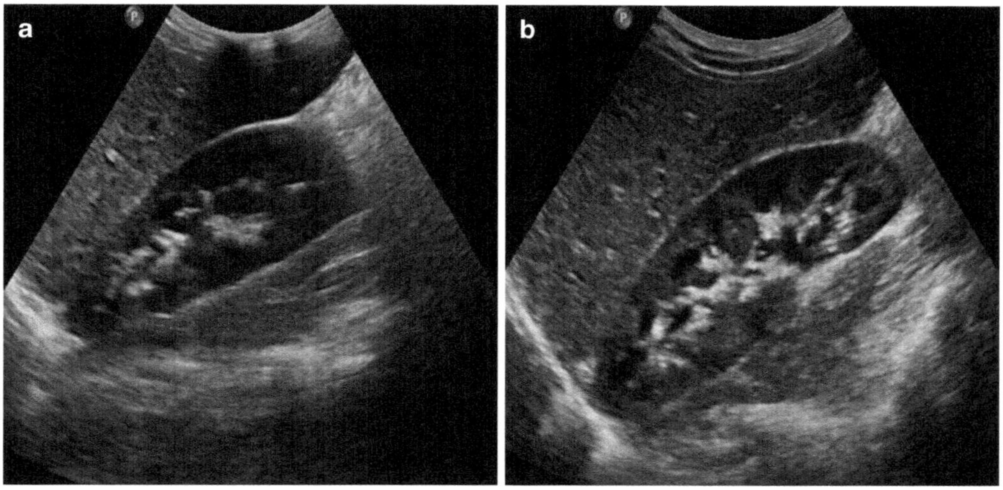

Fig. 2.41 Grayscale ultrasound image demonstrating an image artifact visible as a hypoechoic band at the liver surface generated by the rupture of the transducer elements (**a**) that disappear after changing the probe (**b**)

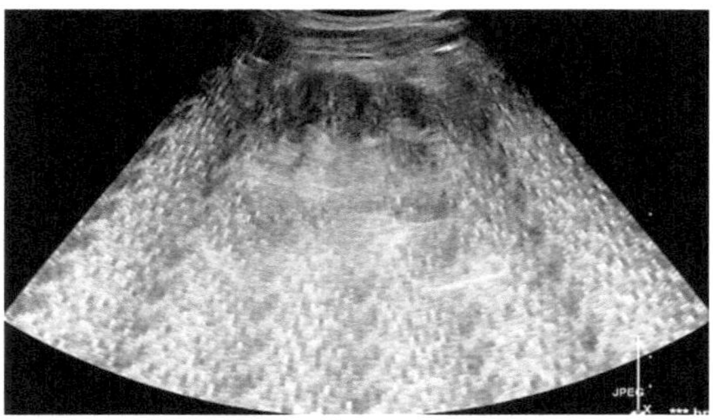

Fig. 2.42 Grayscale ultrasound image which highlights some vertical bands caused by electrical interference

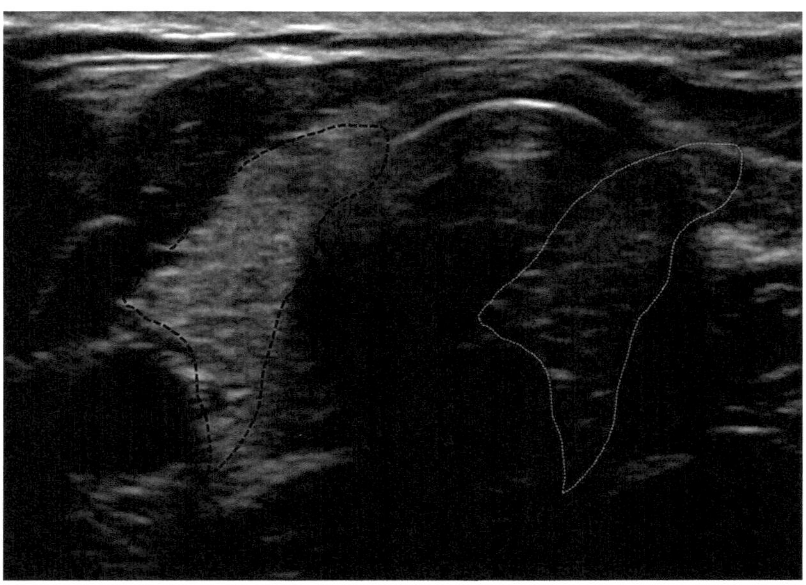

Fig. 2.43 Grayscale ultrasound image demonstrating an artifact caused by the erroneous summary of the lines of view in which the right thyroid lobe is projected near the left thyroid lobe (the delimitation on the right image)

2.3.5 Artifacts Produced by the Adaptive Filtering (Artifacts from Poor Resolution)

2.3.6 The Dragging Artifact (Cigar Effect)

This artifact is not modifiable by the operator [2].

2.3.7 Hyperbolic Artifacts

References

1. Abu-Zidan FM, Hefny AF, Corr P. Clinical ultrasound physics. J Emerg Trauma Shock. 2011;4(4):501–3.
2. Ziviello MBE, Ferrari F, Maresca G, Rubaltelli L. Ecotomografia, vol. II. Napoli: Oliva; 1990. p. 407.
3. Kirberger RM. Imaging artifacts in diagnostic ultrasound—a review. Vet Radiol Ultras. 2005;36(4):297–306.
4. Prabhu SJ, et al. Ultrasound artifacts: classification, applied physics with illustrations, and imaging appearances. Ultrasound Q. 2014;30(2):145–57.
5. Feldman MK, Katyal S, Blackwood MS. US artifacts. Radiographics. 2009;29(4):1179–89.
6. Hindi A, Peterson C, Barr RG. Artifacts in diagnostic ultrasound. Rep Med Imaging. 2013;6:29–48.
7. Scanlan KA. Sonographic artifacts and their origins. AJR Am J Roentgenol. 1991;156(6):1267–72.
8. Huang J, et al. Imaging artifacts of medical instruments in ultrasound-guided interventions. J Ultrasound Med. 2007;26(10):1303–22.
9. Lichtenstein D, et al. The comet-tail artifact. An ultrasound sign of alveolar-interstitial syndrome. Am J Respir Crit Care Med. 1997;156(5):1640–6.
10. Nelson TR, et al. Sources and impact of artifacts on clinical three-dimensional ultrasound imaging. Ultrasound Obstet Gynecol. 2000;16(4):374–83.
11. Sorensen MD, et al. B-mode ultrasound versus color Doppler twinkling artifact in detecting kidney stones. J Endourol. 2013;27(2):149–53.

Color Doppler and CEUS Artifacts

3

Orlando Catalano

3.1 Introduction

An ultrasound artifact is any error in the perception or representation of the sonography information, potentially leading to a diagnostic misinterpretation. The error occurs because of assumptions that do not completely correspond with the reality involved in generating the image [1, 2]. Artifacts are inherent to sonography and occur to some extent in every image, despite any optimal scanner setting [3]. Though many artifacts are readily recognizable as such, occasionally, these misleading images may obstacle the diagnosis or may even create false abnormalities. As a matter of fact, artifacts have a twofold interest in the sonography practice. From one side, artifact may confound the image interpretation, mimicking or masquerading true abnormalities. Had the artifact article not been recognized for its real nature, the findings may have been misinterpreted, leading to further, unnecessary, imaging or intervention. For the other side, however, appropriate knowledge of these changes is important since they may be employed to better understand the nature of the normal and abnormal structures being imaged and, consequently, to improve diagnosis [1, 2, 4].

Despite the recent advances, the potential to encounter imaging artifacts still remains. Some artifacts, such as the twinkling artifact, are even more common with digital technology than with older systems using an analog technology [5]. Artifacts can be classified into those resulting from body structure anatomy and physiology and those caused by the sonography scanner properties and setting [6, 7]. In this chapter we review the artifacts seen during Doppler imaging (both native and contrast-enhanced Doppler techniques) as well as during grayscale contrast-enhanced sonography. We illustrate the common artifacts that can be encountered in the practice of urinary tract imaging, analyze the factors leading to their formation, and discuss the strategies useful to recognize and minimize these images.

3.2 Doppler Imaging Artifacts

Doppler techniques are largely employed in the sonography imaging of the urinary tract. Appropriate assessment of the renal pedicle, starting from the search of renal artery stenosis in hypertensive subjects, required mandatorily the use of Doppler. The same applies to a wide range of renal parenchyma abnormalities, including infarctions, intrarenal fistulas and pseudoaneurysms, complex cysts, and solid masses (characterization, detection of renal vein involvement, etc.). In this subsection we illustrate the main

O. Catalano (✉)
Department of Radiology, Varelli Diagnostic Institute, Naples, Italy

A. Granata, M. Bertolotto (eds.), *Imaging in Nephrology*, https://doi.org/10.1007/978-3-030-60794-4_3

artifacts that can be encountered using native Doppler techniques, i.e., spectral Doppler, color Doppler, and/or power Doppler. Some artifacts are related to inappropriate equipment setting, or at least a setting that is not adequate to correctly display the normal or abnormal vascular flows present in the body area investigated. This includes choosing an inappropriate Doppler transmission frequency, pulse repetition frequency, Doppler angle, Doppler sample volume, Doppler gain, and wall filter [4, 7]. In this case the system may fail to detect flow signals within a vessel (pseudothrombosis artifact), may cause the representation of signal where there is no flow, or may display findings simulating the turbulent flow seen at the level of a stenosis (aliasing artifact). Correction of the parameter or parameters regulated inappropriately is sufficient to demonstrate the artifactual nature of the Doppler finding in these cases. Other artifacts are not related to the equipment, being basically due to atypical anatomical or physiological conditions. In many of these cases, however, a typical location and appearance are sufficient to allow differentiation between an artifact and a true abnormality. However, if any uncertainty persists, evaluation of the spectral Doppler analysis usually allows a definitive clarification, by demonstrating no signal, noise, or signal that in no case resembles that of true vascular flow (normal or abnormal).

3.2.1 Aliasing Artifact

Aliasing is an inaccurate display of spectral or color velocity and occurs when the velocity range exceeds the scale available to display it [4]. Since Doppler techniques use a pulsed beam, the aliasing artifact is observed if the frequency of the Doppler signal exceeds one-half of the pulse repetition frequency (i.e., exceeds the Nyquist sampling rate) [7]. In case of aliasing the display "wraps around" the scale and overwrites the existing data [4]. At spectral analysis, the velocity peak is cut off at the top of the scale and written from the lowest portion of the scale back toward the top. This would cause an incorrect measurement of the flow velocities with the spectrum. At color Doppler, adjacent colors from red to yellow to light blue to dark blue are displayed simultaneously. This resembles somehow the mixture of colors seen at the level of a vascular stenosis. To avoid the aliasing artifact it is usually sufficient to move the spectrum baseline upwards or downwards and/or to increase the pulse repetition frequency. Also, decreasing the Doppler transmission frequency and increasing the Doppler angle result in a correction of the aliasing artifact. Since power Doppler provides no directional information, it does not display ant aliasing artifact. Aliasing is easily seen in conditions where the velocity is particularly high. In the urinary tract this occurs, for example, for spontaneous or post-bioptic arteriovenous fistulas [8].

3.2.2 Twinkling Artifact

The twinkling artifact appears as a rapidly fluctuating mixture of color Doppler signals and is identified at the level of and behind strongly reflecting interfaces [9] (Fig. 3.1). It is somehow similar in appearance to the B-mode comet-tail artifact [10]. The possibility of detecting a twinkling artifact is not significantly influenced by the chosen pulse repetition frequency while it may depend on the focal zone selected that must be

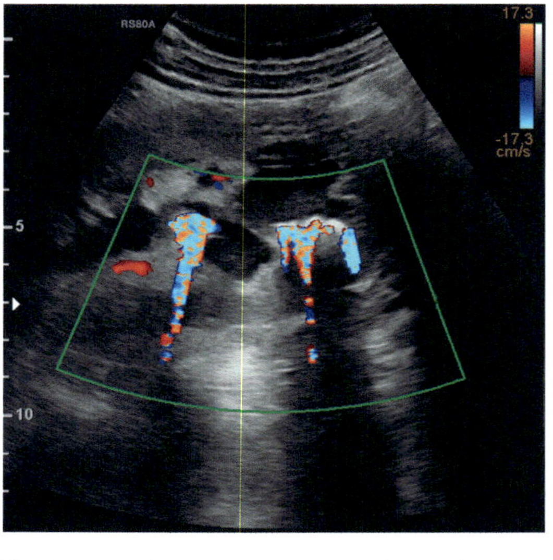

Fig. 3.1 Renal stones, twinkling artifact. Tail-shaped mosaic of Doppler signal distal to intrarenal calculi. Calyx dilatation

placed at the level of the image of interest [10]. The medium must be stationary, irregular, and rough, being composed of small individual reflectors. Examples include calculi, calcifications, stents, medical materials (clips, coils, etc.), and foreign bodies [11]. The twinkling artifact may simulate true vascular flows, and particularly turbulence [12]. As a matter of fact, an echogenic focus in the kidney on grayscale imaging may present a calcified artery or renal stone. A focally increased color signal in the kidney may result from a turbulent flow in a vascular abnormality (arteriovenous fistula, intrarenal artery stenosis, etc.) or a twinkle deep to a renal stone. However, the mosaic of signal due to a twinkling artifact is nondirectional and the Doppler spectrum registered at that level will only show a broadband noise [6, 12]. On the other side, the twinkling artifact is interesting since it can be employed to detect small stones in the kidney or along the urinary tract, as a complementary feature in addition to grayscale findings and color Doppler assessment of the vesicoureteral jet. This sign is found in up to 86% of urinary stones [10] and it has a high positive predictive value (94%) for detecting urolithiasis [5]. As a matter of fact, one of the major limitations of grayscale sonography for identifying renal stones is the presence of small echogenic areas at tissue interfaces, which do not show a well-defined acoustic shadow. According to an *in vitro* study [13], calcium oxalate dihydrate and calcium phosphate stones always produce a twinkling artifact, whereas stones composed of calcium oxalate monohydrate and urate lack this artifact. Consequently, the search of a twinkling artifact may be helpful to chemically characterize the urinary tract calculi, and, in turn, to predict their fragmentability. Use of the twinkling artifact also allows avoiding false-positive misinterpretation of these interfaces. At the same time, use of the twinkling artifact sign allows to confirm a small calculus when sonography only shows subtle echoic foci within the kidney or ureter [5, 14] (Fig. 3.2).

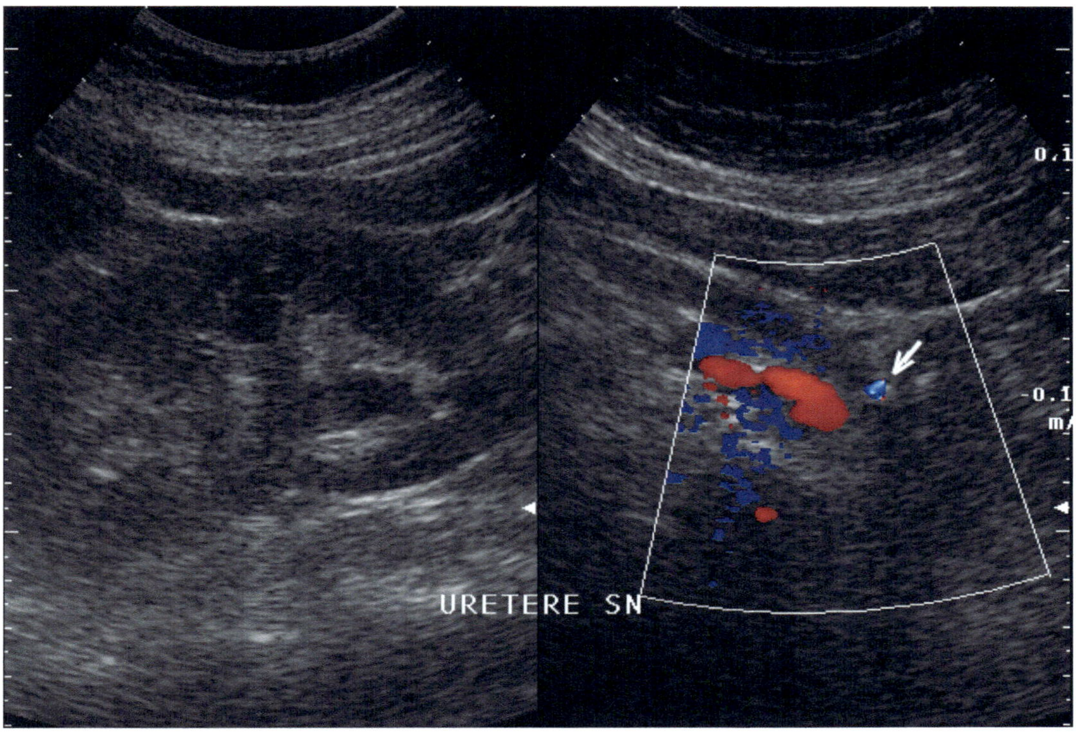

Fig. 3.2 Ureteral stone, twinkling artifact. Subtle dilation of the calyces (left) and ureter (right) due to a small calculus (arrow). The latter was seen also because of generating of a small Doppler twinkle

3.2.3 Edge Artifact

The edge artifact, which is similar but different from the twinkling one, is related to strong, smooth specular reflectors. It appears as a steady color signal generated along the rim of calcified structures such as gallstones or bony cortex [4, 6]. It is rarely encountered in the urinary tract, where it may be noted at the level of bladder stones, bladder encrustations, Foley balloons, or stents. Edge artifact is seen with color Doppler and, even more, with power Doppler imaging (because of the larger dynamic range) [10]. It is more frequently seen with a low pulse repetition frequency setting. In case of edge artifact the Doppler spectrum shows a noisy, straight-line signal on both sides of the baseline and allows for a definitive diagnosis.

3.2.4 Flash Artifact

Flash artifact manifests as a sudden, transitory color signal caused by tissue motion [6, 15]. In the absence of grayscale echoes, color pixels take the priority, so that an apparent random flow is seen in nearly stationary fluid. Flash artifact is usually encountered at the level of cysts (particularly if dense and pseudosolid) or fluid collections (Fig. 3.3). Again, the Doppler spectrum sampling fails to recognize any flow signal. A kind of flash artifact is seen at the level of severe stenoses or high-flow arteriovenous fistulas, because of the perivascular tissue vibration, and is called "color bruit" [4] (Fig. 3.4). The flash artifact may also coincide real movements (transducer motion, respiration, cardiac or vascular pulsation).

3.2.5 Pseudoflow Artifact (Ureteral Jet Phenomenon Included)

Pseudoflow is related to true motion of non-blood fluids, such as ascites, amniotic fluid, and urine [4, 6]. It appears similar to blood flow but is seen in the absence of real vascular structures. Spectral Doppler analysis reveals some kind of flow signals, but that are atypical for a normal vessel. Pseudoflow can be noted, for example, at the neck of a large bladder diverticulum. A kind of pseudoflow is also seen at the level of the ureterovesical junction, the so-called ureteral jet. The jet is an oblique flow signal identified intermittently from the ureteral meatus pointing the bladder midline. The jets from the two sides can be synchronous or not. To detect the ureteral jet, the bladder has to be adequately distended and the scanner must be set to identify slow flows (low pulse repetition frequency, low wall filter, etc.). In clinical practice the jet phenomenon can be employed to assess the ureteral patency. In case of complete obstruction there will be no jet on the side of the abnormality (although some signal may still persist). In case of partial obstruction the jet on the abnormal side will be weaker in intensity and longer in duration compared to the contralateral one [16]. Finally, in case of ureterovesical junction abnormality, such as intramural stone, the jet may be seen as deflected.

3.3 Contrast-Enhanced Doppler Imaging Artifacts

3.3.1 (Color) Blooming Artifact

Blooming is a color and power Doppler artifact resulting in a "bleeding" of signal outside vessel walls, making it difficult to assess the vessel itself and mimicking the presence of flow in areas where there is no actual flow [4] (Fig. 3.5). Blooming can be due to an incorrect scanner section, with an overamplification of the flow signal. However, this artifact is usually seen in the presence of microbubbles, because of the strong increase in backscattering echo signal. Contrast medium-induced blooming artifact results from color signal overload at the moment of contrast arrival in the scanned area [17, 18]. The display of vessels in the color Doppler mode is exaggerated after the injection of the sonography contrast media and where color displays are evident in regions without significant blood flow [19, 20]. This phenomenon is more evident in the early phase following the injection of the microbubbles, particularly when the contrast medium is injected as a quick bolus, because at this time the

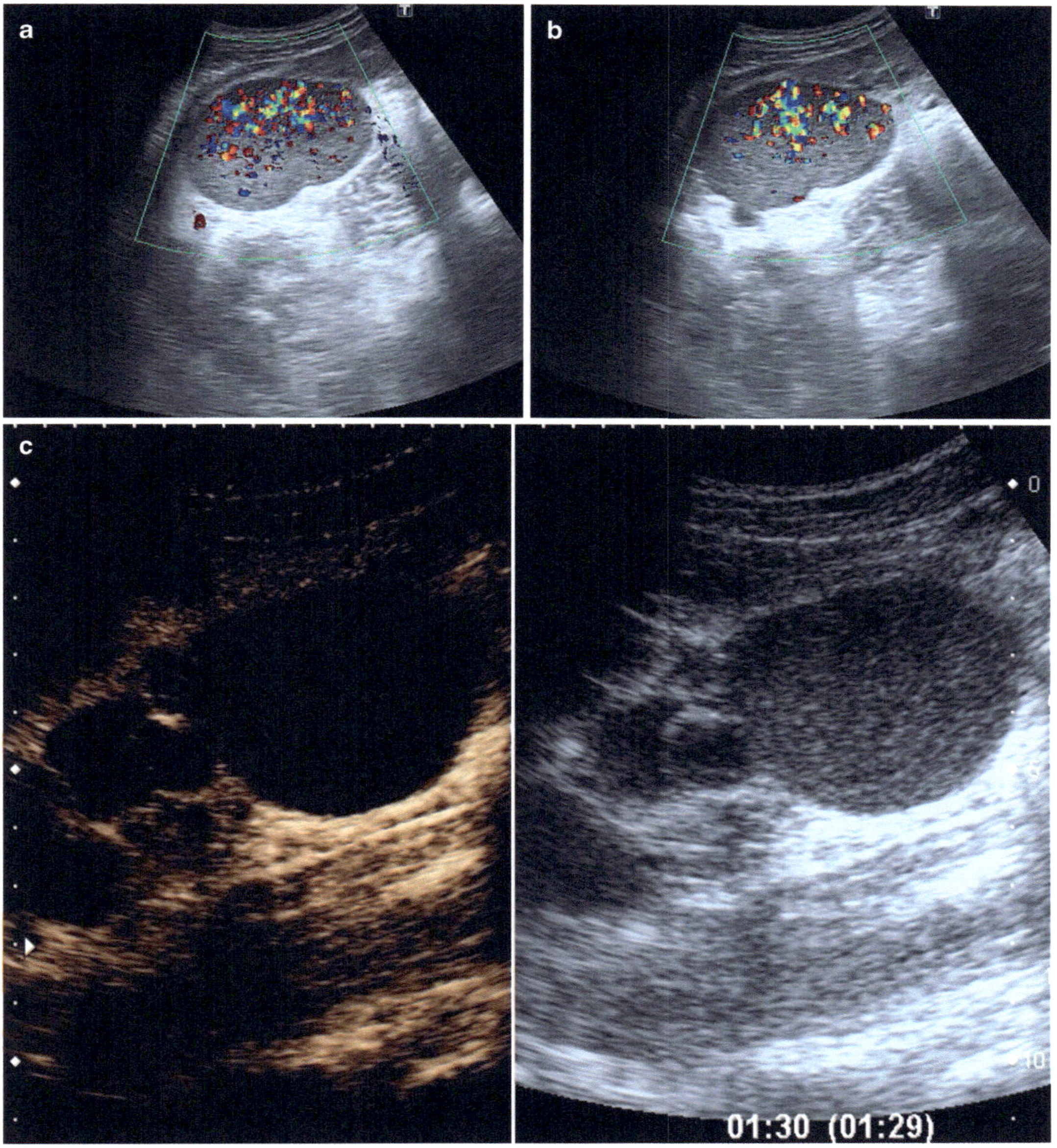

Fig. 3.3 Fluid motion artifacts within a corpusculated renal cyst, in a patient with multicystic renal disease. The artifactual signal changes over time (**a**, **b**). CEUS demonstrates complex lack of enhancement, excluding a solid mass (**c**)

increase in signal strength is the highest [21]. As a consequence of blooming, both normal and pathological structures can be misinterpreted during imaging analysis. Specifically, grayscale pixels are seen changing to color display in regions where flow is not present. To avoid this phenomenon it is necessary to decrease the color gain, increase the wall filter, decrease the output power, or inject the contrast medium in a slower manner [22]. Any of these maneuvers, however, represent an obstacle for an effective imaging of lesions. In the end, blooming is the main obstacle limiting the use of contrast-enhanced Doppler techniques, at least as a dynamic assessment of tumor vascularization after microbubble bolus injection.

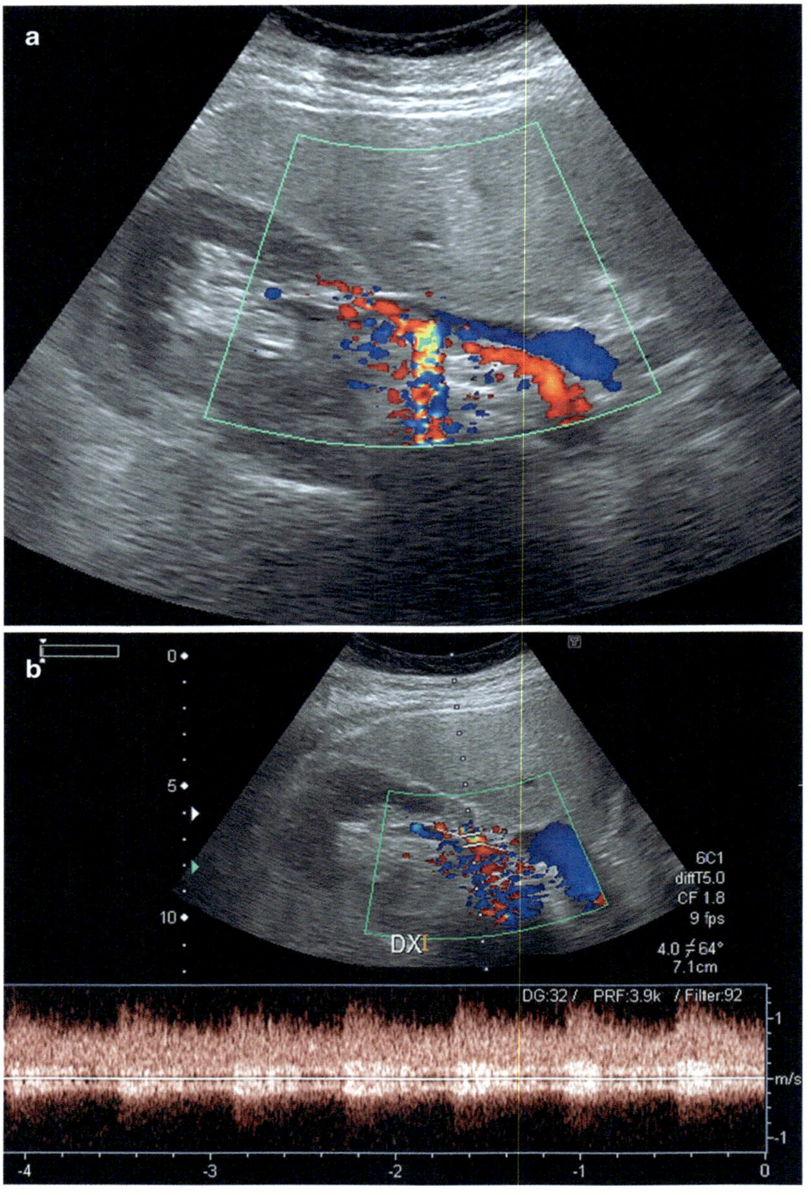

Fig. 3.4 Tissue vibration artifact at the level of a severe, dysplastic stenosis at the level of the distal portion of the right renal artery (**a**). Doppler spectrum shows turbulent flow, confirming the stenosis (**b**)

3.3.2 Jail-Bar Artifact

The jail bar image is represented by a lack of color along some vertical lines of the color box [18, 23]. It is particularly seen in relation with the power Doppler mode. It is determined by an error in image interpolation due to the Doppler signal saturation from backscattering microbubbles.

3.3.3 Systolic Peak Velocity Increase

It is commonly assumed that, because of the intrinsic limited dynamic range of the sonography system, the injection of a contrast medium may determine an increase in the systolic velocity [22]. However, the velocity increase is not significant, usually being around 5 cm/s [24, 25].

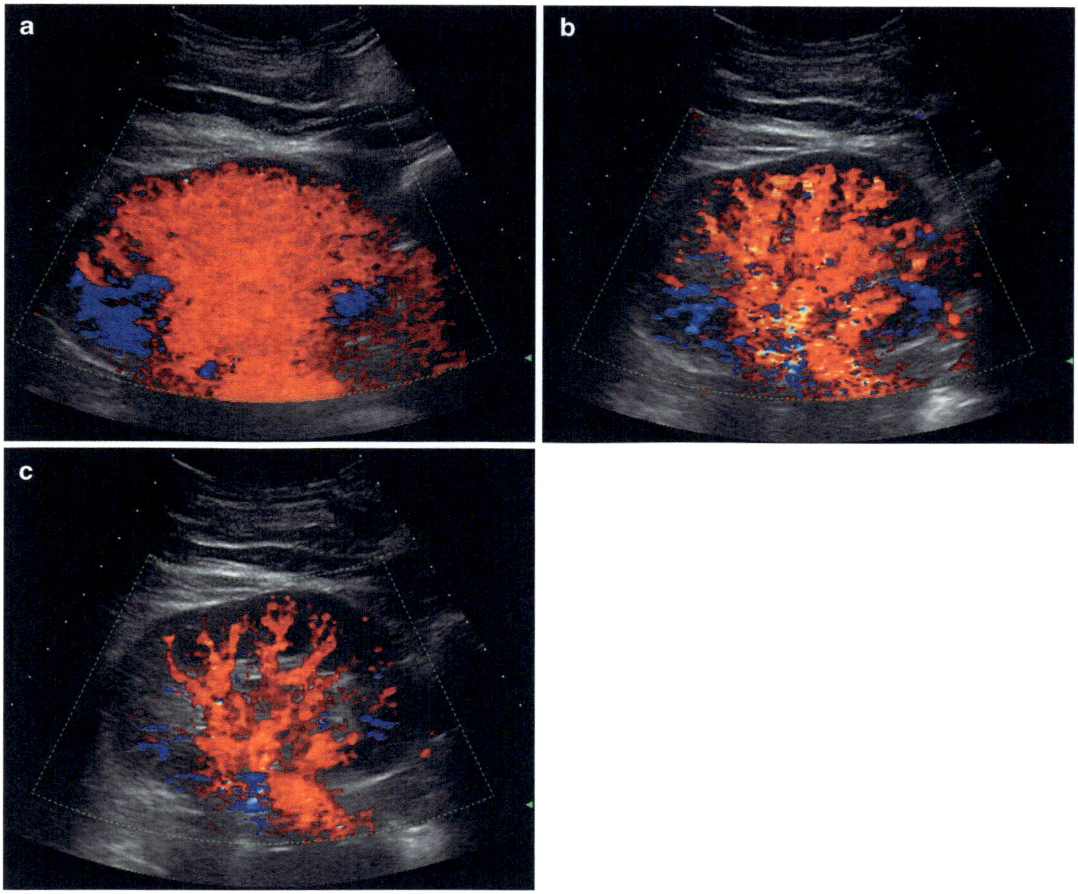

Fig. 3.5 Normal right kidney, post-contrast blooming artifact. After contrast medium bolus injection, there is overamplification of the signal (**a**), making it impossible to explore the organ. After some time, the excessive increase in Doppler signal diminishes progressively, allowing appropriate assessment of renal vascular architecture (**b**, **c**)

This phenomenon may theoretically lead to the overestimation of a stenosis, although no relevant turbulence is seen in combination with the high systolic velocity in these cases. To avoid this pitfall, it is necessary to decrease the Doppler gain or to inject the contrast medium more slowly [22]. However, as a general rule, it is better to sample the vessels before, rather than after, the contrast injection, at least when the color flow signal is already visible at the pre-contrast assessment.

3.3.4 High-Intensity Spikes

High-intensity transient artifacts can be detected with spectral analysis at peak enhancement or during late enhancement [18, 22] (Fig. 3.6). These sharp spikes are evident, because they cover the entire frequency spectrum. Additionally, they are associated with a crackling heard from the machine audio. The source of this artifact is represented by collapsing and/or aggregated microbubbles, detected at high-mechanical-index

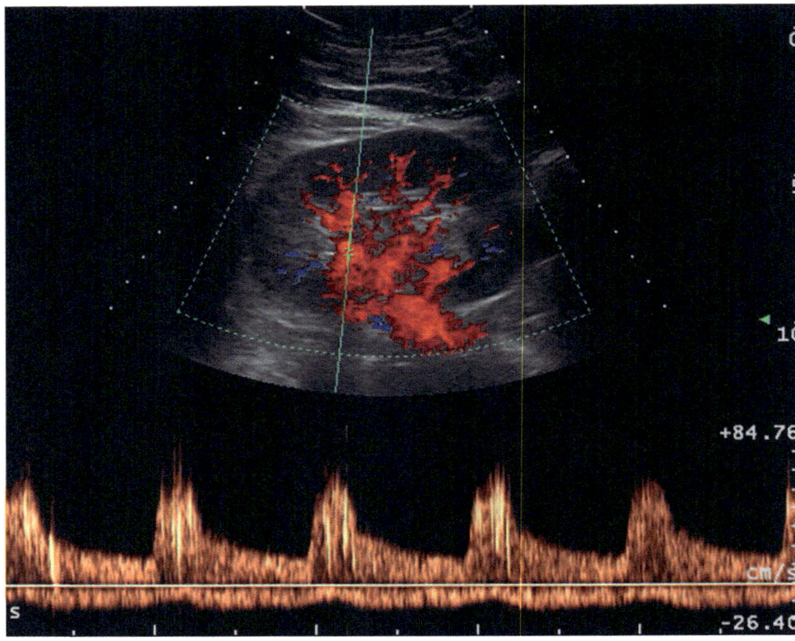

Fig. 3.6 Normal right kidney, spectral sampling after contrast medium injection. The presence of contrast microbubbles determines the presence of spikes within the spectrum, seen as thin vertical lines within the flow signal

spectral Doppler analysis. Noise on the spectrum represents the reason why, if possible, the Doppler analysis should be registered before and not after the contrast medium injection.

3.4 Contrast-Enhanced, Grayscale Sonography Artifacts

The use of contrast-enhanced sonography (CEUS) has consistently grown in the last decade and the kidney is probably the most frequently imaged organ after the liver [26–29]. CEUS is currently performed using low-mechanical-index software, allowing real-time imaging of microbubble circulation. CEUS should be employed, when conventional US is equivocal, in the following clinical situations: (1) suspected vascular disorders, including renal infarction and cortical necrosis; (2) differential diagnosis between solid lesions and cysts; (3) differential diagnosis between renal tumors and anatomical variations ("pseudotumors"); (4) characterization of complex cystic masses; (5) follow-up of nonsurgical complex masses; (6) identification of clinically suspected renal abscesses in patients with complicated infection; and (7) visualization of the lesion and detection of any residual or recurring tumor in patients undergoing renal tumor ablation [30]. Other scenarios may include renal trauma and extravascular, intracavitary contrast medium administration. Several technical and procedural parameters have influence on the quality of CEUS, which requires adequate operator training and proper scanner setting and contrast medium preparation and injection [31]. Atypical microbubble destruction may happen in the area close to the transducer, as a consequence of an excessively high-power output (mechanical index) [32]. Instead, lack of penetration, in combination with weak contrast signal, suggests a too much low mechanical index [32]. Prolonged scanning of an organ, in our case the kidney, during contrast medium circulation may worsen the image quality by decreasing the microbubble concentration, particularly in the late phases. This particularly if not using the ultralow mechanical index required for real-time CEUS. The same happens with an excessive microbubble destruction, as the operator may cause by using an excessive number of high-mechanical-index flashes to reassess the enhancement at contrast arrival [32].

Although much of the experience relates by now liver imaging, in this section we mention those artifacts that may be encountered during renal CEUS.

3.4.1 Slice-Thickness Artifact or Partial-Volume Artifact

CEUS shares with conventional sonography and color Doppler an artifact that is due to volume averaging [1, 33]. Enhancing structures may be partially visualized over adjacent non-enhancing ones (cysts, bladder, dilated renal pelvis, etc.), with the risk of simulating the presence of vascularization within nonvascular structures. This artifact results from a slice thickness that is not infinitely thin [4].

The same concept applies to dorsal enhancement, i.e., presence of a brighter signal deep to fluid-filled structures such as cysts. Also this well-known conventional sonography artifact is seen with CEUS [33].

3.4.2 Background Signal and Pseudoenhancement

A background signal may determine some undesired noise on the CEUS image, requiring to lower the acoustic pressure or the gain [32, 33]. Particularly at the moment of contrast medium arrival, the gain must be kept low, only showing the strongest reflectors.

The pseudoenhancement artifact is pitfall that has been described for the liver [34]. Although there are no specific articles dealing with the kidney, it may be possible to find this image also in the setting of renal CEUS. Hyperechoic lesions at baseline (angiomyolipoma, ablated nodules, etc.) may appear as falsely enhancing in the late phase of contrast medium circulation, only because of the re-emerging of their native reflexivity when the microbubble-related enhancement is going to vanish. However, knowledge of this phenomenon and observation of the poor enhancement in the early phase usually allow to correctly interpret the image.

3.4.3 Overenhancement

Current platforms allow to use a lower dose of contrast medium compared to early CEUS systems. The strength of the CEUS signal is directly dependent on the number of microbubbles present in that given area. If the contrast medium dose is too high, hypervascular regions may glare, with consequent shadowing of the structures below [32, 33]. Additionally, differences in enhancement within a hypervascular regions may merge into a single, uniform hyperechogenicity. Reducing the gain may allow to decrease the impact of overenhancement, when occurring.

3.4.4 Underenhancement

Deep structures, as are frequently the kidneys and their abnormalities, are more difficult to be imaged with CEUS, as well as with any other sonographic modality. To improve their visualization the operator may increase the mechanical index but this may turn into a higher microbubble destruction, artifacts, and loss of spatial resolution [32]. In such cases it is important to increase the depth penetration and to put the beam focus at level or immediately below the area of interest.

References

1. Bönhof JA. Ultrasound artifacts—Part 1. Ultraschall Med. 2016;37:40–53.
2. Bönhof JA. Ultrasound artifacts—Part 2. Ultraschall Med. 2017;38:130–48.
3. Keogh CF, Cooperberg PL. Is it real or is it an artifact. Ultrasound Q. 2001;17:201–10.
4. Rubens DJ, Bhatt S, Nedelka S, Cullinan J. Doppler artifacts and pitfalls. Radiol Clin N Am. 2006;44:805–35.
5. Kielar AZ, Shabana W, Vakili M, Rubin J. Prospective evaluation of Doppler sonography to detect the twinkling artifact versus unenhanced computed tomography for identifying urinary tract calculi. J Ultrasound Med. 2012;31:1619–25.

6. Campbell SC, Cullinan JA, Rubens DJ. Slow flow or no flow? Color and power Doppler US pitfalls in the abdomen and pelvis. Radiographics. 2004;24:497–506.
7. Prabhu SJ, Kanal K, Bhargava P, Vaidya S, Dighe MK. Ultrasound artifacts: classification, applied physics with illustrations, and imaging appearances. Ultrasound Q. 2014;30:145–57.
8. Lubas A, Wojtecka A, Smoszna J, Koziński P, Frankowska E, Niemczyk S. Hemodynamic characteristics and the occurrence of renal biopsy-related arteriovenous fistulas in native kidneys. Int Urol Nephrol. 2016;48:1667–73. https://doi.org/10.1007/s11255-016-1411-z.
9. Rahmouni A, Bargoin R, Herment A, Bargoin N, Vasile N. Color Doppler twinkling artifact in hyperechoic regions. Radiology. 1996;199:269–71.
10. Lee JY, Kim SH, Cho JY, Han D. Color and power Doppler twinkling artifacts from urinary stones: clinical observations and phantom studies. AJR Am J Roentgenol. 2001;176:1441–5.
11. Trillaud H, Pariente JL, Rabie A, Grenier N. Detection of encrusted indwelling ureteral stents using a twinkling artifact revealed on color Doppler sonography. AJR. Am J Roentgenol. 2001;176:1446–8.
12. Gao J, Ng A, Dang MN, Min R. Flow turbulence or twinkling artifact? A primary observation on the intrarenal color Doppler sonography. Clin Imaging. 2010;34:355–60.
13. Chelfouh N, Grenier N, Higueret D, et al. Characterization of urinary calculi: in vitro study of "twinkling artifact" revealed by color-flow sonography. AJR Am J Roentgenol. 1998;171:1055–60.
14. Catalano O, Nunziata A, Altei F, Siani A. Suspected ureteral colic: primary helical CT versus selective helical CT after unenhanced radiography and sonography. AJR Am J Roentgenol. 2002;178:379–87.
15. Pozniak MA, Zagzebski JA, Scanlan KA. Spectral and color Doppler artifacts. Radiographics. 1992;12:35–44.
16. Catalano O, De Sena G, Nunziata A. The color Doppler US evaluation of the ureteral jet in patients with urinary colic. Radiol Med. 1998;95:614–7.
17. Forsberg F, Liu JB, Burns PN, Merton DA, Goldberg BB. Artifacts in ultrasonic contrast agent studies. J Ultrasound Med. 1994;13:357–65.
18. Quaia E. Ultrasound of the kidney. In: Quaia E, editor. Radiological imaging of the kidney. New York: Springer; 2014. p. 83–123.
19. Forsberg F, Liu JB, Merton DA, Rawool NM, Goldberg BB. Parenchymal enhancement and tumor visualization using a new sonographic contrast agent. J Ultrasound Med. 1995;14:949–57.
20. Pugh CR, Arger PH, Sehgal CM. Power, spectral, and color flow Doppler enhancement by a new ultrasonographic contrast agent. J Ultrasound Med. 1996;15:843–52.
21. Wu CY, Lo MT, Tsao J, Chu A, Chou YH, Tiu CM. Factor analysis in both spatial and temporal domains of color blooming artifacts in ultrasound investigations utilizing contrast agents. Comput Med Imaging Graph. 2004;28:129–40.
22. Correas JM, Bridal L, Lesavre A, Méjean A, Claudon M, Hélénon O. Ultrasound contrast agents: properties, principles of action, tolerance, and artifacts. Eur Radiol. 2001;11:1316–28.
23. Catalano O, Migaleddu V, Quaia E, Caruso G. Terminology for contrast-enhanced sonography: a practical glossary. J Ultrasound Med. 2007;26:717–30.
24. Melany ML, Grant EG, Farooki S, McElroy D, Kimme-Smith C. Effect of US contrast agents on spectral velocities: in vitro evaluation. Radiology. 1999;211:427–31.
25. Ressner M, Brodin LA, Jansson T, Hoff L, Ask P, Janerot-Sjoberg B. Effects of ultrasound contrast agents on Doppler tissue velocity estimation. J Am Soc Echocardiogr. 2006;19:154–64.
26. Bertolotto M, Catalano O. Contrast-enhanced ultrasound: past, present, and future. Ultrasound Clinics. 2009;4:339–67.
27. Cantisani V, Bertolotto M, Weskott HP, Romanini L, Grazhdani H, Passamonti M, Drudi FM, Malpassini F, Isidori A, Meloni FM, Calliada F, D'Ambrosio F. Growing indications for CEUS: The kidney, testis, lymph nodes, thyroid, prostate, and small bowel. Eur J Radiol. 2015;84:1675–84. https://doi.org/10.1016/j.ejrad.2015.05.008.
28. Gulati M, King KG, Gill IS, Pham V, Grant E, Duddalwar VA. Contrast-enhanced ultrasound (CEUS) of cystic and solid renal lesions: a review. Abdom Imaging. 2015;40:1982–96.
29. Setola SV, Catalano O, Sandomenico F, Siani A. Contrast-enhanced sonography of the kidney. Abdom Imaging. 2007;32:21–8.
30. Piscaglia F, Nolsøe C, Dietrich CF, Cosgrove DO, Gilja OH, Bachmann Nielsen M, Albrecht T, Barozzi L, Bertolotto M, Catalano O, Claudon M, Clevert DA, Correas JM, D'Onofrio M, Drudi FM, Eyding J, Giovannini M, Hocke M, Ignee A, Jung EM, Klauser AS, Lassau N, Leen E, Mathis G, Saftoiu A, Seidel G, Sidhu PS, ter Haar G, Timmerman D, Weskott HP. The EFSUMB guidelines and recommendations on the clinical practice of contrast enhanced ultrasound (CEUS): update 2011 on non-hepatic applications. Ultraschall Med. 2012;33:33–59.
31. Greis C. Technical aspects of contrast-enhanced ultrasound (CEUS) examinations: tips and tricks. Clin Hemorheol Microcirc. 2014;58:89–95.
32. Dietrich CF, Ignee A, Hocke M, Schreiber-Dietrich D, Greis C. Pitfalls and artefacts using contrast enhanced ultrasound. Z Gastroenterol. 2011;49:350–6. https://doi.org/10.1055/s-0029-1245851.
33. Dietrich CF, Ignee A, Greis C, Cui XW, Schreiber-Dietrich DG, Hocke M. Artifacts and pitfalls in contrast-enhanced ultrasound of the liver. Ultraschall Med. 2014;35:108–25.
34. Yu H, Jang HJ, Kim TK, Khalili K, Williams R, Lueck G, Hudson J, Burns PN. Pseudoenhancement within the local ablation zone of hepatic tumors due to a nonlinear artifact on contrast-enhanced ultrasound. AJR Am J Roentgenol. 2010;194:653–9.

AKI and CIN: Real or Hype?

4

Fulvio Stacul

4.1 Introduction

Nephrotoxicity of contrast media (CM) was considered a significant safety issue since the introduction of these agents. However recently a number of papers questioned or downgraded the risk of contrast-induced nephropathy (CIN), at least following intravenous contrast administration. These new data can substantially change the management of patients at risk for CIN. The Contrast Media Safety Committee (CMSC) of the European Society of Urogenital Radiology (ESUR) updated its guidelines on CIN in 2011 [1]. However these guidelines could be affected by the incoming new data. A personal critical appraisal to this topic will be provided.

4.2 Limitations of Previous Studies on CIN

CIN was always perceived as an important risk for patients referred to contrast-enhanced studies. However several issues confound our knowledge on this topic; that is, early studies on CIN considered high osmolar CM that are no longer used; most clinical studies included patients undergoing cardiac arteriography and much less patients undergoing CT; other concomitant nephrotoxic risk factors that could lead to renal function deterioration were poorly considered; very few clinical studies of CIN included a control group not exposed to CM; such few studies were often confounded by a selection bias of the control population; serum creatinine is a poor marker of renal injury; different definitions of CIN were used; CIN studies were dominated by patients with normal or mildly impaired renal function [2].

4.3 Definition of CIN and PC-AKI

CIN was defined as "a condition in which an impairment in renal function (an increase in serum creatinine by more than 25% or 44 μmol/L) occurs within 3 days following the intravascular administration of a contrast medium in the absence of an alternative etiology" [1]. This definition is widely used but was questioned in the nephrological community. The Acute Kidney Injury Network (AKIN) suggested diagnostic criteria for acute kidney injury (AKI) using both absolute and relative SCr changes [3, 4]. An absolute increase in serum creatinine level of ≥0.3 mg/dL (26.4 μmol/L, or a percentage increase in serum creatinine level of ≥50% (1.5-fold from baseline)) or a reduction in urine output (documented oliguria of <0.5 mL/kg/h for >6 h) within 48 h was included. The serum creatinine

F. Stacul (✉)
Retired, S.C. Radiologia Ospedale Maggiore, Trieste, Italy

A. Granata, M. Bertolotto (eds.), *Imaging in Nephrology*, https://doi.org/10.1007/978-3-030-60794-4_4

threshold of 0.3 mg/dL was based on the evidence that even such slight changes in serum creatinine are associated with worse outcomes (increase in short-term morbidity and mortality and in 1-year mortality). This is probably the new standard to follow, although these criteria may be very sensitive and lead to an increase in the number of false-positive diagnoses.

It should be underlined that post-contrast AKI (PC-AKI) is not the same as CIN. These two terms are not interchangeable, as PC-AKI may occur regardless of whether CM was the cause of renal function deterioration, while CIN is caused by CM. It means that PC-AKI is a correlative diagnosis, while CIN is a causative diagnosis. Only a suitable control group allows distinguishing PC-AKI from CIN. If such a group is not available, the term PC-AKI is to be preferred.

4.4 Risk Factors

A number of patient-related risk factors were investigated and there is general agreement that the most significant among them is chronic kidney disease, particularly in combination with one or more among these factors: diabetic nephropathy, dehydration, congestive heart failure (NYHA grades 3–4) and low LVEF, recent myocardial infarction (<24 h), use of intra-aortic balloon pump, periprocedural hypotension, low hematocrit level, age over 70, and concurrent administration of nephrotoxic drugs. It is intuitive that patients with known or suspected acute renal failure should be considered at risk as well [1].

Procedure-related risk factors include the choice of CM (the CMSC suggested the use of CM with low or iso-osmolarity in patients with risk factors for CIN), dose of CM (the incidence of CIN is related to the dose of CM), multiple studies within a short period of time, and route of CM administration. The CMSC agreed that the risk was lower following i.v. CM injection (patients with eGFR <45 mL/min/1.73 m^2 had to be considered at risk) vs. intra-arterial CM administration (patients with eGFR <60 mL/min/1.73 m^2 had to be considered at risk). Such last issue received much attention in recent literature and deserves special consideration.

Several publications that compare the incidence of PC-AKI after angiocardiography and i.v. contrast administration have found the risk after angiocardiography to be higher [5, 6]. The incidence of PC-AKI following PCI (intra-arterial CM administration) in a large number (n = 1826) of consecutive patients was 14.5%, and the incidence of patients requiring dialysis was 0.7% [7]. On the other side, the overall incidence of PC-AKI in 1075 renal insufficient patients, that is, patients at risk, following CT (intravenous CM administration) was 5.1% and nobody required dialysis [8]. Several reasons can be advocated to justify such different incidences (different populations, in particular fewer hemodynamically unstable patients referred to CT, cholesterol embolization that can mimic CIN following intra-arterial CM administration), but the most convincing reason appears the lower CM dose used in CT, which commonly ranges between 25 and 50 g of iodine compared with reported 40–90 g of iodine in intra-arterial coronary studies [9]. Therefore it appears that the main issue is not the route of CM administration but the dose of CM (less in intravenous studies such as CT vs. intra-arterial procedures). Actually this conclusion is reinforced by researches by Nyman et al. [9] who found roughly the same gram-iodine/GFR ratio (~1:1) as a limit of relatively safe CM doses for both intravenous CT and intra-arterial coronary procedures.

New incoming data in the last 4 years challenged our belief that CM can deteriorate renal function in patients referred to CT. Large studies addressed selection bias in the unenhanced CT population (control groups) through the use of propensity score adjustment and propensity score matching. Actually control groups were biased by intentional clinical avoidance of intravenous contrast administration in patients with nephrotoxic risk factors. With such statistical approach each patient who received CM was matched with another patient who did not receive CM but who had a similar propensity score. McDonald et al. [10] used this approach, reviewed 13 CT trials, and showed similar incidence of AKI, dialysis, and death between the CM group and the control group. The same group performed a retrospective analysis involving 157,140 CT scans and showed that the incidence of PC-AKI was not significantly different from contrast material-independent AKI [11]. They concluded that CM is not a risk factor even in patients with eGFR level less than 30 mL/min/1.73 m^2 and therefore iodine-based CM may not be the causative agent in diminished renal function after intravenous CM administration [11]. Later they showed that intravenous contrast material exposure is not an independent risk factor for dialysis or mortality even among at-risk patients [12]. Another group [13] performed a retrospective analysis involving 20,242 CT scans and got slightly different results: they showed that CM is a risk factor in patients with stable eGFR level less than 30 mL/min/1.73 m^2. Five large (>10,000 patients) retrospective studies utilizing propensity score matching to address selection bias were carried out: the Mayo Clinic group (headed by McDonald) [14] concluded that CIN is nonexistent, or so rare as to be undetectable, while the Michigan University group (headed by Davenport) [13] showed that CIN is real, but rare. Many reasons can explain such slightly different conclusions, namely different covariates chosen for inclusion, the method of controlling baseline renal function instability, the statistical methodology, and possible differences in patient populations or clinical practice [14].

Anyway, if only patients with eGFR less than 30 mL/min/1.73 m^2 are to be considered at risk, we should consider that they represent a low minority of patients referred to CT, that is, 2.1% of inpatients [13] and 0.2% of outpatients [15].

Additionally, assuming the worst-case point estimates, the incidence of PC-AKI in CT would be 2.5% in patients with eGFR 30–44 mL/min/1.73 m^2 and 15% in patients with eGFR less than 30 mL/min/1.73 m^2 [16].

However a careful evaluation of these studies is required. None of them is prospective. It is not possible to conclude that CIN after CT does not exist because many patients in these populations were preselected and may have been given CIN prophylaxis [16]. Additionally, very few patients with eGFR 20–30 mL/min/1.73 m^2 have been enrolled and there is nearly no patient with eGFR below 20 mL/min/1.73 m^2.

Additional data provided by McDonald et al. [14] partially overcame these perplexities. They performed a retrospective analysis of 6902 patients referred to CT, including patients with severe renal impairment (4496 CKD stage III, matched: 1220 contrast and 1220 noncontrast; 2086 CKD stage IV–V, matched: 491 contrast and 491 noncontrast). They refined their methodology, considering only patients with stable baseline renal function, performing a manual chart review and evaluating the amount of i.v. fluid administration, and showed that i.v. contrast administration was not associated with an increased risk of AKI, emergent dialysis, and short-term mortality. The same group [17] considered a cohort of 6877 intensive care unit patients who underwent CT and showed that following propensity score adjustment, the rates of AKI, dialysis, and mortality were not significantly higher in the contrast vs. noncontrast group in the matched eGFR >45 mL/min/1.73 m^2 population, while significantly higher rates of dialysis were observed in the contrast group in the eGFR ≤45 subset.

All such data are clinically very significant. Nevertheless Nyman et al. [18] challenged these studies and argued that they are affected by several methodological concerns, namely the use of relative rather than absolute GFR in risk stratification, the use of unenhanced CT as a control group, the lack of use of contrast material dose in relation to renal function in the risk evaluation, and the limited attention to results stratified according to nonrenal risk factors. Additionally we cannot forget that preclinical data consistently showed that iodine-based contrast media are nephrotoxic and we are fully aware that CIN is a significant clinical problem in the cardiology setting (after PCA and PCI).

Literature on PC-AKI showed that the risk is lower following CT vs. angiocardiography, although some recent studies reported a similar risk [19–22]; proved that there are physiological SCr fluctuations [23, 24]; suggested that risk stratification is required; and showed that probably patients with eGFR >30 mL/min/1.73 m^2 referred to CT are not to be considered at risk.

All these features lead to the advice of being more liberal in our policies in regard to CM administration [25]. Can nephrologists agree with this approach? Nephrologists can argue that AKI definitions based on SCr have distinct limitations. It is well known that a number of nonrenal factors affect creatinine levels, namely factors affecting creatinine generation (such as age, sex, race, muscle mass, diet, and nutritional status), factors affecting tubular secretion of creatinine (bilirubin toxicity, drug-induced inhibition), factors affecting extrarenal elimination of creatinine (inhibition of gut creatininase by antibiotics, fluid overload), and laboratory variability (assay calibration is required) [26–30]. Additionally, GFR levels can be sustained by renal functional reserve, even during kidney injury: we know that with sufficient renal functional reserve, up to 50% of nephrons can be lost with no clinical impact on GFR or SCr levels [31]. It means that kidney injury can affect renal functional reserve without significant changes of GFR or SCr (subclinical AKI) and it means that following repeated kidney injuries, renal functional reserve can be lost with resulting clinical AKI and possible progression to chronic kidney disease [31]. Thus the absence of SCr increase does not imply absence of AKI, and the potential for subclinical disease should always be considered following kidney attacks. Such subclinical AKI can be detected with biomarkers that can allow early AKI diagnosis. It was suggested that a combination of biomarkers can improve prediction of AKI detection [32]. Biomarkers can be combined with functional criteria (SCr, urinary output) in definitions of AKI [32, 33]. All such features suggest that it would not be wise adopting a more liberal approach with CM administration on the basis of retrospective trials that considered SCr changes.

4.5 Management of At-Risk Patients

Before the contrast-enhanced examination, at-risk patients should be identified. Organization issues and economical evaluations favor having a blood sample for SCr (and eGFR) in all patients referred for studies with iodine-based CM. Questionnaires can be used as well and may identify patients with eGFR <45 mL/min/1.73 m^2 with adequate sensitivity. It is disappointing that still some radiologists do not identify patients at risk [34]. In patients at risk for CIN, an alternative imaging method not using iodine-based CM should be considered; additionally, the need to stop nephrotoxic drugs should be discussed with the referring physician; and the most important preventive measure is volume expansion: a suitable protocol is intravenous normal saline, 1.0–1.5 mL/kg/h, for at least 6 h before and after CM. An alternative protocol is intravenous sodium bicarbonate, 3 mL/kg/h for 1 h before CM and 1 mL/kg/h for 6 h after CM [1]. Again, it is disappointing that a significant number of radiologists do not suggest hydration in at-risk patients or advocate oral hydration [34].

It would be important providing advice on the most appropriate contrast-enhanced study (CT or MRI) to be performed in patients with eGFR <30 mL/min/1.73 m^2. The suggestion is that MRI should be preferred when there are no differences in diagnostic capabilities, as MRI with a low-risk agent at the approved dose has a clearer safety margin [16, 35].

4.6 Conclusion

At the end, AKI and CIN, real or hype? It is extremely clear that we are looking for a rare disease with a weak signal using a poor biomarker [2]. We could be tempted to conclude that CIN is extremely rare after enhanced CT, but such a conclusion should be supported by an improved biomarker for CIN (sensitive, specific, and predictive of long-term adverse events). Prospective trials using a combination of SCr level-based assays and novel renal biomarkers are warranted [14].

For the time being, I think it is probably too early to skip volume expansion in patients referred to CT with eGFR between 30 and 45 mL/min/1.73 m^2 and we should keep on taking care of them. There is still a need for guidelines to reduce the risk of PC-AKI [35] (www.esur.org) [36].

References

1. Stacul F, Van Der Molen AJ, Reimer P, Webb JA, Thomsen HS, Morcos SK, Almen T, Aspelin P, Bellin MF, Clement O, Heinz-Peer G, Contrast Media Safety Committee of European Society of Urogenital, R. Contrast induced nephropathy: updated ESUR Contrast Media Safety Committee guidelines. Eur Radiol. 2011;21:2527–41.
2. Davenport MS, Cohan RH, Khalatbari S, Ellis JH. The challenges in assessing contrast-induced nephropathy: where are we now? AJR Am J Roentgenol. 2014;202:784–9.
3. Acute Kidney Injury Work Group, K. D. I. G. O. K. KDIGO clinical practice guideline for acute kidney injury. Kidney Int Suppl. 2012;2:1–138.
4. Mehta RL, Kellum JA, Shah SV, Molitoris BA, Ronco C, Warnock DG, Levin A, Acute Kidney Injury, N. Acute Kidney Injury Network: report of an initiative to improve outcomes in acute kidney injury. Crit Care. 2007;11:R31.
5. Solomon R. Contrast-induced acute kidney injury: is there a risk after intravenous contrast? Clin J Am Soc Nephrol. 2008;3:1242–3.
6. Dong M, Jiao Z, Liu T, Guo F, Li G. Effect of administration route on the renal safety of contrast agents: a meta-analysis of randomized controlled trials. J Nephrol. 2012;25:290–301.
7. McCullough PA, Wolyn R, Rocher LL, et al. Acute renal failure after coronary intervention: incidence, risk factors, and relationship to mortality. Am J Med. 1997;103:368–75.
8. Katzberg RW, Lamba R. Contrast-induced nephropathy after intravenous administration: fact or fiction? Radiol Clin N Am. 2009;47:789–800.
9. Nyman U, Almen T, Jacobsson B, Aspelin P. Are intravenous injections of contrast media really less nephrotoxic than intra-arterial injections? Eur Radiol. 2012;22:1366–71.
10. McDonald RJ, McDonald JS, Bida JP, Carter RE, Fleming CJ, Misra S, Williamson EE, Kallmes DF. Intravenous contrast material-induced nephropathy: causal or coincident phenomenon? Radiology. 2013;267:106–18.
11. McDonald JS, McDonald RJ, Comin J, Williamson EE, Katzberg RW, Murad MH, Kallmes DF. Frequency of acute kidney injury following intravenous contrast medium administration: a systematic review and meta-analysis. Radiology. 2013;267:119–28.
12. McDonald RJ, McDonald JS, Carter RE, Hartman RP, Katzberg RW, Kallmes DF, Williamson EE. Intravenous contrast material exposure is not an independent risk factor for dialysis or mortality. Radiology. 2014;273:714–25.
13. Davenport MS, Khalatbari S, Cohan RH, Dillman JR, Myles JD, Ellis JH. Contrast material-induced nephrotoxicity and intravenous low-osmolality iodinated contrast material: risk stratification by using estimated glomerular filtration rate. Radiology. 2013;268:719–28.
14. McDonald RJ, McDonald JS, Newhouse JH, Davenport MS. Controversies in contrast material-induced acute kidney injury: closing in on the truth? Radiology. 2015;277:627–32.
15. Herts BR, Schneider E, Poggio ED, Obuchowski NA, Baker ME. Identifying outpatients with renal insufficiency before contrast-enhanced CT by using estimated glomerular filtration rates versus serum creatinine levels. Radiology. 2008;248:106–13.
16. Davenport MS, Cohan RH, Ellis JH. Contrast media controversies in 2015: imaging patients with renal impairment or risk of contrast reaction. AJR Am J Roentgenol. 2015;204:1174–81.
17. McDonald JS, McDonald RJ, Williamson EE, Kallmes DF, Kashani K. Post-contrast acute kidney injury in intensive care unit patients: a propensity score-adjusted study. Intensive Care Med. 2017;43:774–84.
18. Nyman U, Aspelin P, Jakobsen J, Bjork J. Controversies in contrast material-induced acute kidney injury: propensity score matching of patients with different dose/absolute glomerular filtration rate ratios. Radiology. 2015;277:633–7.
19. Karlsberg RP, Dohad SY, Sheng R. Iodixanol peripheral computed tomographic angiography study investigator panel. Contrast medium-induced acute kidney injury: comparison of intravenous and intra-arterial administration of iodinated contrast medium. J Vasc Interv Radiol. 2011;22(8):1159–65.
20. Kooiman J, Le Haen PA, Gezgin G, De Vries JP, Boersma D, Brulez HF, Sijpkens YW, Van Der Molen AJ, Cannegieter SC, Hamming JF, Huisman MV. Contrast-induced acute kidney injury and clinical outcomes after intra-arterial and intravenous contrast administration: risk comparison adjusted for patient characteristics by design. Am Heart J. 2013;165:793–9, 799.e1
21. McDonald JS, Leake CB, McDonald RJ, Gulati R, Katzberg RW, Williamson EE, Kallmes DF. Acute kidney injury after intravenous versus intra-arterial contrast material administration in a paired cohort. Investig Radiol. 2016;51:804–9.
22. Nijssen C, Rennenberg R, Nelemans P, Essers B, Janssen M, Vermeeren M, Vanommen V, Wildberger J. Prophylactic hydration to protect renal function from intravascular iodinated contrast material in patients at high risk of contrast-induced nephropathy (AMACING): a prospective, randomised, phase 3, controlled, open-label, non-inferiority trial. Lancet. 2017;389:1312–22.
23. Bruce RJ, Djamali A, Shinki K, Michel SJ, Fine JP, Pozniak MA. Background fluctuation of kidney function versus contrast-induced nephrotoxicity. AJR Am J Roentgenol. 2009;192:711–8.
24. Newhouse JH, Kho D, Rao QA, Starren J. Frequency of serum creatinine changes in the absence of iodinated contrast material: implications for studies of contrast nephrotoxicity. AJR Am J Roentgenol. 2008;191:376–82.

25. Newhouse JH, Roychoudhury A. Quantitating contrast medium-induced nephropathy: controlling the controls. Radiology. 2013;267:4–8.
26. Dunn RS, Gabuzda GM, Superdock KR, Kolecki RS, Schaedler RW, Simenhoff M. Induction of creatininase activity in chronic renal failure: Timing of creatinine degradation and effect of antibiotics. Am J Kidney Dis. 1997;29:72–7.
27. Joffe M, Hsu CY, Feldman HI, Weir M, Landis JR, Hamm LL, Chronic Renal Insufficiency Cohort Study, G. Variability of creatinine measurements in clinical laboratories: results from the CRIC study. Am J Nephrol. 2010;31:426–34.
28. Macedo E, Bouchard J, Soroko SH, Chertow GM, Himmelfarb J, Ikizler TA, Paganini EP, Mehta RL, Program to Improve Care in Acute Renal Disease, S. Fluid accumulation, recognition and staging of acute kidney injury in critically-ill patients. Crit Care. 2010;14:R82.
29. Puzantian HV, Townsend RR. Understanding kidney function assessment: the basics and advances. J Am Assoc Nurse Pract. 2013;25:334–41.
30. Van Slambrouck CM, Salem F, Meehan SM, Chang A. Bile cast nephropathy is a common pathologic finding for kidney injury associated with severe liver dysfunction. Kidney Int. 2013;84:192–7.
31. Sharma A, Mucino MJ, Ronco C. Renal functional reserve and renal recovery after acute kidney injury. Nephron Clin Pract. 2014;127:94–100.
32. Murray PT, Mehta RL, Shaw A, Ronco C, Endre Z, Kellum JA, Chawla LS, Cruz D, Ince C, Okusa MD, Workgroup, A. Potential use of biomarkers in acute kidney injury: report and summary of recommendations from the 10th Acute Dialysis Quality Initiative consensus conference. Kidney Int. 2014;85:513–21.
33. Ronco C, Stacul F, McCullough PA. Subclinical acute kidney injury (AKI) due to iodine-based contrast media. Eur Radiol. 2013;23:319–23.
34. Fishman EK, Reddan D. What are radiologists doing to prevent contrast-induced nephropathy (CIN) compared with measures supported by current evidence? A survey of European radiologists on CIN associated with computed tomography. Acta Radiol. 2008;49:310–20.
35. Thomsen HS, Stacul F. CIN: can we forget it? Acta Radiol. 2014;55:1027–30.
36. WWW.ESUR.ORG. [Accessed].

NSF: Real or Hype? 5

Yousef W. Nielsen and Henrik S. Thomsen

5.1 Introduction

The first magnetic resonance (MR) scanner for imaging (MRI) of the human body became commercially available in the early 1980s. Since then, the number of scanners around the world has increased considerably. From being a rare examination only for a very selected group of patients, it is now an examination that many patients undergo daily. The possibility of having, i.e., 35 examinations or more (due to, e.g., control of a brain tumor) is now high; in the 1980s it was impossible.

Initially it was believed that contrast agents were not necessary for MR imaging. However, it did not take long time before it became obvious that contrast agents were a necessity for visualization of various lesions. The significant increase in capacity increased the risk of being exposed to an MR contrast agent, not only once, but many times. This applies also to patients with reduced renal function or on dialysis. Most of the contrast agents used for MRI underwent phase 2 and phase 3 registration studies when there was only limited capacity and repeated enhanced studies were unlikely. Thus, none of the old agents have been tested under the present situation, where a patient may have multiple MRI examinations. Until 2006 it was believed that the contrast agents used for MRI were the safest agents also for patients with reduced or absent renal function. MRI agents based on macrocyclic chelate must today be considered as rather safe as no clear cases of nephrogenic systemic fibrosis have been reported after exposure to those agents in the peer-reviewed literature and other moderate and severe adverse reactions to those agents are seen infrequently (<0.1%).

Y. W. Nielsen · H. S. Thomsen (✉)
Department of Diagnostic Radiology, Copenhagen University Hospital Herlev-Gentofte, Herlev, Denmark
e-mail: henrik.thomsen@regionh.dk

5.2 MR Contrast Agents

Copper (Cu^{2+}), manganese (Mn^{2+}), and gadolinium (Gd^{3+}) were considered as potential paramagnetic ions to be used in MRI contrast agents in the 1980s. However, gadolinium (atomic number 64 and atomic weight of 157) turned out to be the most powerful with seven unpaired electrons, but unfortunately also the most toxic of those ions. All the current MRI contrast agents contain gadolinium (Gd^{3+}) that affects MR signal properties of surrounding tissues. Gd^{3+} reduces the T1 and T2 relaxation times which increase tissue signal intensity on T1-weighed MR images and has nearly no effect on T2-weighed images. The chemical properties of the contrast agents, including their structure and stability, are important to understand because the risk of gadolinium-related adverse events is determined by the chemistry. The currently used gadolinium-based agents are shown in Table 5.1. Notice that not all agents are authorized for use in Europe.

A. Granata, M. Bertolotto (eds.), *Imaging in Nephrology*,
https://doi.org/10.1007/978-3-030-60794-4_5

Table 5.1 Structures, types, names, and excretion of commercial gadolinium-based contrast media used for MRI

Structure charge	Linear ionic			Linear nonionic
Renal excretion	>99%	96%	50%	>99%
Protein binder	No	Yes	Yes	No
Hepatic excretion	<1%	4%	50%	<1%
Chemical structure	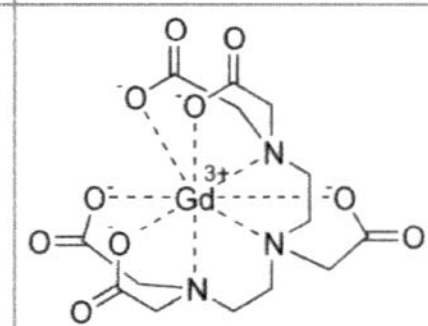	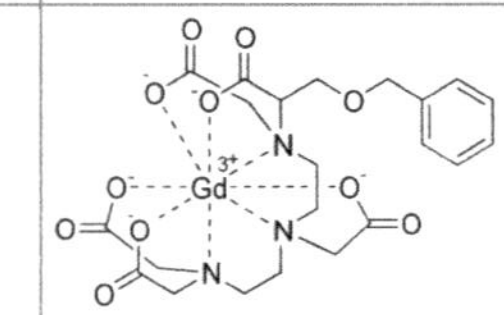	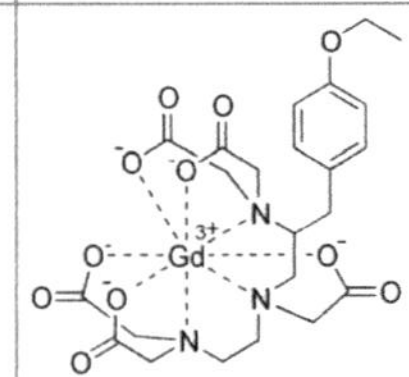	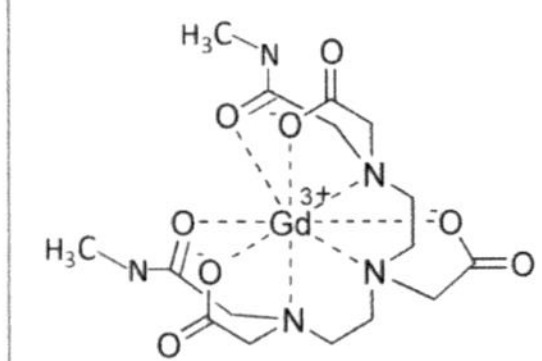
Abbreviation	Gd(DTPA)$^{2-}$	Gd(BOPTA)$^{2-}$	Gd(DTPA-EOB)$^{2-}$	Gd(DTPA-BMA
Generic name	Gadopentetate dimeglumine	Gadobenate dimeglumine	Gadoxetate disodium	Gadodiamide
Trade name	Magnevist	MultiHance	Eovist, Primovist	Omniscan
EMA referral 2017	Authorization suspended	Approved for liver imaging	Approved for liver imaging	Authorization suspended
Risk of NSF (EMA referral 2010)	High	Intermediate	Intermediate	High

Macrocyclic ionic	Macrocyclic nonionic	Macrocyclic nonionic
>99%	>99%	>99%
No	No	No
<1%	<1%	<1%
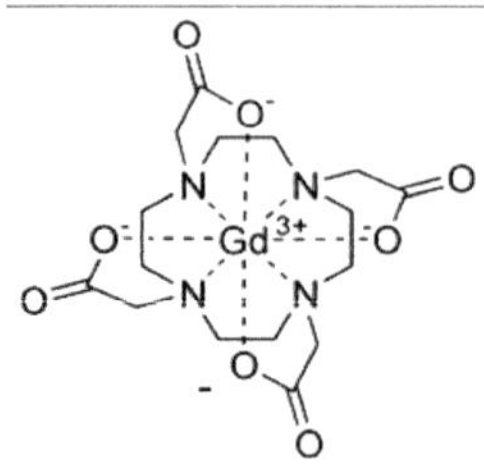	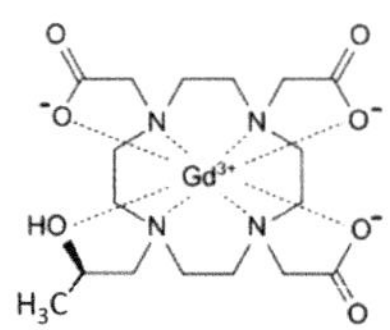	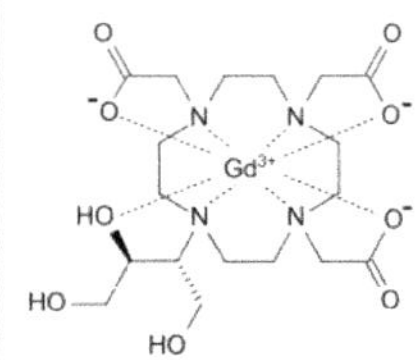
Gd(DOTA)$^{-}$	Gd(HP-DO3A)	Gd(BT-DO3A)
Gadoterate	Gadoteridol	Gadobutrol
Dotarem, Magnescope	ProHance	Gadovist, Gadavist
No restrictions	No restrictions	No restrictions
Low	Low	Low

In solution, each structure also coordinates one water molecule. All agents distribute to extracellular space. The figures shown apply to human beings. Protein binding and excretion vary with species. Trade names are protected by copyright.

5.2.1 Chemistry

Gadolinium cannot be administered as simple inorganic solutions as chlorides and sulfates because the simple salts of gadolinium hydrolyze immediately to form insoluble oxides and hydroxides. At pH 7 these are retained for very long periods in macrophage organs like liver and bone. Mice LD_{50} values for injected raw gadolinium ions are about 0.1–0.3 mmol/kg, or about equal to standard human dose of a current gadolinium-based contrast agent [1]. To be used in a contrast agent, gadolinium must be firmly and stably bound to a carrier molecule that solubilizes it and prevents hydrolysis while still allowing the catalysis of water proton relaxation. Furthermore, it must be rapidly excreted, carrying the heavy metal ion out of the body.

Certain polycarboxylic acids, such as diethylene tetraamine penta-acetate (DTPA), have been known to coordinate metal ions strongly since the 1950s. Gadolinium (III) is a 3+ charged ion with nominally nine sites at which another chemical can bound it. When the DTPA ligand is used, eight of these sites are occupied by three N and five O^- in the carboxyl groups. The ninth gadolinium site is available for fast exchange of water molecules between the "inner sphere" (bonded directly to gadolinium) and the bulk (non-bonded) water. This feature is necessary for strong water proton relaxation. All commercially available gadolinium chelates, except the protein binders, achieve similar effects on proton relaxation and hence visibility in MRIs.

For gadolinium-based contrast agents the choice of ligand structure influences the compound's chemical and biological stability and the colligative properties of its formulations, both of which in turn influence tolerance, pharmacokinetics, clinical uses, and contraindications. Two fundamental structural types are in use:

1. Linear seven-ring structures derived from DTPA
2. Macrocyclic eight-ring structures derived from dodecane tetra-acetic acid (DOTA)

The fundamental difference in these structures is that the chain of nitrogen and carbon atoms making up the backbone of the chelating agent is open on both ends in linear agents and closed into a single loop in macrocycles.

5.2.2 Stability

There are significant differences in the liability to release free gadolinium ions between the various MRI contrast agents [2, 3]. The instability of gadolinium-based contrast agents is an important factor in the pathogenesis of the serious complication of nephrogenic systemic fibrosis (NSF). Coordination sites of gadolinium represent the number of atoms or ligands directly bonded to the metal center such as Gd^{3+}. The bonding between the metal center (Gd^{3+}) and the ligands is through valent bonds in which shared electron pairs are donated to the metal ion by the ligand. In an ionic linear molecule such as Gd-DTPA, Gd^{3+} is coordinated with five carboxyl groups and three amino nitrogen atoms. The three negatively charged carboxyl groups neutralize the three positive charges of the Gd ion and the remaining two carboxyl groups are neutralized by two meglumine cations. In a nonionic linear molecule such as gadodiamide, the number of carboxyl groups is reduced to three because each of the other two carboxyl groups has been replaced by a nonionic methyl amide. Although both amide carbonyl atoms are directly coordinated to Gd^{3+}, the binding is weaker compared to that with carboxyl groups. This weakens the grip of the nonionic chelate on the Gd^{3+} and decreases the stability of the complex.

The other feature influencing the binding between the Gd^{3+} and the chelate is whether the configuration of the molecule is cyclic or linear. The macrocyclic molecule offers better protection and binding of Gd^{3+} because it is a preorganized rigid ring of almost optimal size to cage the Gd ion. In contrast, the linear structure, which is a flexible open chain, provides weaker protection of the gadolinium ion [2, 4].

The in vitro measurements used to assess the stability of the chelate molecules are the following [5]:

1. The *thermodynamic stability constant* (measured under very alkaline conditions (pH ~11); at this pH there are no competing hydrogen ions for the chelate and a theoretical maximum stability for the chelate is obtained)
2. The *conditional stability constant* (measured at physiological pH of 7.4)
3. The *kinetic stability* (dissociation half-life under very acidic conditions (pH 1))

The higher the value of these measurements, the higher the stability of the molecule.

The amount of excess chelate in the gadolinium-based contrast agent preparations is another marker of the stability of these agents. A large amount of excess chelate is present in agents of low stability. The excess chelate is included in the preparation to ensure the absence of free Gd^{3+} in solution. The addition of excess chelate to gadodiamide (nonionic linear chelate) dramatically reduces the acute toxicity of non-formulated preparations (no excess chelate) by a factor of 2.5 as shown by acute toxicity studies (intravenous LD_{50}) [1]. Physical data for commercial gadolinium-based contrast media for MRI at 37 °C are shown in Table 5.2.

The dissociation of gadolinium-based contrast agents incubated in human serum at 37 °C is another suitable method for predicting the stability of these agents in vivo. The examination has been known for many years; the dissociation of gadolinium from gadodiamide with time was already shown in 1995 [6]. A study of dissociation with time showed that the highest release of gadolinium (Gd^{3+}) is observed with the nonionic linear chelate gadodiamide [7]. The addition of phosphate to serum markedly increased the release of Gd^{3+} and the total amount of Gd^{3+} released at day 15 increased from 20% to around 35% of the total dose of these agents. With the ionic linear chelate gadopentetate dimeglumine, phosphate did not increase the total amount of Gd^{3+} released, which remained at 2%, but the speed of the release was increased in day 1–2% and remained at this level up to day 15 [7]. The smaller release of free Gd^{3+} from the ionic linear chelates compared to the nonionic chelates is due to a higher thermodynamic stability of the former. No release of Gd^{3+} was observed with the macrocyclic gadolinium-based contrast agents even after phosphate was added to the serum. As expected from the chemical structure, all the above mentioned stability measurements confirm the superior stability of the macrocyclic chelates and the low stability of the nonionic linear chelates [7].

5.2.3 Transmetallation

Transmetallation of gadolinium-based contrast media leads to release of free gadolinium by replacement of the Gd^{3+} within the chelate molecule by body cations such as iron, copper, zinc, and calcium. It is mainly zinc that displaces a significant amount of Gd^{3+}, due to its high concentration in the blood (55–125 μmol L^{-1}) [2]. Copper is present in very small amounts (1–10 μmol L^{-1}); calcium ions have low affinity to organic ligands. Iron ions are tightly bound by the storage proteins ferritin and hemosiderin and are not available for transmetallation with Gd^{3+}. Transmetallation between Gd^{3+} and zinc results in the formation of zinc chelate, which is excreted in urine. The released Gd^{3+} becomes attached to endogenous anions such as phosphate, citrate, hydroxide, or carbonate, which deposit in the tissues as insoluble compounds. In vivo, in vitro, and human studies have shown that linear chelates, particularly the nonionic ones, cause a large increase in zinc excretion in urine. The nonionic linear chelate gadodiamide induced a decrease of 32% of plasma zinc after a single injection in healthy volunteers [8]. This is thought to be secondary to transmetallation and the presence of excess chelate in the gadodiamide preparation. In patients undergoing contrast-enhanced MRI, gadodiamide caused a large increase in zinc excretion in the urine, which was almost three times greater than that induced by the ionic linear molecule Gd-DTPA. In comparison, the ionic macrocyclic Gd-DOTA had no effect on zinc

Table 5.2 Physical data for commercial gadolinium-based contrast media for MRI at 37 °C (except where noted)

Structure type	Linear				Macrocyclic		
Charge type	Ionic			Nonionic	Ionic	Nonionic	
Trade name	Magnevist	MultiHance	Eovist Primovist	Omniscan	Dotarem Magnescope	ProHance	Gadovist Gadavist
[Gd] in M (commercial preparations)	0.5	0.5	0.25	0.5	0.5	0.5	1.0
Osmolality, mOsm/kg	1960	1970	688	789	1350	630	1603
Viscosity, mPa/s	2.9	5.3	1.2	1.4	2.0	1.3	5.0
Relaxivity, plasma							
r_1—1.5 T mM^{-1} s^{-1}	3.9–4.1	6.3–7.9	6.9	4.3	3.6	4.1	4.7–5.2
r_2—1.5 T mM^{-1} s^{-1}	4.6–5.3	8.7–18.9	8.7	5.2	4.3	5.0	6.1–7.5
r_1—3 T mM^{-1} s^{-1}	3.7–3.9	5.5–5.9	6.2	4.0	3.5	3.7	4.5–5.0
r_2—3 T mM^{-1} s^{-1}	5.2	11.0–17.5	11.0	5.6	4.9	5.7	6.3–7.1
Stability constants							
Log K_{eq}, M^{-1a}	22.5	22.6	23.5	16.9	25.6	23.8	21.8
Log K_{eq}, pH 7[a]	18.4	18.4	18.7	14.9	19.3	17.1	15.5
$T_{1/2}$ dissociation pH 1	<5 s[a]	<5 s[a]	<5 s[a]	<5 s[a]	26 h	2.0 h	7.9 h
Risk of NSF[b]	High	Intermediate	Intermediate	High	Low	Low	Low

Reprinted with permission from the publisher [1]

[a]25 °C

[b]According to the classification approved by the European Medicines Agency (EMA). High-risk agents are contraindicated in patients with a glomerular filtration rate (GFR) <30 mL/min × 1.73 m² and should be used with caution in patients with a GFR between 30 and 60 mL/min × 1.73 m² (ESUR guidelines on Contrast Media version 8.1—www.esur.org (Jan 2014)).

excretion [8]. Ex vivo studies have also confirmed that all macrocyclic gadolinium-based contrast agents are insensitive to transmetallation by zinc ions compared to the open-chain complexes.

5.2.4 Pharmacokinetics

The pharmacokinetics depends on whether the contrast agent is an extracellular agent or an organ-specific agent. The extracellular agents behave in blood just like the well-known iodine-based agents. The protein binders are also excreted via hepatobiliary system. Their pharmacokinetics follow the two-compartment model, where the two compartments are the intravascular plasma space and the other is the interstitial space.

5.3 Adverse Reactions

5.3.1 Acute Adverse Reactions

It is the same reactions that are seen after iodine-based contrast media. They are very infrequent (1–2%), especially the moderate and the severe reactions (<0.2%). Mild reactions which do not require treatment are the most frequent.

5.3.2 Very Late Adverse Reaction

Nephrogenic systemic fibrosis (NSF) is a disease, which was seen for the first time in 1997 [3, 9], at about the time when radiologists began to transfer patients from enhanced radiographic examinations to magnetic resonance imaging and to do magnetic resonance arteriography with double or triple dose of the supposedly "non-nephrotoxic contrast media." The gadolinium-based contrast agents were also used for some radiographic examinations such as conventional arteriography and CT [10]. In 2006 two European groups found a correlation between the occurrence of NSF and exposure to gadodiamide [11, 12]. Very rapidly it became clear that unconfounded (i.e., only one contrast agent ever used in the patient) cases were only seen after exposure to the least stable agents (gadodiamide, and, to a lesser extent, gadopentetate dimeglumine). All the patients had reduced renal function or were on dialysis. It occurred all over the world and in both young and old people. The severity of the disease varied from a single small plaque on a lower extremity to nearly universal disease-causing severe disability, cachexia, and death. The adverse reaction can start hours to several years after the last exposure to the gadolinium-based contrast medium. Not all patients with renal impairment develop NSF after exposure to one of the high-risk agents. Thus, there must be another as of yet not known factor. Most believe that the cause of the disease is transmetallation. The free gadolinium thus liberated (dissociated) localizes in the brain, the skin, the liver, and, in particular, the bone, probably as a complex of calcium and phosphate [13, 14]. This may trigger the circulating fibrocytes and fibrosis may develop. After each intravenous injection of a gadolinium-based contrast medium a tiny amount of unchelated Gd^{3+} is left in the body—more after the nonionic linear chelates than after the ionic linear chelates. The latter leave more than the macrocyclic agents and more in patients with reduced renal function than in patients with normal function as the agents stay longer in the body the poorer the renal function is. Whether the accumulation has any long-term effects even in patients with normal renal function is still unknown. Therefore, it is advisable—independent of renal function—to use an agent that leaves the smallest amount of gadolinium. Furthermore, the lowest dose for sufficient diagnostic workup of the patient should be used. The nonionic linear gadodiamide and the ionic linear gadopentetate dimeglumine are now contraindicated to use in patients with GFR <30 mL/min × 1.73 m^2 and should only be used with caution in patients with GFR between 30 and 60 mL/min × 1.73 m^2. Therefore, it is mandatory to determine the renal function before use of these agents.

We do not know the exact number of patients who got NSF between 1996 and 2007. There has been a significant underreporting due to the large variety in the disease (from a small plaque on a lower extremity to cachexia and death) and due to the fact that the patients contacted a variety of physicians (e.g., dermatologists, nephrologists, rheumatologists, pathologists), but not the radiologists who administered the agent. Furthermore, administration of contrast agents is at several institutions not listed together with the drugs that the patients take daily, weekly, or monthly. With exemption of two studies, all other studies are based on registries (retrospective data). Several may have died during 11 years without any registration of their skin changes. The prevalence of skin changes after gadodiamide in the retrospective studies varies between 3% and 5%, but in the single prospective study, where the skin of all exposed patients was examined, the prevalence was as high as 18%; lower in case of one injection; and higher if more than one dose has been administered [9, 15]. It has been estimated that around 10,000 patients have developed NSF. It seems like the disease has been erased at least in Europe, Japan, and the USA thanks to the guidelines for use of gadolinium-based contrast agents issued by the European Society of Urogenital Radiology (ESUR) [16] and American College of Radiology [17]. It is recommended that if a department continues to use the least stable agents in patients with normal renal functions, the least stable agents are kept from the more stable agents, so one avoids—by a mistake—to give one of the contraindicated agents to a patient with reduced renal function or on dialyses. Mistakes have taken place.

5.4 Discussion

NSF is a horrible adverse reaction that we must avoid. We should not develop gadophobia because of that adverse reaction. The consequence should not be that we refuse giving gadolinium-based contrast agents to patients with reduced renal function or on dialysis as we may overlook series lesions that can be treated. Based on the experience obtained during the last 10 years, it is OK to administer the macrocyclic agents. There is no report of NSF after gadoterate meglumine (Dotarem) both in retrospective and prospective studies. There is a single report in the non-peer-reviewed literature regarding gadoteridol (ProHance); however, the plaque was located at the upper part of the back, but not in the lower extremities, where NSF changes are typically located. The three cases related to gadobutrol (Gadovist) and published in peer-reviewed literature do not fulfill the Yale criteria for NSF. In addition, the environment changed in 2006/2007. One is no longer so liberal regarding referral to contrast-enhanced MRI for patients with reduced renal function or on dialysis as one was before 2006. Therefore, studies done before 2007 cannot be compared with studies performed after 2007. Comparative studies must be undertaken under the same conditions. Would there be any cases of nephrogenic systemic fibrosis after exposure to gadopentetate under current conditions where we do not use Gd contrast agents as liberally as we did before 2006? We will never know. Radiologists (>50%) have switched to macrocyclic agents in all patients in North America and Europe. Anyhow it seems like we have erased the adverse reaction NSF and that we can use macrocyclic agents in patients with reduced renal function or on dialysis safely, when an enhanced MR examination is clinically indicated.

5.5 Conclusion

There is no doubt that the lanthanide gadolinium, which does not occur naturally in the human body, is the cause of nephrogenic systemic fibrosis both in man and animals. It was not a hype; it was a reality and a horror story for those patients who developed severe nephrogenic systemic fibrosis. It was a shock for radiologists as they do their imaging examinations in order to help the patients, not to disable them. It seems like one can get the diagnostic advantages of gadolinium and avoid the development of fibrosis by following the guidelines.

References

1. Thomsen HS, Dawson P, Tweedle M. Chapter 7: MR and CT contrast agents for perfusion imaging and regulatory issues. In: Brammer R, editor. MR and CT perfusion imaging: clinical applications and theoretical principles. Philadelphia, PA: Lippincott Williams and Wilkins; 2015. p. 85–102.
2. Morcos SK. Gadolinium chelates and stability. In: Thomsen HS, Webb JAW, editors. Contrast media: safety issues and ESUR guidelines. 3rd ed. Heidelberg: Springer; 2014. p. 175–80.
3. Thomsen HS. Nephrogenic systemic fibrosis: a serious adverse reaction to gadolinium—1997–2006–2016. Part 1. Acta Radiol. 2016;57:515–20.
4. Morcos SK. Nephrogenic systemic fibrosis following the administration of extracellular gadolinium based contrast agents: is the stability of the contrast agent molecule an important factor in the pathogenesis of this condition? Br J Radiol. 2007;80:72–6.
5. Thomsen HS. Nephrogenic systemic fibrosis and gadolinium-based contrast media. In: Thomsen HS, Webb JAW, editors. Contrast media: safety issues and ESUR guidelines. 3rd ed. Heidelberg: Springer; 2014. p. 207–18.
6. Laurent S, van der Elst L, Muller RN. Comparative study of the physicochemical properties of six clinical low molecular weight gadolinium contrast agents. Contrast Media Mol Imaging. 2006;128–37.
7. Frenzel T, Lengsfeld P, Schirmer H, et al. Stability of gadolinium based magnetic resonance imaging contrast agents in human serum at 37°C. Investig Radiol. 2008;43:817–28.
8. Kimura J, Ishguchi T, Matsuda J, et al. Human comparative study of zinc and copper excretion via urine after administration of magnetic resonance imaging contrast agents. Radiat Med. 2005;23:322–6.
9. Thomsen HS. Nephrogenic systemic fibrosis: a serious adverse reaction to gadolinium—1997–2006–2016. Part 2. Acta Radiol. 2016;57:643–8.
10. Thomsen HS, Leander P. Radiography with gadolinium-based contrast media. In: Thomsen HS, Webb JAW, editors. Contrast media: safety issues and ESUR guidelines. 3rd ed. Heidelberg: Springer; 2014. p. 193–200.
11. Grobner T. Gadolinium—a specific trigger for the development of nephrogenic fibrosing dermopathy and nephrogenic systemic fibrosis? Nephrol Dial Transplant. 2006;21:1104–8.
12. Marckmann P, Skov L, Rossen K, et al. Nephrogenic systemic fibrosis: suspected causative role of gadodiamide used for contrast-enhanced magnetic resonance imaging. J Am Soc Nephrol. 2006;17:2359–62.
13. Thomsen HS. T1-hyperintensity in the brain after multiple intravenous injections of gadolinium-based contrast agents. Acta Radiol. 2016;57:389–91.
14. Stacul F, Thomsen HS. Extracellular contrast media in perfusion imaging. In: Saremi F, editor. Perfusion imaging in clinical practice. A multimodality approach to tissue perfusion analyses. Philadelphia, PA: Wolters Kluwer; 2015. p. 205–16.
15. Rydahl C, Thomsen HS, Marckmann P. High prevalence of nephrogenic systemic fibrosis in chronic renal failure patients exposed to gadodiamide, a gadolinium (Gd) containing magnetic resonance contrast agent. Investig Radiol. 2008;43:141–4.
16. ESUR Contrast media guidelines version 9.0. www.esur-cm.org. Accessed 6 Sep 2017.
17. ACR, American College of Radiology. ACR Manual on Contrast Media Version 10.3; 2017. https://www.acr.org/Quality-Safety/Resources/Contrast-Manual. Accessed 6 Sep 2017.

Gadolinium Retention in Brain and Body: Clinical and Preclinical Evidence

6

Carlo Cosimo Quattrocchi and Aart J. Van Der Molen

6.1 Introduction to Clinical GBCA Use in MRI and Gadolinium Retention in General

6.1.1 Clinical Use of Contrast-Enhanced MRI

Appropriate use of gadolinium-based contrast agents (GBCAs) in contrast-enhanced MRI is indicated for morphologic imaging, lesion characterization, perfusion imaging, and contrast-enhanced angiography [1]. The added diagnostic value of GBCAs consists of (a) increasing differences of T1, T2, and T2* relaxation time constants between different tissues or normal and pathologic tissues; (b) increasing overall MRI sensitivity; (c) increasing MRI diagnostic specificity by allowing evaluation of different patterns of enhancement and perfusion of differently vascularized tissues; and (d) increasing contrast between intra- and extravascular space in cardiac and vascular imaging.

As a heavy metal in the lanthanide group, elemental free gadolinium is toxic to humans and shows a very long excretion rate with only 1–3% eliminated per day and with the remaining deposited in different tissues including liver, kidney, bone, etc. GBCAs have been developed by chelating gadolinium to organic ligands to decrease toxicity and decrease blood half-life down to about 1 h [2, 3]. Free Gd^{3+}, showing a size similar to that of Ca^{2+}, plays the role of a competitive inhibitor of biological processes requiring Ca^{2+}, can bind to Ca^{2+}-binding enzymes, and affects voltage-gated calcium channels, potentially leading to adverse biological effects [4].

6.1.2 Definitions and Terminologies

On a chemical structure point of view, GBCAs are distinct in two main categories: macrocyclic compounds where gadolinium is caged within the cavity of the ligand and open-chain (commonly called linear) compounds in which gadolinium has a lower thermodynamic and kinetic stability [3, 5]. Gadobutrol, gadoterate meglumine, and gadoteridol are macrocyclic GBCAs, and the remaining are linear forms. Also, within each category, molecules may be differentiated into ionic and nonionic GBCAs, according to the presence of opposite charges or covalent bonds, respectively [6], that have an impact on kinetic stability as nonionic compounds result to be less stable than ionic ones. Although GBCAs are considered as they all behave similarly in each category, differences must be taken into account,

C. C. Quattrocchi (✉)
Diagnostic Imaging, Universita Campus Bio-Medico di Roma, Rome, Italy
e-mail: c.quattrocchi@unicampus.it

A. J. Van Der Molen (✉)
Department of Radiology, Leiden University Medical Center, Leiden, The Netherlands
e-mail: a.j.van_der_molen@lumc.nl

A. Granata, M. Bertolotto (eds.), *Imaging in Nephrology*,
https://doi.org/10.1007/978-3-030-60794-4_6

mainly those related to local extracellular concentration as a main consequence of the compound concentration at the injection site and to relaxivity, i.e., the ability to shorten time constants as a main consequence of the molecular mass [1].

Currently approved GBCAs have similar biodistribution patterns, blood half-lives, and mechanisms of action as well as clearance pathway, mostly secreted through the kidneys. Among these, gadoxetic acid and gadobenate dimeglumine are different as a fraction of the injected dose (50% and 3–5%, respectively) is intracellularly taken up by normally functioning hepatocytes and then excreted through the biliary system [2, 3].

6.1.3 Safety and Efficacy of GBCAs: The Role of Gadolinium Retention

Numerous studies have demonstrated the safety and efficacy of the GBCAs approved for contrast-enhanced MRI with a very low prevalence and incidence of adverse events in phase II–IV clinical trials as well as in post-authorization studies [7–10].

The issue of gadolinium retention in tissues emerged with the first description of the nephrogenic fibrosing dermopathy by Cowper in 2000, leading to what was afterwards called nephrogenic systemic fibrosis (NSF) by Grobner in 2006. Indeed, patients with severe renal impairment were at high risk to develop this systemic disease within a period of up to months after last intravenous injection of GBCAs. Despite this being out of the scope of this chapter, physiopathology of NSF has then been related to the retention of gadolinium in tissues and to its ability to stimulate expression and release of cytokines involved in the development of tissue fibrosis [11–13]. The relationship of the disease with the high rate of tissue retention has then been related to the amounts of gadolinium that persist in the body and that may dissociate from their carrier ligands and/or chelates [14]. As a final end product, through transmetallation, gadolinium may then bind with readily available phosphates, carbonates, or citrates, and form insoluble molecules that deposit into tissues [15, 16]. Preexisting renal failure has been the most prevalent patient characteristic associated with NSF as a clinical risk factor that further decreases the excretion rate of gadolinium forms and prolongs the presence of gadolinium in the body tissues. Nevertheless, an overall epidemiologic evaluation demonstrates that the event of the nephrogenic systemic fibrosis is rare even in the entire population of patients with severe renal impairment and exposure to high-risk GBCAs, especially the linear nonionic gadodiamide which represents the most unstable molecule among all. This suggests that other cofactors have still to be identified to distinguish the subpopulation at maximum risk to develop NSF [17].

However, in the last decade the introduction of specific recommendations such as patient prescreening for renal function, the contraindication of the so-called high-risk GBCAs (Magnevist, Omniscan, and Opti-MARK) in patients with stage IV and V chronic kidney disease, and the restriction of the use of GBCAs to the lowest necessary dose have led to a marked drop of new cases of NSF [18].

In fact, the awareness of NSF and its association with the retention of gadolinium associated with some GBCAs in patients with renal failure has led to introduction of screening for the possible presence of renal disease prior to any GBCA intravenous administration. It is now generally accepted across the world that if renal disease is present, the GBCA agent to be administered is chosen among those recognized at low risk of NSF and the dose is kept as small as possible [19].

However, while alerts on NSF of patients with renal failure have decreased down to zero, the use of GBCAs has been unconditioned in patients with normal renal function in the last 10 years. Indeed, the patient who currently undergoes GBCA administration retains gadolinium into his/her body, although this occurs at a lower rate than in patients with renal failure. Therefore, the event of tissue retention and the deposition of non-chelated gadolinium are currently considered potential risk factors to develop gadolinium-related toxicity even without impairment of the renal function. Some studies have reported single cases of patients with NSF and gadolinium deposition in multiple organs (including heart, lungs, spleen, kidney, skeletal muscle, and meninges) [20, 21]. To date, the tissues that have been investigated in most of the patients with normal renal function were the bone, skin, brain, and liver, confirming what had been previously observed in preclinical studies.

6.2 Gadolinium Retention in the Brain

6.2.1 Clinical Studies

In 2014 the work of Kanda et al. suggested that the retrospectively observed hyperintensity of the dentate nucleus and the globus pallidus on unenhanced T1-weighted images of a population of patients with brain primary and secondary tumors was related to repeated administrations of GBCAs [22]. Soon after, Errante et al. [23] reported similar findings on unenhanced T1-weighted brain images after multiple injections of gadodiamide in two different unconfounded patient groups, 38 patients with multiple sclerosis and 37 patients with brain metastases. A progressive increase in SI ratios (dentate nucleus/pons signal intensity ratio) was seen in both patient populations. The study demonstrated that the findings were not related to a specific pathology, in addition to confirming the observations of Kanda and colleagues. Several publications were then published in 2015 and 2016. Kanda et al. [24] compared T1 signal intensity after exposure to linear contrast agent (gadopentetate dimeglumine) to that observed after a macrocyclic agent (gadoteridol). Hyperintensity in the dentate nucleus on unenhanced T1-weighted images was associated with prior administration of gadopentetate dimeglumine but not gadoteridol.

Quattrocchi et al. [25] then showed the results from a study including patients that had multiple follow-up brain MRIs for evaluation of meningiomas. In patients with a history of at least six enhanced studies using gadodiamide, a significant increase in the signal intensity of the dentate nucleus on T1-weighted precontrast studies was noted, clarifying that this finding was not related to medical therapy (as could have been the case with the prior studied patient populations). Radbruch et al. [26] also published a comparison of the linear gadopentetate dimeglumine and the macrocyclic gadoterate meglumine, with 50 patients in each group, demonstrating that a change occurred with the first agent, a linear chelate, and not with the second, a macrocyclic chelate. All patients underwent at least six consecutive MR examinations with exclusive use of either the linear or the macrocyclic GBCA. In June 2015, Ramalho et al. [27] published a study evaluating 23 patients who received linear nonionic gadodiamide (5 ± 2.4 injections) and 46 who received the linear ionic gadobenate dimeglumine (4.6 ± 2.1 injections). They found that a significant increase of T1 signal intensity ratio between the dentate nucleus and the middle cerebellar peduncle was seen after gadodiamide but not gadobenate dimeglumine. The rate of change suggested gadolinium deposition in the dentate nucleus also with gadobenate dimeglumine although less than with gadodiamide [27]. In this regard the other commercially available linear liver-specific GBCA, gadoxetic acid, has been associated with T1 signal intensity of the dentate nucleus after a number of doses that are relatively higher than those reported for general-use linear GBCAs such as gadodiamide and gadopentetate dimeglumine [28, 29].

All these investigations suggested a mechanism of progressive accumulation of gadolinium, detectable at conventional MRI and dependent on the structure of the compound chelating gadolinium ions. The high signal intensity on unenhanced T1-weighted images is related to the number of administrations of GBCAs with lower kinetic inertness and this occurs in patients without any kind of renal disease and with a mechanism that is not related to the physiopathology of the disease nor to systemic interval therapy nor to previous brain radiation therapy [25].

These experimental results radically modified two dominant concepts in the medical community: (a) Gadolinium is not completely eliminated from the body about 24–48 h after, i.v., injection in subjects with normal renal function and (b) gadolinium chelates are not unable to cross an intact blood-brain barrier. McDonald et al. [30] in fact published the first report with data on human postmortem specimens in 13 patients with at least four contrast-enhanced brain examinations (using exclusively gadodiamide) and compared them with patients who had not received intravenous contrast agents. Neuronal tissue from the contrast group demonstrated up to 59 μg gadolinium per gram of tissue (ppm), with a significant dose-dependent relationship correlating with precontrast T1-weighted signal intensity changes. Most of the gadolinium deposits were observed in the endothelial layers of brain vessels and a variable part of them (18–42%) were located in the extracellular interstitium, as an effect of crossing an intact blood-brain barrier. No gadolinium was detectable in the neuronal tissue of control patients. McDonald et al. in fact found gadolinium inside the nervous tissue, not only in the globus pallidus and in the dentate nucleus but also in the pons and in the thalamus at a lower concentration. These findings were then confirmed by a new autopsy study conducted by Kanda et al. [31] on five patients who received at least two total doses of less stable GBCAs. In this last report gadolinium was found not only in the brain gray matter nuclei but also in the frontal lobe cortex, in the frontal lobe white matter, and in the cerebellar white matter (Fig. 6.1).

Investigation on brain MRI scans after more than 35 doses of linear GBCAs confirmed that high signal on T1-weighted images may be observed not only in the dentate nucleus and the globus pallidus but also in many other structures such as the substantia nigra, thalamus, red nucleus, colliculi, superior cerebellar peduncle, caudate nucleus, and putamen [32]. As a counterpart, Radbruch et al. [33] did not observe an increase of T1 signal intensity of the dentate nucleus after more than 20 doses of macrocyclic GBCA.

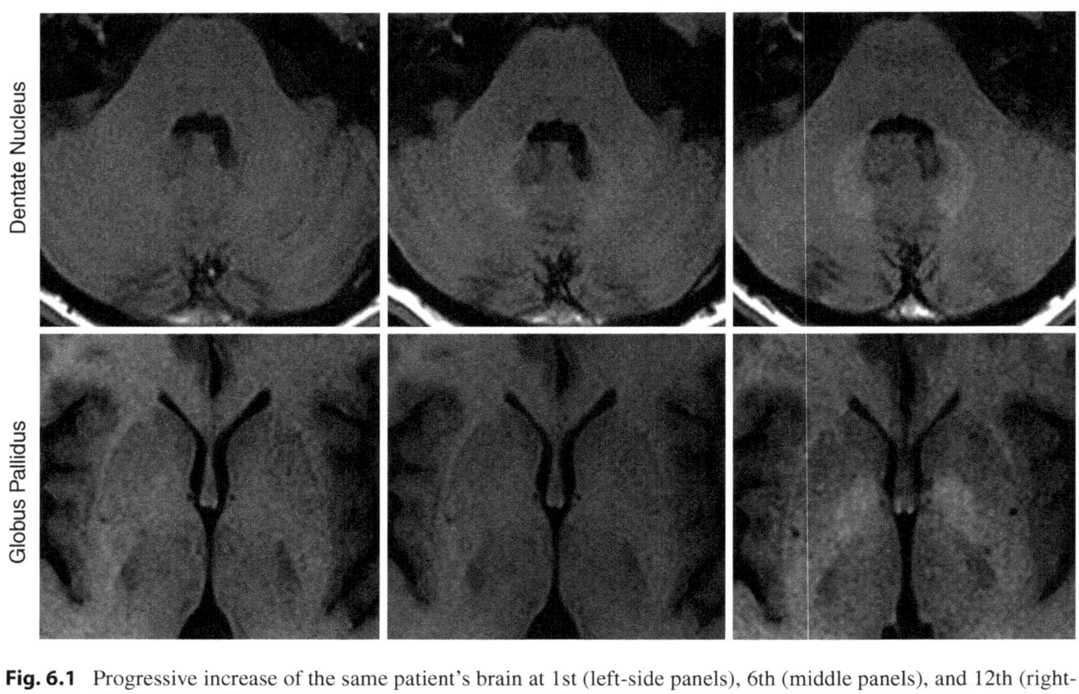

Fig. 6.1 Progressive increase of the same patient's brain at 1st (left-side panels), 6th (middle panels), and 12th (right-side panels) enhanced MRI scan using the linear nonionic gadodiamide

6.2.2 Preclinical Results on Brain Retention (i.e., Animal Studies)

The first preclinical study on gadolinium retention in the brain was published by Robert et al. in 2015 [34]; that work reinforced the idea that T1 high signal intensity and gadolinium retention in the brain are indeed observed only after repeated administrations of a nonionic linear GBCA, but not with similar doses of an ionic macrocyclic agent. They also showed that there is no evidence of a reduction of T1 hyperintensity after a "washout" period of 5 weeks from the last injection, not only in the deep cerebellar nuclei but also in other brain structures [34]. Although the analytical methods used to measure the presence of gadolinium in the brain were not able to distinguish between free and chelated gadolinium, these experimental data highlighted the importance of in vivo dechelation of gadolinium ions from less stable GBCAs and opened questions on the mechanisms of gadolinium ability to progressively concentrate in the brain, regardless of the presence of a renal dysfunction and with a clear dose-effect relationship.

Shortly after, other studies were conducted under preclinical experimental conditions and confirmed that a difference exists in the amount of total gadolinium retained in the brain when comparing different GBCA compounds [35–38]. Recently, evidence from an animal study has shown that gadolinium levels measured in the brain 24 days after the last injection have to be distinguished into three different chemical forms: soluble small molecules, soluble macromolecules, and insoluble forms [38]. The gadolinium contained in the soluble fraction is the component that is slowly secreted and is retained for several weeks; of this, the gadolinium linked to its original molecule or to macromolecules may affect the environment and increase tissue T1 relaxivity, at a sufficient rate to achieve T1 shortening and high signal intensity on T1-weighted images [38]. When comparing different GBCA compounds, Frenzel et al. identified that, although a comparable gadolinium content is present in the soluble fraction of tissue brain homogenates, there is a much higher amount of gadolinium linked to macromolecular complexes for linear than for macrocyclic GBCAs [38].

As it regards the question on the pathway of GBCA entry into the brain, no differences have been found between cerebrospinal fluid penetration and distribution of linear and macrocyclic GBCA compounds [39] and the role of glymphatic circulation has been called out. These data have been supported by the observation of T1 signal intensity increase in the dentate nucleus and globus pallidus after only intrathecal administration of a linear ionic GBCA in a clinical setting [40].

In summary, preclinical evidence is currently available as it regards the mechanisms, amount, and timing of gadolinium retention in the brain. In humans, clinical effects of gadolinium retention in the brain need further research [41].

6.3 Gadolinium Retention in Bone

6.3.1 Clinical Studies

Affinity of most metals and especially lanthanides for the skeleton has been observed via biodistribution studies in the whole body. Nevertheless, to date mechanisms of metal retention and/or deposition in bone are poorly understood mainly because of its structural complexity and dynamic bone tissue remodeling [42].

Non-complexed gadolinium ions and other members of the lanthanide series (e.g., samarium, europium, and cerium) have long been known to deposit in bone tissue of animals and humans.

First observation in humans with a linear GBCA was made by Gibby et al. who studied the retention of gadolinium in human bone tissue collected from patients undergoing hip joint replacement surgery [43]. Further studies compared retention of the nonionic linear gadodiamide and the macrocyclic ProHance [44, 45]. Data confirmed that gadolinium, introduced as its chelated form, is retained for at least 8 years [45]. Also, the demonstration of higher retention in osteoarthritis patients vs. those with osteoporotic fractures suggests the important role of bone resorption and remodeling on gadolinium retention [45]. However, these clinical studies are partly not confirmed by the fact that ovariectomy-induced osteoporosis has shown no significant difference in total Gd concentration between rats receiving gadodiamide and treated with ovariectomy or not [46].

Recently the bone compartment has shown retention of gadolinium not only after exposure to the linear gadobenate dimeglumine but also after the macrocyclic gadoteridol and gadobutrol with levels measured within a median of 23 times higher than the brain (globus pallidus) in a small group of unconfounded patients exposed to GBCAs [47, 48].

6.3.2 Preclinical Results on Bone Retention (i.e., Animal Studies)

In animal studies, gadolinium retention in the femur has been shown to be 25-fold higher with gadodiamide than with gadoteric acid [46]. At least 21 days after the injection of gadopentetate dimeglumine, more than 96% of the released gadolinium ions were deposited in the bone as a result of translocated Gd ions from dechelation of the Gd-DTPA [49].

When comparing different GBCAs, there appears to be four times more gadolinium in the bones of patients with normal renal function after a nonionic linear chelate than after a nonionic macrocyclic chelate [44]. After 7 days, mice with renal impairment that had received the ionic macrocyclic chelate had three times more radioactivity in their bone than control mice. However, mice with renal impairment that had received an ionic linear chelate or a nonionic chelate had 8 times and 24 times more radioactivity in their bone, respectively [50]. From a literature search on bone retention of gadolinium, the bone residence times of ^{153}Gd have been shown to be more prolonged in the groups of animals that received the linear GBCAs, with half-time values varying from 10 days for gadobenate dimeglumine to 158 days for gadodiamide vs. 4–13 days for macrocyclic compounds [2].

The adult human skeleton is composed of 80% cortical bone and 20% trabecular (cancellous) bone [51]. The annual turnover of cortical bone is in the range of 2–3% vs. 20–30% in cancellous bone [51]. As such, long retention times and highly dynamic remodeling have suggested that human bone may serve as a reservoir for gadolinium into the bloodstream [2].

In summary, current knowledge gaps that need further investigation are the state of gadolinium in the bone, if chelated as initially administered to the patient or in a new compound formed after transmetallation, and the role of different pools of gadolinium complexes (trabecular bone, cortical bone, or bone marrow) in affecting the overall bone metabolism.

6.4 Gadolinium Retention in the Skin

6.4.1 Clinical Studies

Gadolinium deposition in skin biopsies was demonstrated shortly after the described association of NSF with GBCA in 2006. Since then, several clinical and preclinical studies have focused on and detected gadolinium in the skin under the condition of chronic kidney disease or with normal renal function.

In patients with normal renal function, deposition of gadolinium in the skin was not expected or expected to be low [52, 53] until recently Murata showed low deposition of gadolinium in the skin of three patients with normal renal function after exposure to the linear gadobenate and the macrocyclic gadoteridol [47]. More recently Roberts described a single case of high levels of gadolinium deposition in the skin of a patient with normal renal function after 61 contrast-enhanced MRI scans. However, no symptoms or histological alterations were detected. Only increased CD34 immunoreactivity was reported in the connective tissue septa of the subcutaneous adipose tissue, indicating inflammation [54].

The clinical event of "gadolinium-associated plaques" in the skin of patients with and without underlying renal insufficiency suggests that, under conditions that are not still understood, retention of gadolinium may lead to clinical features, even with normal renal function [55].

6.4.2 Preclinical Results on Skin Retention (i.e., Animal Studies)

In preclinical models, Sieber et al. have shown a different potential for different GBCAs to release gadolinium into the skin. They observed fibrosis, increased cellularity, and increased cell swelling in 80% of animals treated with linear gadodiamide [56]. Overall, studies in rodents seem to show that in the condition of normal renal function Gd^{3+} tissue retention is greater after injection of a nonionic linear GBCA (gadodiamide) when compared to an ionic linear GBCA (gadopentetate) and that the lowest level of tissue retention occurs with a nonionic macrocyclic agent (gadoteridol). Also, the high concentration of gadolinium deposited was accompanied by more histological changes (e.g., spindle and stellate cells under epidermis layer and thicker epidermis layer) in the skin of rats treated with gadodiamide compared with gadoteric acid-treated rats [46].

Initial investigations in healthy rats treated with high doses of different GBCAs have shown macroscopic and histological skin changes after gadodiamide but not after macrocyclic agents with a significant higher level of gadolinium retention into the skin after gadodiamide than after macrocyclic agents [56]. An experimental model of repeated administrations of GBCAs, despite a high rate of elimination from the skin of gadolinium within a time period of about 2 months, has shown long-term retention with significantly higher values in animals treated with nonionic linear agents than in those rats receiving ionic linear GBCAs. After treatment with macrocyclic compounds, gadolinium levels in the skin were in the same range of controls [57].

Wang et al. showed that Gd^{3+} concentration was 180-fold higher in the skin of rats receiving the linear gadodiamide than rats treated with gadoteric acid. Ultrastructural changes in the skin after gadodiamide exposure included focal Gd^{3+} deposition/incrustation of collagen fibers with a "halo" formation around some fibers [46].

In summary, gadolinium retention/deposition in the skin is higher with linear than with macrocyclic GBCAs; however, there is still need to further understand the relationship between gadolinium exposure and clinical occurrence of skin plaques, if this is dependent on the cumulative doses of gadolinium and, eventually, the underlying physiopathological mechanisms.

6.5 Gadolinium Retention in Splanchnic Organs

6.5.1 Clinical Studies

Quantitation of gadolinium into the liver tissues has been reported in a group of pediatric hematopoietic stem cell transplant recipients [58]. In these patients, with normal liver and renal function and under the condition of iron overload, they found high levels of total retained gadolinium compared to age-matched controls and a positive correlation between liver gadolinium and iron concentration after exposure to the macrocyclic gadoterate meglumine. Moreover, gadolinium liver concentration was reduced after treatment with chelation therapy with deferoxamine [58].

6.5.2 Preclinical Results from Splanchnic Organs (i.e., Animal Studies)

The retention of gadolinium in splanchnic organs is known from preclinical evidence. Tweedle et al. found that gadolinium retention in liver 2 weeks after injection of GBCAs was three times greater following the linear and nonionic GBCA gadodiamide compared to the linear and ionic gadopentetate. In both mice and rats, total gadolinium retention in tissues was minimal with the macrocyclic chelates gadoteric acid and gadoteridol [59].

These results were confirmed by Wang et al. who demonstrated the deposition of gadolinium in the liver of rats exposed to gadodiamide or gadoteric acid [46].

Histopathological and molecular changes (apoptosis) in the liver, lungs, and kidney tissues have been observed in GBCA-treated mice [60]. In Balb/c mice exposed to IV injection of different contrast agents, including gadopentetate dimeglumine, a number of changes including reduction in total white blood cell count, increases in serum levels of inflammatory cytokines (IL-6 and TNF-R), and hepatic histopathologic changes (vacuolar degeneration, disorganized hepatic cords) were observed. One concern regards the possibility that gadolinium might be trapped by the reticuloendothelial system (RES) in splenic macrophages, liver Kupffer cells, and hepatocytes, as reported after administration of a soluble gadolinium salt to rats [61].

Under the condition of impaired renal function, exposure to gadopentetic acid increased short-term (3 days after last injection) Gd retention in the liver, spleen, and kidney but did not affect long-term (45 days after last injection) Gd retention. Gadopentetate showed higher Gd retention than gadoterate meglumine. Although Gd retention of the liver and the spleen in the group exposed to the macrocyclic gadoterate meglumine was generally low, impaired renal function increased only long-term hepatic Gd retention [62].

In summary, although gadolinium retention/deposition is now well established to occur in different organs despite normal renal function, the burden of gadolinium retention in splanchnic organs is not well understood as well as the species of gadolinium present and the link to health consequences.

6.6 Clinical Consequences of Gadolinium Retention

Retention of gadolinium in different tissues of patients with normal renal function is currently under study to exclude any potential deleterious effect of gadolinium species on the cellular functions at low concentrations observed in vivo in clinical and preclinical conditions. The brain is the only organ where MR imaging is able to detect a sign of gadolinium retention, the high signal intensity on unenhanced T1 weighted images of the deep brain structures after exposure to cumulative doses of GBCAs. Only analytical chemistry techniques can be used to detect gadolinium in all other organs. While no associated clinical health consequences have been described until now, health consequences cannot be ruled out, and further preclinical and clinical studies are needed.

There are currently only case reports of patients self-reporting nonspecific complaints such as headache, central torso pain, peripheral leg and arm pain, peripheral leg and arm thickening and discoloration, as well bone pain [63, 64].

The current state of the knowledge (see drawing below) is that stability of the gadolinium-based contrast agents affects the gadolinium chelation state with linear GBCAs that tend to dechelate at higher rates than macrocyclic GBCAs. Both, in patients with either impaired or normal renal function, where differences in excretion times may affect the level of tissue retention are conditioned by the specific environment of different organs. No matter whether the intact compound is retained or transmetallation favors the dechelation of gadolinium, in vivo magnetic resonance imaging is able to detect tissue retention only in the brain depending on the interstitial concentration of paramagnetic forms of gadolinium, their relaxivity, and the technical parameters of the MRI clinical setup. The amount of gadolinium that is retained rarely associates with clinical symptoms as most of the exposed patients remain asymptomatic even after multiple administrations of the most unstable of the

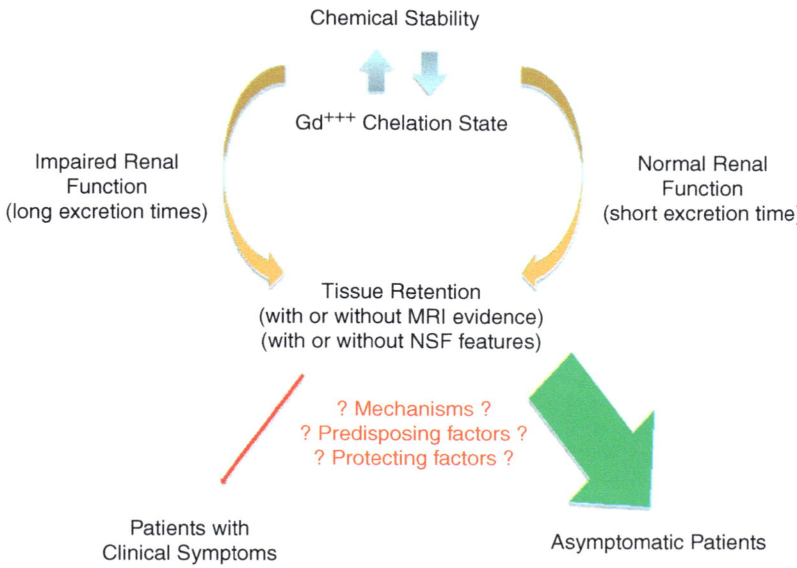

Fig. 6.2 Diagram of the potential link between GBCAs kinetic inertness, renal function and clinical consequences. It should be acknowledged that symptoms have been rarely associated with exposure to gadolinium-based contrast agents while there is no proof that cumulative doses and higher amounts of retained gadolinium are related to a higher risk of clinical consequences

gadolinium-based contrast agents, supporting the idea that genetic vulnerability or other unknown predisposing/protecting factors are involved and need further investigation (Fig. 6.2).

6.7 Concluding Remarks

The use of GBCAs has revolutionized the field of magnetic resonance in the last 25 years. Clinical applications in steady-state parenchymal imaging, MR angiography, and perfusion are now part of routine radiological practice.

There is now evidence that gadolinium can accumulate in tissues regardless of renal function and that linear GBCAs are associated with higher tissue accumulation that is related to their differences in kinetic inertness.

Radiologists as well as nephrologists should be aware of the characteristics of the various agents including chelate stability, relaxivity, and concentration along with the differences in long-term retention in the body and the brain. Further knowledge on this safety issue will be available in the next future and optimization of contrast agent selection and amount to be administered will be a topic of discussion.

References

1. Kanal E, Maravilla K, Rowley HA. Gadolinium contrast agents for CNS imaging: current concepts and clinical evidence. AJNR Am J Neuroradiol. 2014;35(12):2215–26.
2. Lancelot E. Revisiting the pharmacokinetic profiles of gadolinium-based contrast agents: differences in long-term biodistribution and excretion. Investig Radiol. 2016;51(11):691–700.
3. Aime S, Caravan P. Biodistribution of gadolinium-based contrast agents, including gadolinium deposition. J Magn Reson Imaging. 2009;30(6):1259–67.
4. Sherry AD, Caravan P, Lenkinski RE. Primer on gadolinium chemistry. J Magn Reson Imaging. 2009;30(6):1240–8.
5. Frenzel T, Lengsfeld P, Schirmer H, Hütter J, Weinmann HJ. Stability of gadolinium-based magnetic resonance imaging contrast agents in human serum at 37 degrees C. Investig Radiol. 2008;43(12):817–28.
6. Hao D, Ai T, Goerner F, Hu X, Runge VM, Tweedle M. MRI contrast agents: basic chemistry and safety. J Magn Reson Imaging. 2012;36(5):1060–71.
7. de Kerviler E, Maravilla K, Meder JF, Naggara O, Dubourdieu C, Jullien V, Desché P. Adverse reactions to gadoterate meglumine: review of over 25 years of clinical use and more than 50 million doses. Investig Radiol. 2016;51(9):544–51.
8. Endrikat J, Vogtlaender K, Dohanish S, Balzer T, Breuer J. Safety of gadobutrol: results from 42 clinical phase II to IV studies and postmarketing surveillance after 29 million applications. Investig Radiol. 2016;51(9):537–43.

9. Endrikat JS, Dohanish S, Balzer T, Breuer JA. Safety of gadoxetate disodium: results from the clinical phase II–III development program and post-marketing surveillance. J Magn Reson Imaging. 2015;42(3):634–43.
10. Forsting M, Palkowitsch P. Prevalence of acute adverse reactions to gadobutrol—a highly concentrated macrocyclic gadolinium chelate: review of 14,299 patients from observational trials. Eur J Radiol. 2010;74(3):e186–92.
11. Wagner B, Drel V, Gorin Y. Pathophysiology of gadolinium-associated systemic fibrosis. Am J Physiol Ren Physiol. 2016;311(1):F1–F11.
12. Rogosnitzky M, Branch S. Gadolinium-based contrast agent toxicity: a review of known and proposed mechanisms. Biometals. 2016;29(3):365–76.
13. Ramalho J, Semelka RC, Ramalho M, Nunes RH, AlObaidy M, Castillo M. Gadolinium-based contrast agent accumulation and toxicity: an update. AJNR Am J Neuroradiol. 2016;37(7):1192–8.
14. Fretellier N, Poteau N, Factor C, Mayer JF, Medina C, Port M, Idée JM, Corot C. Analytical interference in serum iron determination reveals iron versus gadolinium transmetallation with linear gadolinium-based contrast agents. Investig Radiol. 2014;49(12):766–72.
15. Idée JM, Fretellier N, Robic C, Corot C. The role of gadolinium chelates in the mechanism of nephrogenic systemic fibrosis: a critical update. Crit Rev Toxicol. 2014;44(10):895–913.
16. Bellin MF, Van Der Molen AJ. Extracellular gadolinium-based contrast media: an overview. Eur J Radiol. 2008;66(2):160–7.
17. Khawaja AZ, Cassidy DB, Al Shakarchi J, McGrogan DG, Inston NG, Jones RG. Revisiting the risks of MRI with gadolinium based contrast agents-review of literature and guidelines. Insights Imaging. 2015;6(5):553–8.
18. Bennett CL, Qureshi ZP, Sartor AO, Norris LB, Murday A, Xirasagar S, Thomsen HS. Gadolinium-induced nephrogenic systemic fibrosis: the rise and fall of an iatrogenic disease. Clin Kidney J. 2012;5(1):82–8.
19. Assessment report for Gadolinium-containing contrast agents. EMA/740640/2010. http://www.ema.europa.eu/docs/en_GB/document_library/Referrals_document/gadolinium_31/WC500099538.pdf.
20. Sanyal S, Marckmann P, Scherer S, Abraham JL. Multiorgan gadolinium (Gd) deposition and fibrosis in a patient with nephrogenic systemic fibrosis—an autopsy-based review. Nephrol Dial Transplant. 2011;26(11):3616–26.
21. Swaminathan S, High WA, Ranville J, Horn TD, Hiatt K, Thomas M, Brown HH, Shah SV. Cardiac and vascular metal deposition with high mortality in nephrogenic systemic fibrosis. Kidney Int. 2008;73(12):1413–8.
22. Kanda T, Ishii K, Kawaguchi H, Kitajima K, Takenaka D. High signal intensity in the dentate nucleus and globus pallidus on unenhanced T1-weighted MR images: relationship with increasing cumulative dose of a gadolinium-based contrast material. Radiology. 2014;270(3):834–41.
23. Errante Y, Cirimele V, Mallio CA, Di Lazzaro V, Zobel BB, Quattrocchi CC. Progressive increase of T1 signal intensity of the dentate nucleus on unenhanced magnetic resonance images is associated with cumulative doses of intravenously administered gadodiamide in patients with normal renal function, suggesting dechelation. Investig Radiol. 2014;49(10):685–90.
24. Kanda T, Osawa M, Oba H, Toyoda K, Kotoku J, Haruyama T, Takeshita K, Furui S. High signal intensity in dentate nucleus on unenhanced T1-weighted MR images: association with linear versus macrocyclic gadolinium chelate administration. Radiology. 2015;275(3):803–9.
25. Quattrocchi CC, Mallio CA, Errante Y, Cirimele V, Carideo L, Ax A, Zobel BB. Gadodiamide and dentate nucleus T1 hyperintensity in patients with meningioma evaluated by multiple follow-up contrast-enhanced magnetic resonance examinations with no systemic interval therapy. Investig Radiol. 2015;50(7):470–2.
26. Radbruch A, Weberling LD, Kieslich PJ, Eidel O, Burth S, Kickingereder P, Heiland S, Wick W, Schlemmer HP, Bendszus M. Gadolinium retention in the dentate nucleus and globus pallidus is dependent on the class of contrast agent. Radiology. 2015;275(3):783–91.
27. Ramalho J, Castillo M, AlObaidy M, Nunes RH, Ramalho M, Dale BM, Semelka RC. High signal intensity in globus pallidus and dentate nucleus on unenhanced T1-weighted MR images: evaluation of two linear gadolinium-based contrast agents. Radiology. 2015;276(3):836–44.
28. Kahn J, Posch H, Steffen IG, Geisel D, Bauknecht C, Liebig T, Denecke T. Is there long-term signal intensity increase in the central nervous system on T1-weighted images after MR imaging with the hepatospecific contrast agent gadoxetic acid? a cross-sectional study in 91 patients. Radiology. 2017;282(3):708–16.
29. Ichikawa S, Motosugi U, Omiya Y, Onishi H. Contrast agent-induced high signal intensity in dentate nucleus on unenhanced T1-weighted images: Comparison of gadodiamide and gadoxetic acid. Invest Radiol. 2017;52(7):389–95.
30. McDonald RJ, McDonald JS, Kallmes DF, Jentoft ME, Murray DL, Thielen KR, Williamson EE, Eckel LJ. Intracranial gadolinium deposition after contrast-enhanced MR imaging. Radiology. 2015;275(3):772–82.
31. Kanda T, Fukusato T, Matsuda M, Toyoda K, Oba H, Kotoku J, Haruyama T, Kitajima K, Furui S. Gadolinium-based contrast agent accumulates in the brain even in subjects without severe renal dysfunction: evaluation of autopsy brain specimens with inductively coupled plasma mass spectroscopy. Radiology. 2015;276(1):228–32.
32. Zhang Y, Cao Y, Shih GL, Hecht EM, Prince MR. Extent of signal hyperintensity on unenhanced T1-weighted brain MR images after more than 35

administrations of linear gadolinium-based contrast agents. Radiology. 2017;282(2):516–25.

33. Radbruch A, Haase R, Kieslich PJ, Weberling LD, Kickingereder P, Wick W, Schlemmer HP, Bendszus M. No signal intensity increase in the dentate nucleus on unenhanced T1-weighted MR images after more than 20 serial injections of macrocyclic gadolinium-based contrast agents. Radiology. 2017;282(3):699–707.
34. Robert P, Lehericy S, Grand S, Violas X, Fretellier N, Idée JM, Ballet S, Corot C. T1-weighted hypersignal in the deep cerebellar nuclei after repeated administrations of gadolinium-based contrast agents in healthy rats: difference between linear and macrocyclic agents. Investig Radiol. 2015;50(8):473–80.
35. Robert P, Violas X, Grand S, Lehericy S, Idée JM, Ballet S, Corot C. Linear gadolinium-based contrast agents are associated with brain gadolinium retention in healthy rats. Investig Radiol. 2016;51(2):73–82.
36. Rasschaert M, Idée JM, Robert P, Fretellier N, Vives V, Violas X, Ballet S, Corot C. Moderate renal failure accentuates T1 signal enhancement in the deep cerebellar nuclei of gadodiamide-treated rats. Investig Radiol. 2017;52(5):255–64.
37. Smith AP, Marino M, Roberts J, Crowder JM, Castle J, Lowery L, Morton C, Hibberd MG, Evans PM. Clearance of gadolinium from the brain with no pathologic effect after repeated administration of gadodiamide in healthy rats: an analytical and histologic study. Radiology. 2017;282(3):743–51.
38. Frenzel T, Apte C, Jost G, Schöckel L, Lohrke J, Pietsch H. Quantification and assessment of the chemical form of residual gadolinium in the brain after repeated administration of gadolinium-based contrast agents: comparative study in rats. Investig Radiol. 2017;52(7):396–404.
39. Jost G, Frenzel T, Lohrke J, Lenhard DC, Naganawa S, Pietsch H. Penetration and distribution of gadolinium-based contrast agents into the cerebrospinal fluid in healthy rats: a potential pathway of entry into the brain tissue. Eur Radiol. 2017;27(7):2877–85.
40. Öner AY, Barutcu B, Aykol Ş, Tali ET. Intrathecal contrast-enhanced magnetic resonance imaging-related brain signal changes: residual gadolinium deposition? Investig Radiol. 2017;52(4):195–7.
41. Olchowy C, Cebulski K, Łasecki M, Chaber R, Olchowy A, Kałwak K, Zaleska-Dorobisz U. The presence of the gadolinium-based contrast agent depositions in the brain and symptoms of gadolinium neurotoxicity—a systematic review. PLoS One. 2017;12(2):e0171704.
42. Vidaud C, Bourgeois D, Meyer D. Bone as target organ for metals: the case of f-elements. Chem Res Toxicol. 2012;25(6):1161–75.
43. Gibby WA, Gibby KA, Gibby WA. Comparison of Gd DTPA-BMA (Omniscan) versus Gd HP-DO3A (ProHance) retention in human bone tissue by inductively coupled plasma atomic emission spectroscopy. Investig Radiol. 2004;39(3):138–42.
44. White GW, Gibby WA, Tweedle MF. Comparison of Gd(DTPA-BMA) (Omniscan) versus Gd(HP-DO3A) (ProHance) relative to gadolinium retention in human bone tissue by inductively coupled plasma mass spectroscopy. Investig Radiol. 2006;41(3):272–8.
45. Darrah TH, Prutsman-Pfeiffer JJ, Poreda RJ, Ellen Campbell M, Hauschka PV, Hannigan RE. Incorporation of excess gadolinium into human bone from medical contrast agents. Metallomics. 2009;1(6):479–88.
46. Wáng YX, Schroeder J, Siegmund H, Idée JM, Fretellier N, Jestin-Mayer G, Factor C, Deng M, Kang W, Morcos SK. Total gadolinium tissue deposition and skin structural findings following the administration of structurally different gadolinium chelates in healthy and ovariectomized female rats. Quant Imaging Med Surg. 2015;5(4):534–45.
47. Murata N, Gonzalez-Cuyar LF, Murata K, Fligner C, Dills R, Hippe D, Maravilla KR. Macrocyclic and other non-group 1 gadolinium contrast agents deposit low levels of gadolinium in brain and bone tissue: preliminary results from 9 patients with normal renal function. Investig Radiol. 2016;51(7):447–53.
48. Murata N, Murata K, Gonzalez-Cuyar LF, Maravilla KR. Gadolinium tissue deposition in brain and bone. Magn Reson Imaging. 2016;34(10):1359–65.
49. Kasokat T, Urich K. Quantification of dechelation of gadopentetate dimeglumine in rats. Arzneimittelforschung. 1992;42(6):869–76.
50. Wadas TJ, Sherman CD, Miner JH, Duncan JR, Anderson CJ. The biodistribution of [153Gd]Gd-labeled magnetic resonance contrast agents in a transgenic mouse model of renal failure differs greatly from control mice. Magn Reson Med. 2010;64(5):1274–80.
51. Clarke B. Normal bone anatomy and physiology. Clin J Am Soc Nephrol. 2008;3(Suppl 3):S131–9.
52. Khurana A, Greene JF Jr, High WA. Quantification of gadolinium in nephrogenic systemic fibrosis: re-examination of a reported cohort with analysis of clinical factors. J Am Acad Dermatol. 2008;59(2):218–24.
53. Christensen KN, Lee CU, Hanley MM, Leung N, Moyer TP, Pittelkow MR. Quantification of gadolinium in fresh skin and serum samples from patients with nephrogenic systemic fibrosis. J Am Acad Dermatol. 2011;64(1):91–6.
54. Roberts DR, Lindhorst SM, Welsh CT, Maravilla KR, Herring MN, Braun KA, Thiers BH, Davis WC. High levels of gadolinium deposition in the skin of a patient with normal renal function. Investig Radiol. 2016;51(5):280–9.
55. Gathings RM, Reddy R, Santa Cruz D, Brodell RT. Gadolinium-associated plaques: a new, distinctive clinical entity. JAMA Dermatol. 2015;151(3):316–9.
56. Sieber MA, Lengsfeld P, Frenzel T, Golfier S, Schmitt-Willich H, Siegmund F, Walter J, Weinmann HJ, Pietsch H. Preclinical investigation to compare different gadolinium-based contrast agents regarding their propensity to release gadolinium in vivo and to

trigger nephrogenic systemic fibrosis-like lesions. Eur Radiol. 2008;18(10):2164–73.
57. Pietsch H, Lengsfeld P, Jost G, Frenzel T, Hütter J, Sieber MA. Long-term retention of gadolinium in the skin of rodents following the administration of gadolinium-based contrast agents. Eur Radiol. 2009;19(6):1417–24.
58. Maximova N, Gregori M, Zennaro F, Sonzogni A, Simeone R, Zanon D. Hepatic gadolinium deposition and reversibility after contrast agent-enhanced MR imaging of pediatric hematopoietic stem cell transplant recipients. Radiology. 2016;281(2):418–26.
59. Tweedle MF, Wedeking P, Kumar K. Biodistribution of radiolabeled, formulated gadopentetate, gadoteridol, gadoterate, and gadodiamide in mice and rats. Investig Radiol. 1995;30(6):372–80.
60. Chen R, Ling D, Zhao L, Wang S, Liu Y, Bai R, Baik S, Zhao Y, Chen C, Hyeon T. Parallel comparative studies on mouse toxicity of oxide nanoparticle- and gadolinium-based T1 MRI contrast agents. ACS Nano. 2015;9(12):12425–35.
61. Spencer AJ, Wilson SA, Batchelor J, Reid A, Rees J, Harpur E. Gadolinium chloride toxicity in the rat. Toxicol Pathol. 1997;25(3):245–55.
62. Kartamihardja AA, Nakajima T, Kameo S, Koyama H, Tsushima Y. Impact of impaired renal function on gadolinium retention after administration of gadolinium-based contrast agents in a mouse model. Investig Radiol. 2016;51(10):655–60.
63. Semelka RC, Commander CW, Jay M, Burke LM, Ramalho M. Presumed gadolinium toxicity in subjects with normal renal function: a report of 4 cases. Investig Radiol. 2016;51(10):661–5.
64. Burke LM, Ramalho M, AlObaidy M, Chang E, Jay M, Semelka RC. Self-reported gadolinium toxicity: a survey of patients with chronic symptoms. Magn Reson Imaging. 2016;34(8):1078–80.

Part II

Native Kidney

Acute Kidney Injury: Color Doppler US

7

Anita Spezzacatene, Camilla Sachs, and Irene Campo

7.1 Introduction

Acute kidney injury (AKI) is characterized by sudden loss of kidney function, resulting in the retention of urea and other nitrogenous waste products and the dysregulation of extracellular volume and electrolytes. It manifests by an abrupt increase in serum creatinine level, a reliable estimation of the glomerular filtration rate (GFR) with or without reduced urine output.

AKI can be secondary to renal hypoperfusion (prerenal AKI), acute urinary tract obstruction (postrenal AKI) or it can be the complication of a wide range of parenchymal renal diseases (renal AKI). Correct AKI classification (prerenal, renal or postrenal) is essential in order to select the appropriate treatment. Differential diagnosis is mainly based on patient's clinical and laboratory findings; imaging techniques provide useful information to confirm diagnosis. Ultrasound imaging plays a very important role in the diagnostic workup and color Doppler ultrasound has been extensively used in the evaluation of renovascular diseases because it is a noninvasive, safe, low-cost, and repeatable tool. It allows excellent depiction of renal vasculature. In patients with AKI, a significant, but nonspecific, reduction of intraparenchymal flow signals is usually detected. Furthermore, it provides more specific information in selected cases, such as the presence of focal avascular areas secondary to renal infarction, severe acute pyelonephritis, or embolic disease. More specifically, renal resistive index (RRI) [(peak systolic velocity—end diastolic velocity)/peak systolic velocity], a semi-quantitative index derived by Doppler evaluation of renal vascular bed, plays an important role in the evaluation of AKI [1] as it allows monitoring of renal perfusion in critically ill patients, including those treated with vasoactive agents (Fig. 7.1).

In particular, it allows evaluation of renal perfusion, prediction of renal response to vasoactive agents [2, 3], prediction of onset and recovery in septic shock patients, differential diagnosis between prerenal and renal AKI and prediction of renal obstruction. Furthermore, high RRI values at AKI diagnosis are strong predictors of intensive care unit (ICU) mortality and persistent AKI at ICU discharge [4]. Normally RRI is in the range of 0.47–0.70; it increases with aging and, usually, it shows a difference between the two kidneys less than 5–8% [5].

A. Spezzacatene (✉) · C. Sachs
Radiology Department, Cattinara Hospital, University of Trieste, Trieste, Italy

I. Campo
Department of Radiology, Civile Hospital, Conegliano, Italy

A. Granata, M. Bertolotto (eds.), *Imaging in Nephrology*, https://doi.org/10.1007/978-3-030-60794-4_7

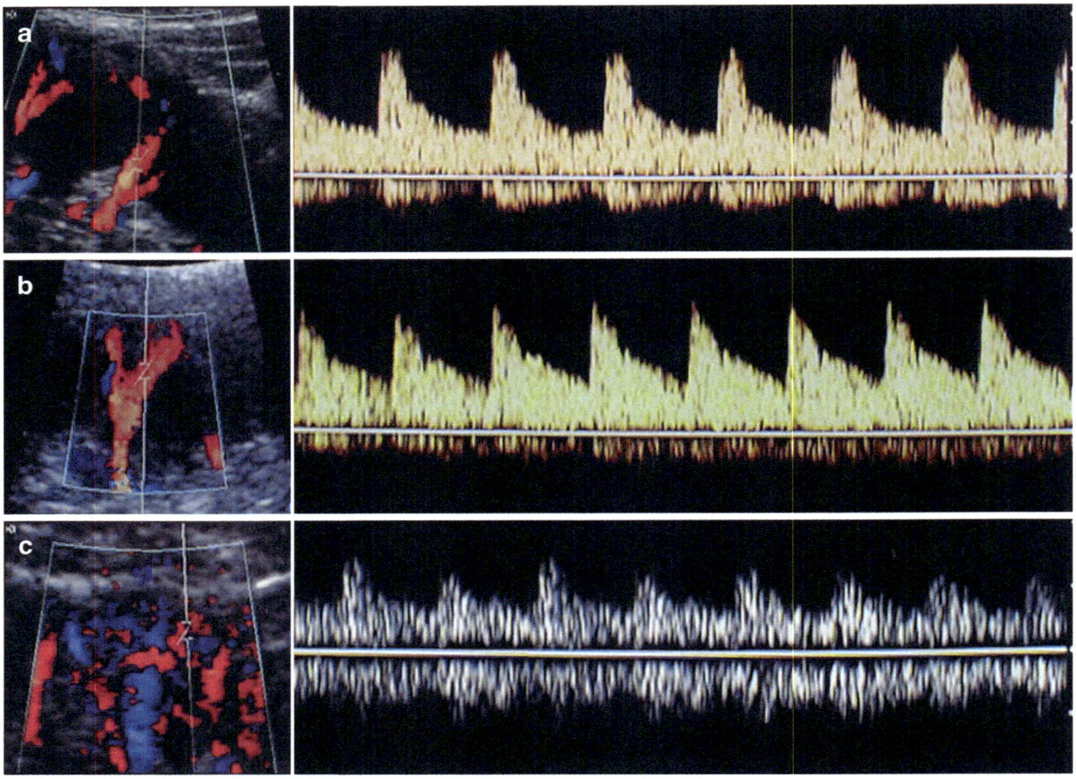

Fig. 7.1 Normal Doppler spectrum: early systolic peak followed by continuous flow during diastole (low-resistance parenchyma): (**a**) segmental artery, (**b**) interlobar artery/arciform, (**c**) interlobular artery

7.2 Prerenal AKI

Prerenal acute kidney injury is a potential reversible functional condition secondary to renal hypoperfusion caused by reduced intravascular volume, reduced cardiac output, systemic vasodilatation or renal vasoconstriction. Prolonged renal hypoperfusion may lead to acute tubular necrosis even though parenchymal damage is still reversible.

The high sensitivity and specificity of color Doppler ultrasound allow a rapid and certain discrimination between prerenal and renal AKI (such as acute tubular necrosis). In the majority of patients with prerenal AKI, RRI is normal, while it is elevated in patients with acute tubular necrosis, with a threshold of 0.75 reported as optimal in the discrimination between renal and prerenal disease [6] (Fig. 7.2). However, the discrimination between these two conditions is difficult in case of drug-induced AKI or dehydration-related AKI, especially in the elderly population and/or diabetic patients with hypertensive nephroangiosclerosis; in these cases, indeed, high RRI values may be related to preexistent parenchymal disease.

The majority of patients with prerenal AKI show normal renal blood flow and RRI, while patients with renal AKI have high RRI values and reduced renal perfusion.

In addition, color Doppler ultrasound is extremely useful during the follow-up of patients treated for prerenal and renal AKI, as it provides early information on organ functional recovery [7].

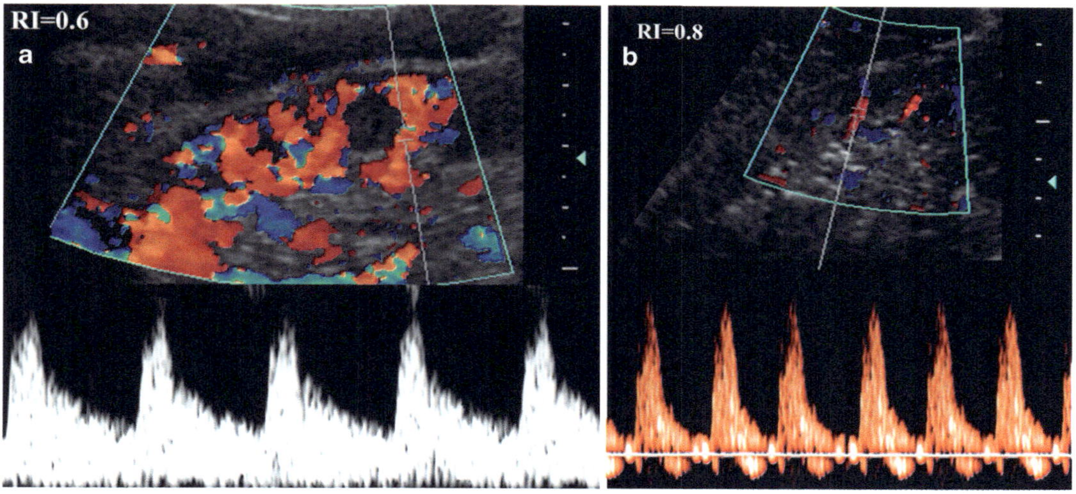

Fig. 7.2 Duplex Doppler US proved valuable in the differential diagnosis between prerenal AKI (**a**) and ATN (**b**). Most patients with prerenal AKI have normal parenchymal flows, whereas patients with ATN reveal markedly abnormal Doppler flow profiles with increased pulsatility or loss of the diastolic flow. A RRI value of 0.75 is considered as optimal in attempting differential diagnosis between ATN and prerenal AKI since 90% of patients with ATN and only 20% of patients with prerenal ARF have parenchymal RRI above this threshold

7.3 Renal AKI

Renal AKI mainly occurs in case of acute tubular necrosis or tubulointerstitial nephropathies secondary to ischemia or nephrotoxic agents. Color Doppler ultrasound cannot distinguish between different causes of renal AKI (sepsis, rhabdomyolysis, drug toxicity, etc.), as the Doppler spectrum can be similar. Generally, RRI is increased in tubulointerstitial diseases, while it tends to be normal in glomerular disease [8]. There are many specific pathologic conditions that can lead to renal AKI.

Hepatorenal syndrome is a particular condition characterized by the development of acute renal failure in patients with decompensated advanced chronic liver disease, in which the value of renal interlobar RRI is used for early detection of renal function impairment, with a cutoff RRI value >0.70 [9]. Generally, patients with overt hepatorenal syndrome show elevated RRI values [10, 11], with normal values in only 1% of cases [12] (Fig. 7.3).

Many forms of vasculitis, such as hemolytic-uremic syndrome, polyarteritis nodosa, and thrombotic thrombocytopenic purpura, can affect small-caliber renal arterioles, leading to AKI.

In hemolytic-uremic syndrome, a rare form of AKI that manifests in children and in the postpartum period, intravascular coagulation and microangiopathy of small-caliber renal arterioles often cause renal failure. Hyperechogenic cortex of the kidney and emphasized corticomedullary differentiation are aspecific findings [13], while marked increase in RRI at color Doppler ultrasound due to reduced parenchymal vascularization is more specific [14]. RRI tends to normalize before patient's clinical improvement, preventing unnecessary dialysis. In acute proliferative glomerulonephritis and in tubulointerstitial nephritis color Doppler ultrasound shows a reduced parenchymal perfusion which correlates to an increase of RRI measured at the level of interlobar-arcuate arteries.

Rarely, severe pyelonephritis may manifest with AKI. Ultrasound imaging is sensitive to detect pyonephrosis. Infected urine or pus within the obstructed collecting system contains diffusely dispersed fine echoes, or the echoes may lay in dependent portions of the dilated pelvis. These features can be difficult to see, especially

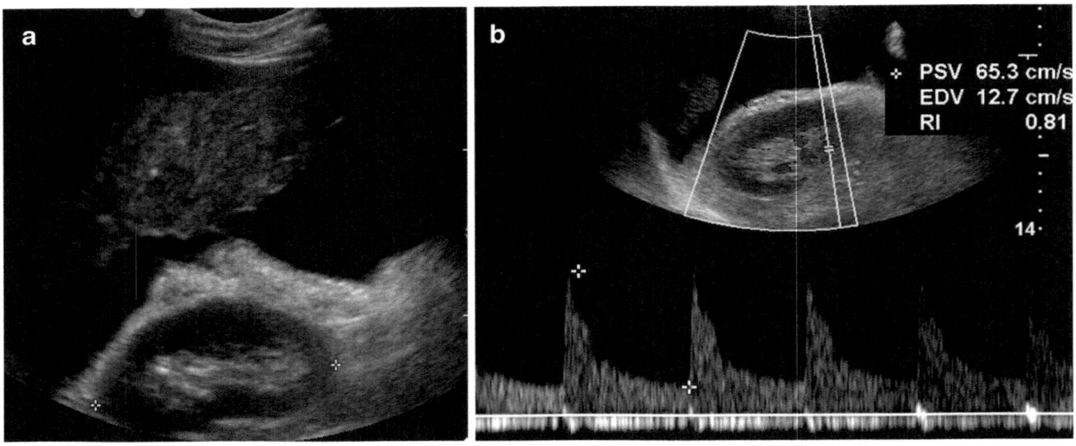

Fig. 7.3 Patient with cirrhosis and ascites. The right kidney has preserved echo structure and dimensions (**a**) but intraparenchymal flows have elevated RRI (**b**)

in obese patients, and are better appreciated with last-generation US equipment, due to better spatial and contrast resolution and using tissue harmonic imaging techniques [15]. Renal abscesses may appear as intrarenal fluid collections or as complex lesions, and presence of intralesional air or layering of content can lead to the diagnosis. Color Doppler can increase the sensitivity of ultrasound, especially in children and young adults [16], by detecting single or multiple perfusion defects; however, the technique remains less sensitive than spiral CT [17].

7.4 Postrenal AKI

Postrenal AKI accounts for 5–10% of AKI cases and it is caused by bilateral urinary tract obstruction (unilateral obstruction in solitary kidney patients or in patients with preexistent compromised renal function) [18].

Urinary tract obstruction may lead to different levels of calicopyelic dilatation. However, early in the course of ureteral obstruction, collecting system dilatation may be absent or only minimal up to 35% of cases. In this situation, color Doppler ultrasound, with renal blood flow analysis and RRI measurement, is helpful in the early diagnosis of urinary tract obstruction, providing functional information [19]. Renal obstruction produces characteristic hemodynamic changes resulting in increased renal vascular resistances and vasoconstriction, reduced renal blood flow, and increased RRI (Fig. 7.4). Many authors, indeed, reported changes in the RRI related to postobstructive renal vasoconstriction after 2 h from acute onset of urinary tract obstruction, with a RRI threshold of 0.70 considered optimal to discriminate between obstructive and nonobstructive pyelocaliectasis [20–23].

Moreover, Doppler diagnosis of obstruction is considered more accurate when the RRI of the potentially obstructed kidney is compared with the RRI of the unaffected contralateral kidney.

Specifically, delta resistive index (delta RI), the difference between left and right kidney mean RRI, is considered predictive of renal obstruction in patients with unilateral renal colic [24], and an RRI difference greater than 0.10 between kidneys is considered a threshold for obstruction [23]. The latter diagnostic criterion is less important in patients with ARF who usually have bilateral obstruction or only one functioning kidney. In obstructed patients with ARF, RRI reduces significantly after nephrostomy, usually before normalization of renal function (Fig. 7.5).

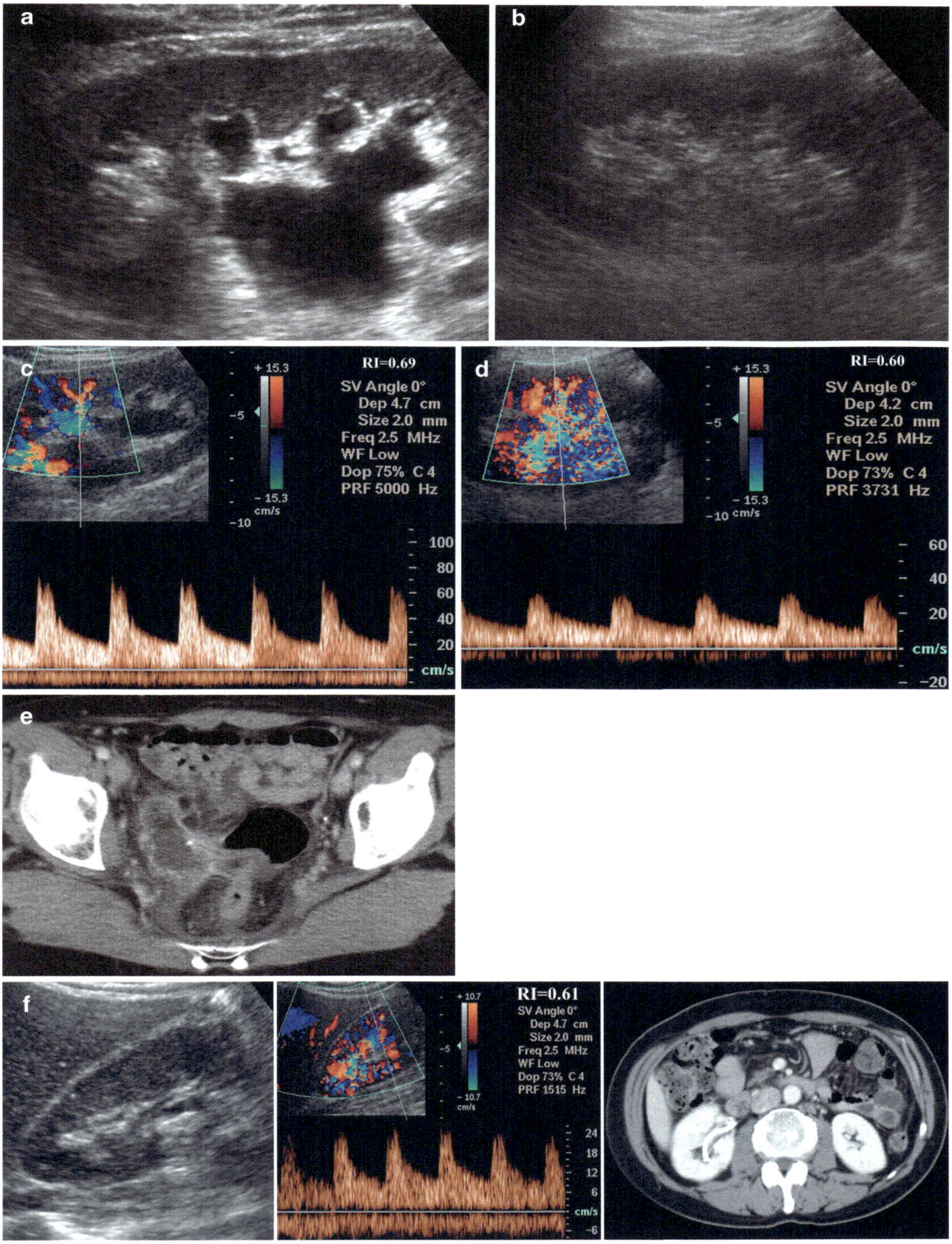

Fig. 7.4 Differences in RRI values between the kidneys, in case of monolateral urinary tract obstruction (right kidney) (**a**). There is no pyelocaliceal dilatation in the left kidney (**b**). Right kidney RRI value (0.69) (**c**) is significantly higher as compared to the contralateral kidney (0.60) (**d**). CT scan demonstrates (**e**) the result of previous intervention of colon neoplasia, the cause of obstruction. After ureteral stenting, the RRI returns to normal values of the right kidney (**f**)

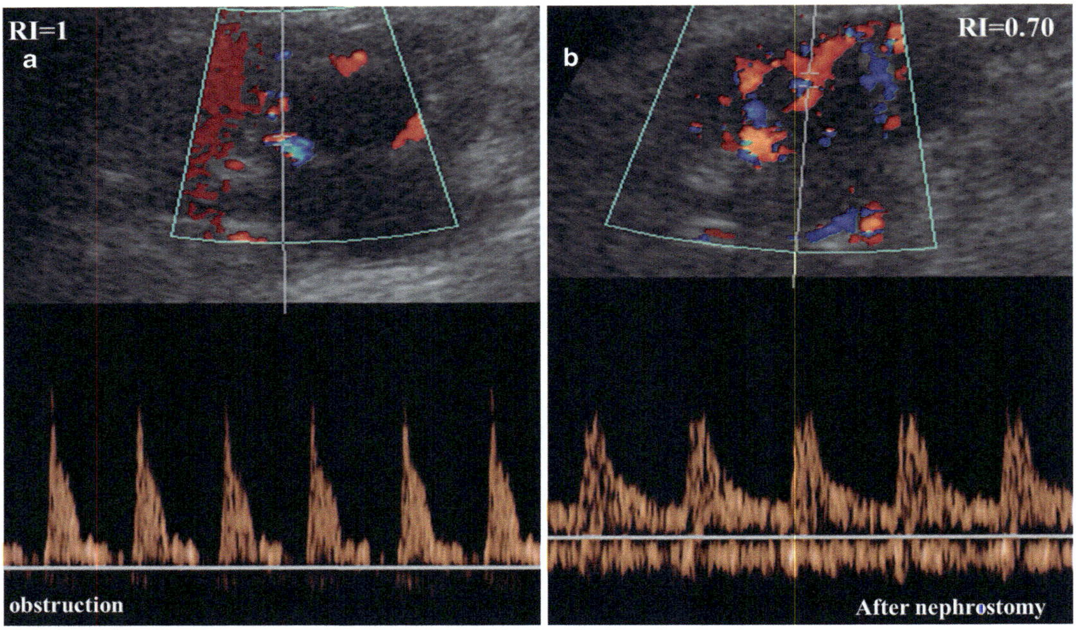

Fig. 7.5 Patient with ARF and bilateral obstruction due to advanced prostatic cancer. There are hydronephrosis and markedly elevated RRI (**a**) which normalize after nephrostomy (**b**)

References

1. Spatola L, Andrulli S. Doppler ultrasound in kidney diseases: a key parameter in clinical long-term follow-up. J Ultrasound. 2016;19:243–50.
2. Lauschke A, Teichgräber UKM, Frei U, Eckardt K-U. 'Low-dose' dopamine worsens renal perfusion in patients with acute renal failure. Kidney Int. 2006;69:1669–74.
3. Deruddre S, et al. Renal arterial resistance in septic shock: effects of increasing mean arterial pressure with norepinephrine on the renal resistive index assessed with Doppler ultrasonography. Intensive Care Med. 2007;33:1557–62.
4. Boddi M, et al. Renal resistive index and mortality in critical patients with acute kidney injury. Eur J Clin Investig. 2016;46:242–51.
5. Darmon M, Schnell D, Zeni F. Doppler-based renal resistive index: a comprehensive review. In: Yearbook of intensive care and emergency medicine. Berlin, Heidelberg: Springer; 2010. p. 331–8. https://doi.org/10.1007/978-3-642-10286-8_31.
6. Pozzi Mucelli R, Bertolotto M, Quaia E. Imaging techniques in acute renal failure. Contrib Nephrol. 2001;132:76–91.
7. Izumi M, et al. Differential diagnosis of prerenal azotemia from acute tubular necrosis and prediction of recovery by Doppler ultrasound. Am J Kidney Dis. 2000;35:713–9.
8. Platt JF, Rubin JM, Ellis JH. Acute renal failure: possible role of duplex Doppler US in distinction between acute prerenal failure and acute tubular necrosis. Radiology. 1991;179:419–23.
9. Kastelan S, Ljubicic N, Kastelan Z, Ostojic R, Uravic M. The role of duplex-Doppler ultrasonography in the diagnosis of renal dysfunction and hepatorenal syndrome in patients with liver cirrhosis. Hepato-Gastroenterology. 2004;51:1408–12.
10. Platt JF. Doppler ultrasound of the kidney. Semin Ultrasound CT MR. 1997;18:22–32.
11. Stevens PE. Doppler ultrasound in renal disease: not quite 'the answer to a maiden's prayer'. Ren Fail. 1995;17:89–100.
12. Platt JF, Ellis JH, Rubin JM, Merion RM, Lucey MR. Renal duplex Doppler ultrasonography: a noninvasive predictor of kidney dysfunction and hepatorenal failure in liver disease. Hepatology. 1994;20:362–9.
13. Lockhart ME, Robbin ML. Renal vascular imaging: ultrasound and other modalities. Ultrasound Q. 2007;23:279–92.
14. Wasserman NF. Principles of genitourinary radiology. 2nd ed. Radiology. 1994;193:246.
15. Bertolotto M, Derchi L. New techniques in uroradiology. Boca Raton, FL: CRC Press; 2006. p. 35–47. https://doi.org/10.3109/9781420016635-4.
16. Sakarya ME, Arslan H, Erkoç R, Bozkurt M, Atilla MK. The role of power Doppler ultrasonography in the diagnosis of acute pyelonephritis. Br J Urol. 1998;81:360–3.

17. Webb JAW. The role of imaging in adult acute urinary tract infection. Eur Radiol. 1997;7:837–43.
18. Mostbeck GH, Zontsich T, Turetschek K. Ultrasound of the kidney: obstruction and medical diseases. Eur Radiol. 2001;11:1878–89.
19. Onur MR, Cubuk M, Andic C, Kartal M, Arslan G. Role of resistive index in renal colic. Urol Res. 2007;35:307–12.
20. Webb JA. Ultrasonography and Doppler studies in the diagnosis of renal obstruction. BJU Int. 2000;86(Suppl 1):25–32.
21. Van Den Noortgate N, et al. The role of ultrasonography in the assessment of renal function in the elderly. J Nephrol. 2003;16:658–62.
22. Platt JF, Rubin JM, Ellis JH, DiPietro MA. Duplex Doppler US of the kidney: differentiation of obstructive from nonobstructive dilatation. Radiology. 1989;171:515–7.
23. Platt JF, Rubin JM, Ellis JH. Distinction between obstructive and nonobstructive pyelocaliectasis with duplex Doppler sonography. AJR Am J Roentgenol. 1989;153:997–1000.
24. Granata A, et al. Predictive role of duplex Doppler ultrasonography in the diagnosis of acute renal obstruction in patients with unilateral renal colic. Clin Nephrol. 2009;71:680–6.

Chronic Kidney Disease: Color Doppler US

8

Anita Spezzacatene, Irene Campo, and Camilla Sachs

8.1 Introduction

Chronic kidney disease (CKD) is a condition characterized by progressive loss of kidney function resulting in waste products and fluids and related multi-organ complications. It is defined according to the presence or absence of kidney damage and level of kidney function (GFR <60 mL/min/1.73 m^2) for ≥3 months. Among individuals with chronic kidney disease, the stages are defined based on the level of kidney function.

The most common causes of CKD are diabetes and hypertension, but many other conditions can be involved, such as glomerulonephritis, chronic tubulointerstitial diseases and polycystic kidney disease.

8.2 Ultrasound Evaluation

In the setting of CKD, the role of ultrasound imaging is to evaluate morphologic parameters (B-mode) and perfusion kidney alterations (color Doppler or contrast-enhanced ultrasound—CEUS) in order to provide useful information to understand the underlying cause. However, correct diagnostic overview with ultrasound imaging is possible in only 50–70% of patients. As in acute kidney injury, so in chronic kidney disease conventional ultrasound imaging parameters consist of longitudinal diameter, parenchymal thickness and echogenicity and urinary tract state.

In patients with CKD, longitudinal diameter and parenchymal thickness are reduced [1, 2], with a progressive increase of cortical echogenicity [3].

Color Doppler ultrasound integrates B-mode morphologic analysis providing some useful parameters (parenchymal perfusion, presence/absence of blood flow, and venous and arterial vessel patency), even though these are not decisive for diagnosis.

Spectral Doppler registers the *V*/*t* curve in the renal artery and the interlobar arteries; a reduced amplitude of spectral Doppler *V*/*t* curve reflects the fall of renal blood flow in CKD that can be related to the progressive loss of nephronic mass.

Furthermore, renal resistive index (RRI) measurement allows indirect evaluation of renal microcirculation state.

A. Spezzacatene (✉) · C. Sachs
Radiology Department, Cattinara Hospital, University of Trieste, Trieste, Italy

I. Campo
Department of Radiology, Civile Hospital, Conegliano, Italy

A. Granata, M. Bertolotto (eds.), *Imaging in Nephrology*, https://doi.org/10.1007/978-3-030-60794-4_8

8.3 Pathological Modifications

Morphologic kidney changes in the setting of CKD may involve different structures: the microcirculation, the glomerulus or the tubulointerstitial structures.

In CKD with predominant microcirculation damage (atherosclerotic remodeling, atheroembolic disease, and vasculitis) vascular compliance reduces and total impedance increases, with consequent increase of intrarenal Renal Resistive Index (RRI) (RRI >0.75). RRI progressively increases with vascular stiffness [4] and it is directly correlated to atherosclerotic damage [5].

Tubulointerstitial nephropathies are related to a variety of conditions, such as nephrotoxic drugs, chronic pyelonephritis, vesicoureteral reflux nephropathy, renal tuberculosis and urinary tract recurrent infections. In these situations, the kidneys are characterized by morphologic alterations involving renal parenchyma (scars, irregular profiles, hypertrophic compensatory areas, hyperechogenicity) or calicopyelic system (architectural distortion and dilatation). In CKD with predominant tubulointerstitial involvement (fibrotic alterations), vascular transmural pressure increases and compliance reduces. Intrarenal RRI increases but in a lesser extent and rarely exceeds 0.75. However, RRI is considered as a useful tool to early identify patients with chronic tubulointerstitial disease [6].

CKD with predominant glomerular alterations, such as in primary glomerulonephritis, is characterized by progressive reduction of kidney dimensions, with irregular margins and ill-defined corticomedullary differentiation (Fig. 8.1). However, the kidneys are symmetric and still well recognizable in the renal loggia even in the late stages of disease [7]. With progressive sclerotic glomerular damage, volume and pressure load moves from afferent arterioles to efferent arterioles, without any significant change in total vascular impedance; therefore, RRI rarely exceeds 0.70–0.72 [8, 9]. This finding helps to differentiate glomerulonephritis from other forms of CKD (secondary inflammatory nephropathies, interstitial nephropathies, vasculitis, and nephroangiosclerosis).

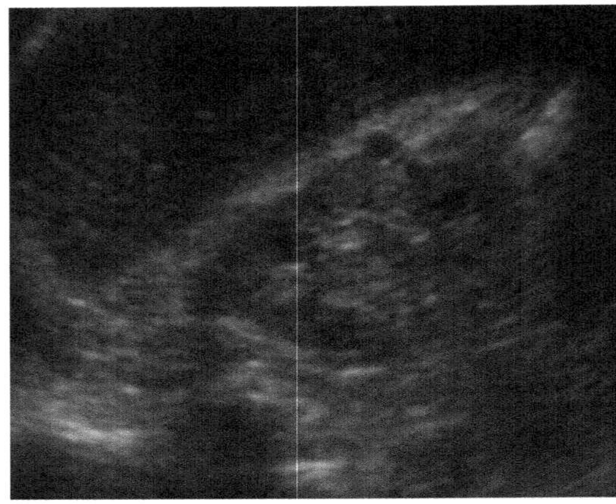

Fig. 8.1 End-stage kidney in primary glomerulonephritis. The kidney appears contracted with subverted architecture

Glomerulonephritis secondary to vasculitis, amyloidosis, nephropathy related to multiple myeloma, or lymphoproliferative disease is characterized by discrepancy between morphologic parameters and renal function [10]. Indeed, morphologic alterations can be aspecific and RRI values are generally increased and cannot distinguish between different etiologies.

In CKD related to diabetic nephropathy, morphologic and functional parameters are variable and depend on the clinical stage of disease.

In the early phase the kidney is characterized by volume increase and hypoechogenicity, with increased parenchymal thickness. Hyperfiltration, increased GFR and fall of vascular resistance (IR <0.55–0.60) may coexist (Fig. 8.2) [11].

In the overt nephropathy phase (proteinuria, hypertension, and retinopathy), RRI progressively increases, while there is a marked morpho-functional discrepancy (volume increase, hypoechogenicity, and fall of GFR).

In stages 4–5 of CKD longitudinal diameters are still normal but RRI is markedly increased (>0.80–0.85) [12].

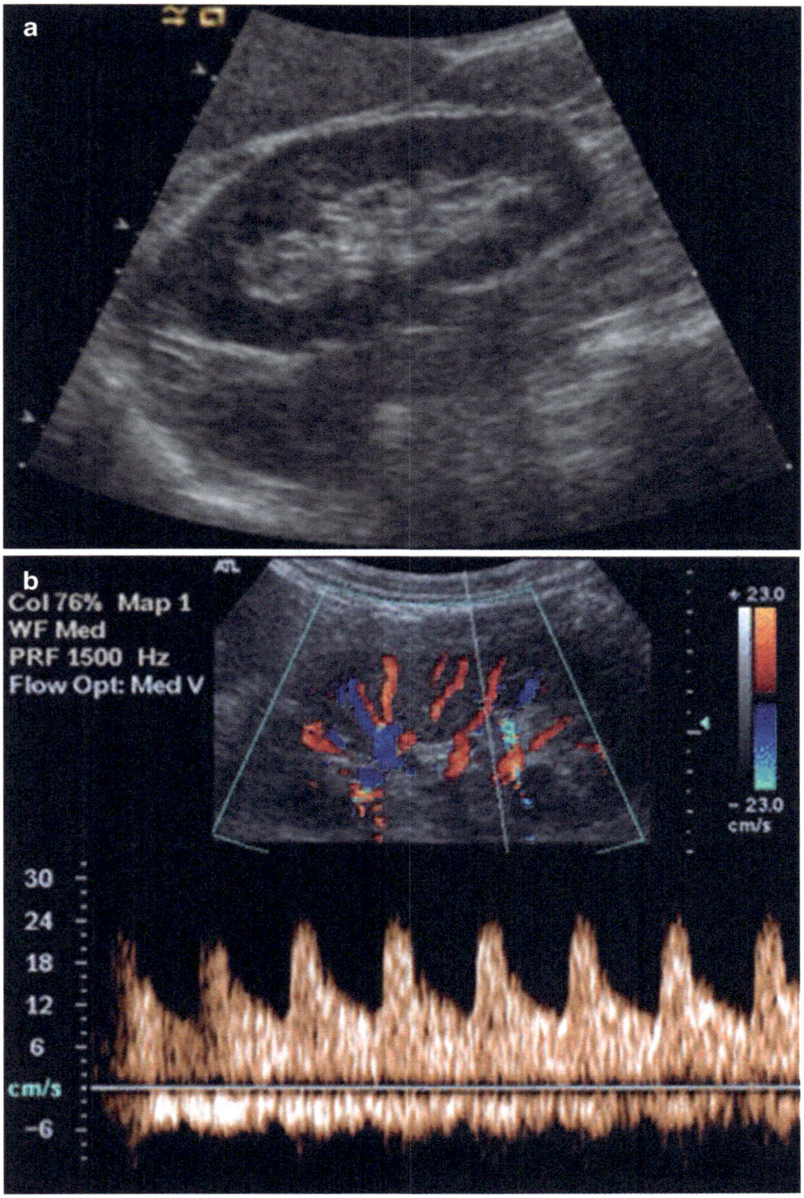

Fig. 8.2 Diabetic nephropathy. The kidney appears hypoechogenic, globular, with volume and parenchymal thickness increase (**a**). Marked decrease of RRI coexists (**b**)

In general, RRI values ≥0.70 are considered predictors of unfavorable evolution of CKD, regardless of GFR [13] and RRI is the parameter that best correlates with renal function, CKD stages (Fig. 8.3) [14] and long-term disease prognosis. For these reasons, together with proteinuria and hypertension, RRI value should be considered as an independent risk factor for disease progression in CKD [14, 15].

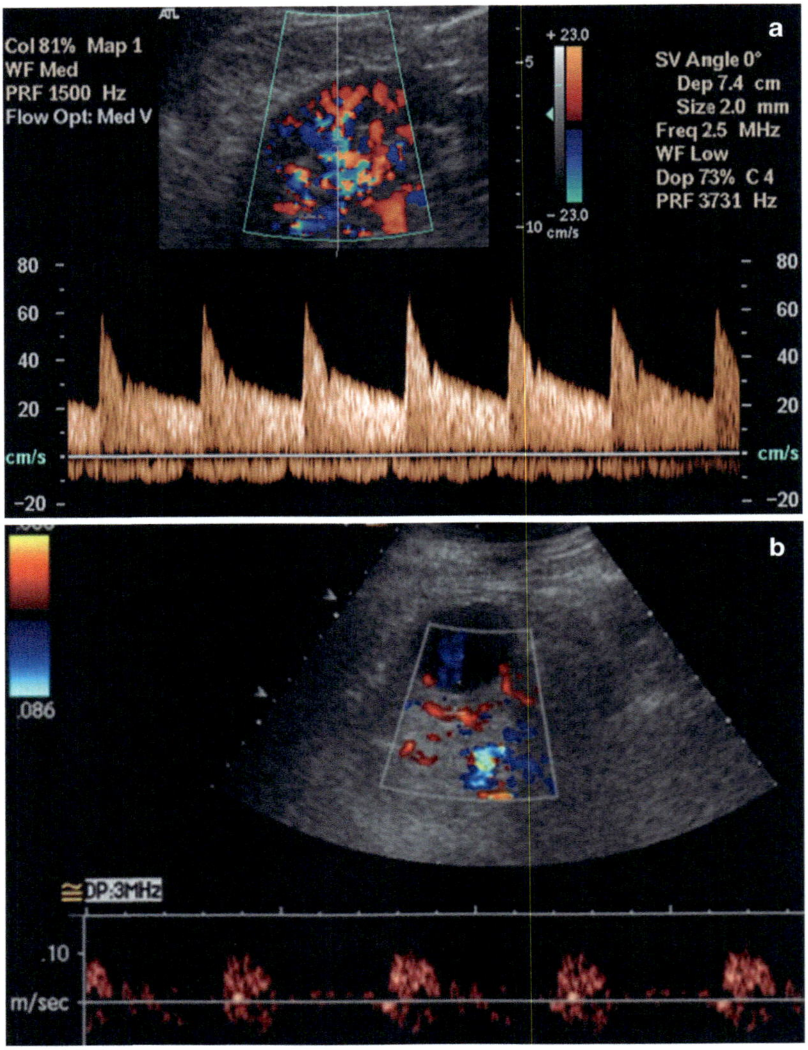

Fig. 8.3 The RRI index based on CKD stages. An ultrasonographic image of a healthy control with CKD stage 1 (**a**) and of a patient with end-stage renal disease (ESRD) with CKD stage 5 (**b**). RRI increased with CKD progression

References

1. AIUM Practice. Guideline for the performance of an ultrasound examination of the abdomen and/or retroperitoneum. J Ultrasound Med. 2012;31:1301–12.
2. Moghazi S, et al. Correlation of renal histopathology with sonographic findings. Kidney Int. 2005;67:1515–20.
3. Khati NJ, Hill MC, Kimmel PL. The role of ultrasound in renal insufficiency: the essentials. Ultrasound Q. 2005;21:227–44.
4. Bude RO, Rubin JM. Relationship between the resistive index and vascular compliance and resistance. Radiology. 1999;211:411–7.
5. Ikee R, et al. Correlation between the resistive index by Doppler ultrasound and kidney function and histology. Am J Kidney Dis. 2005;46:603–9.
6. Boddi M, et al. Renal resistive index and mortality in critical patients with acute kidney injury. Eur J Clin Investig. 2016;46:242–51.
7. Platt JF, Rubin JM, Ellis JH, DiPietro MA. Duplex Doppler US of the kidney: differentiation of obstructive from nonobstructive dilatation. Radiology. 1989;171:515–7.
8. Watanabe S, et al. Valsartan reduces serum cystatin C and the renal vascular resistance in patients with essential hypertension. Clin Exp Hypertens. 2006;28:451–61.
9. Leoncini G, et al. Changes in renal resistive index and urinary albumin excretion in hypertensive patients under long-term treatment with lisinopril or nifedipine GITS. Nephron. 2002;90:169–73.
10. Quaia E, Bertolotto M. Renal parenchymal diseases: is characterization feasible with ultrasound? Eur Radiol. 2002;12:2006–20.

11. Christiansen JS, Gammelgaard J, Frandsen M, Parving HH. Increased kidney size, glomerular filtration rate and renal plasma flow in short-term insulin-dependent diabetics. Diabetologia. 1981;20:451–6.
12. Ishimura E, et al. Intrarenal hemodynamic abnormalities in diabetic nephropathy measured by duplex Doppler sonography. Kidney Int. 1997;51:1920–7.
13. Parolini C, et al. Renal resistive index and long-term outcome in chronic nephropathies. Radiology. 2009;252:888–96.
14. Hanamura K, Tojo A, Kinugasa S, Asaba K, Fujita T. The resistive index is a marker of renal function, pathology, prognosis, and responsiveness to steroid therapy in chronic kidney disease patients. Int J Nephrol. 2012;2012:139565.
15. Izumi M, et al. Differential diagnosis of prerenal azotemia from acute tubular necrosis and prediction of recovery by Doppler ultrasound. Am J Kidney Dis. 2000;35:713–9.

The Diabetic Kidney

9

Boris Brkljačić and Iva Biondić

9.1 Introduction

According to the International Diabetes Federation in the year 2015 415 million adults worldwide were affected by diabetes. They estimate this number to rise to 642 million by 2040. Diabetic nephropathy occurs in patients with diabetes mellitus [1]. Some studies showed prevalence of diabetes mellitus of 13% for both males and females in all age groups [2]. More than half of these cases are undiagnosed which consequently leads toward progression and development of microvascular and macrovascular complications such as nephropathy, retinopathy, neuropathy, stroke, or coronary heart disease [3]. Vascular complications are unusual in childhood and adolescence [4]. Diabetic nephropathy refers to certain structural and functional changes in kidneys within both types of diabetes and has become one of the leading causes of chronic renal failure and end-stage renal disease in developed countries (Western Europe, the USA, Japan). In both diabetes types—insulin dependent (type 1) and non-insulin dependent (type 2)—20–40% of patients will progress to nephropathy, so early diagnosis and starting with treatment as well as early detection of microalbuminuria are necessary [4–6]. The peak rate of the incidence is approximately after 15 years of duration of the illness. Most affected are patients suffering from diabetes mellitus type 2 because of growing prevalence of this type, and more importantly, care for patients is much better. Consequently they live longer and develop micro- and macrovascular complications, including diabetic nephropathy [6]. Risk factors for developing and progression of diabetic nephropathy are hyperglycemia, increased blood pressure, genetic predisposition, elevated serum lipids, and smoking habits [7]. Hypertension is crucial for progression of chronic renal failure in diabetic nephropathy patients [6].

Screening for microalbuminuria should be performed yearly, starting 5 years after diagnosis in type 1 diabetes or earlier in the presence of puberty or poor metabolic control. In patients with type 2 diabetes, screening should be performed at diagnosis and yearly thereafter [7].

Treatment interventions in diabetic nephropathy include glycemic and blood pressure control, cessation of smoking, protein restriction, and renal replacement therapy. Multifactorial approach includes combined therapy targeting hyperglycemia, hypertension, microalbuminuria, and dyslipidemia [8].

B. Brkljačić (✉) · I. Biondić
Division of Ultrasound, Department of Diagnostic and Interventional Radiology, University Hospital Dubrava, University of Zagreb School of Medicine, Zagreb, Croatia
e-mail: boris.brkljacic@zg.htnet.hr

A. Granata, M. Bertolotto (eds.), *Imaging in Nephrology*, https://doi.org/10.1007/978-3-030-60794-4_9

9.2 Pathophysiology and Natural History

Diabetic nephropathy is a microvascular complication of diabetes mellitus marked by albuminuria and renal impairment. The pathophysiology of diabetic nephropathy is a multifactorial and complex cascade of numerous reactions between metabolic (glucose, advanced glycation end products, polyols) and hemodynamic (components of renin-angiotensin system, endothelin) factors interacting with each other and with various reactive oxygen species. Their interactions influence gene regulation and activation of transcription factors, growth factors, and cytokines. Diabetic nephropathy is a complex genetic disease; more genes may be involved in the development of nephropathy. Consequently kidneys undergo several structural and functional changes stimulated by the exposure to the hyperglycemia and advanced glycation end products, increased activity of growth factors, and activation of cytokines. Therefore, pathologically in kidneys there appear expansion of mesangial matrix with diffuse and nodular glomerulosclerosis (Kimmelstiel-Wilson nodules), glomerular basement membrane thickening, proliferative changes, and tubular atrophy resulting in interstitial fibrosis, arteriosclerosis, and hyalinosis of afferent and efferent arterioles. Over time hyaline entirely replaces vessel wall structure that is highly specific for diabetes mellitus. All these changes result in glomerular hyperfiltration, glomerular hypertension, renal hypertrophy at early stage, and renal sclerosis at the advanced stage, which manifest clinically as albuminuria, declining renal function and hypertension [9–11].

Natural history of diabetic nephropathy in patients with type 1 is identical to that in patients with type 2 diabetes mellitus. Timing of the onset of type II is difficult to assess; therefore a patient may present with proteinuria and on kidney biopsy have diabetic nephropathy before even diabetes is diagnosed. Another major difference between these two types is cardiovascular morbidity and mortality which can occur at any point in patients with type 2 and in patients with type 1 risk elevates when kidney disease is at the advanced stage [9].

Stages of diabetic nephropathy depend on the presence of albuminuria and the stage of renal failure. Microalbuminuria and increased glomerular filtration (usually doubled) are hallmarks of early stage, also known as hyperfiltration phase of nephropathy. Microalbuminuria is defined as urinary albumin excretion of 30–299 mg/24 h in a 24-h urinary collection, 20–199 µg/min in a timed urine collection, or 30–299 µg/mg creatinine in a spot urine collection on at least two occasions within a 3–6-month period [8]. Initially, there are constriction of the efferent arterioles and dilation of afferent arterioles, which leads to glomerular capillary hypertension and hyperfiltration [12]. It is enormously important to recognize this early stage, because with treatment of hypertension and hyperglycemia, progression of diabetic nephropathy can be delayed [13]. GFR increases because of increased renal plasma flow and reduction in serum albumin resulting in decreased glomerular oncotic pressure. If metabolic factors are well controlled GFR decreases [12, 13]. In the absence of treatment interventions, approximately 80% of patients with type 1 diabetes mellitus progress to the stage of overt nephropathy. Early stage occurs approximately 5–10 years after the onset of diabetes mellitus. In diabetes type 2 greater proportion of patients have microalbuminuria and overt nephropathy at or shortly after the diagnosis of diabetes. Overt nephropathy usually occurs after 10–15 years characterized by macroalbuminuria, declining of GFR, and rising of blood pressure and mortality. Last phase of diabetic nephropathy is end-stage renal disease [8, 12].

9.3 Ultrasound Imaging

Undoubtedly, ultrasound examination is the first imaging technique used in pathologic changes of urogenital system. Conventional grayscale (B-mode) provides important information about morphology of kidney, its size, parenchymal thickness and echogenicity, presence of masses, collecting system dilatation, and many others, but it does not give any functional information (Fig. 9.1). The information about renal blood supply is given by colored duplex and power Doppler (Figs. 9.2 and 9.3) of renal and intrarenal segmental, interlobar, and arcuate arteries and veins. It is possible to noninvasively estimate renal vascular resistance and measure it.

For correct estimation of renal vascular resistance it is necessary to obtain clear spectral analysis on at least three different intrarenal arteries in different parts of kidney, but spectral analysis is most commonly performed at the level of interlobar arteries. RI (resistance index) and PI (pulsatility index) calculated from the blood flow velocities can be used for spectral quantification of vascular resistance, and RI is used almost exclusively in clinical practice [14]. Resistance index is the difference of peak systolic velocity and end diastolic velocity, divided with peak systolic velocity. The higher the end diastolic velocity the lower the RI, and vice versa. Different studies showed that normal RI values are in the range from 0.58 to 0.64. For adults all values of RI equal or above 0.70 refer to increased renal vascular resistance [15–17]. Recent study showed a normal range of 0.47–0.7 [18]. RI physiologically increases with aging and elders have 10–15% higher values of RI and PI in comparison with youngers [14, 18].

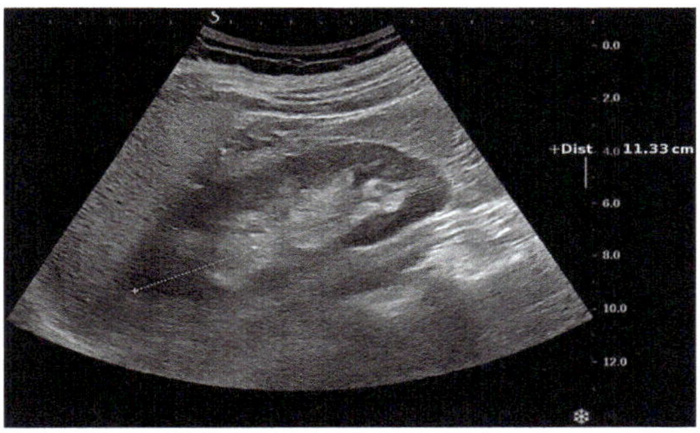

Fig. 9.1 Longitudinal section of the kidney on B-mode of a 64-year-old patient with long-lasting type 2 diabetes mellitus

Renal changes in diabetic patients are detectable by conventional ultrasound usually in advanced stage of diabetic nephropathy [19, 20]. Detection and follow-up of the progressing diabetic nephropathy are generally based on clinical and laboratory examinations, while imaging techniques have a secondary role, especially in the early phase of the disease [19].

In the early stage of diabetic nephropathy at conventional B-mode kidneys may be enlarged because of hyperfiltration [19, 20]. Hyperfiltration and nephromegaly are the first abnormalities seen in kidneys in both types of diabetes mellitus and can be ideal parameters for intervention because they represent reversible stage of renal involvement in diabetes mellitus in which glomerular filtration rate (GFR) is still preserved. With the progression of disease, at the advanced stage kidney size reduces because of glomerulo-

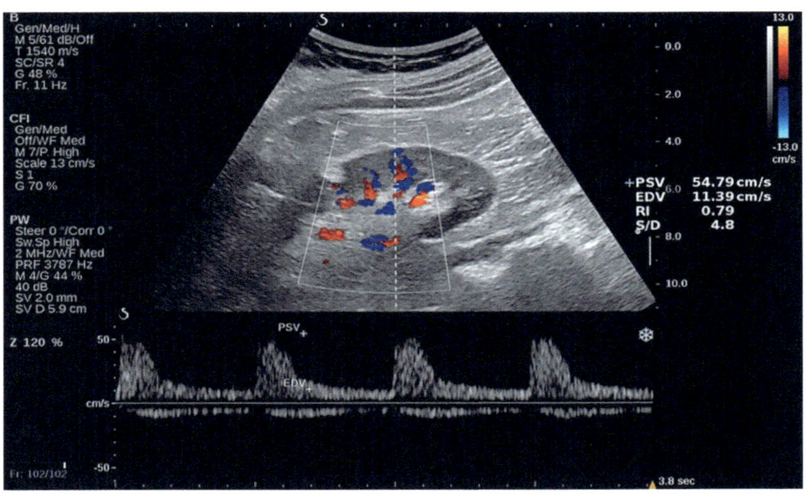

Fig. 9.2 Color Doppler and spectral analysis of the same patient's kidney showing increased resistance index RI of 0.79

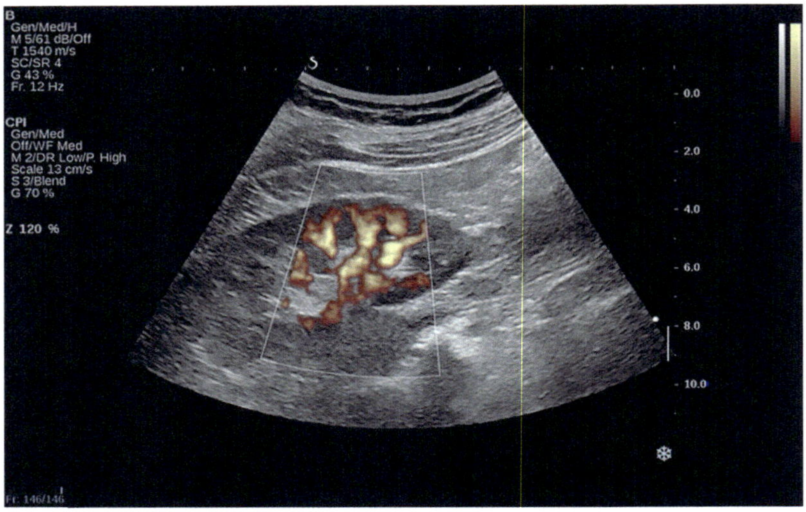

Fig. 9.3 Power Doppler ultrasound is also of clinical value in evaluating the renal vasculature showing areas of decreased renal flow

sclerosis and tubular atrophy with increasing interstitial fibrosis [5].

Renal cortical hyperechogenicity particularly can be seen only in advanced nephropathy, correlating well with the severity of interstitial changes and being a reliable sign of renal functional impairment at conventional B-mode [19, 21].

In diabetic kidneys pathologic changes are predominantly found in vascular structures, which can explain why an increase of renal vascular resistance may be found earlier than changes in morphology [19].

Measuring RI with duplex Doppler ultrasound may identify nephropathy at early stage because some patients may present with elevated indices at early, preclinical stage of nephropathy and therefore contribute to early diagnosis and prevention of disease progression. At the advanced stages of nephropathy indices are higher in comparison with early stages and the highest values are measured in patients at the end stage of renal impairment. Also, atherosclerotic changes in intrarenal arteries develop faster in patients with diabetes and contribute to the increase of the RI. Therefore, RI increase reflects increased renal vascular resistance in diabetic nephropathy and indicates the progression of disease with renal scarring which precedes the appearance of albuminuria and shows positive correlation with laboratory and clinical parameters, but offers no advantages over these in disease progress or in patient care [5, 17, 19, 21–25] (Fig. 9.2).

References

1. International Diabetes Federation. IDF Diabetes Atlas Seventh Edition. 2015.
2. Soriguer F, Goday A, Bosch-Comas A, Bordiu E, Calle-Pascual A, Carmena R, et al. Prevalence of diabetes mellitus and impaired glucose regulation in Spain: the Diabetes Study. Diabetologia. 2012;55:88–93.
3. Fowler M. Microvascular and macrovascular complications of diabetes. Clin Diabetes. 2008;26:77–82.
4. Saif A, Soliman NA, Abdel-Hameed AA. Early evaluation of renal hemodynamic alterations in Type I diabetes mellitus with duplex ultrasound. Saudi J Kidney Dis Transpl. 2010;21(2):295–9.
5. Mancini M, Masulli M, Liuzzi R, Mainenti PP, Ragucci M, Maurea S, Riccardi G, Vaccaro O. Renal duplex sonographic evaluation of type 2 diabetic patients. J Ultrasound Med. 2013;32:1033–50.
6. Rychlik I. Epidemiology of diabetic nephropathy. Vnitr Lek. 2008;54(5):488–93.
7. Gross JL, De Azevedo MJ, Silveiro SP, Canani LH, Caramori ML, Zelmanovitz T. Diabetic nephropathy: diagnosis, prevention and treatment. Diabetes Care. 2005;28(1):164–76.
8. Ayodele OE, Alebious CO, Salako BL. Diabetic nephropathy—a review of the natural history, burden, risk factors and treatment. J Natl Med Assoc. 2004;96(11):1445–54.
9. Umanath K, Lewis JB. Update on diabetic nephropathy: core curriculum 2018. Am J Kidney Dis. 2018;S0272-6386(17):31102.

10. Cao Z, Cooper ME. Pathogenesis of diabetic nephropathy. J Diabetes Investig. 2011;2(4):243–7.
11. Schena FP, Gesualdo L. Pathogenic mechanisms of diabetic nephropathy. JASN. 2005;16(3 suppl 1):S30–3.
12. Ismail N, Becker B, Strzelczyk P, Ritz E. Renal disease and hypertension in non-insulin-dependent diabetes mellitus. Kidney Int. 1999;55(1):1–28.
13. Toriu N, Yamanouchi M, Hiramatsu R, Hayami N, Hoshino J, Sekine A, Kawada M, Hasegawa E, Suwabe T, Sumida K, Ueno T, Sawa N, Ohashi K, Fujii T, Takaichi K, Yanagita M, Kobayasi T, Ubara Y. Preservation of renal function by intensive glycemic control. Endocrinol Diabetes Meab Case Rep. 2018;2018:17–0136.
14. Brkljačić B, Castellani S, Deane C, Dietrich CF. Doppler ultrasound of renal vessels. In: Dietrich CF, editor. EFSUMB–European Course Book; 2012. p. 715–36.
15. Knapp R, Ploetzender A, Frauscher F, et al. Variability of Doppler parameters in healthy kidney: an anatomic-physiologic correlation. J Ultrasound Med. 1995;14:427–9.
16. Brkljačić B, Drinković I, Delić-Brkljačić D, Hebrang A. Age related changes of renal vascular resistance in normal native kidneys: color duplex Doppler US assessment. Radiol Oncol. 1995;29:102–6.
17. Brkljačić B, Mrzljak V, Drinković I, Soldo D, Sabralj-Matovinović M, Hebrang A. Renal vascular resistance in diabetic nephropathy: duplex-Doppler US evaluation. Radiology. 1994;192:549–54.
18. Spatola L, Andrulli S. Doppler ultrasound in kidney diseases: a key parameter in clinical long-term follow-up. J Ultrasound. 2016;19(4):243–50.
19. Soldo D, Brkljačić B, Božikov V, Drinković I, Hauser M. Comparison of conventional and duplex Doppler ultrasonographic findings. Acta Radiol. 1997;38:296–302.
20. Elgyoum AM, Osman H, Elzaki A, Elrahim EA. Ultrasonographic renal size in individuals with known diabetes mellitus. Sch J App Med Sci. 2013;1(6):690–2.
21. Shaw M, Bhagat S, Panda BB, Nisa S, Das B, Panda A. Diabetic nephropathy: ultrasound, color Doppler and biochemical correlation—a 2 year study. JMSCR. 2016;4:12025–34.
22. El Dayem SA, El Megd El Bohy A, Hamed M, Ahmed S. Follow up of value of the intrarenal resistivity indices and different renal biomarkers for early identification of diabetic nephropathy in type 1 diabetic patients. MJMS. 2017;5(2):188–92.
23. Hamano K, Nitta A, Ohtake T, Kobayashi S. Associations of renal vascular resistance with albuminuria and other macroangiopathy in type 2 diabetic patients. Diabetes Care. 2008;31(9):1853–7.
24. Viazzi F, Leoncini G, Derchi LE, Baratto E, Storace G, Vercelli M, Deferrari G, Pontremoli R. Subclinical functional and structural renal abnormalities predict new onset type 2 diabetes in patients with primary hypertension. J Hum Hypertens. 2013;27:95–9.
25. Bruno RM, Daghini E, Landini L, Versari D, Salvati A, Santini E, Di Paco I, Magagna A, Taddei S, Ghiadoni L, Solini A. Dynamic evaluation of renal resistive index in normoalbuminuric patients with newly diagnosed hypertension or type 2 diabetes. Diabetologia. 2011;54(9):2430–9.

Renal Vessels

10

Maria Vittoria Raciti, Elena Turpini, Ilaria Fiorina, Elena Belloni, Chandra Bortolotto, and Fabrizio Calliada

10.1 Normal Anatomy

10.1.1 Renal Arteries

Renal arteries usually arise from the lateral surface of the abdominal aorta at the level of the first or second lumbar vertebral body, below the origin of superior mesenteric artery. The right renal artery (RRA) orifice is typically more superior to the left and usually a single renal artery supplies each kidney. They run in the retroperitoneum covered by the correspondent veins; the right renal artery, which is also the longest, crosses anteriorly the inferior vena cava. Both arteries lean posteriorly on the medial diaphragmatic arch at its insertion on the spine.

Renal arteries are about 4–6 cm long and 5–6 mm large, since the kidney gets around one-fifth of the cardiac output [1]. The right renal artery usually has a downward course posterior to the inferior vena cava, whereas the left renal artery (LRA) has a more horizontal course [2].

Near the hilum the main renal artery divides into a ventral and dorsal branch; the ventral branch has the biggest caliber and runs anteriorly; it enters the renal hilum between the branches of the renal vein and the renal pelvis; at the hilum the anterior division branches into four segmental arteries: apical, upper, middle, and lower anterior. The dorsal branch runs posteriorly to the renal pelvis and the posterior division supplies a large portion to the dorsal part of the kidney. A relative hypovascular plane is between the anterior and posterior arterial divisions of the kidney (Brodel's line).

The segmental arteries then branch into the lobar, interlobar, arcuate, and interlobular arteries [3]. Furthermore the renal artery gives off the inferior adrenal, capsular, and proximal ureter branches.

The most common renal vascular variant is the accessory renal artery. It is seen in up to one-third of individuals and is bilateral in about 12% of patients.

Most commonly accessory renal artery originates from the abdominal aorta and supplies the inferior pole of the kidney, but occasionally can arise from the thoracic aorta, iliac, lumbar, or mesenteric artery [4].

Accessory renal arteries are categorized into hilar arteries, if entering in the kidney at the

M. V. Raciti (✉) · E. Turpini · C. Bortolotto
F. Calliada
Radiology Department, Fondazione IRCCS Policlinico San Matteo Pavia, Pavia, Italy

I. Fiorina
Radiology and Neuroradiology Diagnostic and Interventional Department, Fondazione IRCSS Policlinico San Matteo, Pavia, Italy

E. Belloni
Radiology Department, Civil Hospital, Vigevano (PV), ASST, Pavia, Italy

A. Granata, M. Bertolotto (eds.), *Imaging in Nephrology*,
https://doi.org/10.1007/978-3-030-60794-4_10

hilum, or polar arteries, if directly piercing the pole of the kidney.

The early branching of the main renal artery is a normal variant in which the LRA branches within 1.5–2.0 cm from the lateral wall of the aorta and the RRA branches in retrocaval segment. This variant is important in renal transplantation, because most surgeons usually require at least a 1.5–2.0 cm length of renal artery before first branching for successful anastomosis [5].

10.1.2 Renal Veins

The renal veins are short and thick venous trunk and they originate from the hilum from around 3–5 smaller renal parenchymal branches. The right vein is more oblique than the left one (since the right kidney is generally in a lower position compared to the left kidney). The left renal vein normally receives the left adrenal vein superiorly, the left gonadal vein inferiorly, and a lumbar vein posteriorly [6].

The left renal vein is longer than the right renal vein and usually courses between the aorta anteriorly and the superior mesenteric artery posteriorly before entering into the medial side of the inferior vena cava (IVC) [7]. The right renal vein enters into the lateral side of the IVC and usually receives no tributaries [6].

The average lengths of the renal veins are approximately 6.8–7.5 cm on the left and 2.5–2.6 cm on the right.

At the hilum, the renal vein commonly lies anterior to the renal artery [5]. Variation of renal venous anatomy is less common than the arteries. Anomalies of the renal veins can lead to significant morbidity during surgical exploration if unidentified presurgically [8].

Multiple renal veins are the most common venous variant and are seen in about 15–30% of patients, mainly on the right side [5–9].

The *left renal vein* in 2–3% of the population may course posterior to the aorta (retroaortic left renal vein; Fig. 10.1) or may bifurcate into two limbs (ventral and dorsal) that encircle the abdominal aorta (circumaortic renal vein) [4, 5].

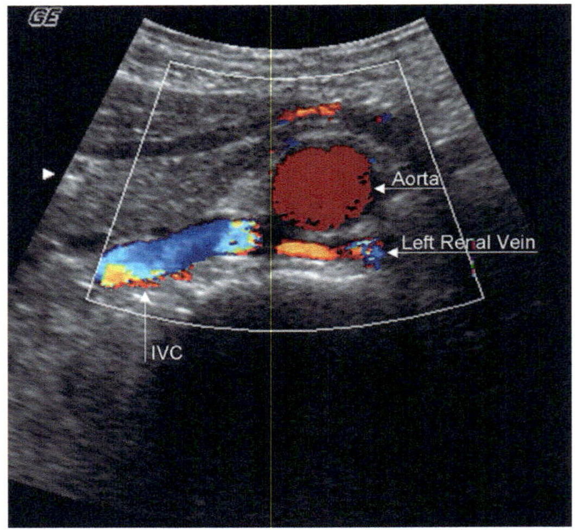

Fig. 10.1 Color Doppler ultrasound of retroaortic left renal vein

In the presence of a circumaortic left renal vein, the adrenal vein enters the preaortic limb and the gonadal vein enters the retroaortic limb [4, 10].

Rarely, left renal vein drains into azygos-hemiazygos system especially in the presence of IVC anomalies [11].

In about 59–88% of the population, the retroperitoneal veins (e.g., lumbar and hemiazygos veins) drain into the left renal vein.

On the right side, the gonadal and adrenal veins enter the right renal vein in only 7% and 31% of cases, respectively [5].

10.2 Ultrasound Examination

Ultrasound is the first-line technique to study renal pathology being well known by performing healthcare professionals and tolerated by patients [12]. Conventional B-mode ultrasound is not capable of studying renal vessels and their pathology while it is capable of giving lots of information about renal morphology and proximal urinary tract.

Vessel analysis relies on a slightly more advanced US technique such as Doppler which allows obtaining data on main and intraparenchymal vessels.

Doppler analysis can be both quantitative and qualitative. From a qualitative point of view it gives information about vessel patency/occlusion, and allows us to distinguish between vein and arteries (continuous vs. pulsed flow) and between incoming and outcoming flow (red vs. blue) and to identify turbulence (reverse flow) and acceleration (aliasing).

Quantitative analysis, with the spectral Doppler, is capable of delivering lots of information starting from peak systolic velocity to end diastolic velocity and other more complex parameters and indexes.

10.2.1 Technique

The approach to renal vessels is not optimal using a classic oblique transverse approach with the patient supine (those generally used to study the kidney with B-mode imaging) both because the patient's habitus and intestinal gas can mask the region of interest and because it is a very unfavorable situation for Doppler angle, especially on the right side. We must bear in mind that angles more than 60° are not acceptable because the percentage of error in the measurements is more than 30%.

The optimal approach is a coronal scan on the abdominal aorta, with the patient lying on the left side (Fig. 10.2) which allows us to obtain, in the most favorable condition, a pseudo-angiographic image of both renal arteries' origin ("banana peel") (Fig. 10.3).

If this approach is not possible because of intestinal gas progressively posterior approaches are possible, still with a longitudinal orientation of the probe. With those progressively posterior approaches, the depth of the vessel progressively increases.

These approaches guarantee an angle of around 0°–30° between the aorta and the renal artery which is perfect for Doppler studies.

The visualization of the whole length of the main renal artery can be difficult because of physical habitus, intestinal gas, and cutaneous scars; the reported percentage of complete visualization is very variable.

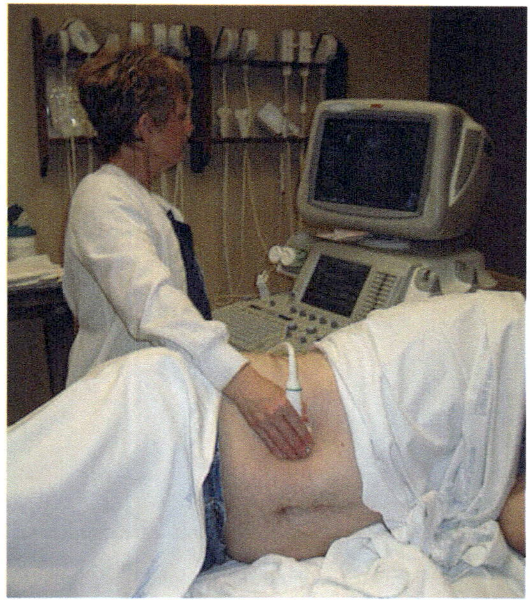

Fig. 10.2 *Ultrasound* approach to study renal arteries. The optimal approach is a coronal scan on the abdominal aorta with the patient lying on the left side

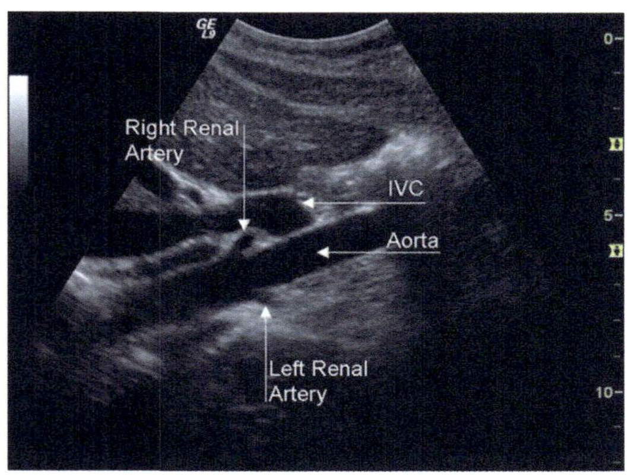

Fig. 10.3 *Conventional B-mode ultrasound* of renal arteries with coronal approach allowing to obtain a pseudo-angiographic image of both renal arteries' origin ("banana peel"). IVC: inferior vena cava

It is possible to identify supernumerary arteries, especially if of good caliber and if near the origin of the main artery (Fig. 10.4). A clue of the presence of a supernumerary artery can be an eccentric approach to the renal hilum of the main artery.

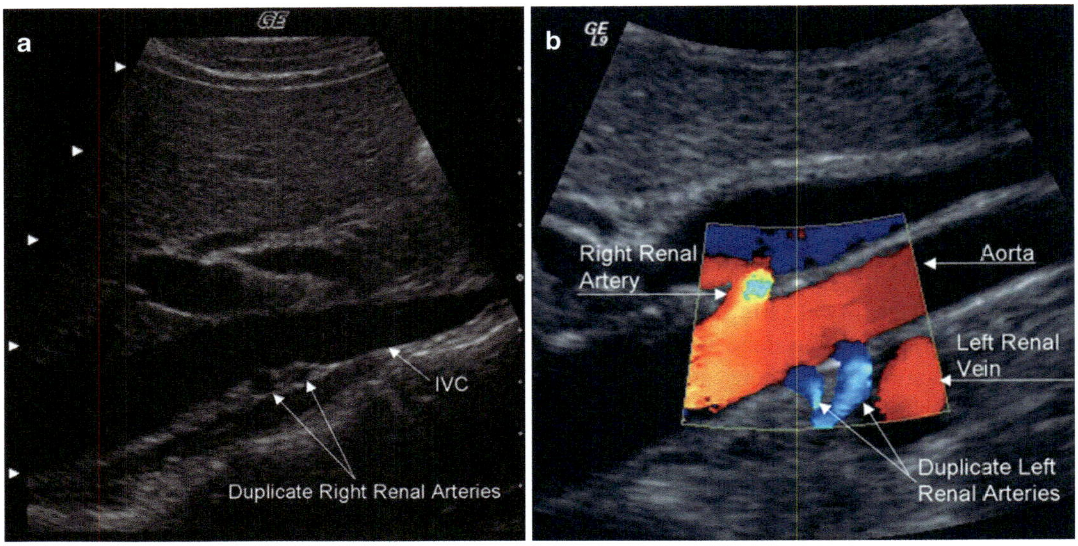

Fig. 10.4 B-mode (**a**) and Color Doppler ultrasound (**b**) of double-left renal artery

On the left side, the renal artery must not be confused with the inferior mesenteric artery. The simplest way to identify the renal artery is to follow it straight to the renal hilum which, unluckily, is not possible in all patients. The inferior mesenteric artery generally shows a high-resistance waveform different from that of the renal artery. Also it originates from the very distal portion of the abdominal aorta; nonetheless also the renal arteries can have abnormal origins.

Spectral Doppler analysis must follow and deepen the color Doppler evaluation since color Doppler is essential to identify the vessel in unfavorable conditions; the correct placement of spectral Doppler box makes measurement more accurate.

The Doppler waveform of the renal arteries reflects that of the vessels directed to a parenchymal organ: a rapid systolic rise, without a particularly elevated rise; the absence of a "reverse" wave; and a continuous diastolic flow (low-resistance flow). Frequently a small "spike" can be seen on the wave of a main renal artery or on the proximal portion of a smaller branch right at the end of the systolic phase ("early systolic peak").

In normal conditions the maximum peak systolic velocity lies between 60 and 120 cm/s; being a high-velocity flow the pulse repetition frequency on the ultrasound scanner must be adequate (generally must be increased from the standard). The diastolic velocity is around or a little lower than the half of the peak systolic velocity.

The identification of an area with aliasing can guide the operator to correctly place the measurement box; in the most severe cases a "mosaic effect" can also be seen characterized by the presence of pixels of various colors dispersed even out of the vessel margins.

Generally speaking, when no aliasing is visible, three measurements must be taken: one at the origin of the vessel, one in the intermediate third, and one at the distal third, right before the hilum.

The evaluation of the proximal portion is essential since most of the atheromatous alterations can be found on this portion and only the spectral evaluation can detect the less severe and more successfully treatable stenosis. Evaluating the artery only at the level of the hilum can lead to underdiagnosed proximal precritical stenosis. Nonetheless evaluating the renal artery at the level of the hilum is essential to detect distal stenosis; since dysplastic lesions are generally located at the intermediate-distal third of the main artery this evaluation has become extremely important in younger patients.

Doppler analysis must be integrated with a B-mode evaluation of the kidneys with coronal and axial scans, measurements of the renal coronal diameter, parenchymal thickness, and evaluation of focal and diffuse lesions. Medium coronal diameter for the right kidney is 10.74 ± 1.35 cm and for the left kidney is 11 ± 1.15 cm; the lower cutoff for normality can be set at 9 cm. A small kidney or an asymmetry between the two kidneys, as well as parenchymal thickness reduction or asymmetries, can be an indirect sign of the presence of a renal artery stenosis.

Intrarenal arterial flow must be studied; at this level the peak systolic velocity is obviously inferior to that of the main renal artery.

In the intrarenal vessel evaluation the color assignment is the opposite of the expected when evaluating the closest half of the kidney in comparison to the most distant half of the kidney.

When a stenosis is present, as in all other vascular districts, an increase in flow velocity and the presence of turbulences are proportional to the degree of stenosis with increase of both systolic and diastolic velocity.

Proximal and subcritical proximal stenosis can produce no or minimal flow alterations at the level of the hilum while in severe stenosis a post-stenotic flow can be detected even at the level of the hilum. Post-stenotic flow is characterized by a reduction in the steep systolic rise and a reduction in systolic-diastolic difference (the shape of the wave becomes more similar to the shape of a "bell"). This kind of waveform is called "tardus et parvus" ("slow and small") and is the typical indirect sign of a more proximal stenosis even if the presence of a distal normal flow cannot rule out the presence of a proximal stenosis. "Tardus" (slow) refers to the deceleration of the systolic rise leading to an increased time to reach the peak systolic velocity. "Parvus" (small) refers to the fact that the peak systolic velocity is significantly lower as a result of a lower peak systolic velocity.

In complete occlusions no flow can be identified along the renal artery; if a collateral circulation is present a very slow flow can be detected at the hilum or in the intraparenchymal vessels.

10.3 Computed Tomography: Technique and Indications

The state-of-the-art multidetector (MD) CT scanners allow volumetric data acquisition with submillimeter isotropic voxels and subsecond gantry rotation, with high temporal and spatial resolution. These parameters are important for angiographic evaluation.

Modern MD scanners can simultaneously acquire up to 0.5 mm collimations thick 320 multidetector sections in 16 cm detector width, with gantry rotation time as low as 280–350 ms [6].

Thinner section thickness allows isotropic voxels, which is essential in order to obtain high-resolution 3D reconstruction (Fig. 10.5) and other post-processing displays, such as maximum intensity projection (MIP) reformatting (Fig. 10.6) [6].

Conventional phase acquisitions are arterial and venous phases, but a delayed pyelographic phase imaging should be added.

CT is the modality of choice for the patients with pacemakers, automatic implantable cardioverter defibrillator, or other non-MR-compatible devices and is mostly preferred to MRA for screening of potential renal donors [6].

CT should also be selected for patients with severe claustrophobia and limited breath-hold capacity because of shorter acquisition time.

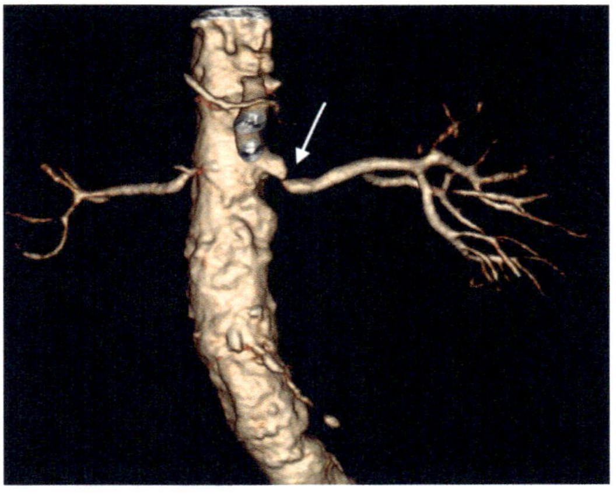

Fig. 10.5 *Computed tomography* angiography of the renal arteries, in volume rendering, shows a high-grade stenosis of left renal artery (*white arrow*)

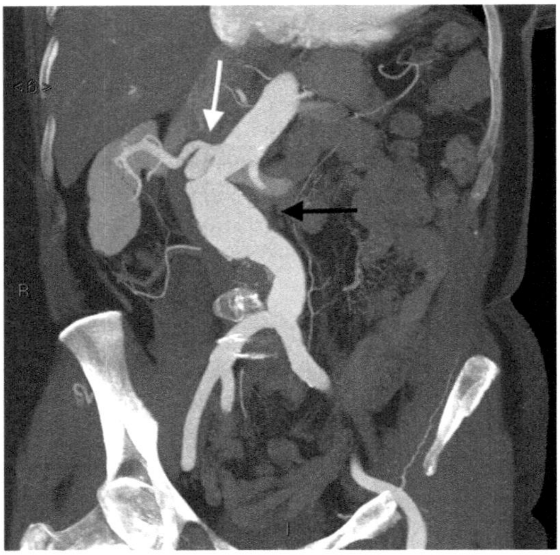

Fig. 10.6 *Computed tomography* angiography of the renal arteries, in coronal plane, with maximum intensity projections (MIP), demonstrates saccular macro-aneurysm of right renal artery (*white arrow*) in the presence of a sub-renal abdominal aortic aneurysm (*black arrow*)

CT is generally preferred when very high spatial resolution is required or when it is particularly important to demonstrate peripheral renal arteries [6].

10.4 MRI: Technique and Indications

MRI techniques have recently expanded and they are now suitable not only for providing excellent depiction of kidney anatomy, but also for studying several functional aspects of kidney physiology. In particular, using different sequences, it is possible to adopt MRI techniques addressed to study renal structure and anatomy, renal blood flow, glomerular filtration rate (GFR), renal perfusion, and renal tissue oxygenation.

In almost all these evaluations, MRI techniques provide the same results of CT and they may be even preferred over it, thanks to the lack of ionizing radiation and iodinated contrast-induced nephropathy. In particular this is true in those cases in which MRI can be performed without contrast medium: for this reason NCE-MRI techniques are now progressively spreading, even if there is still lack of standardization.

Using conventional catheter angiography as reference, 3-dimensional (3D) gadolinium MRA is accurate for diagnosing renal artery stenosis, comparable to CTA and superior to ultrasound and captopril renography [13]. The median sensitivity and specificity, calculated considering different studies and compared to conventional catheter angiography, are, respectively, 92% and 93.5% without contrast, and 96% and 93% with contrast.

The variety of pulse sequences in MRI that assess organ function complement anatomic information for diagnosing renal artery stenosis and help determine which patients/kidneys can benefit from renal revascularization. This combined MRA-based examination thus has the potential to increase sensitivity and specificity, so MRA can become a highly effective screening exam for renovascular disease [13].

Gadolinium contrast-enhanced magnetic resonance angiography (CE-MRA) is a valuable, noninvasive tool for evaluation of renal vasculature in potential live kidney donors. Precise detail of the renal arterial and venous vasculature enables the surgeon decide whether a kidney is suitable for the transplantation and helps to predict any problems that may arise during vascular anastomosis.

In particular, multiple renal arteries, presence of large accessory artery (especially lower polar artery), or early branches increase the complication rate of donor nephrectomy and in all these cases the surgeon may opt for right nephrectomy instead of the usual left one [14].

Similarly, detection of renal artery stenosis, parenchymal disease, or collecting system anomalies may preclude surgery [14]. Variants of renal venous anatomy are also important to recognize, in particular before laparoscopic donor nephrectomy because in this case a retroaortic configuration may preclude surgery too [14, 15].

CE-MRA offers an accurate evaluation of all these anatomical aspects, with an accuracy comparable to digital subtraction angiography (DSA), which has long been considered the gold standard (Fig. 10.7) [15, 16].

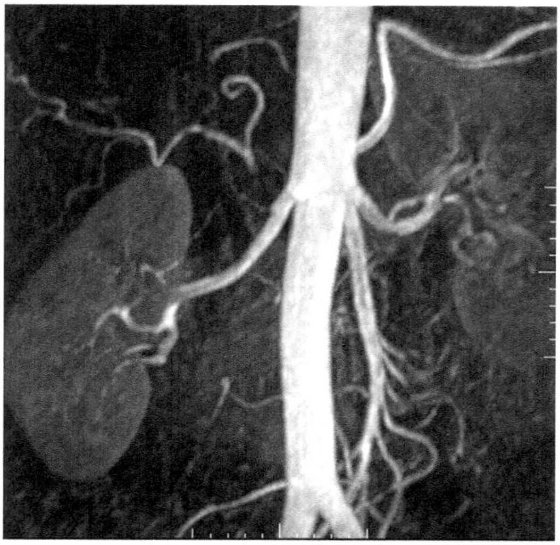

Fig. 10.7 *Contrast-enhanced-magnetic resonance angiography* (CE-MRA) offers an accurate evaluation of all these anatomical aspects, with an accuracy comparable to digital subtraction angiography (DSA), which has long been considered the gold standard

CE-MRA has significant advantages over other MRI techniques: both phase-contrast (PC) and time-of-flight (TOF) imaging are hampered by long acquisition time, limited volume coverage in the axial plane respiratory artifacts, and difficulties in visualizing flow in both directions of aorta and renal artery [14]. CE-MRA can be performed in coronal plane avoiding the problem of flow direction and in the last years has been improved by the introduction of breath-hold techniques with reduction of breathing artifacts. CE-MRA is particularly suited to obtaining information on venous anatomy, as a simple second breath-hold acquisition directly after the arterial first pass will show venous enhancement.

In the field of NE-MRA techniques we know that TOF and PCA are limited because of the reasons explained above, but in a recent study Xu et al. [16] have evaluated the results obtained with inflow invasion recovery (IFIR) magnetic resonance angiography, compared to CE-MRA. They concluded that IFIR MRA provided better quality images than CE-MRA and superior visualization of branch renal arteries and accessory renal artery, with highly homogenous signal intensity within the vessel lumen and better declination of the vessel border, as compared to CE-MRA [16]. IFIR MRA allows high diagnostic confidence for more accurate quantitative hemodynamic analysis. It may be helpful to improve visualization of disease in the more distal branches of the renal arteries, such as fibromuscular dysplasia, vasculitis, and renal arteriovenous malformations [16, 17].

These results are promising but strictly subordinated to stable respiratory rate and they should be further examined and confirmed on a larger population.

10.5 Renal Angiography: Indications and Technique

Renal arteriography is nowadays performed for interventional purposes, instead of diagnostic scope, because of improvements of renal artery imaging. Technological developments allowed many different kinds of interventional procedures in the last decades, such as percutaneous transluminal angioplasty, stent placement, renal embolization, and renal denervation. Tools used for percutaneous renal artery interventions have in fact recently improved with pre-mounted, low-profile stents and balloons, and steerable guiding catheters.

Impaired renal function may limit the use of iodinated contrast medium for angiography, so carbon dioxide is recently employed to perform endovascular renal procedures.

Endovascular procedures are usually performed via local anesthesia. Femoral artery access is an established standard approach, but in the cases of severe kinking or untreated stenosis/occlusion of the iliac arteries or abdominal aorta, a brachial or radial access is preferred.

The guidewire is then advanced into the abdominal aorta and a preliminary aortography is performed placing a pigtail or straight-tip catheter at the level of the body of L1 through a contrast medium injection with a power injector pump.

Many different kinds of catheters may be used in selective renal angiography; usually it is preferable to manage it with "Cobra 2," "Simmons 1 or 2," and "Renal Double Curve." In order to select the renal artery origin in a stable position, it is possible to apply different selective techniques:

- ***"No-touch technique"*** *[18]* that corresponds to the selective renal artery with a steerable stiff 0.014 in. guidewire, placing a guiding catheter into the abdominal aorta, using a second guidewire within the guiding catheter to minimize the contact between the guiding catheter and the atherosclerotic plaques
- ***"Telescoping technique,"*** which consists of the cannulation of the renal artery with a 5F diagnostic catheter and a guidewire: then the guiding catheter is advanced across the diagnostic catheter, which is pulled out thereafter
- Direct selective with a pre-shaped long sheath

10.6 Renal Artery Stenosis

10.6.1 Introduction

Renovascular disease is the most common cause of potentially curable secondary hypertension, and is found in up to 5% of the general hypertensive population. In patients with symptoms (e.g., poorly controlled hypertension), the prevalence of renal artery stenosis rises to 20–40%. The two most common causes of renal artery stenosis are atherosclerosis (60–70%) and fibromuscular dysplasia (FMD). Ostial atherosclerotic lesions are the most common cause of renal artery stenosis, representing about 90% of the cases, due to the plaque formation in the aortic wall with the progressive involvement of renal artery origin. It is a progressive disease that may cause renal hypoperfusion, development of renal artery occlusion, and kidney atrophy.

10.6.2 Renal Artery Stenosis: Ultrasound

Numerous diagnostic criteria can be used to identify a renal artery stenosis and generally are divided into "indirect" and "direct."

Direct parameters can be obtained by evaluating the main renal artery or accessory renal arteries and can be defined as "proximal criteria" [19].

The difficulties related to the evaluation of the stenosis, the long time needed to obtain a diagnostic confidence, and the difficulties in the evaluation of smaller accessory renal arteries had led many authors to the identification of alterations in the waveform of distal, and more accessible, vessels such as hilar, intraparenchymal, and perforating vessels ("distal criteria"). Such alterations are generally all related to the "tardus et parvus" waveform.

Distal criteria make it easier, especially for less experienced authors, to identify the presence of a renal artery stenosis even with the downside of the lack of anatomical correspondence and lower sensitivity and specificity.

Also, a stenosis on a small supernumerary artery or a small branch is a diagnostic challenge [20] but can be suspected if a significant difference in waveform or intraparenchymal resistance between superior, middle, and inferior third of the kidney is present.

10.6.3 Direct (Proximal) Criteria

1. Qualitative: presence of a small aliasing spot, of a post-stenotic turbulence with a "mosaic effect," or of a post-stenotic dilatation.
2. Quantitative:
   (a) Peak systolic velocity (PSV): can be easily calculated from the spectral Doppler of an arterial flow. In literature mainly two historical cutoffs, respectively, of 180 cm/s and 200 cm/s can be found with little differences in sensitivity and specificity which generally are around 90% (Fig. 10.8a) [21]. The only possible limitation of the PSV is related to a certain variability with age [22]. An attempt to reduce this variability was tried with the "aortic-renal ratio."
   (b) Aortic-renal ratio: Is the ratio between the peak systolic velocity in the renal artery and the peak systolic velocity in the abdominal aorta, measured just proximal

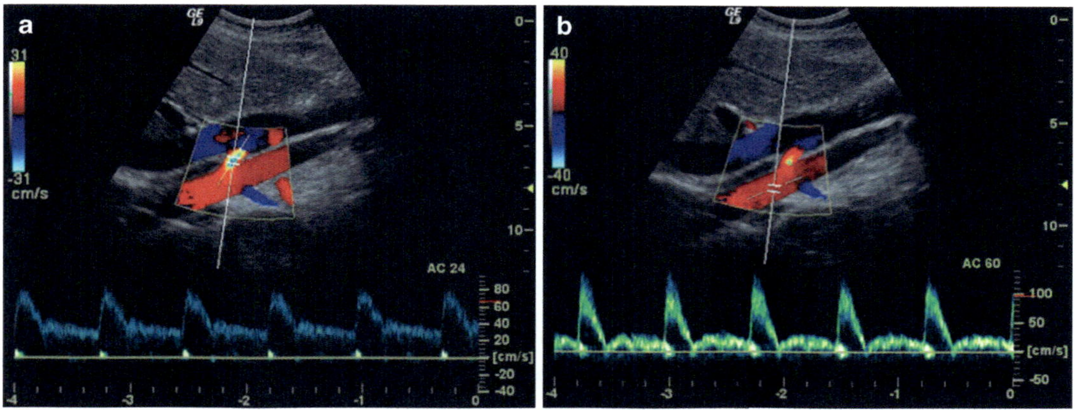

Fig. 10.8 *Color and spectral Doppler ultrasound* of proximal renal arteries. (**a**) The color Doppler image shows qualitative criteria of proximal renal artery stenosis, and the presence of a small aliasing spot in the right renal artery. The spectral Doppler in the site of aliasing spot shows a normal peak systolic velocity (PSV) <180 cm/s. (**b**) Spectral Doppler of the abdominal aorta measured just proximal to the renal artery origin and the calculation of aortic-renal ratio confirm the absence of stenosis (<2.5)

to the renal artery origin. In literature variable cutoffs can be found. In the very first work from Hoffman and colleague [23] a ratio of 3.5 was proposed with sensitivity and specificity of, respectively, 92% and 62%. In a more recent work from Staub and colleague the cutoff was lowered to 2.5 with a sensitivity of 92% and a specificity of 79% (Fig. 10.8b) [21]. This criterium is nowadays receiving new attention [19].

(c) End diastolic velocity (DV): Easily calculated on the Doppler curve which represents the waveform of the flow in the renal artery which is the less significant direct criterium. A velocity higher than 150 cm/s is highly specific for a stenosis but sensitivity is very low. The most significant application is that an end diastolic velocity lower than 70 cm/s allows to exclude high-grade stenosis [21].

10.6.4 Indirect (Distal) Criteria

1. Qualitative:
   (a) Identification of a "tardus et parvus" waveform
   (b) Absence of the early systolic peak is an index of renal artery stenosis [24]
2. Quantitative:
   (a) Intrarenal resistivity index (RRI): measures the impedance between intrarenal arteries (Fig. 10.9):

   RRI = PSV–DV/PSV [25].

   The normal values range between 58% and 64%. Newborn and children have higher RRI which progressively decreases to reach the "adult" values at around 4–5 years of age.

   In a "tardus et parvus" waveform the RRI is decreased.

   (b) Difference between RRI on two sides: The cutoff reported in the literature and almost unanimously well accepted is 0.05. When the ratio increases it is highly specific (unfortunately with a low sensitivity) for a significant renal artery stenosis [26].
   (c) Acceleration time (AT): It is the time between the beginning of the systole and the peak systolic velocity. A post-stenotic peak is rounded, with an increase in the duration of the systolic rise which translates into a deceleration in AT. Pathological values are higher than 0.07 s.

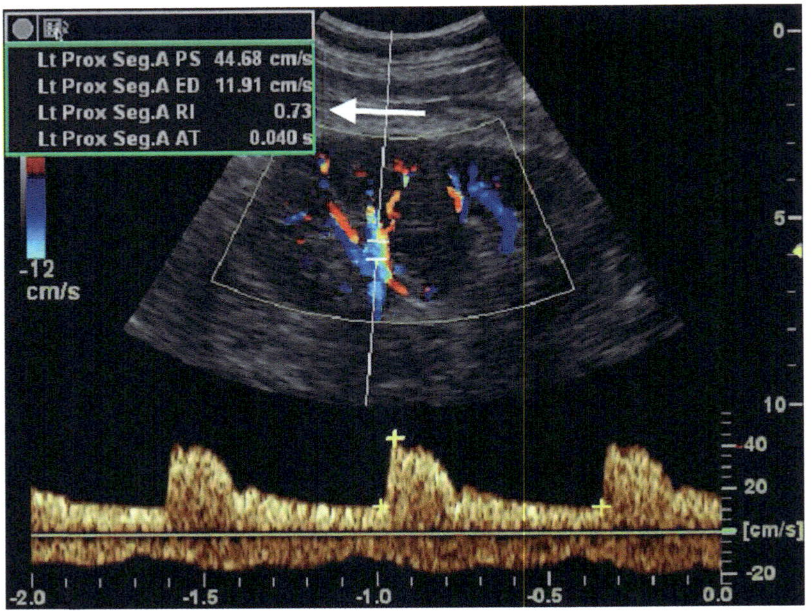

Fig. 10.9 *Spectral Doppler ultrasound* of intrarenal arteries shows an intrarenal resistivity index of 73% (white arrow)

(d) Acceleration index (AI): It is the velocity to reach the systolic peak. Pathological values are higher than 3 m/s^2 [24].

Several intrinsic factors can influence the systolic acceleration (AT and AI) making these parameters not much specific: cardiac aortic valve pathology (e.g., aortic and mitral valve), left ventricle dysfunction, and drugs affecting the cardiovascular system. Several factors affect the vascular compliance such as age, hypertension, and diabetes. These influences can explain why several studies had difficulties in reproducing the results obtained with some of these criteria and indexes.

(e) Evaluation of perforating arteries: Perforating arteries are small vessels that link the parenchymal arteries to the arteries of the capsular plexus. A reliable index of renal artery stenosis is an inversion of the flow direction in these arteries [27].

Sensibility of all these parameters increases after the administration of ACE inhibitors. These drugs inhibit the vasoconstrictive effect of the angiotensin II, increasing the compliance of the vessel wall and lowering the intrarenal vascular resistance. This mechanism, around 1 h after the administration of these kind of drugs, increases the possibility to detect a "tardus et parvus" waveform with an increased diagnostic accuracy (sensitivity increases from 69% to 100%) [28].

A well-known meta-analysis [29] had considered all the previously mentioned parameters to try to figure out their accuracy in the diagnosis of renal artery stenosis. The conclusions are that Doppler analysis is an accurate tool in the diagnosis of renal artery stenosis and that the measurement of PSV delivers the best performance with a sensitivity of 85% and a specificity of 92%. The addition of other parameters does not increase the diagnostic accuracy.

10.7 Prognostic Value of Doppler Measurements

Once the stenosis is identified and its entity is considered hemodynamically significant the next step is to assess its relation with the hypertension and to get prognostic information.

The analysis of intrarenal parenchymal arteries, with the evaluation of the AI and the morphology of the waveform, may respond to this question with a 95% overall diagnostic accuracy in the evaluation of the stenosis and a 100% in foreseeing the clinical response [30]. As a feasible prognostic criterium the RRI after captopril administration was also evaluated [28].

An increase in RRI correlates with the alterations of small renal artery and arterioles distal to the stenosis, factors that contribute to establishing the irreversibility of the hypertension/renal insufficiency, even after a successful revascularization.

It had been demonstrated over the years that in patients with a stenosis more than 50% in at least one renal artery, a RRI of more than 80% is highly specific and sensitive in predicting a failure in the functional recovery after stenting or surgery. RRI also correlates with the stability of the pressure value after intervention and even with the lack of survival of the organ [31]. Conversely, low RRI values correlate with a prompt response to treatment of pressure values and renal function.

It must be taken into account that other conditions, aside from the renal artery stenosis, lead to an increase in RRI [32]: tubulointerstitial renal disease, nephroangiosclerosis, hypertension, hydronephrosis, subcapsular and perirenal collections, and severe bradycardia.

10.8 Technological Improvements Over the Years

When studying renal arteries with Doppler sampling issues are always one of the challenges. A 15% of technical failure of the examination is related to the lack of individuation or sampling of the renal artery at its origin frequently related to mixed factors (related to the ultrasound scanner but also to the habitus and the intestinal gas).

Over the years a solution that had several coming and going is the use of contrast medium. Ultrasound contrast medium enhances the Doppler signal inside the vessels and was initially developed as echo amplifiers to be used in all vascular districts. The constant amelioration of the Doppler technology makes them useless in most of the situations but in the study of renal artery stenosis this use had somehow survived over the decades [33]. A positive aspect is the ability to enhance also supernumerary vessels making it more easy to study and sample their Doppler signal. The main downsides are related to an increase in cost and invasiveness.

In literature, the first studies underline that curves are more reproducible and the time to perform the exam significantly decreases [34]. Conversely, sensitivity and specificity do not increase significantly.

Another possible use of ultrasound contrast medium is to quantify renal enhancement using Doppler signal after the administration of a contrast medium bolus (sono-scintigraphy) [33]. This technique allows to create time-intensity curves and some authors demonstrated an AUC wider in renal artery stenosis than in healthy volunteers [35]. In severe stenosis, a delay in the wash-in phase was also underlined. Nowadays, even after almost a decade of study, these methods seem to be far from being adopted in the clinical practice.

As already mentioned the most up-to-date ultrasound scanners had reduced the necessity of contrast medium as an echo enhancer almost to zero thanks to B-mode and Doppler frequency decoupling. B-mode imaging uses a relatively high harmonic frequency (4–6 MHz) while Doppler imaging had a lower frequency (less than 1.75 MHz). Motion and wall filters reduced artifacts increasing the diagnostic confidence and the ability to detect supernumerary arteries. Microconvex or vectorial low-frequency probe had been proposed to sample deeper vessels or increase the effectiveness of the abdominal compression but this dedicated probe is not used routinely.

10.9 Follow-Up After Revascularization

The velocity assessment after revascularization generally shows a decrease in PSV and a reduction in turbulence. Even after stenting, ultrasound has no limitation or artifacts impairing its ability to study renal vessels before, inside the stent, and distal to it.

Doppler may also find a sectorial but important application when a cholesterinic embolization is suspected (generally after a radiological interventional procedure or after a surgical intervention on the renal artery). This complication, generally found in patients with severe atherosclerosis, is characterized by a partial occlusion of the peripheral vascular bed. Doppler velocimetry shows a global reduction in the velocity of the flow with a characteristic disappearance or severe reduction in the diastolic component.

10.10 Atherosclerotic Stenosis

10.10.1 CT

The typical feature of an *atherosclerotic stenosis* is an eccentric and irregular stricture of the renal artery by atherosclerotic plaque. CT allows to distinguish calcified hard plaques from hypoattenuating soft plaques and the distinction between ostial and truncal stenosis that may be useful for planning angiographic interventions [35].

CT gives an accurate grading of stenosis on a five-point scale: grade 0: no stenosis (<30%); grade I: nonsignificant (30–50%); grade II: moderate (50–70%); grade III: high grade (70% low to 100%); and grade IV: occlusion (100%) [35].

A significant stenosis is often associated with post-stenotic dilatation and collateral vessels also indicate a long-standing high-grade stenosis or an occlusion.

Indirect sign can be observed on standard CT examinations. Asymmetry in kidney size (right kidney 2 cm smaller than the left, or left kidney 1.5 cm smaller than the right), cortical thinning, different level of enhancement, and time to excretion between two kidneys may suggest unilateral significant renal artery stenosis.

For computed tomography the overall sensitivity, specificity, and positive and negative predictive accuracy in the detection of atherosclerotic stenosis are 94%, 93%, 71%, and 99% [36]. But it is essential to know that extensive calcifications can obscure the blood flow in RA on MIP reformations and lead to an overestimation of the stenosis. In this case a careful evaluation of source or volume-rendered images is needed not to overestimate the degree of stenosis [37, 38]. If the cross-sectional images are disregarded and only the MIP is considered the diagnostic accuracy of CT declines to 80–90% [35].

CT should not be used for screening of all hypertensive patients related to the low prevalence of RA stenosis. CT is a screening tool in patients who have high clinical suspicion of renovascular hypertension and, given the high negative predictive value, a normal CT can exclude a significant stenosis [35].

CT is a reliable tool for pre-interventional assessment of vascular condition; it can demonstrate vessel variants such as accessory vessels or an unusual shift in vascular origin, can quantify the degree of stenosis, and can distinguish hard or soft plaque and ostial or truncal stenosis [35].

10.10.2 MRI

Typical findings of MRI in renal artery stenosis are the following:

- Loss of cortico-medullary differentiation in unenhanced T1-weighted images: Although this finding is a nonspecific marker of renal dysfunction, it is expected in ischemic nephropathy because of the reduction of blood flow, which is more pronounced in the cortex than in the medulla [39].
- Delayed and decreased medullary enhancement: The transit time of contrast medium from cortex to medulla is longer in case of renal artery stenosis and decreased function. As a result, dysfunctional kidneys present delayed medullary enhancement during the tubular phase (1–4 min) instead of the first 20 s [39].
- For the same reason explained above, a delayed scan (10 min after contrast administration) shows asymmetrical signal intensity in collecting systems, caused by decreased renal excretory function [39].

- Acceleration of blood flow at stenosis, detectable using 3D phase-contrast (PC) MRA: This sequence shows normal-flowing blood bright; in case of severe stenosis (>75% narrowing) a black jet is observed. This sequence is characterized by underestimation of mild stenosis and overestimation of severe ones [39].
- Loss of parenchymal volume/renal atrophy as a result of long-term ischemia: A difference of more than 1 cm in kidney size should be considered as a sign of ischemia of kidney [39].

When there is bilateral renal artery stenosis, both kidneys reduce in size, making this criterion less useful. Atrophic kidneys are less likely to benefit from revascularization because the parenchyma has been destroyed.

10.10.3 Nuclear Medicine

Renal artery stenosis and renovascular hypertension had always been evaluated also with nuclear medicine. While functional problems in several settings are no longer evaluated with nuclear medicine renovascular hypertension remains an indication for those studies after more than 40 years and after all the technological improvement over imaging techniques.

The understanding of the mechanism behind the nuclear medicine studies needs a full understanding of the functioning of the renin-angiotensin-aldosterone (RAA) system. A drop in renal perfusion (such as one tied to a renal artery stenosis) causes the release by the glomerular structures of renin. Renin is an enzyme that converts circulating angiotensinogen in angiotensin I. Angiotensin-converting enzyme (ACE) converts angiotensin I into angiotensin II. Angiotensin II causes an increase in renal perfusion both directly (causing peripheral vasoconstriction) and indirectly (stimulating the release of aldosterone which increases extracellular fluids by increasing the sodium reabsorption).

Because of these compensatory systems if a renal scintigraphy was performed in a patient with a renal artery stenosis no difference would be spotted. But if the RAA system is temporarily shorted out a difference can be easily detected. For this reason the "captopril test" (Fig. 10.10) is a simple and elegant way to detect a unilateral drop in renal perfusion (generally tied to a renal artery stenosis). The captopril is a drug able to interrupt the RAA cascade. After captopril administration the renal scintigraphy clearly demonstrates the difference between the normally/increased perfused kidney (without stenosis) and the one with a lower perfusion (likely caused by a renal artery stenosis) (Fig. 10.11). A decrease of more than 40% in the relative GFR in the stenotic kidney and a delayed peak uptake of more than 10 min are the two main diagnostic criteria [40].

The positive aspects of the renal scintigraphy after captopril administration are the high sensi-

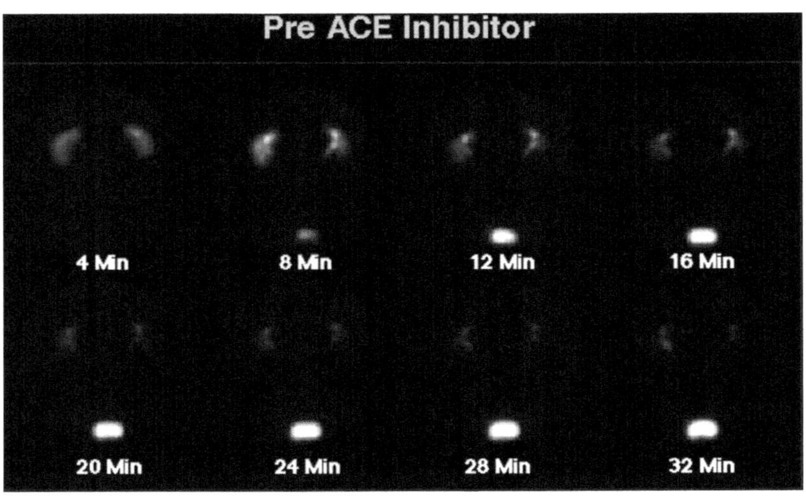

Fig. 10.10 *Captopril test*: Renal scintigraphy after ACE inhibitor administration shows a non-pathological condition with normally perfused kidneys

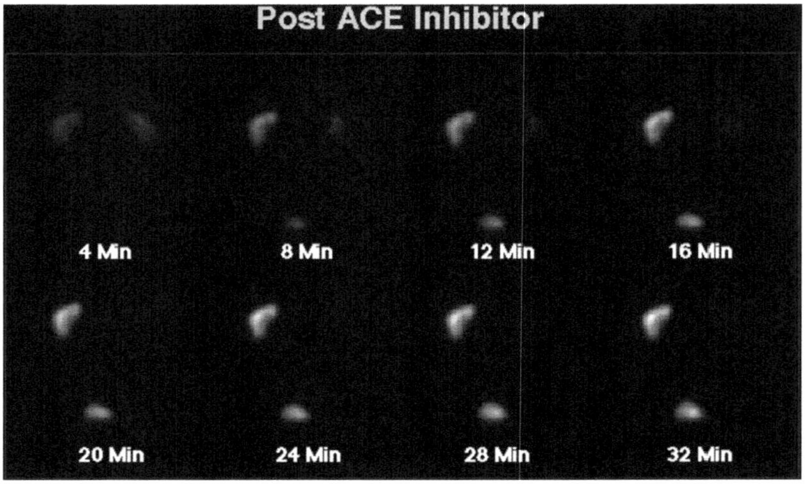

Fig. 10.11 *Captopril test*: Renal scintigraphy after ACE inhibitor administration shows a pathological condition with normally perfused right kidney, without renal artery stenosis, and left kidney with a lower perfusion caused by a renal artery stenosis

tivity and specificity, respectively, of 93–100% and 80–95% [41]. The main downside is the absence of standardization: several factors from the agent used for scintigraphy in the dose and timing of its administration are extremely variable from a center to another. Other downsides are related to the possibility of a bilateral stenosis (with the same or a different degree of obstruction) and the loss of efficiency in patients with renal insufficiency. Since captopril is an ACE inhibitor some patients may not be suitable for the exam (e.g., aortic stenosis).

A particular warning must be put on the sensitivity/specificity data for renal scintigraphy; these data vary during the decades and are influenced by several factors such as the advancement done with other imaging technologies. Unfortunately the trend in sensitivity/specificity reports seems to be a negative one: from the first report of Muller (sensitivity/specificity 100/95%) in 1986 to the slightly worst 93–100/80–95% in 1998. Newest comparison seems to more markedly downgrade the ability of renal scintigraphy to detect abnormalities to a poor 52/63% [42]; because of this poor performance, the authors do not recommend renal scintigraphy to assess renal artery stenosis. Although these last data may be lower than the reality, they clearly depict nowadays a trend to put aside renal scintigraphy in favor of other imaging techniques such as MR and CT. This poor performance had been confirmed also in the pediatric population (48–73%) [43].

To overcome the problem of the lack of standardization several attempts had been made. One of the most thorough evaluations had been published in 1999 [44]. Several aspects such as patient preparation (and especially hydration), radiopharmaceutical types and dose, and patient and camera positioning (including quality control and correction) had been evaluated and recommendations were issued.

One of the most complex aspects to regulate is surely radiopharmaceutical selection among those available for this study. The first choices are ^{123}I orthoiodohippurate (^{123}I OIH) and ^{99m}Tc MAG_3. ^{99m}Tc-DTPA must be avoided particularly in patients with impaired renal function. In addition the superiority of ^{99m}Tc MAG_3 over ^{99m}Tc-DTPA has been demonstrated in several papers, thus discouraging the use of ^{99m}Tc-DTPA [45]. Nonetheless some papers suggest that a combined use of more agents (with different properties, e.g., ^{99m}Tc-DTPA and ^{99m}Tc-MAG3) may be helpful [46].

As already stated other imaging techniques (such as US, CT, and MR) had undergone several technological improvements over the years. While renal scintigraphy had not undergone a profound technological improvement several improvements were nonetheless introduced. Among them it is important to underline the importance of the introduction of deconvolution methods to differentiate both normal kidney from those with renal artery stenosis and kidney with renal artery stenosis from those with parenchymal insufficiency [47].

In pediatric patients all imaging methods seem to be fairly useless since the fibromuscular dysplasia causing the renal artery stenosis affects mainly small branches. Not only nuclear medicine but almost all the imaging methods are therefore severely impaired in their diagnostic power since the involvement of one or several small branches is very difficult to be detected also with MR and CT and not only by US or nuclear medicine. In the pediatric population some studies suggest a primary role for angiography [48], in patients with a strong suggestion for stenosis, being both diagnostic and therapeutic. Nonetheless along the pathologies causing renal artery stenosis in pediatric patients there are some uncommon such as the Moya-Moya disease. Moya-Moya disease can cause bilateral stenosis but nonetheless captopril renal scintigraphy seems to show a good performance [49]. Also Page kidney, caused by microvascular ischemia inducing hypertension through an improper activation of RAA system caused by parenchymal compression, may show a significant value not only monitoring the renal function but also determining the appropriate treatment (among medical and surgical ones).

10.10.4 Angiography

The common angiographic aspect of an atherosclerotic lesion is an eccentric narrowing within 1 cm to the renal ostium, usually associated with a post-stenotic dilatation (Fig. 10.12). A 70% degree of stenosis is usually considered significant, with a systolic pressure gradient >20 mmHg between the aorta and the renal artery distally to the lesion or >10% of mean arterial pressure.

Other indirect signs suggesting a renal stenosis are slow distal flow to the lesion, the presence of collateral circulation, and the reduced size of the kidney.

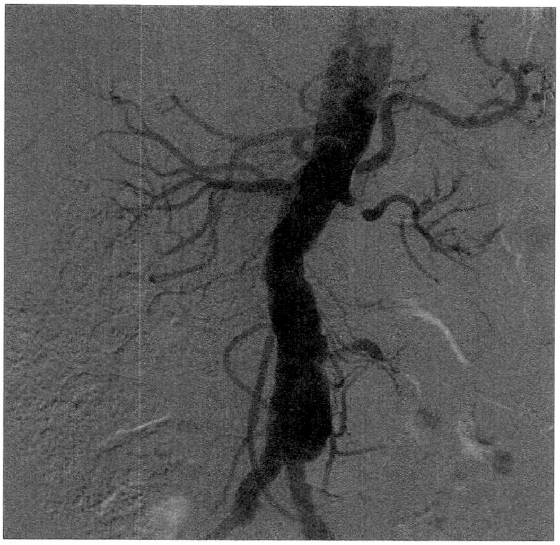

Fig. 10.12 Pigtail catheter *arteriography* of the aorta shows a sub-occlusive stenosis of the left renal artery

Comparisons of angioplasty with or without stenting for atheromatous disease showed increased long-term renal artery patency with the use of stents [50]. But the management of atherosclerotic renal artery stenosis is still on debate, because some recent randomized trials have failed to show any benefit of revascularization over the best medical therapy (STAR, CORAL, ASTRAL) [51–53], probably due to population selection bias [54]. In fact it is well demonstrated in case reports and case series that renal stenting has an impact on blood pressure control, renal function, and left ventricular hypertrophy on a group of patients.

The management of renovascular hypertension is still problematic and controversial.

Pre-interventional translesional pressure gradient measurement can provide information about the hemodynamic relevance of the stenosis, but is not recommended as a routine procedure.

Distal embolic protection devices are used to reduce the peri-interventional risk of renal atheroembolism, but its usefulness is still on debate.

In cases of highly calcified tight lesions, predilatation should be performed to allow full stent expansion. Balloon-expandable stents are usually used with a stent-to-vessel ratio of 1.1:1 and with the minor length possible to cover the lesion, with a dilation time of at least 23–30 s to permit full stent expansion. The role of drug-eluting stents and covered stents is still uncertain.

Post-interventional angiogram, without the guidewire in place, should be performed to evaluate the treated lesion and to exclude peripheral embolism, renal perforation, or dissection.

10.11 Fibromuscular Dysplasia

Fibromuscular dysplasia (FMD) is the second most common cause of renovascular hypertension. In almost one-third of the patients, it occurs mainly in young women between 30 and 55 years of age.

FMD is classified into six different types in relation to the layer of the arterial wall involved and histopathologic findings: medial fibroplasia (60–70%), perimedial fibroplasia (20%), medial hyperplasia (5–15%), medial dissection (5–10%), intimal fibroplasia (1–2%), and adventitial fibroplasia (<1%) [55].

FMD typically affects both renal arteries, most frequently mid and distal segments of the arteries [3, 56]. Renal artery branches are rarely affected without concomitant disease in extrarenal arteries and such cases of isolated intrarenal FMD are extremely hard to detect.

Association of FMD with Ehlers-Danlos syndrome, Alport syndrome, pheochromocytoma, Marfan syndrome, and Takayasu arteritis has been described [57]. Complications of FMD include aneurysm formation dissection and renal artery occlusion.

10.11.1 Fibromuscular Dysplasia

10.11.1.1 CT

FMD is seen as a unifocal or multifocal stenosis with alternating areas of short segmental strictures and aneurysmal dilations called string-of-pearls appearance.

The sensitivity of CT in FMD is lower at 75–80%.

10.11.1.2 Angiography

The typical angiographic feature is the presence of multifocal string of beads at the medial-distal portion of the renal artery and small focal stenosis in the distal segments of the renal arteries [58]. There are other uncommon variants, such as the following:

- Perimedial FMD, with fewer beads of smaller diameter and collateral arteries around the stenosis
- Medial hyperplasia, with a concentric focal band
- Intimal FMD, with a focal concentric stenosis due to a long smooth narrowing or a focal band-like narrowing
- Adventitial FMD, with a perimedial collar of focal stenosis

Percutaneous transluminal angioplasty (PTA) is the gold standard treatment for stenosis of fibromuscular disease origin [59] in case of symptomatic disease (renovascular hypertension or renal atrophy). Stent placement, which is the common endovascular treatment for atherosclerotic stenosis, is not advised in FMD and has been reserved for cases with complications, such as dissection or restenosis or persistent hypertension. Angioplasty alone results in reduction of blood pressure in few weeks, with good acute and long-term results with restenosis rate of about 10%.

10.12 Renal Artery Aneurysm

Renal artery aneurysm is a dilated segment of renal artery that exceeds twice the diameter of a normal renal artery, with preservation of all three layers of the vessel wall (intima, media, and adventitia) [60].

Renal artery aneurysm is an uncommon disease in the general population (0.1%), accounts for 22% of all visceral aneurysms, and is mainly asymptomatic [61, 62]. In rare cases a spontaneous rupture might complicate RA aneurysm, leading to perinephric or retroperitoneal hematoma.

Renal artery aneurysms can be classified according to their location, morphology, and dimension in extraparenchymal or intraparenchymal, saccular or fusiform, and macro- (>1 cm) or microaneurysms (<1 cm), respectively.

Saccular extraparenchymal ones are the most diffused. The most common etiologies are atherosclerosis and FMD [4, 6]. In 20% of patients with renal artery aneurysms, the pathology is bilateral and in 30% they have multiple aneurysms [63].

RA aneurysms have also been reported in association with vasculitis, connective tissue disease, neurofibromatosis, infection, and trauma. CT with MPR and MIPs allows to measure the aneurysm neck and to distinguish between saccular and fusiform aneurysms (Fig. 10.13). These findings are essential to choose between a percutaneous endovascular and open surgical approach for intervention [55].

A different kind of abnormal vessel dilatation is the pseudoaneurysm. The *pseudoaneurysm* arises from direct arterial injuries (inflammatory or traumatic) which result in disruption of arterial wall continuity. Under the influence of arterial pressure, blood extravasates and dissects through the injured arterial wall and it is contained by the media or adventitia or by extravascular surrounding tissues.

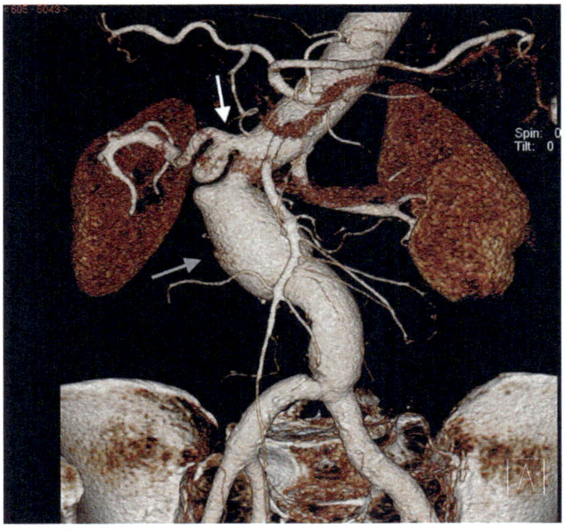

Fig. 10.13 *Computed tomography* angiography of the renal arteries, in volume rendering, shows saccular macroaneurysm of right renal artery (*white arrow*) in the presence of a sub-renal abdominal aortic aneurysm (*grey arrow*)

The pseudoaneurysms are usually acquired, especially for iatrogenic causes such as surgical or percutaneous procedures, and have a saccular shape, or are secondary to phlogistic (mycotic) causes [64] or Kawasaki disease [65].

Instead the causes of multiple intraparenchymal pseudoaneurysms include vasculitis and amphetamine use [60].

10.12.1 Endovascular Embolization of Renal Artery Aneurysm

Treatment is indicated for aneurysms larger than 2 cm or for aneurysms of any size in women of childbearing age [66] because spontaneous rupture of a renal artery aneurysm is more likely to occur during pregnancy due to increased blood flow and intra-abdominal pressure, and vascular changes secondary to increased steroid production [67]. Other indications for intervention are an enlarging or symptomatic renal artery aneurysm (hypertension, pain, renal ischemia, or infarction) or its rupture.

On the basis of the anatomy and location, Rundback et al. proposed an angiographic classification system [68] with different modality managements:

- Type I: saccular aneurysm, which arises either from the main renal artery trunk or proximally from a large segmental artery. It can be treated with exclusion through stent-graft (Fig. 10.14) or stent/balloon coil embolization (Fig. 10.15).
- Type II: fusiform aneurysm, which occurs at the main renal artery or proximal segmental arteries. Surgical treatment is the best option.
- Type III: intraparenchymal aneurysms, affecting the small segmental or accessory arteries. Coil embolization allows minimal loss of parenchyma, preserving the distal perfusion of the normal parenchyma. Embolization of intraparenchymal aneurysms can be achieved with regular nondetachable coils, detachable coils, N-butyl cyanoacrylate, ethylene vinyl copolymer, or gelfoam.

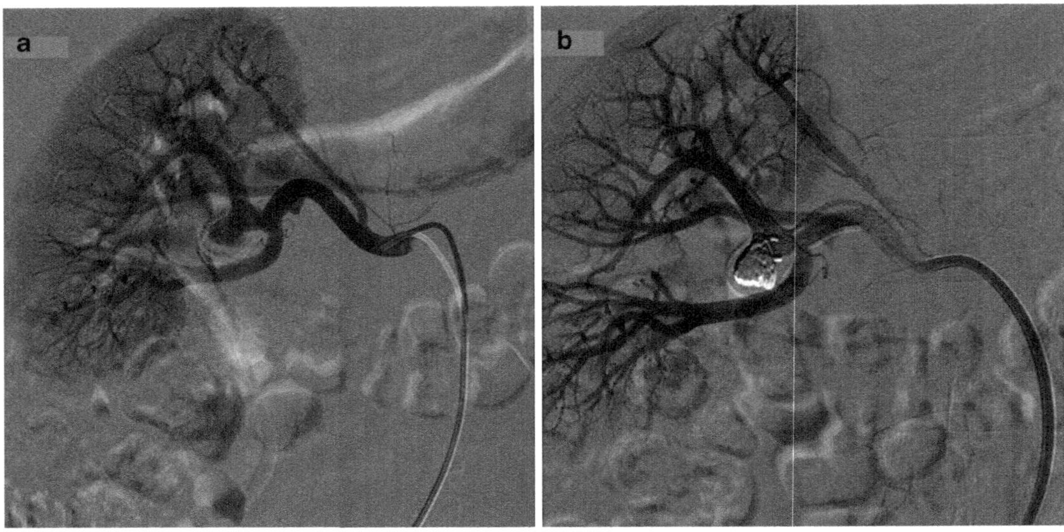

Fig. 10.14 Pigtail catheter *arteriography* of the aorta (**a**) shows an aneurysm of the right renal artery and subsequent exclusion of the aneurysm by stent-graft placement (**b**)

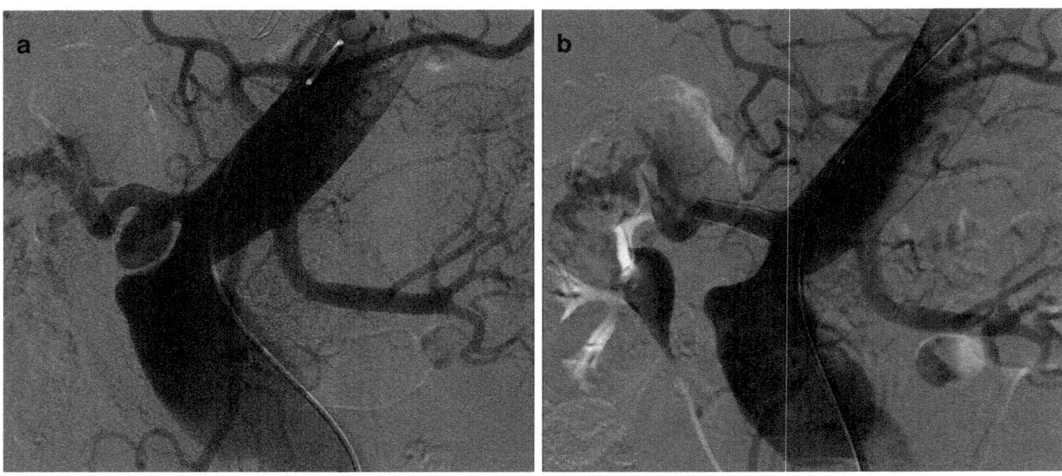

Fig. 10.15 Selective right renal *arteriography* (**a**) shows a renal hilum aneurysm and subsequent superselective embolization with metal coils (**b**)

10.13 Arteriovenous Malformations

Renal arteriovenous malformation (AVM) is a very rare abnormal communication between artery and vein; they may be congenital or acquired, and often iatrogenic. Renal AVMs are usually identified during evaluation of hematuria and hypertension, flank pain, and high cardiac output failure, primarily depending on the size and location [69].

There are two subtypes of congenital AVMs [70]:

- Cirsoid, which is characterized by multiple tortuous and dilated communications between the arteries and veins, usually larger than 1 cm in diameter and located adjacent to the collecting system.
- Cavernous, when a single artery feeds into a single cystic chamber, with a single draining

vein; they are usually less than 1 cm in diameter and located near the periphery.

On CTA renal AVM is shown as abnormal tortuous vascular channels in the renal sinus and surrounding the pelvic calyceal system with enlarged feeding renal artery, and draining renal vein [71].

Angiographic embolization is the preferred treatment for symptomatic AVMs.

10.14 Renal Artery Dissection

The most common cause of renal artery dissection is the extension of an aortic dissection [72, 73].

Spontaneous isolated dissection of the renal artery without aortic dissection is rare and the etiology includes blunt injury, iatrogenic trauma, atherosclerosis, and fibromuscular dysplasia [74].

Iatrogenic dissections are increasing with more frequent use of interventional treatment techniques and usually during catheter manipulation or balloon dilation [75].

In dissection, renal artery flow can be compromised either by direct extension of the aortic aneurysm into the renal artery or by collapsed or thrombosed true or false lumen from which RA arises.

The visualization of the intimal flap is the most specific finding for the diagnosis of renal dissection; however, it may not be always demonstrated in all cases and the parenchymal effects (cortical hypoperfusion) can be the only findings [55].

Treatment remains controversial; revascularization is usually reserved for cases refractory to medical therapy, based on a combination of antihypertensive drugs and systemic anticoagulation. Renal artery dissection that leads to renal dysfunction or recalcitrant hypertension may be treated through endovascular revascularization with stent placement or surgical treatment.

10.15 Acute Renal Artery Occlusion: Renal Artery Thrombosis

Acute renal artery occlusion can be secondary to thrombosis (traumatic or iatrogenic) or thromboembolism, most frequently cardiogenic embolism due to atrial fibrillation, myocardial infarction (postinfarction thrombi), and rheumatic mitral stenosis [76].

Acute renal artery occlusion can be symptomatic (acute flank pain, hematuria, proteinuria), and it should be suspected in patients with a history of atrial fibrillation, valvular heart disease, endocarditis, or previous embolic episodes.

Contrast-enhanced CT is able to identify the arterial filling defect and partial or complete lack of cortical enhancement [66].

10.16 Vasculitis

Takayasu disease is a rare nonspecific arteritis of unknown etiology and affects most frequently young Asian women. The disease commonly involves the aorta, its proximal branches, and the pulmonary arteries [77]. Rarely, it may involve the abdominal aorta and renal arteries, resulting in renovascular hypertension.

The early phase of the disease is characterized by inflammation of the involved vessels and mural thickening.

In the early and active phase of the disease, contrast-enhanced CT can demonstrate arterial wall thickening and hyperenhancement [78, 79].

This disease leads to progressive arterial stenosis, occlusion, and aneurysm formation [55].

Polyarteritis nodosa is a medium and small artery vasculitis and commonly involves the kidneys [80].

Arterial alterations include vessel irregularity, microaneurysms, dissection, stenosis, and occlusion.

Microaneurysms often are multiple and intraparenchymal, and the diagnostic utility of CT in assessing them is limited [61]. However CT can show perirenal and subcapsular hematomas in case of aneurysm rupture and wedge-shaped hypoenhanced areas in renal infarcts [81].

Radiation arteritis of renal artery tends to present years after irradiation and is an occlusive disease within the irradiated field with characteristic sparing of no irradiated arteries [82, 83].

10.17 Renal Vein Thrombosis

Renal vein thrombosis can result from a variety of conditions like glomerulonephritis, collagen vascular disease, dehydration, sepsis trauma, and malignancy [7, 84].

It involves the left side more frequently and can cause either incomplete or complete obstruction.

Contrast-enhanced CT shows directly a filling defect of renal vein and, in complete obstruction, secondary signs such as enlargement of the kidney and delay in the cortical nephrogram may be present.

If the obstruction is long-standing, extensive collaterals may develop [85, 86].

Renal cell carcinoma may grow into renal vein and cause a tumor thrombus, which can extend into the inferior vena cava and further into the right side of the heart.

CE CT shows the tumor thrombus as a hypodense filling defect and, unlike the bland thrombus, that enhances on delayed phase and causes venous distension [87].

10.18 Spontaneous Splenorenal Shunt

Spontaneous portosystemic shunts or varices are a common complication of severe liver disease and portal hypertension, including gastro-renal and splenorenal shunts.

In the latter case enlarged and tortuous collateral veins extend from the splenic hilum to the left renal vein.

Gastro-renal shunts originate from the left gastric vein and reach the left renal vein.

With a routine abdominal CT it is possible to detect the shunts but 3D or MPR images are useful for better understanding of complex vascular anatomy that may not be adequately evaluated in two dimensions.

Such venous mapping is mandatory for surgical planning in liver transplantation and it is also useful for surgery involving left upper quadrant organs [88].

10.19 Renal Varix

Isolated renal vein varices are abnormal renal vein dilation within the renal hilum or a dilated venous network adjacent to the renal pelvis, upper ureter, or convex surface of the kidney.

They usually present without symptoms (or rarely with recurrent hematuria), are easily detectable on routine CT, and often are incidental findings.

Renal varices can occur as a result of an increase in venous pressure due to various reasons including renal vein compression, thrombosis, and inherent weakness of the vessel wall [89].

10.20 Nutcracker Syndrome

The nutcracker syndrome or left renal vein entrapment syndrome is a compression of the left renal vein between the aorta and the superior mesenteric artery.

The compression causes left renal vein outflow obstruction, which results in renal venous hypertension, collateral veins, and gonadal vein reflux.

In most patients this phenomenon has no clinical relevance, but in some cases may cause abdominal pain, hematuria, pelvic congestion syndrome in women, and varicoceles in male [90, 91].

The nutcracker syndrome has a prevalence of 27% in asymptomatic population; it is not a radiologic diagnosis but rather a diagnosis based on a comprehensive review of clinical, laboratory, and radiologic data [92].

10.21 Miscellaneous

Primary renal carcinomas or other *retroperitoneal malignancies* can involve the renal arteries and veins, causing compression, displacement, stenosis, or even occlusions.

Retroperitoneal fibrosis is an inflammatory fibrosing disorder of unknown etiology, included in the diseases called periaortitis, which affects the infrarenal great vessels and the surrounding retroperitoneal structures [55, 93].

Retroperitoneal fibrosis most frequently causes ureteral obstruction, but rarely can involve the renal arteries and veins producing stenosis.

The *median arcuate ligament* (MAL) *syndrome* is an extrinsic compression of abdominal arteries, including renal arteries, due to a low insertion of the MAL or to a high origin of the arteries involved [94].

Segmental arterial mediolysis (SAM) is a rare nonarteriosclerotic, noninflammatory vascular disease of unclear etiology, characterized by vacuolization and lysis of arterial smooth muscle, that causes vessel dissection, dilation, occlusion, or rupture [95, 96].

References

1. Hazirolan T, Oz M, Turkbey B, et al. CT angiography of the renal arteries and veins: normal anatomy and variants. Diagn Interv Radiol. 2011;17:67–73.
2. Beregi JP, Mauroy B, Willoteaux S, et al. Anatomic variation in the origin of the main renal arteries: spiral CTA evaluation. Eur Radiol. 1999;9:1330–4.
3. Quaia E. Radiological imaging of the kidney. Berlin: Springer; 2011.
4. Kadir S. Angiography of the kidneys. Diagnostic angiography. Philadelphia: Saunders; 1986. p. 445–95.
5. Turkvatan A, Ozdemir M, Cumhur T, Olcer T. Multidetector CT angiography of renal vasculature: normal anatomy and variants. Eur Radiol. 2009;19:236–44.
6. Tuna IS, Tatli S. Contrast-enhanced CT and MR imaging of renal vessels. Abdom Imaging. 2014;39:875–91.
7. Urban BA, Ratner LE, Fishman EK. Three-dimensional volume-rendered CT angiography of the renal arteries and veins: normal anatomy, variants, and clinical applications. Radiographics. 2001;21:373–86.
8. Mathews R, Smith PA, Fishman EK, Marshall FF. Anomalies of the inferior vena cava and renal veins: embryologic and surgical considerations. Urology. 1999;53:873–80.
9. Harrison LH Jr, Flye MW, Seigler HF. Incidence of anatomical variants in renal vasculature in the presence of normal renal function. Ann Surg. 1978;188:83–9.
10. Beckmann CF, Abrams HL. Circumaortic venous ring: incidence and significance. AJR. 1979;132:561–5.
11. Matsuoka S, Antoniou EE, Mori K, Hayabuchi Y, Kuroda Y. The first report of a patient with interrupted inferior vena cava, multiple post-renal veins and azygos–hemiazygos continuation. Acta Paediatr Jpn. 1995;37:514–7.
12. Al-Katib S, Shetty M, Jafri SM, Jafri SZ. Radiologic assessment of native renal vasculature: a multimodality review. Radiographics. 2017;37:136–56.
13. Zhang HL, Sos TA, Winchester PA, Gao J, Prince MR. Renal artery stenosis: imaging options, pitfalls, and concerns. Prog Cardiovasc Dis. 2009;52:209–19.
14. Subramaniam M, Mizzi A, Roditi G. Magnetic resonance angiography in potential live renal donors: a joint radiological and surgical evaluation. Clin Radiol. 2004;59:335–41.
15. Israel GM, Lee VS, Edye M, et al. Comprehensive MR imaging in the preoperative evaluation of living donor candidates for laparoscopic nephrectomy: initial experience. Radiology. 2002;225:427–32.
16. Xu X, Lin X, Huang J, Pan Z, Zhu X, Chen K, et al. The capability of inflow inversion recovery magnetic resonance compared to contrast-enhanced magnetic resonance in renal artery angiography. Abdom Radiol. 2017;2:2479–87.
17. Safian RD, Textor SC. Renal- artery stenosis. N Engl J Med. 2001;344:431–42.
18. Feldman RL, Wargovich TJ, Bittl JA. No-touch technique for reducing aortic wall trauma during renal artery stenting. Catheter Cardiovasc Interv. 1999;46(2):245–8.
19. Zachrisson K, Herlitz H, Lönn L, Falkenberg M, Eklöf H. Duplex ultrasound for identifying renal artery stenosis: direct criteria re-evaluated. Acta Radiol. 2017;58:176–82.
20. Andersson Z, Thisted E, Andersen UB. Renal branch artery stenosis: a diagnostic challenge? A case report with review of the literature. Urology. 2017;100:218–20.
21. Tafur-Soto JD, White CJ. Renal artery stenosis. Cardiol Clin. 2015;33:59–73.
22. Staub D, Canevascini R, Huegli RW, et al. Best duplex-sonographic criteria for the assessment of renal artery stenosis--correlation with intra-arterial pressure gradient. Ultraschall Med. 2007;28:45–51.
23. Hoffmann U, Edwards JM, Carter S, et al. Role of duplex scanning for the detection of atherosclerotic renal artery disease. Kidney Int. 1991;39:1232–9.
24. Stavros AT, Parker SH, Yakes WF, et al. Segmental stenosis of the renal artery: pattern recognition of tardus and parvus abnormalities with duplex sonography. Radiology. 1992;184:487–92.

25. Boddi M. Renal ultrasound (and Doppler sonography) in hypertension: an update. Adv Exp Med Biol. 2017;956:191–208.
26. Schwerk WB, Restrepo IK, Stellwaag M, Klose KJ, Schade-Brittinger C. Renal artery stenosis: grading with image-directed Doppler US evaluation of renal resistive index. Radiology. 1994;190:785–90.
27. Bertolotto M, Quaia E, Galli G, Martinoli C, Locatelli M. Color Doppler sonographic appearance of renal perforating vessels in subjects with normal and impaired renal function. J Clin Ultrasound. 2000;28:267–76.
28. René PC, Oliva VL, Bui BT, et al. Renal artery stenosis: evaluation of Doppler US after inhibition of angiotensin-converting enzyme with captopril. Radiology. 1995;196:675–9.
29. Williams GJ, Macaskill P, Chan SF, et al. Comparative accuracy of renal duplex sonographic parameters in the diagnosis of renal artery stenosis: paired and unpaired analysis. AJR Am J Roentgenol. 2007;188:798–811.
30. Gottlieb RH, Lieberman JL, Pabico RC, Waldman DL. Diagnosis of renal artery stenosis in transplanted kidneys: value of Doppler waveform analysis of the intrarenal arteries. AJR Am J Roentgenol. 1995;165:1441–6.
31. Radermacher J, Chavan A, Bleck J, et al. Use of Doppler ultrasonography to predict the outcome of therapy for renal-artery stenosis. N Engl J Med. 2001;344:410–7.
32. Schäberle W, Leyerer L, Schierling W, Pfister K. Ultrasound diagnostics of renal artery stenosis: Stenosis criteria, CEUS and recurrent in-stent stenosis. Gefässchirurgie. 2016;21:4–13.
33. Missouris CG, Allen CM, Balen FG, Buckenham T, Lees WR, MacGregor GA. Non-invasive screening for renal artery stenosis with ultrasound contrast enhancement. J Hypertens. 1996;14:519–24.
34. Lencioni R, Pinto S, Napoli V, Bartolozzi C. Noninvasive assessment of renal artery stenosis: current imaging protocols and future directions in ultrasonography. J Comput Assist Tomogr. 1999;23:S95–100.
35. Prokop M, Galanski M, van der Molen AJ, Schaefer-Prokop CM. (ed) Spiral and multislice computed tomography of the body. Stuttgart: Thieme; 2003.
36. Rountas C, Vlychou M, Vassiou K, et al. Imaging modalities for renal artery stenosis in suspected renovascular hypertension: prospective intraindividual comparison of color Doppler US, CT angiography, GD-enhanced MR angiography, and digital subtraction angiography. Ren Fail. 2007;29:295–302.
37. Tatli S. Magnetic resonance angiography of the aorta and peripheral arteries. In: Kwong RY, editor. Cardiovascular magnetic resonance imaging. Totowa: Humana Press; 2007. p. 567–612.
38. Baskaran V, Pereles FS, Nemcek AA Jr, et al. Gadolinium-enhanced 3D MR angiography of renal artery stenosis: a pilot comparison of maximum intensity projection, multiplanar reformatting, and 3D volume-rendering postprocessing algorithms. Acad Radiol. 2002;9:50–9.
39. Zhang LJ, Wu X, Yang GF, et al. Three-dimensional contrast-enhanced magnetic resonance venography for detection of renal vein thrombosis: comparison with multidetector CT venography. Acta Radiol. 2013;54:1125–13.
40. Kallistratos MS, Giannakopoulos A, German V, Manolis AJ. Diagnostic modalities of the most common forms of secondary hypertension. Hell J Cardiol. 2010;51:518–29.
41. Karasch T, Rubin J. Diagnosis of renal artery stenosis and renovascular hypertension. Eur J Ultrasound. 1998;7:S27–39.
42. Eklöf H, Ahlström H, Magnusson A, et al. A prospective comparison of duplex ultrasonography, captopril renography, MRA, and CTA in assessing renal artery stenosis. Acta Radiol. 2006;47:764–74.
43. Abdulsamea S, Anderson P, Biassoni L, et al. Pre- and postcaptopril renal scintigraphy as a screening test for renovascular hypertension in children. Pediatr Nephrol. 2010;25:317–22.
44. Prigent A, Cosgriff P, Gates GF, et al. Consensus report on quality control of quantitative measurements of renal function obtained from the renogram: International Consensus Committee from the Scientific Committee of Radionuclides in Nephrourology. Semin Nucl Med. 1999;29:146–59.
45. Kiratli PO, Caner B, Altun B, Cekirge S. Superiority of tc-99m MAG3 to tc-99m DTPA in treating a patient with mild renal artery stenosis. Ann Nucl Med. 2001;15:45–8.
46. Itoh K, Matsui Y, Kato C, Mochizuki T, Kitabatake A. Differences between 99mTc-DTPA and 99mTc-MAG3 captopril renographies in renovascular hypertension. Ann Nucl Med. 1996;10:251–5.
47. Kempi V. Renogram and deconvolution parameters in diagnosis of renal artery stenosis. Variants of background subtraction and analysis techniques. Nuklearmedizin. 2007;46:281–90.
48. Reusz GS, Kis E, Cseprekál O, Szabó AJ, Kis E. Captopril-enhanced renal scintigraphy in the diagnosis of pediatric hypertension. Pediatr Nephrol. 2010;25:185–9.
49. Choi Y, Kang BC, Kim KJ, et al. Renovascular hypertension in children with moyamoya disease. J Pediatr. 1997;131:258–63.
50. Van de Ven PJG, Kaatee R, Beutler JJ, et al. Arterial stenting and balloon angioplasty in ostial atherosclerotic renovascular disease: a randomised trial. Lancet. 1999;353(9149):282–6.
51. Cooper CJ, Murphy TP, Cutlip DE, et al. Stenting and medical therapy for atherosclerotic renal-artery stenosis. N Engl J Med. 2014;370(1):13–22.
52. Wheatley K, Ives N, Gray R, et al. Revascularization versus medical therapy for renal-artery stenosis. N Engl J Med. 2009;361(20):1953–62.
53. Bax L, Woittiez AJ, Kouwenberg HJ, et al. Stent placement in patients with atherosclerotic renal artery

stenosis and impaired renal function: a randomized trial. Ann Intern Med. 2009;150:840–8.
54. Mousa AY, AbuRahma AF, Bozzay J, et al. Update on intervention versus medical therapy for atherosclerotic renal artery stenosis. J Vasc Surg. 2015;61(6):1613–23.
55. Flors L, Leiva-Salinas CL, Ali Ahmad E, et al. MD CT angiography and MR angiography of nonatherosclerotic renal artery disease. Cardiovasc Intervent Radiol. 2011;34:1151–64.
56. Das CJ, Neyaz Z, Thapa P, Sharma S, Vashist S. Fibromuscular dysplasia of the renal arteries: a radiological review. Int Urol Nephrol. 2007;39:233–8.
57. Slovut DP, Olin JW. Fibromuscular dysplasia. N Engl J Med. 2004;350:1862–71.
58. Persu A, Touze E, Mousseaux E, et al. Diagnosis and management of fibromuscular dysplasia: an expert consensus. Eur J Clin Investig. 2011;42(3):338–47.
59. Trinquart L, Mounier-Vehier C, Sapoval M, et al. Efficacy of revascularization for renal artery stenosis caused by fibromuscular dysplasia. A systematic review and meta-analysis. Hypertension. 2010;56:525–32.
60. Working Group on Renovascular Hypertension. Detection, evaluation, and treatment of renovascular hypertension. Final report. Arch Intern Med. 1987;147:820–9.
61. Dieter RS, Schmidt WS, Pacanowski JP, Jaff MR. Renovascular hypertension. Expert Rev Cardiovasc Ther. 2005;3:413–22.
62. Eskandari MK, Resnick SA. Aneurysms of the renal artery. Semin Vasc Surg. 2005;18:202–8.
63. Stanley JC, Rhodes EL, Gewertz BL, et al. Renal artery aneurysms. Significance of macroaneurysms exclusive of dissections and fibrodysplastic mural dilations. Arch Surg. 1975;110(11):1327–33.
64. Ohebshalom MM, Tah JA, Coll D, et al. Massive hematuria due to right renal artery mycotic pseudoaneurysm in a patient with subacute bacterial endocarditis. Urology. 2001;58(4):607.
65. Yacoe ME, Dake MD. Development and resolution of systemic and coronary artery aneurysms in Kawasaki disease. AJR. 1992;159(4):708–10.
66. Kawashima A, Sandler CM, Ernst RD, et al. CT evaluation of renovascular disease. Radiographics. 2000;20:1321–40.
67. Love WK, Robinette MA, Vernon CP. Renal artery aneurysm rupture in pregnancy. J Urol. 1981;126:809–11.
68. Rundback JH, Rizvi A, Rozenblit GN, et al. Percutaneous stent-graft management of renal artery aneurysms. J Vasc Interv Radiol. 2000;11:1189–93.
69. An HS, Kang TG, Yun HJ, et al. Hypertension caused by renal arteriovenous fistula. Korean Circ J. 2009;39:548–50.
70. Munoz IA, Bustos GA, Pardal AG, et al. Heart failure and severe pulmonary hypertension secondary to a giant renal arteriovenous malformation. J Ultrasound Med. 2006;25:933–7.
71. Riedlinger WF, Kissane JM, Gibfried M, Liapis H. Congenital bilateral renal arteriovenous malformation: an unrecognized cause of renal failure. Pediatr Dev Pathol. 2004;7:285–9.
72. Tatli S, Yucel EK, Lipton MJ. CT and MR imaging of the thoracic aorta: current techniques and clinical applications. Radiol Clin N Am. 2004;42:565–85.
73. Kanofsky JA, Lepor H. Spontaneous renal artery dissection. Rev Urol. 2007;9:156–60.
74. Katz-Summercorn AC, Borg CM, Harris PL. Spontaneous renal artery dissection complicated by renal infarction: a case report and review of the literature. Int J Surg Case Rep. 2012;3:257–9.
75. Bostwick DG, Chang L. Non-neoplastic diseases of kidney. Urologic surgical pathology. 2nd ed. Edinburgh: Mosby Elsevier; 2008. p. 39.
76. Amilineni V, Lackner DF, Morse WS, Srinivas N. Contrast-enhanced CT for acute flank pain caused by acute renal artery occlusion. AJR. 2000;174:105–6.
77. Sharma S, Saxena A, Talwar KK, et al. Renal artery stenosis caused by nonspecific arteritis (Takayasu disease): results of treatment with percutaneous transluminal angioplasty. AJR. 1992;158:417–22.
78. Canyigit M, Peynircioglu B, Hazirolan T, et al. Imaging characteristics of Takayasu arteritis. Cardiovasc Intervent Radiol. 2007;30:711–8.
79. Nastri MV, Baptista LP, Baroni RH, et al. Gadolinium-enhanced three-dimensional MR angiography of Takayasu arteritis. Radiographics. 2004;24:773–86.
80. Ozaki K, Miyayama S, Ushiogi Y, et al. Renal involvement of polyarteritis nodosa: CT and MR findings. Abdom Imaging. 2009;34:265–70.
81. Liu PS, Platt JF. CT angiography of the renal circulation. Radiol Clin N Am. 2010;48:347–65. viii–ix
82. Modrall JG, Sadjadi J. Early and late presentations of radiation arteritis. Semin Vasc Surg. 2003;16:209–14.
83. Spira D, Kotter I, Ernemann U, et al. Imaging of primary and secondary inflammatory diseases involving large and medium-sized vessels and their potential mimics: a multitechnique approach. AJR Am J Roentgenol. 2010;194:848–56.
84. Gonzalez R, Schwartz S, Sheldon CA, Fraley EE. Bilateral renal vein thrombosis in infancy and childhood. Urol Clin North Am. 1982;9:279–83.
85. Si-Hoe CK, Thng CH, Chee SG, Teo EK, Chng HH. Abdominal computed tomography in systemic lupus erythematosus. Clin Radiol. 1997;52:284–9.
86. Zhang LJ, Wu X, Yang GF, et al. Three-dimensional contrast-enhanced magnetic resonance venography for detection of renal vein thrombosis: comparison with multidetector CT venography. Acta Radiol. 2013;54:1125–31.
87. Smith PA, Marshall FF, Urban BA, Heath DG, Fishman EK. Three-dimensional CT stereoscopic visualization of renal masses: impact on diagnosis and patient treatment. AJR. 1997;169:1331–4.
88. Henseler KP, Pozniak MA, Lee FT Jr, Winter TC 3rd. Three-dimensional CT angiography of spontaneous portosystemic shunts. Radiographics. 2001;21:691–704.

89. Beckmann CF, Abrams HL. Idiopathic renal vein varices: incidence and significance. Radiology. 1982;143:649–52.
90. Rudloff U, Holmes RJ, Prem JT, et al. Mesoaortic compression of the left renal vein (nutcracker syndrome): case reports and review of the literature. Ann Vasc Surg. 2006;20:120–9.
91. Venkatachalam S, Bumpus K, Kapadia SR, et al. The nutcracker syndrome. Ann Vasc Surg. 2011;25:1154–64.
92. Lars JG, Bjorn IE, Rendon CN, et al. Incidental detection of nutcracker phenomenon on multidetector CT in an asymptomatic population: prevalence and associated findings. J Comput Assist Tomogr. 2013;37:415–8.
93. Scheel PJ Jr, Feeley N. Retroperitoneal fibrosis: the clinical, laboratory, and radiographic presentation. Medicine (Baltimore). 2009;88:202–7.
94. Ilica AT, Kocaoglu M, Bilici A, et al. Median arcuate ligament syndrome: multidetector computed tomography findings. J Comput Assist Tomogr. 2007;31:728–31.
95. Soulen MC, Cohen DL, Itkin M, et al. Segmental arterial mediolysis: angioplasty of bilateral renal artery stenoses with 2-year imaging follow-up. J Vasc Interv Radiol. 2004;15:763–7.
96. Michael M, Widmer U, Wildermuth S, et al. Segmental arterial mediolysis: CTA findings at presentation and follow-up. AJR Am J Roentgenol. 2006;187:1463–9.

Renal Traumas in Nephrologic Patients

11

Mario Scuderi, Maurizio Mannino, Elena Schembari, Walter Terranova, and Valeria Urzia

11.1 Introduction

Although modern driving safety standards have reduced mortality caused by cranial trauma, they have not significantly changed the incidence of abdominal trauma, particularly of renal trauma (representing 10% of all abdominal traumas).

This is due to the modality of impacts, frequently lateral, and often destructive [1].

Car accident represent the major cause of abdominal trauma (61% of the total), while accidental injuries, pedestrian injuries, and sports injuries are, respectively, the second, third, and fourth major causes representing 11%, 9%, and 7% of the total [1].

Male sex is more involved in abdominal trauma (M.F = 3:1) mostly in the second and third decades. Pediatric age is however the most prevalent one due to the higher vulnerability of the natural anatomic protection systems.

Relating to the last aspect, kidneys are situated in a deep anatomic space well protected by bone structures (thoracic bones, vertebra, hip bone).

Capsula, peritoneal fascia, and interposed soft-tissue amortized trauma reduce kinetic energy.

Kidneys do not have a real sustainable system. The vascular pedicle and the urinary tract are the only anchorage structures which the enormous pressures generated by high-velocity trauma vent on.

The susceptibility of the renal parenchyma to traumatic insult grows in parallel to the increase of speed, impact power, and energetic absorption [1].

The relative mobility of the kidneys and the possibility of collisions with the adjacent stiffer organs such as iliac crest, last ribs, and spinal column are the principal causes of renal damage due to crash, deceleration, and backlash.

For example, the compression of the kidney with the spinal column causes an increase in pressure until the development of blast injuries.

During a sudden deceleration, kidney moves faster and more widely than the aorta and the ureter, tearing the renal artery and the ureter-pelvic junction.

More than 90% of the lesions intersect the renal parenchyma and segmentary vascular branches.

M. Scuderi (✉)
III Level Emergency Department, Operative Unit of Emergency Ultrasound, Hospital School SIUM "Urgency-Emergency", Cannizzaro Hospital for vv, Catania, Italy
e-mail: mscuderi@tiscali.it

M. Mannino · E. Schembari
Graduation School of General Surgery, University of Catania, Catania, Italy

W. Terranova
General Medicine, Siracusa ASP, Siracusa, Italy

V. Urzia
Graduation School of Catania, Catania, Italy

A. Granata, M. Bertolotto (eds.), *Imaging in Nephrology*,
https://doi.org/10.1007/978-3-030-60794-4_11

A correlation has been observed between the hydrostatic pressure during the trauma and the involvement of pelvis and/or renal junction.

Hydronephrosis, subcortical or parapelvic cysts, and renal masses determine a higher vulnerability of the kidney and of the urinary tract [2, 3].

The mechanisms of development can be classified as "closed" or "penetrating." Generally, closed traumas are more common, representing 90–95% of the total [4].

In a penetrating trauma, kidney is involved in 4–8% of the cases.

Particularly, penetrating traumas of the basis of the thorax, of the superior abdomen, or of the flank or the back frequently involve kidney although the protection system is constituted by many anatomical structures and fascial systems (last ribs, abdominal organs, retroperitoneal fat, oblique muscle, psoas, transversalis fascia).

Bilateral lesions are extremely rare, while kidney lesions are frequently associated with lesions of other organs or districts (polytrauma).

11.2 Clinical Evaluation

During the anamnesis, whenever possible, the mechanism of trauma, eventual presence of preexistent pathology, and/or genitourinary malformation (such as lithiasis, hydronephrosis, pyelo-ureteral joint stenosis, or eventual previous renal surgery) that could cause major damages even in minor trauma should be investigated.

The objective exam follows that phase. Airway, breathing, and hemodynamic situation must be checked monitoring vital parameters (respiratory rate, cardiac output rate, systolic pressure) and, if necessary, life support maneuvers should be performed.

The objective exam of the abdomen with skin inspection is fundamental to detect bruising on the flank or on the back. Palpation can detect rib fractures and/or swelling in the lumbar area that could be a sign of a huge perirenal hematoma [1–4].

Hematuria is one of the most important clinical signs to be considered during the initial evaluation of a patient with a genitourinary system trauma.

Hematuria is positive in 80% of the cases, but in the case of a major trauma it could be only transitory or absent. Generally, microhematuria is related to minor severity trauma, while macrohematuria is related to major trauma. However, it has been demonstrated that the level of hematuria is not related to the severity of the trauma.

In those traumas involving the pyelo-ureteral joint or those provoking the avulsion or the thrombosis of the vascular pedicle, hematuria could be totally absent.

At the same time, a bio-humoral monitoring with hemochrome, coagulation markers, and renal functionality parameters is performed.

11.3 Type and Classification of Renal Trauma

Many classifications of renal damage based on pathogenesis, morphologic characteristics, and clinical parameters were proposed over the past [5].

Two of the most important classifications are the one based on radiological findings and, more recently, the one AAST (American Association for the Surgery of Trauma) proposed.

The last one, based on surgical experiences, is useful to predict the outcome of patients suffering from a renal damage [6, 7]. Its severity score comprehends five grades relating to the seriousness of the damage, to the vascular involvement, and to the secretory system involvement [8] (Table 11.1).

1st grade: It is the most common form of renal damage (75–85% of the cases). It includes the organ contusion associated with micro- or macro-hematuria and the subcapsular hematoma without parenchymal tearing.

2nd grade: It matches to the situation of a non-effusive perirenal hematoma confined in the retroperitoneum space, with a laceration of the cortical surface no deeper than 1 cm and with no involvement of the secretory system [5].

The perirenal hematoma is often not well defined and it *mitigates* the collection between

Table 11.1 AAST kidney injury scale (2011)

Grade[a]	Description or injury
1	Contusion or non-expanding sub-capsular haematoma No laceration
2	Non-expanding peri-renal haematoma Cortical laceration <1 cm deep (without urinary extravasation)
3	Cortical laceration >1 cm deep (without urinary extravasation)
4	**Laceration:** through corticomedullary junction into collecting system or **Vascular:** segmental renal artery or vein injury with contained haematoma, or partial vessellaceration, or vessel thrombosis
5	**Laceration:** shattered kidney or **Vascular:** renal pedicle avulsion

[a]Advance one grade for bilateral injuries up to grade 3

the kidney and the Gerota [9, 10]. It is possible to observe also the thickening of the intestinal walls, the kidney dislocation, and the compression on the colon.

3rd grade: It includes the lacerations of the cortical surface deeper than 1 cm, but with no involvement of the excretory system [5].

4th grade: It includes the deep lacerations of the parenchyma extending from the cortical and from the medullary to the excretory system; damages of the renal vein with limited hemorrhage; and segmental infarctions without associated tearing [5].

Thrombosis of the principal renal artery is the most serious vascular consequence of a closed abdominal trauma.

The deceleration causes stretching and laceration of intima, which is the starting point of the thrombosis that then extends distally.

5th grade: It is the most serious grade and it includes massive lacerations that destroy kidney with a complete tearing or a thrombosis of the principal artery or vein, causing the devascularization of the organ.

Multiple infarction areas are visible in the context [5–9].

The Peters Classification ranks the damage of the kidney in a more simplified way, including a subdivision in minor and major lesions [11].

Simplified classification of the kidney damage according to Peters (1997):

- Minor kidney lesions: Contusion, hematoma, simple parenchymal laceration
- Major kidney lesions: Parenchymal rupture with perirenal hematoma, excretory system laceration, lesion of the renal artery or the vein
  - **Minor lesions** are to be inserted in a clinical ultrasound follow-up: contusions, parenchymal and subcapsular hematoma, parenchymal fissures with or without subcapsular hematoma, segmentary ischemic stroke.
  - **Major lesions**, which represent a real surgical emergency: rupture of the capsula with renal and perirenal hematoma formation, parenchymal fractures; excretory system fractures mostly identified by the presence of urinomas; vascular pedicle laceration; renal vein thrombosis and renal ischemia due to a thrombosis of the renal artery.

11.4 Imaging

A correct and immediate diagnosis of renal trauma using imaging techniques is extremely important; any diagnostic delay could slow down an effective treatment and increase the mobility and mortality risk [12].

The four most important objectives of radiologic exams in renal trauma are:

- To carefully determine the grade of damage
- To identify any preexisting pathology of the damaged kidney
- To ascertain the functionality of the other kidney
- To recognize any possible lesion to other organs

Not all the patients with a renal trauma need a radiological evaluation. The decision on the diagnostic follow-up has to consider the history of the patient, objective examination, and laboratoristic findings.

A clinical evaluation mixed with a careful analysis of the mechanism of trauma is fundamental to establish if the patient needs an immediate CT scan, or if he/she can be submitted to a US/clinical follow-up [13].

The target of imaging is indeed to differentiate damages needing an immediate surgery from damages which can be conservatively managed [14].

Intravenous urography and renal arteriography were historically used as the first-line diagnostic tools for hemodynamically stable patients, while, by now, abdominal and pelvic CT scan with contrast enhancement is considered the gold standard.

In hemodynamically unstable conditions, a CT scan cannot be performed immediately, so an alternative technique such as US becomes fundamental [15], because it can be performed in the emergency room, it is safe and repeatable, and it allows to evaluate also the hemodynamic situation of the patient [16].

US, in the form of EFAST (Extended Focused Assessment with Sonography for Trauma), is the first step for the management of trauma in many important institutes for emergency, being the first-line approach for closed abdominal trauma [1].

Most precisely, the goal of EFAST protocol is to identify rapidly in traumatic patients pericardial, peritoneal, and pleural collections (liquid or gas) by 6–8 US scans that in order examine:

1. Peri-cardiac space examination
2. Right subphrenic and Morrison space
3. Apex of the thorax (right)
4. Left subphrenic space and splenic space
5. Apex of the thorax (left)
6. Douglas pouch
7. Right parietal-colic space
8. Left parietal-colic space [17]

In EFAST protocol, the examination of the two subphrenic space has to include an, albeit rapid, evaluation of the kidneys, even if symptoms are not specific (Fig. 11.1) [18].

The diagnostic management of patients who suffered a low-energy trauma is still unclear.

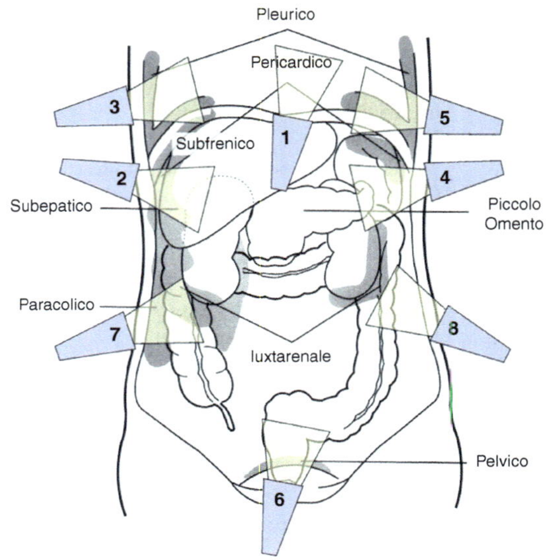

Fig. 11.1 Thoracic and abdominal scans for EFAST protocol

Many imaging methods could be used (CT, conventional X-ray, or US) related to clinical presentation and laboratoristic findings.

US evaluation of renal trauma can highlight:

- Renal contusion, characterized by lumbar pain and microhematuria: A US scan could be fully negative or it could show in the initial phases intraparenchymal areas of enhanced echogenicity that mean hematic extravasation in the parenchyma. After this phase, a little fluid subcapsular collection not well defined appears, due to colliquative events.

  In the damaged zone, edema and vasospasm generate a minor vascularized area visible to the color and power Doppler. If the trauma were a penetrating one, arteriovenous fistula could be present and identified by color Doppler due to the turbulence of the bloodstream [19].
- Partial tearing of the capsula can be identified as an anechogen or a hypoechogen perirenal collection (Fig. 11.2), not well defined with unimportant modification in the parenchyma. The presence of the capsula and of the perirenal space, bounded by the Gerota fascia, is

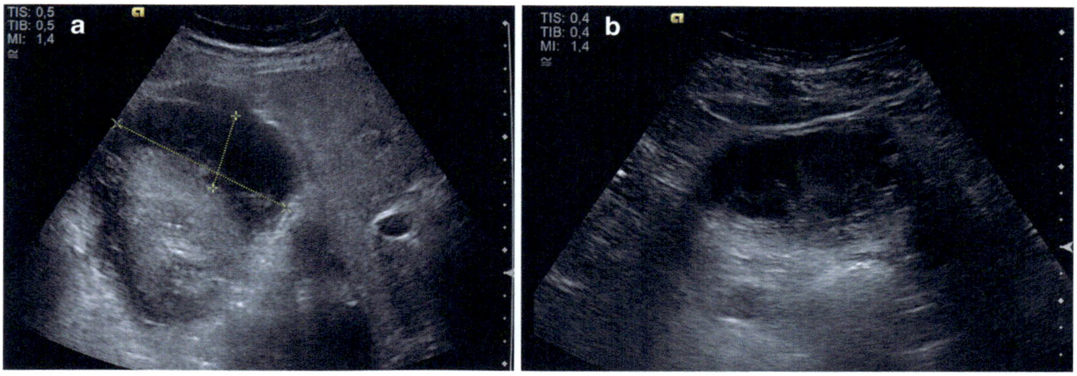

Fig. 11.2 Lacero-contusion: Tearing of the parenchyma (**a**) associated to an anechogen perirenal collection (**b**), not well defined with mild changes in the parenchyma

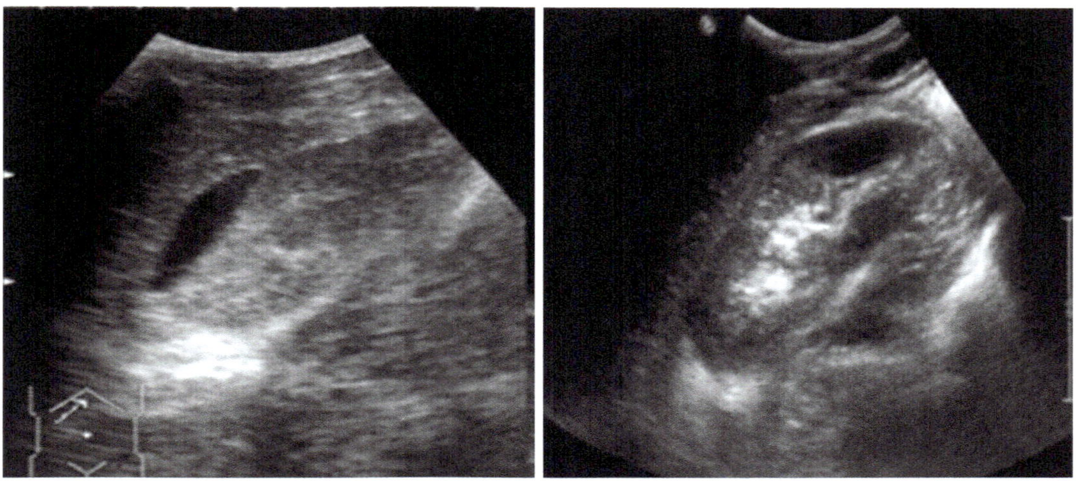

Fig. 11.3 Subcapsular hematoma: hypo-anechoic lenticular area, the external surface deforms the profile (bulging)

the cause of the quick organization of the renal hematoma due to a compression mechanism. This is the explanation for the spontaneous resolution of even mildly severe lesions.

An extra reason for no extravasation of a perirenal hemorrhage could be the presence of thin trabecular structures made of connective tissue situated in the perirenal fat. Those structures are easily recognizable in CT and US scan, particularly in obese patients. They tend to form a texture contrasting the hemorrhagic infiltration and, at the same time, plugging the active bleeding [16].

- The renal hematoma, as a consequence of the segmental vascular distribution, tends to be better delimited in a single site or in several contiguous districts with consequent lower organ compromise (Fig. 11.3).

However, such segmental involvement can often result in renal scars (wedge-shaped and cyst-like lesions). Furthermore, it must be considered that the ultrasound semiology of the traumatic renal lesions is not always the same as that of the other parenchymal organs. In fact, the presence of a particularly complex and branched vascular network, with small vessels with thin walls, immediately adjacent to the excretory system, almost always determines a mixture of blood, urine, and transudate. These make the ultrasound images of parenchymal damage extremely polymorphous. When the lesion is predominantly vascular, the hyperechogenic pattern prevails, due to the reflective properties of the blood which flows to the extravascular site (this is probably consequent to the presence of microclots and/or big clots, which determine larger and more complex interfaces with increased reflections and echoes). Otherwise, when a lesion of the collecting duct system occurs and the urinary leakage is predominant, the area has less or no reflectivity (non-infected urine is completely anechoic). Finally, when the edematous component is significant, the ultrasound findings are characterized by greater heterogeneity. Moreover, the difficulties increased with the passage of time. In fact, after the degradation of hemosiderin, the fluid blood becomes anechoic, so the hematomas tend to reduce their reflectivity, becoming hyperechoic [1].

- Multiple lacerations become evident when the normal renal structure is difficult to recognize: the profiles are poorly defined and around the kidney there is an extensive urine-hematic collection in part anechoic and partly echogenic.
- Renal or excretory system ruptures are difficult to identify with ultrasound because the loss of urine is not shown [20]. In these cases, ultrasound shows the severity of renal damage, but it fails to assess the extension of the trauma.
- Vascular complications (AV fistulas, pseudoaneurysms, complete or segmental infarcts) are more frequent in kidney than in other organs due to the complexity of the renal excretory perfusion. When vascular damage is present in renal traumas, such as thrombosis (Fig. 11.4) or vascular pedicle avulsion, renal morphology is generally preserved (Fig. 11.5), but Doppler shows the absolute absence of intraparenchymal flow, which is the principal sign of renal ischemia.

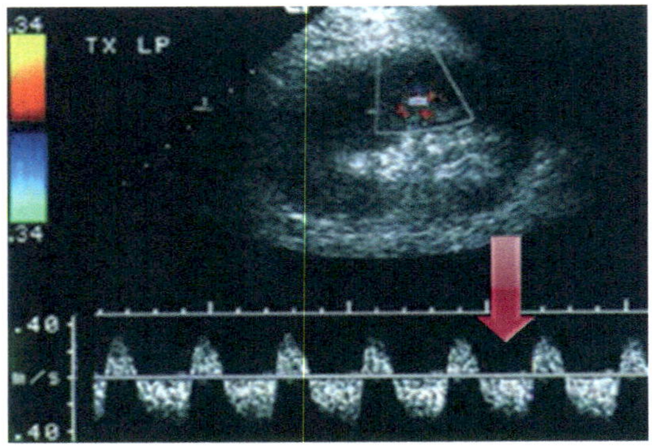

Fig. 11.4 Renal vein thrombosis: enlarged and hypoechoic kidney, acoustic silence in the Doppler of the renal vein, renal artery with reverse flow

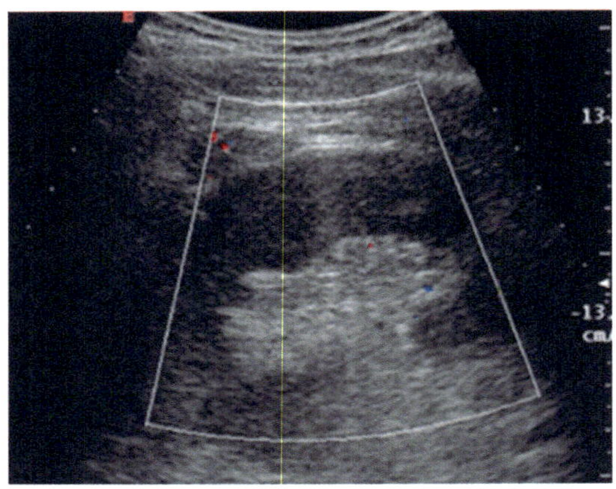

Fig. 11.5 Parenchymal ischemia. The renal parenchyma has a normal corticomedullary differentiation without vascular signal to color Doppler

- Rupture of the excretory tracts without vessel injury is identified by enlarged excretory pathways associated with a medial perirenal fluid collection that extends along the edge of the iliopsoas muscle [21]. In the bladder, the unilateral absence of the jet phenomenon can be detected. Furthermore, as a result of penetrating traumas, arteriovenous (AV) fistulas can also be created; they are easily identifiable with the color Doppler due to turbulent blood flow phenomena [19].

11.5 Second-Level Imaging with Contrast

Thanks to the possibility of using second-generation contrast agent (or sulfur hexafluoride), in the algorithm for the diagnosis of renal traumas, there is a two-level approach that concerns ultrasound; this technique is commonly called contrast-enhanced ultrasound (CEUS).

Compared to traditional sonography, CEUS is more accurate in the assessment of renal trauma, in the evaluation of the number and size of traumatic lesions, and in the detection of vascular involvement, showing an excellent correlation with CT findings [22, 23]. Moreover, the absence of ionizing radiation, the lack of nephrotoxicity, and the low cost of the technique give CEUS the potential to become a first-approach imaging method [24]. This is due to its high sensitivity and specificity of, respectively, 96% and 99%, with a high positive and negative predictive value of 98% [17].

The ultrasound contrast medium is administered intravenously with a slow bolus, lasting a few seconds, with subsequent bolus infusion of 10 mL of saline solution. The microbubbles have a renal cortical phase at about 10–15 "from the injection, while the medullary vessels gradually fill up after about 25–35." This happens because the medulla has a lower speed to achieve complete perfusion than the cortex. The washout begins in the medulla and then extends more slowly to the cortex.

In CEUS, we can distinguish three contrast phases:

- Early arterial phase, where arterial vessels are clearly visible
- Late arterial phase, or cortical phase, characterized by an intense and uniform enhancement of cortex (from 12 to 35 s after the infusion), where corticomedullary differentiation is evident
- Medullary or late phase (from 40 to 12 s), where the pyramids gradually fill with contrast until they become isoechoic with the cortical

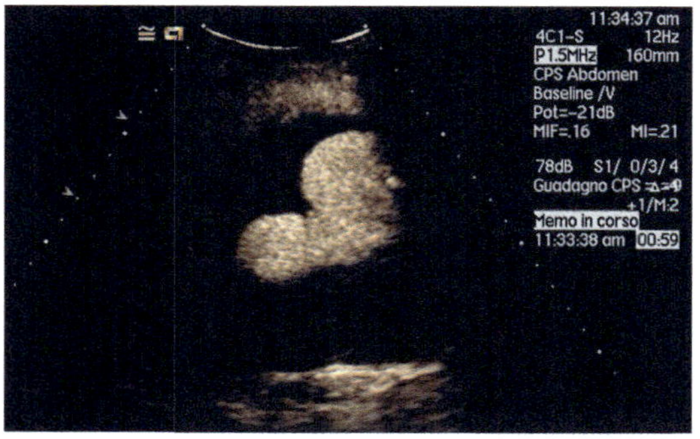

Fig. 11.6 CEUS allows to show better the perirenal hematoma and it allows to evaluate eventual parenchymal lesions

There is no collecting system phase (secretory and/or excretory) since, unlike iodinated contrast or gadolinium, the microbubbles remain in the circulatory system [25].

Using the ultrasound according to the modalities listed above, the traumatic lesions appear as enhancement defects, which are surrounded by healthy renal parenchyma [26, 27]. In particular:

- Contusions appear as tenuously hypoechoic areas, with poorly defined margins.
- Lacerations appear as striae or anechoic bands that reach the surface of the organ (filling defects that interrupt the renal profile).
- Hematomas are areas of more or less marked intraparenchymal or subcapsular hypoechogenicity (Fig. 11.6).
- Infarcts have the appearance of clear and defined avascular areas [28].

Active bleedings should be detected by microbubble extravasation.

Since microbubbles are not filtered through the glomeruli or secreted in the tubules, only indirect signs (abdominal effusion) of bladder and ureteral damage or of insufficiency of the excretory system can be detected through the CEUS. Consequently, this method could not be used to evaluate lesions of the excretory pathways in patients with renal trauma [29, 30].

11.6 Conclusions

The advent and introduction of modern and sophisticated methods of "imaging" (US–CT) in the emergency area have led to a radical modification of the attitude towards the traumatic abdominal pathology. In particular, there has been a lot of change due to the development of clinical protocols for the diagnosis and management of renal traumas. These have positively influenced the prognostic index of these pathologies.

The association of US and CT can currently be considered the gold standard in the diagnostic management of renal traumas.

In the previous years, the surgeon was pushed to perform the operation, initially with an exploratory purpose, even if after … it often became unnecessarily demolitive! … Today, both imaging techniques provide accurate diagnostic information about the conditions of parenchyma, minimizing the risk of misdiagnosing renal injuries. Consequently, they guide the type of treatment and allow follow-up of the sequelae!

In particular, on the one hand the ultrasound investigation involves many advantages already well known in the study of abdominal trauma (low cost, wide availability, repeatability, noninvasiveness [4, 20], possibility of association with resuscitation maneuvers, ability to define the diagnostic workup) [17] with high ability to detect the presence of free fluid in the abdominal cavity [31] and high sensitivity for perirenal effusions (63–96%). On the other hand, it does not allow to differentiate bleedings from extravasation of urine or other biological liquids [32, 33]. It presents further limitations related to the fact of being an operator-dependent technique and, above all, it is characterized by low sensitivity in the direct visualization of the lesions of parenchymatous organs and *retroperitoneal hemorrhage* [34, 35].

Using Doppler imaging combined with B-mode US gives more information about the vascularization of the organ, improving the diagnostic accuracy and also allowing to monitor the evolution of the lesion itself, which usually represents an unstable and changeable situation over time [36]. Vascular evaluation with color and power Doppler is not always easy in case of renal contusions and fractures, although the visualization of normal-pulsating artery and vein at the hilum allows to rule out a lesion of the peduncle.

However, the ultrasound method is less reliable than CT and MRI [37] in the evaluation of the damage suffered by the excretory pathways, in particular by the ureters and vascular pedicle.

For patients who have undergone low-energy abdominal trauma, the use of CEUS appears to be advisable, especially after a negative traditional ultrasound, because of the possibility of reducing the observation time and need for CT [17].

In case of negative CEUS, patients could be discharged advising clinical-laboratory monitoring, without the need to resort to CT.

On the contrary, patients who present a positive CEUS should continue the diagnostic tests with CT scan with contrast to exclude the presence of negative prognostic elements such as active bleeding and injuries of the urinary tract [17].

However, to this day, the future use of CEUS will be more likely to occur in the follow-up of nonsurgical renal traumas or in nonoperative management (NOM), especially in young patients [22], rather than in the first evaluation of the traumatized patient [30].

References

1. Romano L, Di Nuzzo L, Russo G, et al. Traumi renali. Imaging Dell'apparato Urogenutale. 2010;6:71–102.
2. Schimidlin FR, Schmid P, Kurtyka T, et al. Force transmission and stress distribution in a computer-simulated model of kidney: an analysis of the injury mechanisms in renal trauma. J Trauma. 1996;40:791–6.
3. Traub KB, Hua V, Broman S, et al. Introduction of a genitourinary trauma database for use as a multi-institutional urologic trauma registry. J Trauma. 2001;51:336–9.
4. Chouhan JD, Winer AG, Johnson C, Weiss JP, Hyacinthe LM. Contemporary evaluation and management of renal trauma. Can J Urol. 2016;23(2):8191–7.
5. Alonso RC, Nacenta SB, Martinez PD, et al. CT findings of blunt and penetrating renal trauma. Radiographics. 2009;21:2033–53.
6. Master VA, McAninch JW. Operative management of renal injuries: parenchymal and vascular. Urol Clin North Am. 2006;33(1):21–31, v–vi

7. Malcolm JB, Derweesh IH, Mehrazin R, et al. Non operative management of blunt renal trauma: is routine early follow-up imaging necessary? BMC Urol. 2008;8:11.
8. Buckley JC, McAninch JW. Revision of current American Association for the Surgery of Trauma Renal Injury grading system. J Trauma. 2011;70(1):35.
9. Harris AC, Zwirewich CV, Lyburn ID, et al. Ct findings in blunt renal trauma. RadioGraphincs. 2001;21:S2010–4.
10. Park SJ, Kim JK, Kim KW, et al. MDCT findings of renal trauma. Am J Roentgenol. 2006;187(2): 541–7.
11. Scrinivasa RN, Akbar SA, Jafri S, et al. Genitourinary trauma. A pictorial essay. Emerg Radiol. 2009;16:21–33.
12. Cetti NE. Blunt renal trauma. Some personal thoughts. Scand J Urol Nephrol. 2000;34:5–9.
13. Catalano O, Aiani L, Barozzi L, et al. CEUS in abdominal trauma: multicenter study. Abdom Imagng. 2009;34:225–34.
14. Santucci RA, Wessells H, Bartisch G, et al. Evaluation and management of renal injuries: consensus statement of the renal trauma subcommittee. BJU Int. 2004;93:937–54.
15. Szmigielski W, Kumar R, Al Hilli S, Ismail M. Renal trauma imaging: diagnosis and management. A pictorial review. Pol J Radiol. 2013;78(4):27–35.
16. Farina RO, Gagliardi N, Rizzo A, Romano L. Gestionee diagnostica integrata del paziente emodinamicamente stabile. Ecografia clinica nelle urgenze emergenze. Scuderi M. 2015;12:135–42.
17. Sessa B, Trinci M, Ianniello S, Menichini G, Galluzzo M, Miele V. Blunt abdominal trauma: role of contrast-enhanced ultrasound (CEUS) in the detection and staging of abdominal traumatic lesions compared to US and CE-MDCT. Radiol Med. 2015;120:180–9.
18. Ma OJ, Maater JR. Emergency ultrasound. New York: McGraw-Hill; 2003. p. 67–88.
19. Noble VE, Brown DF. Renal ultrasound. Emerg Med Clin North Am. 2004;22:641–59.
20. Korner M, Krotz MM, et al. Current role of emergency US in patient with major trauma. Radiographics. 2008;28:225–44.
21. Kamel IR, Berkowitz JF. Assessment of the cortical rim sign in post-traumatic renal infarction. J Comput Assist Tomogr. 1996;20(5):803–6.
22. Valentino M, Serra XC, Zironi G, De Luca C, Pavlica P, Barozzi L. Blunt abdominal trauma: emergency contrast-enhanced sonography for detection of solid organ injuries. AJR. 2006;186:1361–7.
23. Miele V, Piccolo CL, Pallottino AA, Galluzzo M, Iannello S, Trinci M. Ruolo dell'ecografia e della CEUS nelle urgenze traumatiche dell'addome. Radiol Med. 2016;3:632–40.
24. Granata A, Floccari F, Logias F, Insalaco M, et al. L'imaging ecocontrastografico nella patologia renale. G Ital Nefrol. 2012;29(S57):S25–35.
25. Granata A, Zanoli I, Inasalaco M, Scuderi M, Valentino M, et al. Contrast-enhanced ultrasound (CEUS) in nephrology: has the time come for its widespread use? Clin Exp Nephrol. 2015;19(4):606–15.
26. Israel GM, Bosniak MA. How do it: evaluating renal masses. Radiology. 2005;236:441–50.
27. Xu ZF, Xu HX, Xie XY, et al. Renal cell carcinoma and renal angiomyolipoma: differential diagnosis with real-time contrast-enhanced ultrasonography. J Ultrasound Med. 2010;29(5):709–17.
28. Meloni MF, Bertolotto M, Alberzoni C, et al. Follow-up after percutaneous radiofrequency ablation of renal cell carcinoma: contrast-enhanced sonography versus contrast-enhanced CT or MRI. Am J Roentgenol. 2008;191:1233–8.
29. Cagini L, Gravante S, Malapsima CM, Cesarano E, et al. Contrast enhanced ultrasound (CEUS) in blunt abdominal trauma. Crit Ultrasound J. 2013;5(Suppl 1):S9.
30. Scialpi M, Scaglione M, Angelelli G, et al. Emergencies in the retroperitoneum: assessment of spread of disease by helical CT. Eur J Radiol. 2004;50:74–83.
31. Dolich MO, McKenney MG, Varela JE, et al. Ultrasound for abdominal trauma. J Trauma. 2001;50:108–12.
32. Jankowski JT, Spirnak JP. Current recommendations for imaging in the management of urologic traumas. Urol Clin North Am. 2006;33(3):365–76.
33. Smith JK, Kenney PJ. Imaging of renal trauma. Radiol Clin N Am. 2003;41(5):1019–35.
34. Poletti PA, Wintermark M, Schneyder P, et al. Traumatic injuries: role of imaging in the management of polytrauma victim (conservative expectation). Eur Radiol. 2002;12:969–78.
35. Clevert DA, Wackbach S, Minaifar N, et al. Contrast-enhanced ultrasound versus MS-CT in blunt abdominal trauma. Clin Hemorheol Microcirc. 2008;39:155–69.
36. Lee GPC, Chung KL, Kan CW. Ultrasonography for acute blunt renal trauma: does it help? Hong Kong J Emerg Med. 2006;13:57–60.
37. Bezzi M, Andreoli G, Miele V, Andreoli C. Imaging and intervention in abdominal trauma. Berlin: Springer; 2010. p. 237–65.

12 The Elderly Kidney

Francesco M. Drudi

12.1 Introduction

It is estimated that after the age of 30 years, GFR progressively declines at an average rate of 8 mL/min/1.73 m/decade [1]. Structural and functional changes affect all components of the kidney. These variations tend to reduce renal functional reserve. Many factors affect kidney changes in the elderly: genetic factors, genomic alterations, oxidative stress, nutrition, drugs, and infections. In addition, elderly patients are frequently affected by clinical conditions such as arterial hypertension, diabetes mellitus, and cardiovascular diseases that can play an additive role in age-related changes, tending to amplify these abnormalities [1].

12.2 Structural Changes

In the elderly, a progressive reduction of renal mass is described; the weight of the kidneys is reduced from about 250–270 g in the young adult to 180–200 g in the eighth decade of life with preferential loss of cortical parenchyma, with relative spare of the medullary one.

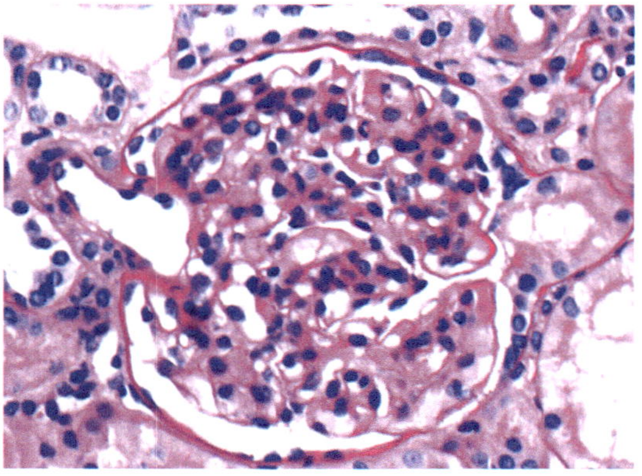

Fig. 12.1 Focal and segmental glomerulosclerosis

On a microscopic level, this atrophy coincides with a reduction in the number of functioning nephrons [2].

In particular glomeruli undergo focal and segmental glomerulosclerosis, thickening of the glomerular basement membrane, and compensatory hypertrophy of the surviving glomeruli [3] (Fig. 12.1).

The tubules encounter dilatation, atrophy, and diverticula, which in turn are possible sites of bacterial colonization and precursors of parenchymal cysts [4].

Interstitium undergoes fibrosis with "patchy" inflammation.

About vessels, we can see hyaline arteriosclerosis (especially in the presence of diabetes), hyperplastic sclerosis of arterioles (especially in

F. M. Drudi (✉)
Departiment of Radiological Sciences, University La Sapienza of Rome, Rome, Italy
e-mail: Francescom.Drudi@uniroma1.it

A. Granata, M. Bertolotto (eds.), *Imaging in Nephrology*,
https://doi.org/10.1007/978-3-030-60794-4_12

the presence of malignant hypertension), and middle-intimal hypertrophy (especially in the presence of hypertension) [5].

12.3 Functional Changes

In the elderly there is a progressive reduction in creatinine clearance of about 50% between 30 and 80 years, as well as a reduction in glomerular filtration rate (VGF) [6].

A problem of advanced age concerns the evaluation of renal function, unreliable on the basis of widely available and economic indicators, valid in young and adult age, such as creatininemia [6].

The renal function in humans can be evaluated by a variety of equations, one of the most used of which is the Cockcroft-Gault equation.

The parameters used in this formula are age, sex, body weight, serum creatinine levels (Scr), and constant values [7]:

$$\frac{\text{COCKROFT GAULT-EQUATION}}{\left[(140-\text{age})\times \text{weight}/72\times \text{Scr}\right](\times 0.85 \text{if female})}$$

Unfortunately, predictive value of the Cockcroft-Gault formula is not optimal in the elderly patient (age >70 aa).

Serum creatinine levels depend on muscle mass that usually reduces with aging. Furthermore, patients with chronic renal insufficiency go on a hypoproteic diet.

Therefore, plasma creatinine levels may not be sensitive markers of actual renal function in chronic renal failure; in fact, many patients may have serum creatinine levels within the normal range even if they have a significant reduction in renal function [8].

As a consequence, for a more accurate evaluation of renal function, the clearance of creatinine with urine collection in 24 h is recommended [9].

Moreover, in the elderly, in addition to a reduction of the lean mass, there is often an increase in fat mass, which induces a pro-inflammatory state [10].

Oxidized LDLs are able to stimulate the production of inflammatory and fibrogenic cytokines, which are responsible for apoptosis of mesangial cells and for increase in the production of reactive O_2 species, creating a self-perpetuating mechanism.

This results in a higher production of matrix and collagen proteins as well as an increased apoptosis of endothelial cells.

In addition, oxidized LDLs increase the production of vasoactive substances such as endothelin and thromboxane and increase renin release from juxtaglomerular cells [10].

A reduction of vasodilating factors, such as NO (nitric oxide), has also been reported [10].

12.4 Ultrasound and Color Doppler Evaluation of Kidney in Elderly

Renal ultrasound in the elderly can provide information related to response to specific clinical questions or can be considered as an extension of the objective examination. The integration with anamnestic, objective, and laboratory data permit fast and reliable clinical, diagnostic, and therapeutic classification.

12.4.1 Ultrasound

Renal ultrasound (US) has become a routine investigation in kidney disease.

It is able to determine the number, location, size, and shape of kidneys.

Size of kidneys and parenchymal echogenicity are considered markers of renal function, so US can be considered useful to assess the presence and degree of renal failure (Figs. 12.2 and 12.3). US can show a reduction of the longitudinal diameter (15% between the third and the ninth decades of life) and a reduction of the volume (mainly due to loss of the parenchymal component) [2].

A renal longitudinal diameter of 9 cm and an average parenchymal thickness of 12 mm are considered within the lower limits of the standard; lower values are considered pathological. However, an accurate evaluation of ultrasound

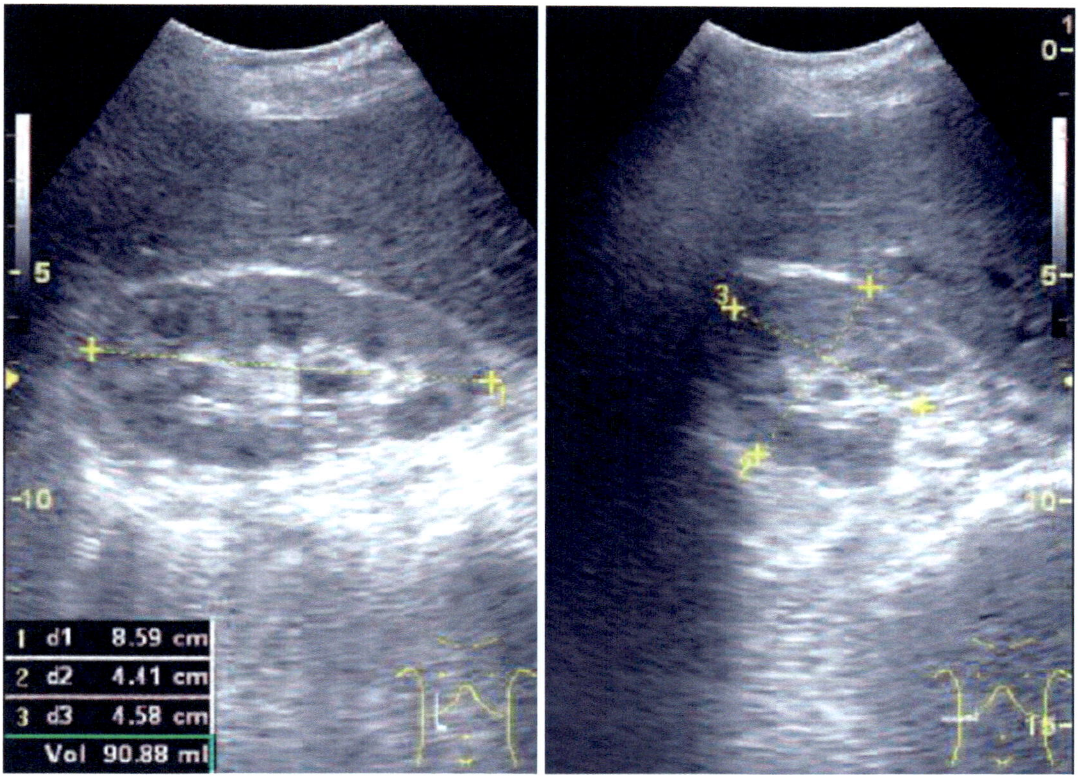

Fig. 12.2 Reduction of the longitudinal diameter and volume

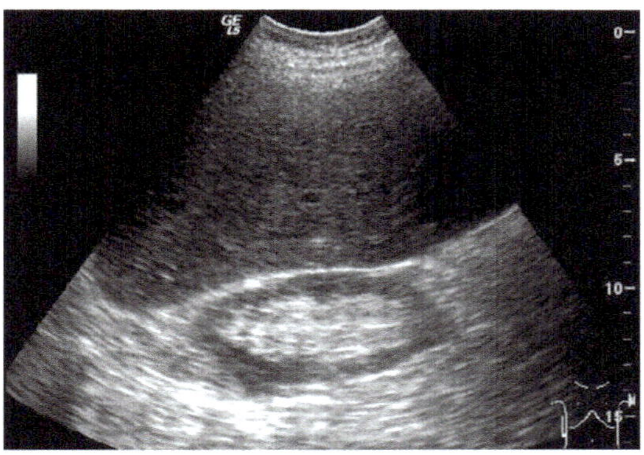

Fig. 12.3 Change in parenchymal (cortical) echogenicity

information must provide for a "correction" for some constitutional parameters (age, sex, body weight, height, blood pressure, sex) [11].

A hiding effect on the reduction of renal size is the apparent normality of the latter in the presence of pathological conditions that increase renal size, as inflammatory processes, infiltration, or accumulation, which can hide a preexisting dimensional reduction; conversely, the latter can mask the increase in dimensional parameters when clinically expected (Fig. 12.4) [12].

Mancuso et al. measure renal diameters, volume, and cortical thickness in association with functional parameters (creatinine and creatinine clearance) in patients with varying degrees of chronic renal failure and in a population of control showing a correlation between size parameters seen with US and decline of GFR during chronic renal failure [11].

Beyond dimensional aspects, senile kidney shows frequent morphological-qualitative ultrasound changes. Cortical-medullary differentiation of the parenchyma is reduced with age and is evident only in about 1/3 of the elderly subjects (Fig. 12.2).

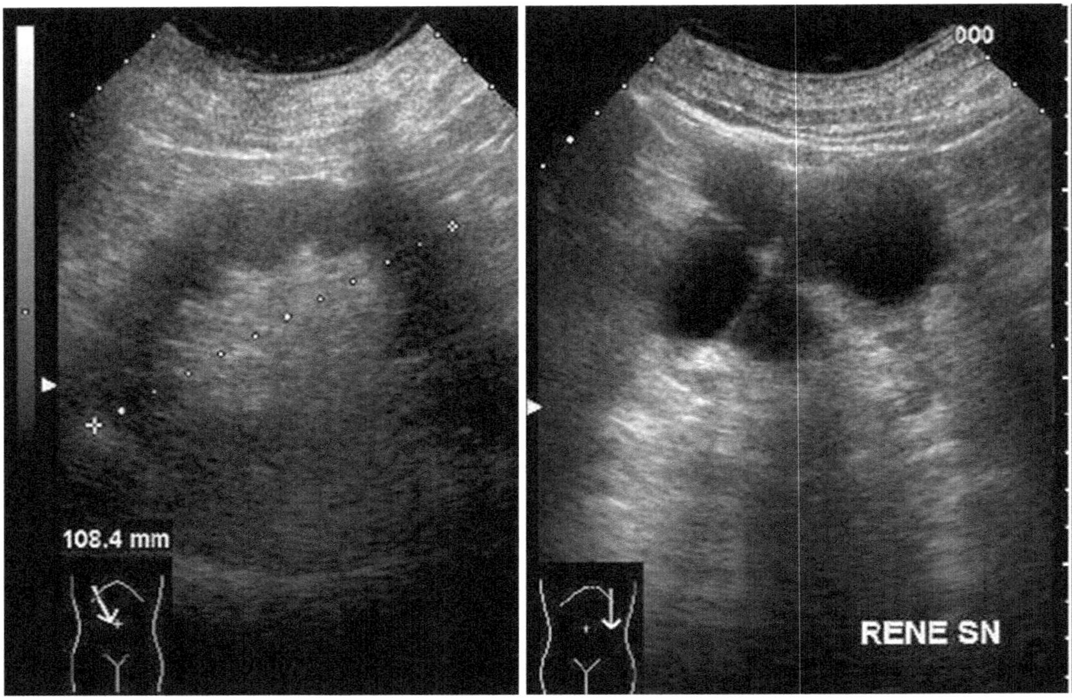

Fig. 12.4 Right kidney: normal size and parenchymal thickness. Left kidney: disappearance of parenchyma, represented exclusively by pyelocaliceal sacs

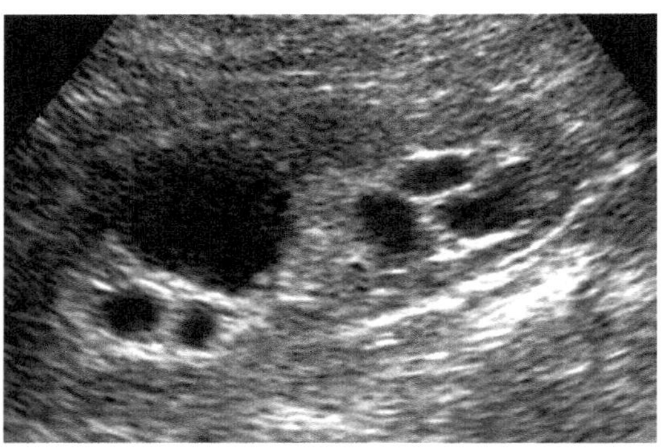

Fig. 12.5 Multiple cystic formations of variable sizes

The finding of cystic formations of variable sizes is frequent on parenchyma and renal sinus [12] (Fig. 12.5).

Moreover, there is frequent finding of a relative hypertrophy of the sinus component, with a reduced parenchyma-sinus ratio.

Increase in sinus share could morphologically compensate for parenchymal loss, so that the volumetric maintenance of the whole organ does not necessarily express the preservation of the functional renal mass, that is, the parenchymal mass; this, therefore, should be measured specifically, subtracting the sinus volume from the total renal volume.

Both volumes can be calculated through the simplified formula of the ellipsoid, i.e., from the product of the three main diameters of the kidney (longitudinal, transversal, and anterior-posterior) for 0.52 [13].

12.4.2 Color Doppler

Senile alterations are evaluable with ecocolor and ecoDoppler. In the elderly, distribution of color signals and expression of the renal vascular tissue appear more attenuated compared to the young or young-adult population, limited to intersegmental and interlobar districts [14] (Fig. 12.6).

Among the ecoDoppler parameters, the one considered most reproducible and less influenced by methodological factors is the **resistance**

index. It is higher in the elderly population; however, it is influenced by various physiological and pathological conditions both intra- and extrarenal, so its modifications or alterations, especially its increase, are not very specific. In elderly an upper limit of 0.70 is usually considered [15] (Figs. 12.7 and 12.8).

According to Tublin et al., a correct sampling must provide the measurement of at least 3/5 waves of dimensions overlapping in three different areas of each kidney; the final value of IR considered corresponds to the arithmetic mean of the values obtained [16]. However, a correct IR can be difficult to evaluate in some conditions such as tachycardia, bradycardia, arrhythmia, and presence of perirenal or subcapsular liquid collections [17].

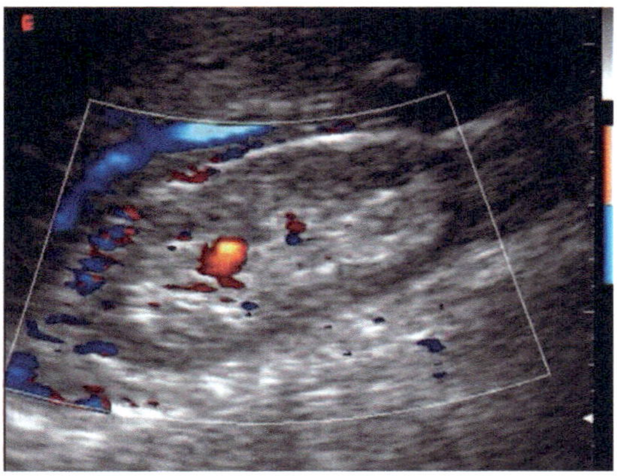

Fig. 12.6 Reduced vascular representation, due to scarcity of color signals (PRF 1 KHz). Using a lower PRF the increase in vascular signals would be affected by the appearance of artifactual motion signals, such as those already evident at the periphery of the kidney

12.5 Renal Disorders in the Elderly

Kidneys in elderly lose the ability to repair itself after a damage, the ability to react to any stress condition, the ability to react to hemodynamic alterations, and the ability to maintain body homeostasis (water, electrolytes, pH) because adaptation mechanisms are reduced.

So kidneys are more susceptible to nephrotoxic factors.

As life expectancy continues to improve worldwide, there is a rising prevalence of comorbidities and risk factors such as hypertension, diabetes, and cardiovascular disease [18]. Several diseases that afflict kidneys in young-adult population have more incidence or worse consequences in the elderly.

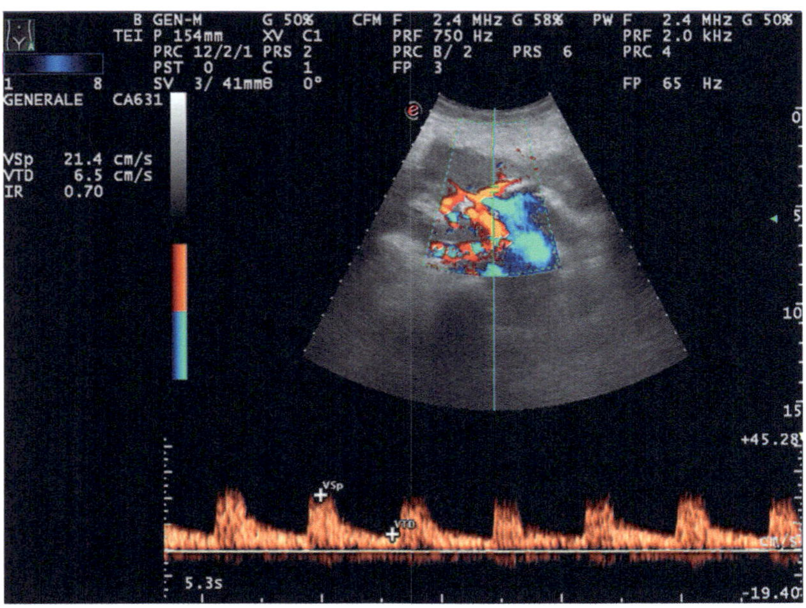

Fig. 12.7 IR = 0.70 in 65-year-old woman

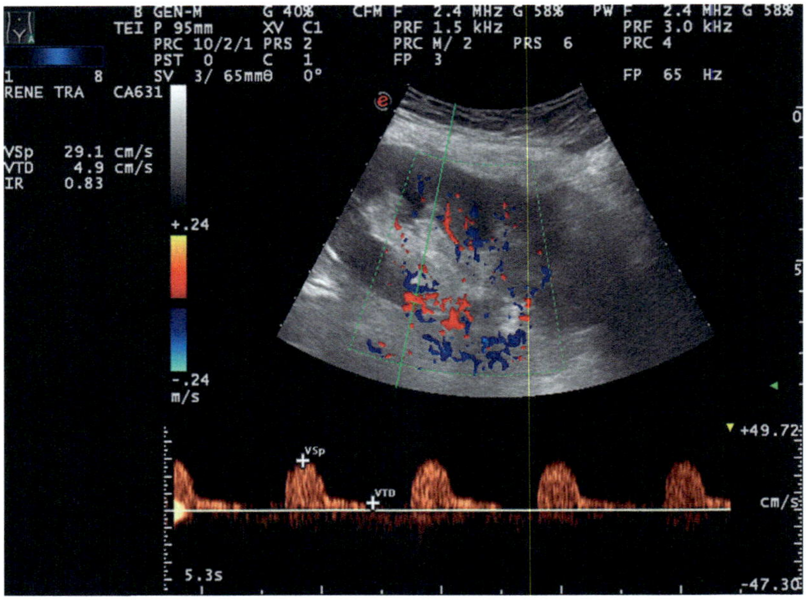

Fig. 12.8 IR = 0.83 in 70-year-old woman

12.5.1 Chronic Kidney Disease (CKD)

Chronic kidney disease (CKD) is a very common clinical problem in elderly patients and is associated with increased morbidity and mortality. CKD definitions are kidney damage evidenced by abnormal renal markers or a reduction of the absolute eGFR to less than 60 mL/min/1.73 m^2 for at least 3 months. Abnormal renal markers are proteinuria, abnormal radiology, abnormal cells in the urine, or renal pathology on biopsy. In addition, a history of renal transplantation is included in the definition [18].

In the elderly, frequent etiopathogenic causes of chronic renal failure are nephrovascular pathologies. In uremic patients, in fact, cardiovascular events represent the largest cause of death, which is about 20 times greater than the general population. In these patients, cerebrovascular accidents appear ten times more frequently than in the general population. In particular, it has been reported that about 50% of patients starting hemodialysis have coronaropathies on atherosclerotic basis; 80% of these patients have dyslipidemia [19]. Atherosclerosis is often present in the uremic patient in a very advanced phase. In fact, it has been shown that the mean intimal thickness of the carotid and femoral arteries, as a marker of atherosclerosis, is higher in patients on hemodialysis compared to healthy controls of the same age and sex [20]. Arterial hypertension, obesity, and diabetes mellitus are also common causes of chronic renal failure in the elderly patient [18].

12.5.1.1 US/Color Doppler

US shows increased echogenicity of the cortex, decreased renal size, and cortical thinning, findings rather frequent in the kidney of the elderly and therefore nonspecific [12].

IR value can be considered a marker of renal damage progression paying attention to possible concomitant confounding factors (renal compression, Valsalva maneuver, cardiac rhythm abnormalities, various extrarenal causes of altered vascular elasticity, etc.) [17]. High IR value ≥0.80 (Fig. 12.8) represents a point of no return in the diagnosis of IRC, being associated with a reduced probability of improvement of renal function after percutaneous transluminal angioplasty (PTA). In transplanted kidney it is predictive of a reduced graft survival. A correlation between IR >0.70 and percentage increase in serum creatinine values has been reported, so an

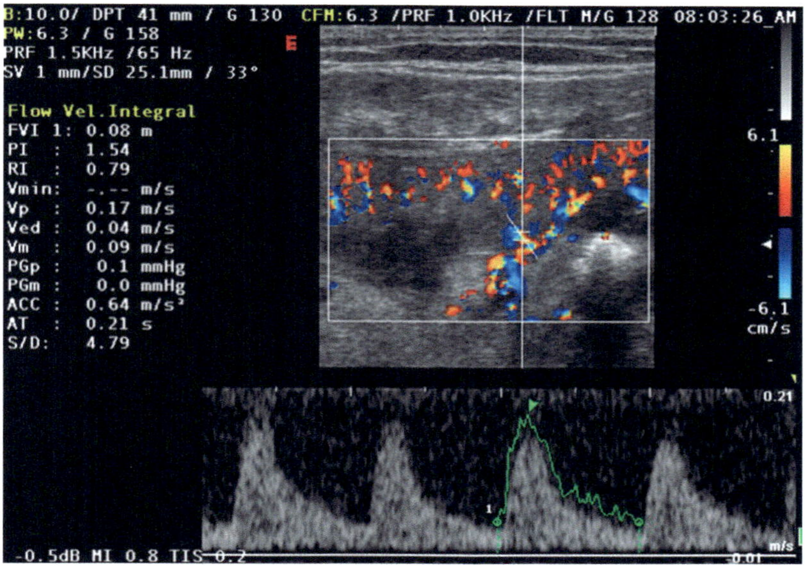

Fig. 12.9 IR increase in chronic kidney disease

IR value >0.70 (Fig. 12.9) may be considered an independent risk factor for worsening renal function in the IRC [17].

12.5.2 Occult Renal Insufficiency (ORI)

It is characterized by normal creatinine and reduced glomerular filtration rate (VFG), frequent in the elderly population and associated with greater risk of adverse pharmacological events.

A ClCr <60 mL/min with creatinine <1.1 mg/dL was identified as ORI.

In clinical practice, the 24-h creatinine clearance (ClCr24h) or the predictive equations of VFG (EP) are used to evaluate renal function. The main EPs are the Cockcroft-Gault equation, the modification of diet in renal disease (MDRD), and the CKD-EPI (chronic kidney disease epidemiology collaboration).

In the hospitalized elderly the prevalence of ORI (ClCr <60 mL/m) was 50.9% [21].

Among the EPs, the estimate of VFG using the Cockcroft-Gault formula seems to provide results that are more similar to those of ClCr24h [21].

12.5.3 Diabetic Nephropathy

Diabetes type 2 has a high incidence among the elderly. Forty percent of type 2 diabetics are at risk of chronic renal disease [22].

Diabetic nephropathy consists of sclerosis and glomerular fibrosis caused by metabolic and hemodynamic changes in diabetes mellitus: thickening of glomerular basement membrane, and capillary and tubular basement membrane thickening. Other glomerular changes include loss of endothelial fenestrations, mesangial matrix expansion, and loss of podocytes [22]. The exudative lesions result from subendothelial deposits of plasma proteins, which form periodic acid-Schiff-positive and electron-dense deposits and accumulate in small arterial branches, arterioles, and glomerular capillaries as well as microaneurysms. Similar subepithelial deposits are seen in Bowman's capsule (capsular drop lesion) and proximal renal tubules [22] (Fig. 12.10).

Diabetic nephropathy manifests as a slowly progressive albuminuria, with a worsening of hypertension and renal failure. Diagnosis is based on anamnesis, physical examination, urinalysis, and urinary albumin/creatinine ratio. Treatment consists of strict glycemic control

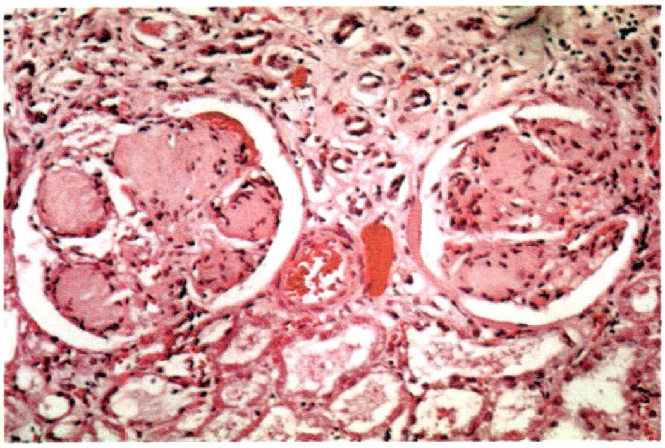

Fig. 12.10 Diabetic glomerulopathy

(using ACE inhibitors and/or angiotensin II receptor inhibitors) and controlling of blood pressure and lipids [22].

Patients are routinely tested for urine detection of proteinuria; if present, the test for microalbuminuria is not necessary because the patient already has a suggestive macroalbuminuria for diabetic nephropathy. In patients without proteinuria, the albumin/creatinine ratio should be measured on a urine sample of the first morning urination. A creatinine ratio ≥0.03 mg/mg (≥30 mg/g) indicates microalbuminuria if it is present in at least two of the three measurements performed within 3–6 months and if it cannot be explained by the presence of infections or exercise [22].

12.5.3.1 US/Color Doppler

IRs are useful indicators of the presence of nephropathy in patients with type 2 diabetes mellitus, even in the absence of microalbuminuria: increased IR represents a risk factor for the development of albuminuria and higher IR is also reported in the presence of macroalbuminuria, even after adjusting for GFR values. In type 2 diabetic patients without microalbuminuria, the increase in IR is predictive of renal involvement.

12.5.4 Acute Renal Failure

Acute renal failure (ARF) is a common problem in older adults. As compared to younger adults, elderly have a greater prevalence of ischemic ARF. Relevant structural and functional changes in the aging kidney predispose to ARF: arteriosclerotic lesions at the level of interlobular and arcuate arteries that causes increase in vascular resistances; decreased ability to retain sodium, due to decreased reabsorptive tubular capacity and impaired aldosterone secretion; tendency to dehydration, due to decreased urinary concentrating ability and deficit in thirst; greater use of drugs that alter intrarenal hemodynamics, such as ACE inhibitors and NSAID; and higher incidence of cardiovascular comorbidity [23].

Obstructive ARF is also more frequent in older people, as well as some intrinsic causes, such as acute cryoglobulinemia, vasculitis, acute interstitial nephritis, acute tubular necrosis, light-chain cast nephropathy, and vascular diseases [23].

Diagnosis is based on the monitoring of creatinine, associated or not with urine production [24].

12.5.4.1 US/Color Doppler

Ultrasound of the urinary tract within 24 h is indicated in all patients in whom the cause of IRA cannot be identified and in those at risk of urinary tract obstruction [24].

In fact urinary tests, normally used in clinical practice, often result to be not useful in the differential diagnosis between the functional (prerenal) and the organic (intrarenal) form due to the presence of confounding factors (use of diuretics, antihypertensive drugs, urinary tract infections, sepsis, etc.) [17].

Intrarenal IRs may be useful for differential diagnosis: mean IR values are significantly higher in patients with organic IRA than those with functional IRA (0.74 ± 0.13 vs. 0.67 ± 0.09, $p < 0.0$) [17] (Figs. 12.11 and 12.12).

Finally, it has been demonstrated that renal IRs predict the onset of IRA in the immediate postoperative period in patients undergoing cardiac surgery with discrete sensitivity (85%) and high specificity (94%) [17].

12.5.5 Vasculitis

Primary and secondary glomerulonephritis, renal vasculitis, and interstitial nephropathies are com-

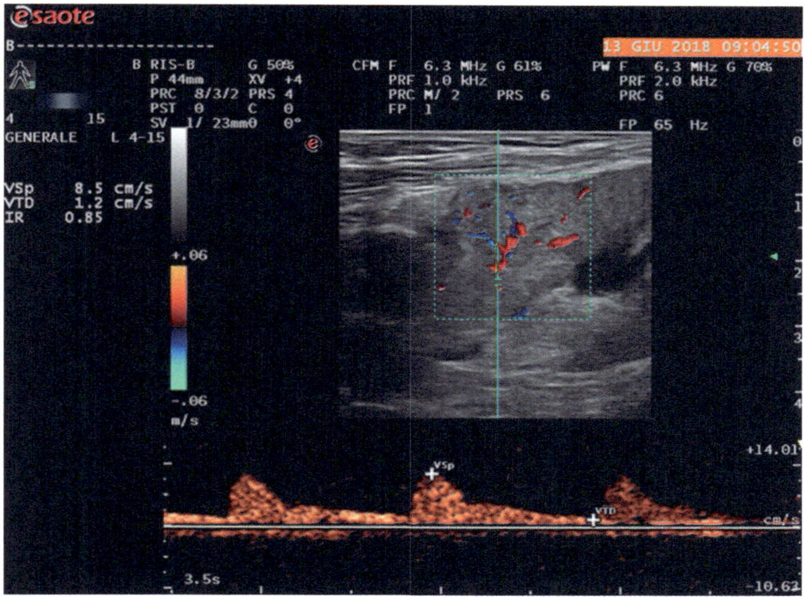

Fig. 12.11 Patients with organic IRA

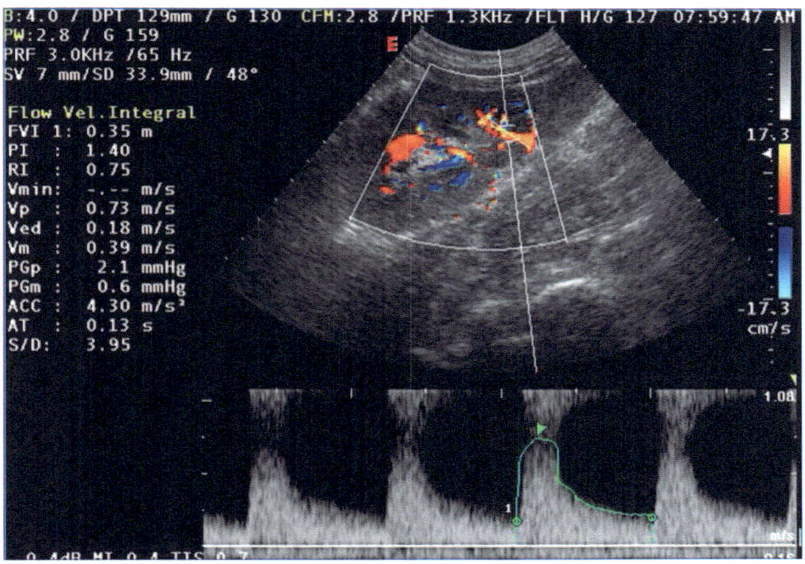

Fig. 12.12 Patients with functional IRA

mon groups of diseases among the elderly. The gold standard is the biopsy. For acute pyelonephritis, instead, the suspicion is placed on a clinical-laboratory basis, but the assessment is based on radiological criteria [25].

12.5.5.1 US/Color Doppler

Patients with vasculitis have higher values of IR (mean IR 0.82 ± 0.05) than those suffering from a pathological process limited to glomeruli (mean IR 0.58 ± 0.05). There is also an anomalous morphology of the Doppler wave in which there is a reduction of the diastolic component rather than the systolic [17].

In patients with lupus nephritis, the detection of IR >0.70 represents an important risk factor of chronicity and correlates with higher creatinine values compared to patients with normal resistance indexes, which appear to have a better renal prognosis [17].

12.5.6 Acute Obstructive Uropathy

Obstructive uropathy is the blockage of urinary flow, which can affect one or both kidneys. Obstructive uropathy becomes more prevalent with increasing age so the diagnosis and management of obstructive uropathy are particularly relevant to the geriatric population [25].

If only one kidney is affected, urinary output may be unchanged and serum creatinine can be normal. When kidney function is affected, this is termed obstructive nephropathy [25].

Main causes of obstructive renal disease in the elderly are benign prostatic hyperplasia and neurological bladder [26]; other common causes are urolithiasis, intrinsic or extrinsic ureteral obstruction, severe bladder ptosis (prolapse and tumors of the uterus, appendages, and vagina), and abdominal aortic aneurysm.

Acute or chronic obstruction of the urinary tract determines renal ischemia, tubular atrophy, and interstitial and glomerular fibrosis, worsening degenerative processes that already afflict senile kidney.

12.5.6.1 US/Color Doppler

Ultrasound, in the suspicion of obstructive nephropathy, should explore kidney, ureters, retroperitoneal space, and pelvic excavation.

It can differentiate acute and chronic obstructive nephropathies: in the first case, kidney has normal or increased dimensions and preserved thickness of parenchyma with accentuated echogenicity; in the second case kidney is small with thinning of parenchyma and hyperechogenic structure.

A mean IR value of 0.69 was reported in obstructed kidneys, while mean IR values of 0.67 and 0.59 were found, respectively, in acutely obstructed kidneys and in unobstructed kidneys with ΔIR (the difference between the mean value of the IR sampled in the two kidneys) significantly high, equal to 0.076. ΔIR has a predictive value of obstruction with 94% sensitivity and 95% specificity.

An IR value >0.70 is correlated with acute renal obstruction and precedes ectasia pyelocaliceal.

References

1. McClure M, Jorna T, Wilkinson L, Taylor J. Elderly patients with chronic kidney disease: do they really need referral to the nephrology clinic? Clin Kidney J. 2017;10(5):698–702.
2. Granata A, Fiorini F, D'Amelio A, et al. L'ecocolorDoppler nella pratica clinica nefrologica. Aggiornamenti in Tema Di Nefrologia. 2010;17:192.
3. McLachlan MS. The ageing kidney. Lancet. 1978;2:143–5.
4. Nasr SH, Fidler ME, Valeri AM, Cornell LD, Sethi S, Zoller A, Stokes MB, Markowitz GS, D'Agati VD. Postinfectious glomerulonephritis in the elderly. JASN. 2011;22(1):187–95.
5. Martin JE, et al. The pathology of ageing: concepts and mechanisms. J Pathol. 2007;211:198–205.
6. Macunluoğlu B, Gökçe I, Atakan A, Demirci M, Arı E, Topuzoğlu A, Borazan A. A comparison of different methods for the determination of glomerular filtration rate in elderly patients with chronic renal failure. Int Urol Nephrol. 2011;43(1):257–63.
7. Cockcroft DW. Gault MH Prediction of creatinine clearance from serum creatinine. Nephron. 1976;16(1):31–41.
8. Roubenoff R. Sarcopenia: effects on body composition and function. J Gerontol Ser A Biol Sci Med Sci. 2003;58:1012–7.
9. Bostom AG, et al. Hyperhomocysteinemia in chronic renal disease. JASN. 2002;13:2140–4.
10. Quaschning T, et al. Abnormalities in uremic lipoprotein metabolism and its impact on cardiovascular disease. Am J Kidney Dis. 2001;38(4 Suppl 1):S14–9.
11. Mancuso D, Comi N, Andreucci M, Donato C, Presta P, Fuiano G. Parametri ecografici renali predittivi di outcome nei pazienti con insufficienza renale cronica. Giornale Italiano di Nefrologia. 2007;24:S-39.
12. Donadio C, Abdelkawy H, Grassi G. Echographic renal dimensions can predict glomerular filtration rate of potential living kidney donors. Transplant Proc. 2010;42(4):1035–9.
13. Afsar B, Elsurer R. Sudden cardiac death and mineral metabolism in chronic kidney disease. Kidney Int. 2010;77(7):648; author reply 648–9
14. Parenti GC, Basteri V, Bucchi E, Sturani A, Degli Esposti E. Colour-Doppler US evaluation of patients with hypertension and nephropathy. Radiol Med. 2006;111(8):1115–23.
15. Parolini C, Noce A, Staffolani E, Giarrizzo GF, Costanzi S, Splendiani G. Renal resistive index

and long-term outcome in chronic nephropathies. Radiology. 2009;252(3):888–96.
16. Tublin ME, Bude RO, Platt JF, et al. The resistive index in renal Doppler sonography: where do we stand? AJR Am J Roentgenol. 2003;180(4):885–92.
17. Fiorini F, Granata A, Noce A, Durante O, Insalaco M, Di Daniele N. Gli indici di resistenza ecografici in nefrologia: quale significato clinico? G Ital Nefrol. 2013;30(2):1.
18. Mallappallil M, Friedman EA, Delano BG, McFarlane SI, Salifu MO. Chronic kidney disease in the elderly: evaluation and management. Clin Pract (Lond). 2014;11(5):525–35.
19. Chrysochou C, Kalra PA. Epidemiology and natural history of atherosclerotic renovascular disease. Prog Cardiovasc Dis. 2009;52(3):184–95.
20. Rogowicz-Frontczak A, Araszkiewicz A, Pilacinski S, Zozulinska-Ziolkiewicz D, Wykretowicz A, Wierusz-Wysocka B. Carotid intima-media thickness and arterial stiffness in type 1 diabetic patients are dependent on age and mean blood pressure. Exp Clin Endocrinol Diabetes. 2011;119(5):281–5.
21. Romano G, Zanoli L, Romano M, et al. Prevalenza di insufficienza renale occulta e valutazione delle equazioni predittive della VFG in anziani ospedalizzati. Abstract Book XXII. Torino: Congresso Nazionale SIUMB; 2010.
22. Alicic RZ, Rooney MT, Katherine R. Tuttle diabetic kidney disease, challenges, progress, and possibilities. CJASN. 2017;12(12):2032–45.
23. Fuiano G, Caglioti A, Marino F, Mancuso D, Comi N, Natale G, Mangiacapra S, Iodice C. L'insufficienza renale acuta nell'anziano. Giorn It Nefrol. 2001;18:469–81.
24. Cartabellotta A, Di Iorio B. Diagnosi e valutazione dell'insufficienza renale acuta. Evidence. 2014;6(2):e1000068. https://doi.org/10.4470/E1000068.
25. Cammarota T, Piccoli G, Sarno A, Rabbia C, Bonenti G. Gilda Olivieri Rene senile: Insufficienza renale nell'anziano. Radiologia geriatrica. Editore: Springer Verlag Anno edizione; 2006. p. 445–59.
26. Tseng TY, Stoller ML. Obstructive uropathy. Clin Geriatr Med. 2009;25(3):437.

13 Intraparenchymal Renal Resistive Index: The Basic of Interpretation and Common Misconceptions

Pierpaolo Di Nicolò, Michele Prencipe, Paolo Lentini, and Antonio Granata

13.1 Introduction

Doppler ultrasonography is a noninvasive, low-cost, and high-sensitive tool for studying the renal circulation. The Doppler spectrum analysis from segmental or interlobar arteries allows us to calculate the renal resistive index (RRI) (Fig. 13.1) that represents the percentage of blood flow reduction at the end of the diastole in renal vessels related to the maximum systolic flow [1]. It is calculated by the following formula: peak systolic velocity (VPS) − telediastolic velocity (VTD)/peak systolic velocity (VPS).

To minimize the intra- and interoperator variability of the RRI and to turn it into a highly reproducible test [2], Doppler sampling must be performed in three different areas of the kidney (i.e., upper, mid, or lower pole) for obtaining a mean value at the end of the examination. The normal RRI value is considered <0.70 but in particular populations such as children up to 6 months old or newborn babies a RI value >0.70 should not necessarily be considered pathological [3]. Several studies have shown that Doppler ultrasound parameters, particularly the RRI, are correlated with biopsy parameters such as vascular and tubulointerstitial lesions [4], but the mechanisms of these correlations remain unknown. In other words RRIs cannot be considered as only markers of renal damage or indicators of renal functional prognosis but they more properly express a clear link between micro- and macro-circulation; moreover RRIs are not always acquired but a possible heritability independently from other proven heritable factors has recently been proved. The purpose of this chapter is to explain the pathophysiological aspects which leads to the bases of this new interpretation providing elements to the nephrologist for a more accurate global vision of the nephropathic patients.

13.2 Examination Technique

A correct measurement of RRI needs a standardized study protocol. First of all a correct detection of the B-mode acoustic window with a precise regulation of focus and gain is required; subsequently, the regulation of the color box is

P. Di Nicolò (✉)
Nephrology and Dialysis Unit, S. Maria della Scaletta Hospital, Imola (Bo), Italy
e-mail: p.dinicolo@ausl.imola.bo.it

M. Prencipe
Nephrology and Dialysis Unit, IRCCS "Casa Sollievo della Sofferenza", San Giovanni Rotondo, Foggia, Italy

P. Lentini
Nephrology and Dialysis Unit, Ospedale "San Bassiano", Bassano del Grappa, VI, Italy

A. Granata
Department of Nephrology and Dialysis, "Cannizzaro" Emergency Hospital, Catania, Italy

A. Granata, M. Bertolotto (eds.), *Imaging in Nephrology*,
https://doi.org/10.1007/978-3-030-60794-4_13

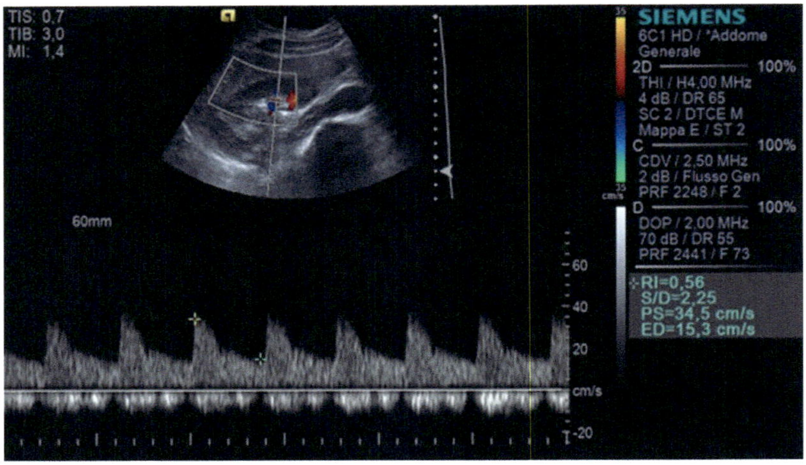

Fig. 13.1 Renal resistive index (RRI) sampled at the level of an interlobar artery. For a more accurate measure multiple Doppler sampling in upper, mid, and lower pole of the kidney is performed and a mean RRI value is obtained

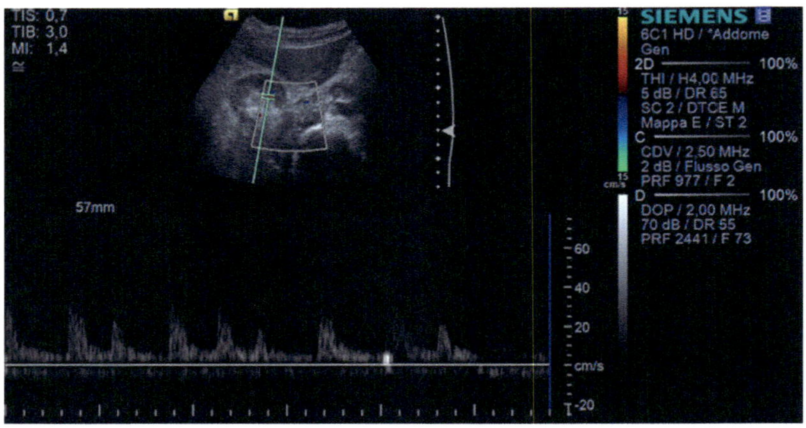

Fig. 13.2 Renal resistive index (RRI) in arrhythmic patient. In these cases the RRI is obtained from average and the diagnostic utility is very limited

basic operation, to facilitate the Doppler analysis and to improve the sensitivity and the frame rate. The color Doppler settings are aimed at the study of interlobar arteries that includes the highest gains possible, the use of the lowest filters, and a low pulse repetition frequency (PRF) of 1–1.5.

After these regulations, the sample volume of the pulsed-wave Doppler module is placed in the lumen of interlobar arteries and the speed–time curve is recorded. To obtain a correct sampling, a careful setting of pulsed-wave Doppler functions (PRF 1.5–3 kHz, gain, depth, filter wall, and Doppler frequency) is a crucial step. The RRI is calculated through the measure of the VPS and the VTD, according to the following formula: VPS − VTD/VPS.

Multiple Doppler sampling in three different areas of the kidney (i.e., upper, mid, or lower pole) at the interlobar or arcuate artery level has been shown to be more effective than a single sampling: by increasing the number of samples, minimizing the intra- and interoperator variability, and considering the RI to be a highly reproducible test [5].

A correct measurement of renal RI can be very difficult in various clinical conditions or in the presence of several confounding factors such as severe hypotension, heart rhythm disorders including tachy–brady arrhythmias (Fig. 13.2), renal compression for perirenal or subcapsular fluid collections, various extrarenal causes of impaired vascular elasticity, and during the Valsalva maneuver.

13.3 Renal Resistive Index Main Determinants

The term RRI is sometimes used as a synonym of "vascular resistance" and this erroneous simplification narrows the number of components in play to only one, which is probably the less important [6, 7], while, actually, systemic and renal parameters both affect the RRI analysis. In fact, evidences obtained from in vitro and in vivo studies prove that vascular resistance and RRI are connected only with dramatic (and probably nonphysiologic) increases of the former while vascular distensibility and pulsatile flow are far more important determinants in the RRI composition [8, 9].

From O'Neill's mathematical analysis we know that RRI is a pulsatility measure with the inverse function of pulse pressure (PP) as the most important parameter in RRI determination [10] and, as a consequence, pulse pressure, cardiac function, vascular compliance, and renal capillary wedge pressure are the most important hemodynamic factors to be considered to understand RRI clinical meaning (Fig. 13.3). Among them a crucial role is played by the PP that is strictly related to extrarenal factors like the cardiac function (CF) and the arterial vascular compliance (VC). The CF and its components (i.e., left ventricular outflow and heart rate) are critical factors in RRI determination in many clinical settings and for example in case of bradycardia, because of a prolonged diastolic duration in the cardiac cycle, the RRI value will result to be elevated showing the inverse relationship between heart rate and RRI that has been largely reported

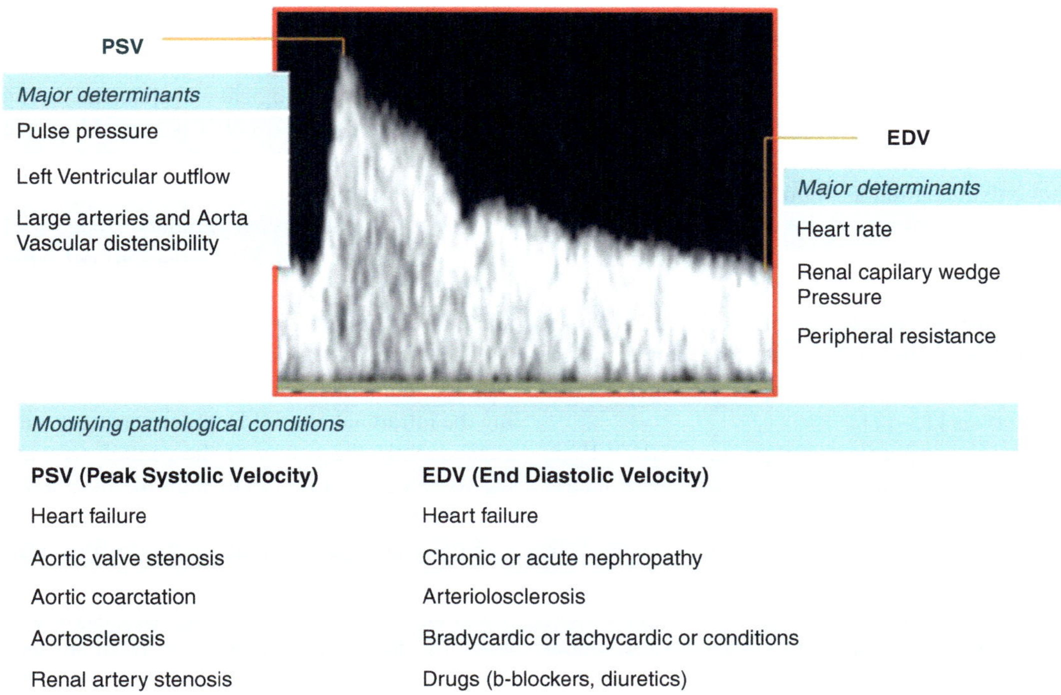

Fig. 13.3 Factors which mainly affect peak systolic velocity and end diastolic velocity in parenchymal renal arteries are here described. The pathological conditions which, acting through one (or more) of the above parameters, are able to modify the renal Doppler spectrum are listed. *PSV* peak systolic velocity, *EDV* end diastolic velocity [47]

in literature [11]. Likewise the left ventricular outflow reduction can have a great impact on RRI and clear demonstrations in this sense can be found in clinical cases of severe valvulopathy (for example aortic valve stenosis) or thoracic aortic coarctation.

Just like it happens in case of a renal artery stenosis the cause for this finding is commonly attributed to the lowering of the PP distal to a stenosis [12] but this explanation is probably incomplete and the independent role of the left ventricular systolic and diastolic function in modifying RRI measure has been proven [13].

The *vascular compliance* (VC) of the aorta and of large arteries determines the blood pressure pulsatility degree by expanding vascular walls during systolic phase of cardiac cycle and by consequently relaxing during the diastole one.

In conditions of systemic VC decreasing such as in the presence of arterial stiffness (physiological or pathological) along with PP modifications, RRI results are strongly affected and this shows an important link between micro- and macrocirculation [14].

Thanks to the wall elasticity of the arterial tree not only a continuous blood flow can be obtained from the heart to the distal vascular bed but also a protection can be offered from microvascular damage to high-resting flow organs (i.e., brain and kidneys). A further confirmation of this phenomenon is the tight connection between RRI and aortic stiffness and between RRI and arteriolosclerosis [15–17].

Renal capillary wedge pressure (RCWP) is another contributing factor in RRI determination and it derives from the combination of renal interstitial and venous pressure. Its variation can also be a consequence of alteration in the systemic hemodynamic: given that in heart failure the decreased cardiac output leads to systemic venous congestion with subsequent elevation of renal venous pressure and kidney impairment, we can suppose that augmented RRI indexes, common in cases of cardiorenal syndrome, probably express increases in the RCWP [18].

Moreover, age, smoking, or other pathological conditions such as atherosclerosis, arterial hypertension, and chronic kidney disease cause reductions in vessel compliance (namely increases in micro- and macro-vascular impedance) and increases in pulse pressure and consequently bring modifications of RRI (Fig. 13.4).

13.4 Cardiovascular System and Resistive Renal Index

In patients with heart failure and preserved ejection function RRI was shown to be elevated compared to control group of hypertensive patients without HF and the severity of these intrarenal vascular hemodynamic alterations was associated with a poor outcome [19].

In another work the RRI prognostic value was evaluated in patients with stable chronic heart failure (CHF). It showed an independent and incremental role in predicting HF progression and it suggested the usefulness of RRI in better defining renal impairment in cardiorenal syndrome [20].

The pathophysiological mechanism is not completely understood but it is probably correlated to the elevated central venous pressure (CVP) [21] that causes renal venous congestion, leading to increased renal capillary wedge pressure (with consequent RRI elevation) determining reduction of the glomerular filtration pressure and consequently worsening of kidney function.

Therefore, it appeared clear that cardiac hemodynamic factors could be crucial in modifying the intrarenal arterial Doppler waveforms and consequently the action of the central pressures has to be kept in mind to explain the mechanism at the basis of this finding [22].

In physiological conditions the central pressures are transmitted unchanged to renal arteries with the pressure reduction occurring beyond the level of the afferent arterioles: if small renal arteries are persistently exposed to high blood flow and high pulsatile pressure the result could be a microvascular damage with a parallel elevation in RRI [23].

Aging can be considered another example of this pathological process and major determinant of RRI, which determines a progressive rigidity of the aorta with a great increase in the arterial

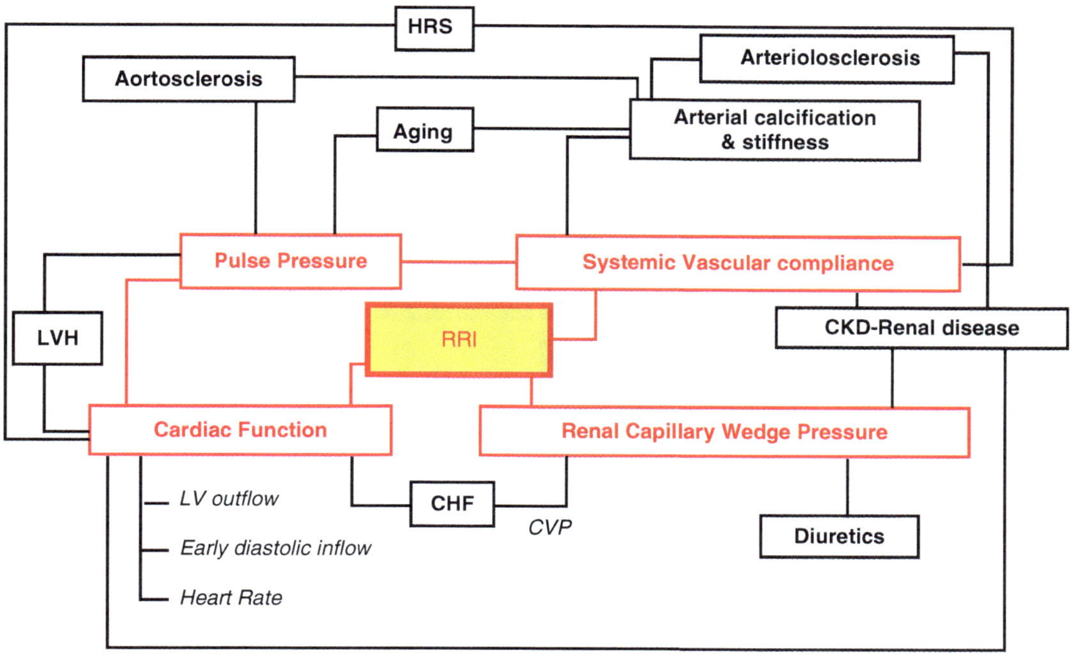

Fig. 13.4 Main hemodynamic factors affecting RRI determination (red rectangles), their reciprocal relationships (red lines), and the most common clinical settings strongly associated with RRI reported in the literature (black rectangles) are depicted. *RRI* renal resistive index, *LV* left ventricle, *LVH* left ventricular hypertrophy, *CHF* chronic heart failure, *CVP* central venous pressure, *CKD* chronic kidney disease, *HRS* hepatorenal syndrome [47]

pulse pressure (which is considered a surrogate parameter of systemic arterial stiffness) and a remarkable exposure of the highly perfused renal arterial bed to pulsatile circumferential stress [24, 25].

Peripheral arterial resistance is strictly connected with intrinsic physical features of the arterial tree; for this reason in the past it was not considered surprising that, as a consequence of renal diseases leading to microvascular damage, RRI was modified.

But after the growing awareness of the small part played by renal arterial resistance in favor of other extrarenal RRI-determining factors [22], new explanations were searched to understand more deeply the pathophysiological link between intrarenal Doppler spectrum profile and vascular system.

In chronic kidney disease (CKD) patients with elevated RRI were strictly related to the presence and extent of abdominal aortic calcification and to systemic atherosclerotic burden indices such as ankle brachial index (ABI) <0.9 and intima media thickness (IMT) >0.1 cm [1].

The strong association between RRI and atherosclerosis in other vascular territories evokes a similar concept raised previously by the following demonstration; in essential hypertensive patients with normal renal function, increased RRI was associated with classical signs of target organ damage such as microalbuminuria, increased IMT, and left ventricular hypertrophy (LVH).

In these patients, the presence of at least two signs of target organ damage was significantly increased in parallel with RRI elevation [26, 27] (Fig. 13.5a–c).

An additional support to these findings derives from a publication by Calabia et al., in which RRI was found to be significantly correlated with all macrovascular damage parameters such as arterial stiffness (carotid-femoral pulse wave velocity, 24-h pulse pressure, and others) and atherosclerotic burden (intended as ABI and IMT),

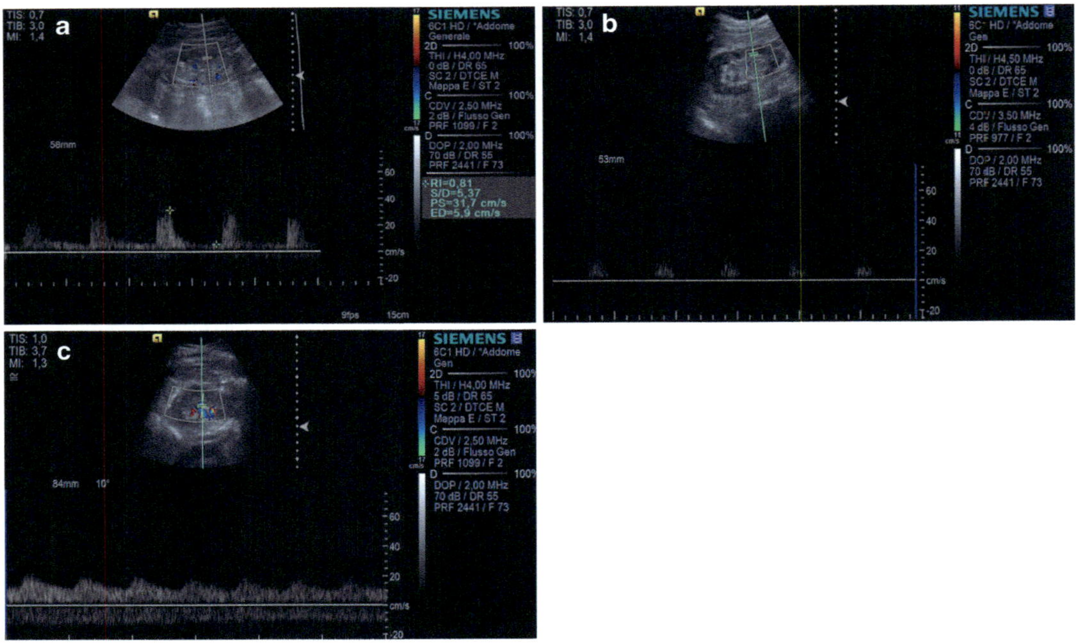

Fig. 13.5 (**a**–**c**) Example of different RRI samples in renal pathologies. (**a**) High RRI value in a patient with widespread and severe atherosclerosis and chronic kidney disease secondary to nephroangiosclerosis. (**b**) Extremely high RRI in a case of acute renal failure (ARF) secondary to tubule interstitial nephritis. Note that no diastolic flow is detectable in renal parenchyma. (**c**) Low RRI value and classic "tardus parvus" waveform pattern distal to a severe renal artery stenosis

with the levels of asymmetric dimethylarginine serum (ADMA) used as a marker of endothelial dysfunction [11].

According to these data, RRI, showing its direct correlation with target organ damage and vascular impairment, seems more as a marker of systemic atherosclerosis than only a specific marker of renal disease.

In addition, it shows its usefulness in the assessment and stratification of cardiovascular risk in hypertensive patients.

13.5 Renal Resistive Index in Acute Kidney Injury

The RRI can be useful to make a differential diagnosis between types of acute kidney injury (AKI): the functional (prerenal) AKI and the organic (renal) AKI. The first one is characterized by reduction in renal perfusion and is a rapidly reversible condition if treated promptly. For this reason, it is generally associated with normal RRI. Differently, organic AKI is more frequently characterized by increased RRI [5].

Platt et al. studied Doppler ultrasound of 91 patients with acute renal failure. They showed that morphological changes were present in only 11% with AKI, while increased RRI (>0.75) occurred in 91% of patients with organic AKI against only 20% of patients with functional AKI. Moreover, the average value of RRI was higher in the group with organic AKI than in the functional AKI group with statistical significance ($p < 0.01$) [28].

RRI is also a good predictor of the onset of AKI in the early postoperative period of patients undergoing cardiac surgery. In fact, AKI is a common complication of cardiac surgery and its incidence ranges from 3 to 30% [29]. A prospective cohort study demonstrated that patients with increased RRI in the immediate postoperative period had an increased risk of developing AKI but the preoperative RRI was not associated with the development of the same risk [30]. Otherwise, Hertzberg et al. showed that a preoperative RRI >0.70 was associated with an increased risk of developing AKI after cardiac surgery [31].

A recent meta-analysis based on 10 studies, including a total number of 911 patients, showed that AKI was associated with higher renal resistive index values preoperatively, immediately after surgery and 24 h postoperatively. Therefore, renal resistive index represents a useful marker with fair performance in the prediction of postoperative acute kidney injury. Future cohorts should establish the optimal timing of measurement and evaluate the most appropriate cutoff value that should be used in the clinical setting [32].

Finally, thanks to its high specificity and sensitivity (85% and 92%, respectively), an RI 0.80 is a more reliable indicator of persistent AKI than that of common urinary markers, and as it does not require blood or urine samples, it is unaffected by changes in Na or Cl in urine or serum after diuretics or hemodialysis and can be performed at the bedside; it could be a promising tool to predict the reversibility of AKI in critically ill patients [32, 33].

13.6 Renal Resistive Index in Chronic Kidney Disease

In chronic kidney disease a renal Doppler ultrasound is a very useful tool because its measurements can provide valid information on therapy and prognosis of these patients.

Several studies showed that increased RRI (≥0.70) is an independent risk factor for the progression of renal failure [34, 35]. Sugiura et al. found a significative correlation between RRI values of 0.70 or higher in chronic nephropathies and parenchymal irreversible damage [36]. In patients with renal artery stenosis, RRI values >0.80 or >0.73 (in the contralateral kidney) were associated to a reduced improvement of renal function after revascularization [37, 38].

Moreover, RRI may be used not only to evaluate the risk for progression to end-stage renal disease, but also to predict the survival rate. In fact, in 162 CKD patients without renal artery stenosis, RRI >0.80 was associated but also to a lower survival rate [39]. The same results were obtained from a large population of patients (n = 1962) with eGFR 15–59 mL/min. In this study RRI ≥0.70 was associated to an increase in all-cause mortality in a median follow-up of 2 years [40].

More recently in patients with moderate renal dysfunction it was observed that a RRI value ≥0.79 was a valid predictor for the annual decline in estimated glomerular filtration rate and a negative prognostic indicator for cardiovascular events [41].

Thus, the use of Doppler ultrasound in CKD should take on a wider role in the nephrologist's daily life but there is certainly a need for further developments in this direction.

13.7 Renal Resistive Index in Transplanted Kidney

The studies carried out on renal allograft recipients can be considered important "in vivo" models useful to verify the hypothesis that if RRIs are so strictly connected with the systemic cardiovascular properties they have to be greatly modified by a complete change in the vascular environment.

The confirmation arrives from the work of Naesens who, in a study involving more than 300 renal allograft recipients, found that RRI was not related to graft features such as function or intrarenal histologic disease pattern but reflected the characteristics of the host and was connected with the recipient age [39].

In other works allograft RRIs were barely related to donor parameters such as age or allograft function while they were well associated with host-related factors such as PP, IMT, and ABI [42].

A recent meta-analysis evaluated the efficacy of RRI in the prediction of delayed graft function in the posttransplant period. Fourteen studies were included with a total of 2741 patients [43].

So we can consider plausible the idea that graft RRIs are "mirror index" of the cardiovascular status of the recipient and they can be considered recipient's survival indicators.

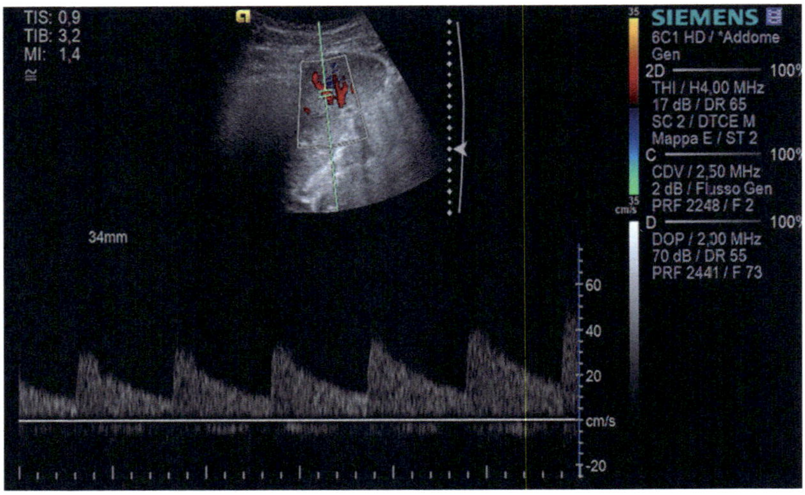

Fig. 13.6 Splenic resistive index (SRI), measured at the level of splenic artery segmental branches. After multiple sampling a mean SRI value is obtained. The DI-RISK is calculated by subtracting the mean SRI from the mean RRI

13.8 Renal Resistive Index and Splenic Resistive Index

In healthy subjects and in patients with chronic kidney disease, RRI and SRI (Fig. 13.6) are mutually connected and both are associated with IMT [44].

Moreover, both RRI and SRI show a strong association with PP, higher LV mass, and Doppler indexes of diastolic dysfunction leading to the conclusion that RRI and SRI can likewise be influenced by cardiovascular risk factors and systemic vascular diseases.

In order to calibrate RRI only in kidney-specific damage, avoiding the effect of other extrarenal factors, a new index called DI-RISK derived from the formula (DI RISK = mean RRI – mean SRI) was introduced.

DI-RISK has shown an independent association with eGFR (but not with systemic hemodynamic factors) and it appears a promising tool in overcoming the limits of the RRI in the evaluation of renal pathology, although its usefulness in prognostic evaluation of CKD is still under discussion [45].

13.9 Renal Resistive Index Heritability

The role of anthropometric factors such as age, female sex, body weight, and height in determining RRI has been clearly shown in literature but a recent family-based population study has raised the possible heritability of RRI and not only as an index of other proven heritable factors.

In particular in subjects of European ancestry and without diabetes mellitus, hypertension, or CKD, RRI was confirmed to be a heritable trait [46].

Additional studies are needed to identify the gene (or multiple genes) which act in the determination of RRI but the future chance of identification of families with lower RRI and therefore with lower risk of renal functional worsening with age appears as an interesting scenery.

The contingency of a genetic pattern involved in RRI control strengthens the conviction that RRIs are not only numbers and that their real hemodynamic value and clinical significance are yet to be discovered.

13.10 Conclusions

RRI determination involves renal and extrarenal factors not always distinguishable in the common clinical practice where a more critical analysis of RRI is recommended; however, the idea that RRI and vascular resistance are synonymous terms can be considered substantially erroneous while the leading role of pulse pressure in RRI determination has always to be stressed [47].

The acknowledgement of all the pathophysiological factors at the basis of the intrarenal

Doppler waveform composition sheds a light on the link between the renal microcirculation and the cardiovascular system and can lead the clinician to valuable information on both the hemodynamic status and the cardiovascular profile of the patient.

References

1. Stefan G, Capusa C, Stancu S, Petrescu L, Nedelcu ED, Andreiana I, Mircescu G. Abdominal aortic calcification and renal resistive index in patients with chronic kidney disease: is there a connection? J Nephrol. 2014;27(2):173–9.
2. Granata A, Zanoli L, Clementi S, Fatuzzo P, Di Nicolò P, Fiorini F. Resistive intrarenal index: myth or reality? Br J Radiol. 2014;87:1038.
3. Andriani G, Persico A, Tursini S, Ballone E, Cirotti D, Lelli Chiesa P. The renal-resistive index from the last 3 months of pregnancy to 6 months old. BJU Int. 2001;87:562–4.
4. Gigante A, Barbano B, Di Mario F, Rosato E, Simonelli M, Rocca AR, Conti F, Ceccarelli F, Giannakakis K, Valesini G, Cianci R. Renal parenchymal resistance in patients with biopsy proven glomerulonephritis: correlation with histological findings. Int J Immunopathol Pharmacol. 2016;29(3):469–74.
5. Fiorini F, Granata A, Noce A, Durante O, Insalaco M, Di Daniele N. Index resistance in renal ultrasound: what is the clinical significance? G Ital Nefrol. 2013;30(2):gin/30.2.4.
6. Tublin ME, Bude RO, Platt JF. The resistive index in renal Doppler sonography: where do we stand? AJR Am J Roentgenol. 2003;180(4):885–92.
7. Chirinos JA, Townsend RR. Systemic arterial hemodynamics and the "renal resistive index": what is in a name? J Clin Hypertens (Greenwich). 2014;16(3):170–1.
8. Bude RO, Rubin JM. Relationship between the resistive index and vascular compliance and resistance. Radiology. 1999;211:411–7.
9. Tublin ME, Tessler FN, Murphy ME. Correlation between renal vascular resistance, pulse pressure, and the resistive index in isolated perfused rabbit kidneys. Radiology. 1999;213:258–64.
10. O'Neill WC. Renal resistive index: a case of mistaken identity. Hypertension. 2014;64(5):915–7.
11. Calabia J, Torguet P, Garcia I, Martin N, Mate G, Marin A, Molina C, Valles M. The relationship between renal resistive index, arterial stiffness, and atherosclerotic burden: the link between macrocirculation and microcirculation. J Clin Hypertens (Greenwich). 2014;16(3):186–91.
12. Kuznetsova T, Cauwenberghs N, Knez J, Thijs L, Liu YP, Gu YM, Staessen JA. Doppler indexes of left ventricular systolic and diastolic flow and central pulse pressure in relation to renal resistive index. Am J Hypertens. 2015;28(4):535–45.
13. Ciccone MM, Iacoviello M, Gesualdo L, Puzzovivo A, Antoncecchi V, Doronzo A, Monitillo F, Citarelli G, Paradies V, Favale S. The renal arterial resistance index: a marker of renal function with an independent and incremental role in predicting heart failure progression. Eur J Heart Fail. 2014;16(2):210–6.
14. Hashomoto J, Ito S. Central pulse pressure and aortic stiffness determine renal hemodynamics: pathophysiological implication for microalbuminuria in hypertension. Hypertension. 2011;58(5):839–46.
15. Kirkpatrick AW, Colistro R, Laupland KB, et al. Renal arterial resistive index response to intraabdominal hypertension in a porcine model. Crit Care Med. 2007;35:207–13.
16. Pozniak MA, Kelcz F, Stratta RJ, Oberley TD. Extraneous factors affecting resistive index. Investig Radiol. 1988;23:899–904.
17. Mullens W, Abrahams Z, Francis GS, Sokos G, Taylor DO, Starling RC, Young JB, Tang WH. Importance of venous congestion for worsening of renal function in advanced decompensated heart failure. J Am Coll Cardiol. 2009;53:589–96.
18. Ohuchi H, Ikado H, Noritake K, Miyazaki A, Yasuda K, Yamada O. Impact of central venous pressure on cardiorenal interactions in adult patients with congenital heart disease after biventricular repair. Congenit Heart Dis. 2013;8(2):103–10.
19. Ennezat PV, Maréchaux S, Six-Carpentier M, Pinçon C, Sediri I, Delsart P, Gras M, Mounier-Véhier C, Gautier C, Montaigne D, Jude B, Asseman P, Le Jemtel TH. Renal resistance index and its prognostic significance in patients with heart failure with preserved ejection fraction. Nephrol Dial Transplant. 2011;26(12):3908–13.
20. Mostbeck GH, Gössinger HD, Mallek R, Siostrzonek P, Schneider B, Tscholakoff D. Effect of heart rate on Doppler measurements of resistive index in renal arteries. Radiology. 1990;175:511–3.
21. Rozemeijer S, Haitsma Mulier JLG, Röttgering JG, Elbers PWG, Spoelstra-de Man AME, Tuinman PR, de Waard MC, Oudemans-van Straaten HM. Renal resistive index: response to shock and its determinants in critically ill patients. Shock. 2019;52(1):43–51.
22. Boddi M, Natucci F, Ciani E. The internist and the renal resistive index: truths and doubts. Intern Emerg Med. 2015;10(8):893–905.
23. O'Rourke MF, Hashimoto J. Mechanical factors in arterial aging: a clinical perspective. J Am Coll Cardiol. 2007;50(1):1–13.
24. Boddi M, Sacchi S, Lammel RM, et al. Age-related and vasomotor stimuli-induced changes in renal vascular resistance detected by Doppler ultrasound. Am J Hypertens. 1996;9:461–6.
25. O'Rourke MF, Safar ME. Relationship between aortic stiffening and microvascular disease in brain and kidney: cause and logic of therapy. Hypertension. 2005;46(1):200–4.
26. Pontremoli R, Viazzi F, Martinoli C, Ravera M, Nicolella C, Berruti V, Leoncini G, Ruello N, Zagami P, Bezante GP, Derchi LE, Deferrari G. Increased renal resistive index in patients with essential hyper-

tension: a marker of target organ damage. Nephrol Dial Transplant. 1999;14(2):360–5.
27. Doi Y, Iwashima Y, Yoshihara F, Kamide K, Takata H, Fujii T, Kubota Y, Nakamura S, Horio T, Kawano Y. Association of renal resistive index with target organ damage in essential hypertension. Am J Hypertens. 2012;25(12):1292–8.
28. Platt JF, Rubin JM, Ellis JH. Acute renal failure: possible role of duplex Doppler US in distinction between acute prerenal failure and acute tubular necrosis. Radiology. 1991;179(2):419–23.
29. Vives M, Wijeysundera D, Marczin N, et al. Cardiac surgery-associated acute kidney injury. Interact Cardiovasc Thorac Surg. 2014;18:637–45.
30. Bossard G, Bourgoin P, Corbeau JJ, et al. Early detection of postoperative acute kidney injury by Doppler renal resistive index in cardiac surgery with cardiopulmonary bypass. Br J Anaesth. 2011;107:891–8.
31. Hertzberg D, Ceder SL, Sartipy U, et al. Preoperative renal resistive index predicts risk of acute kidney injury in patients undergoing cardiac surgery. J Cardiothorac Vasc Anesth. 2017;31:847–52.
32. Bellos I, Pergialiotis V, Kontzoglou K. Renal resistive index as predictor of acute kidney injury after major surgery: a systematic review and meta-analysis. J Crit Care. 2019;50:36–43.
33. Nori G, Granata A, Leonardi G, Sicurezza E, Spata C. The US color Doppler in acute renal failure. Minerva Urol Nefrol. 2004;56(4):343–52.
34. Parolini C, Noce A, Staffolani E, Giarrizzo GF, Costanzi S, Splendiani G. Renal resistive index and long-term outcome in chronic nephropathies. Radiology. 2009;252(3):888–96.
35. Sugiura T, Wada A. Resistive index predicts renal prognosis in chronic kidney disease. Nephrol Dial Transplant. 2009;24(9):2780–5.
36. Sugiura T, Wada A. Resistive index predicts renal prognosis in chronic kidney disease: results of a 4-year follow-up. Clin Exp Nephrol. 2011;15(1):114–20.
37. Radermacher J, Chavan A, Bleck J, Vitzthum A, Stoess B, Gebel MJ, Galanski M, Koch KM, Haller H. Use of Doppler ultrasonography to predict the outcome of therapy for renal-artery stenosis. N Engl J Med. 2001;344(6):410–7.
38. Bruno RM, Daghini E, Versari D, Sgrò M, Sanna M, Venturini L, Romanini C, Di Paco I, Sudano I, Cioni R, Lerman LO, Ghiadoni L, Taddei S, Pinto S. Predictive role of renal resistive index for clinical outcome after revascularization in hypertensive patients with atherosclerotic renal artery stenosis: a monocentric observational study. Cardiovasc Ultrasound. 2014;12:9.
39. Heine GH, Gerhart MK, Ulrich C, Köhler H, Girndt M. Renal Doppler resistance indices are associated with systemic atherosclerosis in kidney transplant recipients. Kidney Int. 2005;68:878–85.
40. Toledo C, Thomas G, Schold JD, Arrigain S, Gornik HL, Nally JV, Navaneethan SD. Renal resistive index and mortality in chronic kidney disease. Hypertension. 2015;66(2):382–8.
41. Kim JH, Lee SM, Son YK, Kim SE, An WS. Resistive index as a predictor of renal progression in patients with moderate renal dysfunction regardless of angiotensin converting enzyme inhibitor or angiotensin receptor antagonist medication. Kidney Res Clin Pract. 2017;36(1):58–67.
42. Naesens M, Heylen L, Lerut E, Claes K, De Wever L, Claus F, et al. Intrarenal resistive index after renal transplantation. N Engl J Med. 2013;369:1797–806.
43. Bellos I, Perrea DN, Kontzoglou K. Renal resistive index as a predictive factor of delayed graft function: a meta-analysis. Transplant Rev (Orlando). 2019;33(3):145–53.
44. Grün OS, Herath E, Weihrauch A, Flügge F, Rogacev KS, Fliser D, Heine GH. Does the measurement of the difference of resistive indexes in spleen and kidney allow a selective assessment of chronic kidney injury? Radiology. 2012;264:894–902.
45. Lennartz CS, Pickering JW, Seiler-Mußler S, Bauer L, Untersteller K, Emrich IE, Zawada AM, Radermacher J, Tangri N, Fliser D, Heine GH. External validation of the kidney failure risk equation and re-calibration with addition of ultrasound parameters. Clin J Am Soc Nephrol. 2016;11(4):609–15.
46. Ponte B, Pruijm M, Ackermann D, Vuistiner P, Eisenberger U, Guessous I, Rousson V, Mohaupt MG, Alwan H, Ehret G, Pechere-Bertschi A, Paccaud F, Staessen JA, Vogt B, Burnier M, Martin PY, Bochud M. Reference values and factors associated with renal resistive index in a family-based population study. Hypertension. 2014;63(1):136–42.
47. Di Nicolò P, Granata A. Renal resistive index: not only kidney. Clin Exp Nephrol. 2017;21(3):359–66.

Contrast-Enhanced Ultrasound (CEUS) in Nephrology

14

Antonio Granata, Luca Zanoli, Irene Campo, Rosario Maccarrone, and Michele Bertolotto

14.1 Introduction

During last years, a major step in the evolution of clinical ultrasound, the contrast-enhanced ultrasonography (CEUS), has been developed. CEUS imaging can easily integrate a Doppler echography examination [1] and be a potential competitor of heavy imaging techniques for both functional and morphological studies of several pathological processes. The main advantages of this new technique in kidney imaging compared to heavy imaging techniques are the absence of ionising radiations and nephrotoxicity, rapidity of execution and immediate feedback, excellent repeatability, as well as possibility to perform the test at the patient's bed and the contained costs [2]. However, there are clinical situations in whom the use of heavy imaging techniques with contrast media would be preferred but the presence of comorbidities and renal dysfunction, highly common in the elderly, and the use of contrast media in these subjects could be highly problematic due to the risk of inducing a further deterioration of the renal function.

Recently, the usefulness of CEUS in nephrology has been reviewed [2]. In particular, CEUS is useful for the evaluation of focal ischemic lesions and traumatisms, as well as for the control of the native kidney and the transplanted one [3, 4]. However, as well as for any innovative medical technique associated with the infusion of pharmacological substances, the potential advantages of CEUS and the possible risks and side effects need to be critically evaluated and clearly codified. In this regard, the International Contrast Ultrasound Society (ICUS) has been recently founded to define the safe, effective use of CEUS imaging [5].

Here we performed an updated overview of the potential nephrological applications of CEUS imaging, reporting some indications and possible risks connected to its use.

14.2 The Chemical Structure of Echo Amplifiers

The two components of the ultrasound contrast media consist of (a) a gas incorporated in microbubbles and (b) the coating membrane (known also as shell). Their composition of the echo

A. Granata (✉) · R. Maccarrone
Nephrology and Dialysis Unit, A.O. per l'Emergenza "Cannizzaro", Catania, Italy

L. Zanoli
Section of Nephrology, Department of Medical and Pediatric Sciences, University of Catania, Catania, Italy

I. Campo
Department of Radiology, Civile Hospital, Conegliano, Italy

M. Bertolotto
Department of Radiology, Cattinara Hospital, University of Trieste, Trieste, Italy

A. Granata, M. Bertolotto (eds.), *Imaging in Nephrology*,
https://doi.org/10.1007/978-3-030-60794-4_14

amplifiers is properly set in order to increase the stability and persistence in the patient's circulatory system. The improvements gradually introduced over time have thus concerned both the gas contained inside the microbubbles and the coating membrane.

Echo amplifiers of the first generation used air as gas enveloped by a coating membrane of lipids and proteins. The first-generation ultrasound contrast media SH U 454 (Echovist, Schering, Berlin) and SH U 508 A (Levovist, Schering, Berlin) are no longer available in the European Union. An analogous first-generation product in the United States was Albunex (Molecular Biosystems Inc., San Diego). Differently to the European version, the coating membrane of Albunex was human albumin. These products had a short persistence in the circulatory system for the high instability of the bubbles that were destroyed too rapidly, with the consequent immediate release of the air contained inside. Therefore, the contrastographic effect was thus short-lasting and hard to manage.

Taking in mind the limits of the first generation of ultrasound contrast media, a second contrast media generation was developed. These echo amplifiers are formed by microbubbles of an inert gas (organic sulphurs) with a lower solubility in the blood and greater stability. The capsule of these microbubbles has a variable chemical structure depending on the commercial product, but it is mainly formed by phospholipids. Consequently, these products have a greater persistence in the circulatory system than the first generation and allow an easier study of the different organs. Of these media, the only one authorised in Europe, sulphur hexafluoride (SonoVue, Bracco Imaging, Milan), has a coated surface of phospholipids and ethylene glycol. This echo amplifier is authorised by the European Medicines Agency for the study of liver, breast, and vascular macro- and microcirculation. Using an extensive interpretation of the latter indication, it is possible to study the kidney and the urogenital system. In the opposite hypothesis that this configures an off-label use of sulphur hexafluoride, it is possible to obtain a specific informed consent from the patient and an authorisation from the company's ethical committee for the clinical use of this media in the context of renal ultrasound. It is also important to verify that the insurance covers both the staff and the hospital in case of accident. The use in paediatric subjects and pregnant women and during breastfeeding is not discussed in the technical notes and thus should always be considered off-label.

14.3 Tolerance and Side Effects

The evaluation of the tolerance and side effects of the CEUS imaging is complex because it is necessary to take into account not only the possible effects of the drug administration, but also the effects of the interaction between the microbubbles and the energy of the ultrasound band. Due to the optimal tolerance of the ultrasound contrast media, its use in the clinical field is authorised by the health authorities of different countries (AIFA, NEMA, FDA, etc.). As highlighted by the studies performed before the authorisation for clinical use, minor side effects (transitory pain at the injection point, altered taste, or hypotension for vasovagal response) were observed in less than 5% of the subjects. More serious adverse reactions were reported in the post-marketing during echocardiographic studies. The onset of ventricular arrhythmia was related to the use of high mechanical index (a safety metric which lets the operator know how much energy is being transmitted into the patient during sonography), and the consequent massive rupture of the bubbles in the telesystolic phase. This side effect on the myocardium has been reproduced in animal models, so that the use of CEUS imaging in cardiology demands particular attention, in particular when large volumes of elevated mechanical bubbles are used [6]. The main contraindications are recent acute myocardial infarction (<7 days), class III/IV cardiac failure, right-to-left shunts, severe pulmonary hypertension, pregnancy, and breastfeeding. A retrospective study on CEUS imaging safety in the abdominal field performed on 23,188 patients reported no fatal event [7]. Adverse reactions were reported in 29 patients (0.009%). Of these adverse reactions, two were classified as severe and four required a medical treatment [7]. The authors concluded that the contrast medium used in Italy (sulphur hexafluoride, Bracco Imaging, Milan, Italy) is highly safe for the study of abdominal disease, with an incidence of adverse reactions extremely lower than that observed following the administration of radiological or gadolinium contrast media [7].

Episodes of rupture of the glomerular capillaries, small intra-glomerular haemorrhages and petechiae on the surface of the kidney, and transitory microhaematuria (reverted in around 24 h) were reported using drug doses, frequencies, mechanical indexes, and exposure durations extremely higher than those actually used in clinical practice [5, 8–10]. These side effects, started from a mechanical index >0.4 KPa, increased in number and size according to the power and the frequency used during sonography [11].

The widely accepted conclusions and the recommendations of the national and international scientific companies confirm the significant safety of the commercially available contrast media used and advise to use a mechanical index lower than 0.2 KPa to minimise the rupture of the bubbles and the consequent phenomenon of cavitation, responsible for the release of energy that can damage the cellular structures. Taking in mind that our current understanding cannot exclude subclinical damage and bio-effects at a distance from the use of the echo amplifiers, the use of these techniques should always be based on valid indications and a correct evaluation of the clinical risk/benefit.

14.4 Clinical Applications of CEUS Imaging in Nephrology

14.4.1 Study Methods

The echo-contrastographic study of the kidney is performed in B-mode with a standard-resolution (3.5–5.0 MHz) convex probe. In order to obtain a harmonic signal useful for the construction of the image, the microbubbles need to be insonated with their specific fundamental frequency, known as *resonance*, which falls in the frequency range usually used for the abdominal ultrasound examination (3.0–5.0 MHz). The second-generation echo-contrastographic tests with microbubbles require a lower insonation power (mechanical index <0.2 kPa) to avoid a rapid destruction. These microbubbles require slow bolus intravenous injection, lasting a few seconds, using 18 gauge needle-cannula, to avoid the Venturi effect or "hydrodynamic paradox," potentially determined by the reduced gauge of the needles and/or an excessively elevated infusion, which would determine the massive destruction of the microbubbles for the turbulence created at the extremity of the needle exit. The bolus is classically followed by a further bolus of 10 mL of physiological solution. The CEUS images were obtained using sulphur hexafluoride (SF_6) microbubbles (Bracco Imaging, Milan, Italy). The gas of these microbubbles is eliminated by the breathing and does not interfere with renal or hepatic excretion.

We performed our studies using the Siemens-Acuson S3000 ultrasound system (Acuson-Siemens, Mountain View, CA, USA) with a 6C2 probe for the US detection of renal parenchymal changes, including the Cadence™ CPS technology, a low-mechanical-index technique with a transmission frequency of 2.0 MHz. Following intravenous bolus injection of 2.4 mL of contrast agent, images were acquired for 3 min using contrast harmonic imaging (CHI) and stored as cine clips and volume data set.

14.4.2 Normal Kidney

The microbubbles reached the kidneys after 10–15″ from the infusion and are first distributed in the cortical (cortical phase), while the medullar vessels are progressively filled after 25–35″. This happens because the medullar presents a lower perfusion than the cortical (190 vs. 400 mL/min/100 g of texture). The *washout* starts in the medullar and then extends slowly to the cortical. Because there is not a tubular phase (secretory and/or excretory) in the echo-contrastographic imaging, it is correct to distinguish (a) early

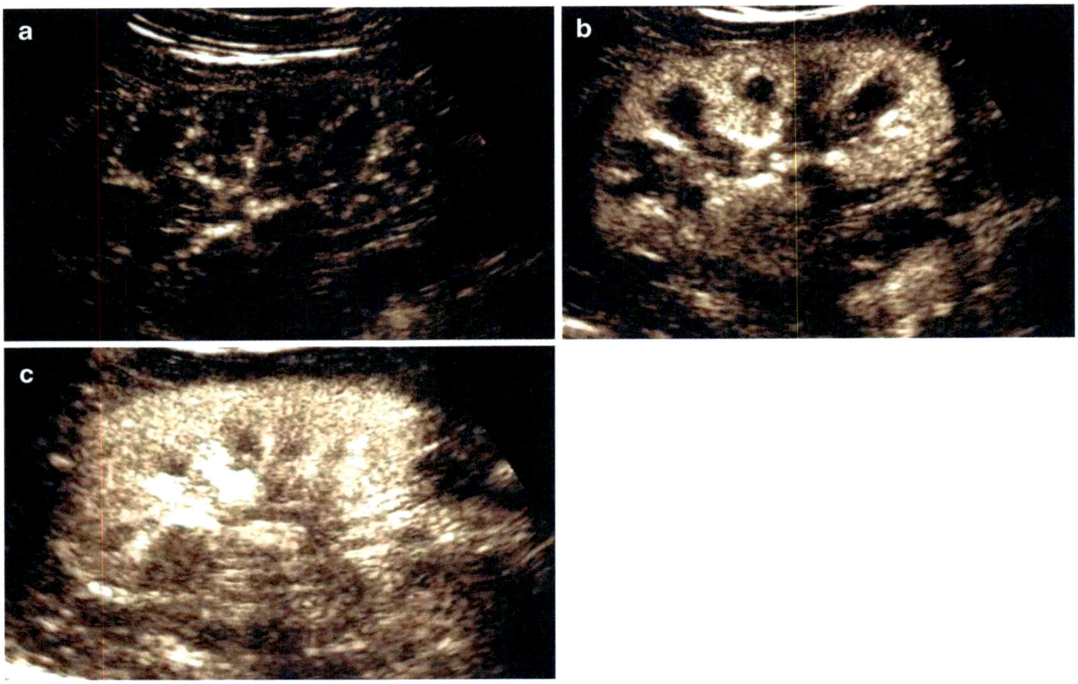

Fig. 14.1 After the administration of the contrast agent. (**a**) The arterial vessels of the vascular peduncle and the interlobar arterial vessels are recognised. (**b**) Subsequently follows the cortical phase with medulla savings. (**c**) Then follows the parenchymal phase characterised by both cortical and medullary enhancement

arterial phase, where arteries are highly evident; (b) late arterial (or cortical) phase, characterised by intense and uniform enhancement of the renal cortex (from 12″ to 35″ after infusion), where the cortico-medullary differentiation is evident; and (c) medullary phase or late phase (from 40″ to 120″), where pyramids gradually fill with contrast until they are isoechoic with the cortex (Fig. 14.1). Unlike iodinated contrast media, CEUS microbubbles remain in the circulatory system and there is no pyelographic phase.

14.4.3 Pseudo-Lesions

Irrespective of the vascularisation, the renal malignancies present different enhancement compared with the surrounding parenchyma. It is possible to differentiate between morphological variants of the parenchyma (hypertrophy of the Bertin column, persistence of fetal lobulation, presence of humps) or pseudo-lesions and renal lesions by observing the enhancement in all the vascular phases, because the former are characterised by an enhancement comparable to the surrounding parenchyma in all the phases (iso-in and iso-out) (Fig. 14.2). It is also important to underline that in many small-sized renal malignancies, after an intense and precocious enhancement in the arterial phase, there is a late enhancement analogous to the parenchyma or, inversely, an early enhancement analogous to the parenchyma in the arterial phase and an early washout in the remaining vascular phases [12].

14.4.4 Differential Diagnosis Between Solid Lesions and Cysts

The differentiation between cystic and solid lesions probably represents, at the current state, the most important application of CEUS imaging in nephrology [4].

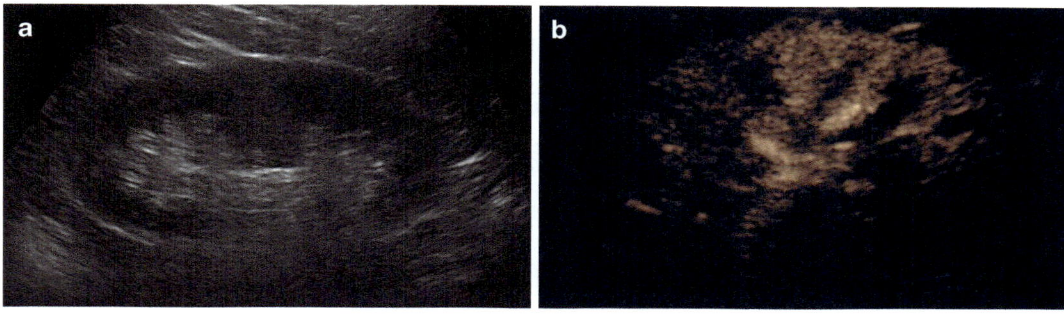

Fig. 14.2 Echo-contrastographic characterisation of the renal pseudo-lesions. (**a**) Basic echographic image of the left kidney showing a focal thickening of the parenchyma. (**b**) Echo-contrastographic image after the administration of the contrast showing how the pseudo-lesion presents the same vascular characteristics of the surrounding renal parenchyma, with visualisation of the renal medulla

Ultrasound criteria of benignity of the cysts are the total anechogenicity of the content, presence of reinforcement of the posterior wall, clear and regular margins, absence of thickened walls, and colour Doppler signal in the context of the cyst.

The simple cysts (type I according to Bosniak) or the minimally complicated ones (type II) appear in B-mode as unilocular, completely anechogenous, without internal echoes even after infusion of the microbubbles. Inversely, in complicated cysts the microbubbles allow to clearly distinguish, with high accuracy, the thin capillaries around the cystic walls, the possible internal septum, and/or vascularising micronodules.

Similarly to CT scan, taking advantage of the wall enhancement, CEUS imaging can detect the septum or the parietal nodules and differentiate cystic lesions (Fig. 14.3) [12] according to the criteria of Bosniak (the Bosniak classification weights the malignancy potential of a cystic lesion [13]). The diagnostic accuracy of CEUS imaging is at least analogous to that of CT and MR, with the undoubted advantages of the low cost and the low biological risk (absence of nephrotoxicity of the echographic contrast and absence of ionising radiation). Also, unlike the MR which is highly dependent on the degree of patient collaboration, CEUS imaging is often useful also in scarcely collaborative patients. Consequently, it can be considered a valid alternative to CT and MR, especially in the follow-up of the complex non-surgical cystic lesions (class IIF according to Bosniak) to exclude their aggressive nature. At this regard, surgery is recommended for class III and IV, whereas class IIF requires follow-up to show stability over time and class II and I are benign. Internal echoes of a cyst can be dense and can therefore mimic a solid tumour on greyscale ultrasonography. CEUS imaging can differentiate between a complicated cyst and solid tumour. A further role of imaging is to differentiate these solid renal masses into benign and malignant lesions. Imaging features of both plain and contrast-enhanced CT and MRI can be applied to CEUS imaging to study the solid renal masses. The tumour echogenicity on grey scale, enhancement patterns, and degree of enhancement at different phases are used to differentiate between benign and malignant solid renal mass lesions. The solid kidney tumours in general have an intense arterial precocious enhancement, equal or greater than that of the surrounding renal parenchyma. Intralesional areas are often detectable without enhancement for the presence of necrosis, while late enhancement is highly variable. Often, once the arterial phase has passed, the lesions may result almost totally isoechogenous in respect to the surrounding parenchyma (Fig. 14.4) [12, 14]. Contrast-enhanced ultrasonography is valuable in differentiating angiomyolipoma (AML) and renal cell carcinoma (RCC) [15]. CEUS features of homogeneous and prolonged enhancement are suggestive of AML whereas an early washout, heterogeneous enhancement, and an enhanced

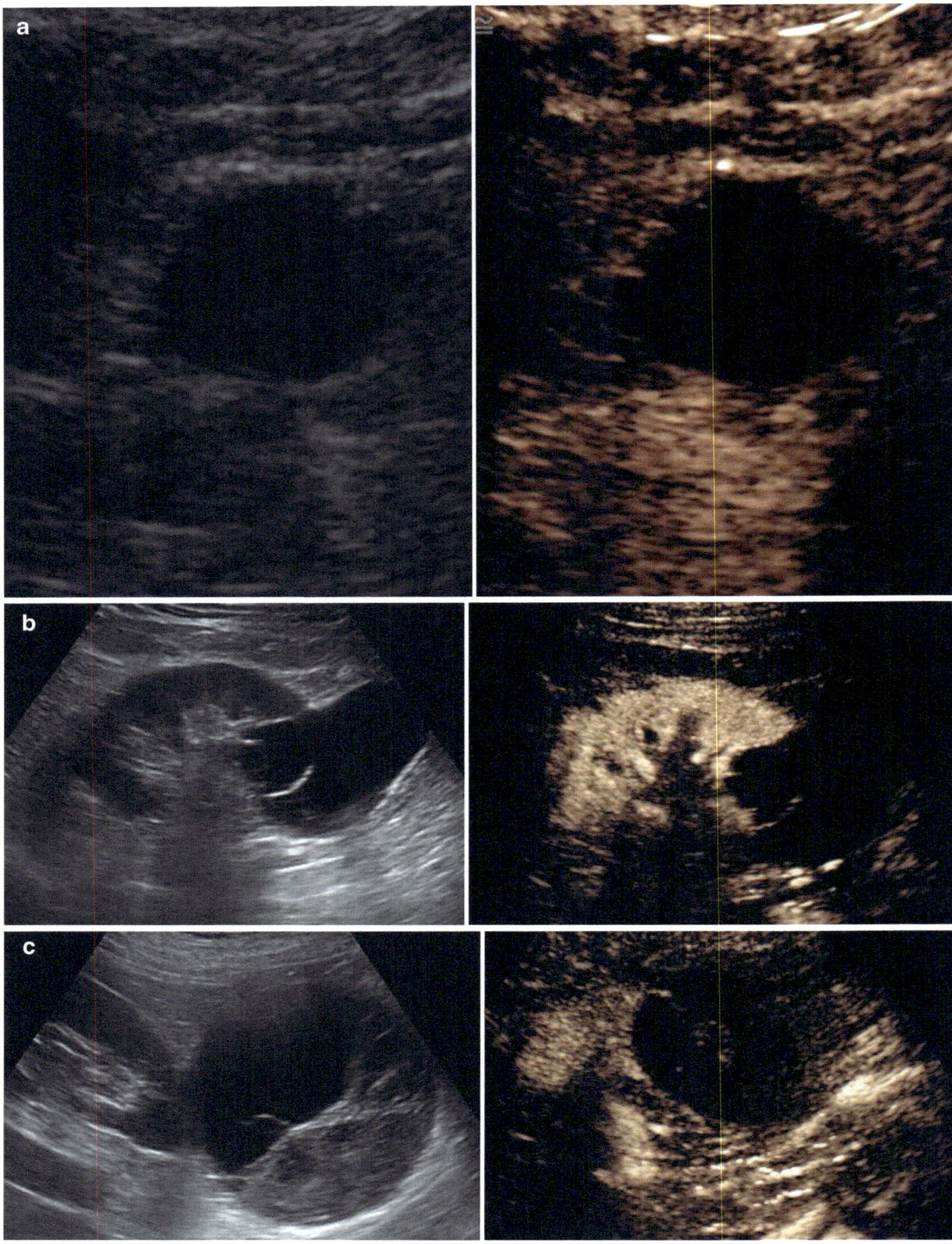

Fig. 14.3 Characterisation of the kidney's complex cystic lesions with echo-contrastography. (**a**) Bosniak category I. Cyst with minimal intralesional echoes, which after the contrast does not present septa, vegetation, or wall thickening. (**b**) Bosniak category II. Cyst with thin calcific septum with absence of intralesional enhancement and parietal irregularities at echo-contrastographic examination. (**c**) Bosniak category IIF. Benign cysts need follow-up examination for the presence of minimally thickened and regular wall with enhancement. (**d**) Bosniak category III. Indeterminate renal cyst for the presence of multiple sects with enhancement with some irregularities of thickness. (**f**) Bosniak category IV. Cysts of malignant appearance for the presence of intralesional vegetations

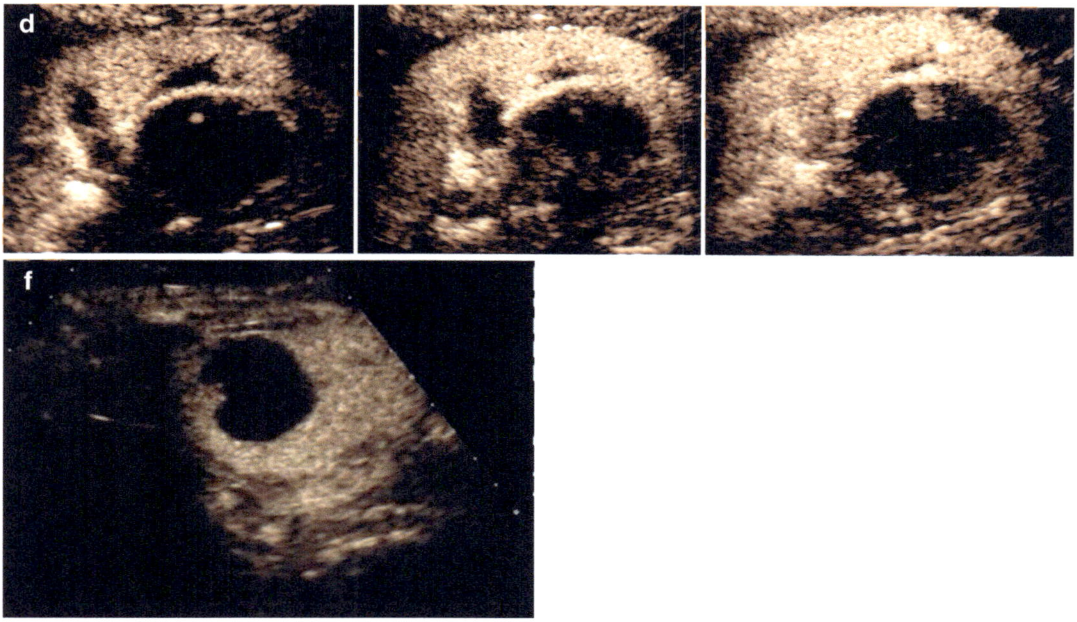

Fig. 14.3 (continued)

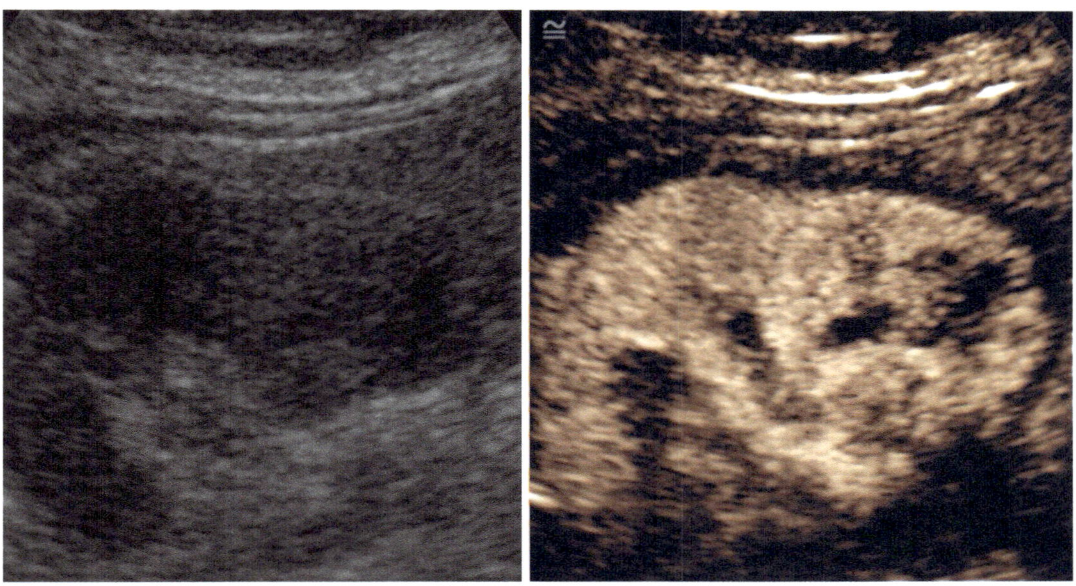

Fig. 14.4 Solid kidney lesion. In the middle third of the right kidney, a lesion is visible characterised by iso-echogenic echogenicity, minimally exophytic, which after administration of the contrast shows an intense, homogeneous vascularisation delimited by the surrounding parenchyma

peritumoral rim or pseudo-capsule is highly suggestive of RCC [7, 8]. Finally, CEUS imaging can also be used to differentiate between malignancies and inferior vena cava thrombus related to renal cell carcinoma.

14.4.5 Lesions with Dubious Enhancement at CT

With the increasing use of CT, the detection of renal lesions characterised by density differences of 10–20 HU between the direct and the nephrographic phase has become relatively common. The lesions that are often not clearly differentiable between solid and cystic using CT alone [14] are often papilliferous or chromophobic malignancies, less vascularised with clear cells. In these situations, ultrasound B-mode and colour Doppler do not provide additive useful diagnostic information, also for the relatively scarce vascularisation of the lesions. Inversely, CEUS imaging, thanks to its high sensitivity in recognising the enhancement also in poorly vascularised lesions and to the excellent spatial resolution, allows to differentiate between solid and cystic lesions, which do not present a vascular signal [14].

14.4.6 Traumatic Pathology

The use of CEUS imaging allows a significant improvement in the diagnostic performance of the ultrasound also in renal traumatism. The traumatic lesions are evident as enhancement defects in the context of the healthy surrounding parenchyma. In particular, the contusions appear as tenuously hypoechogenic areas with poorly defined margins, the laceration as striae or anechogenous bands that reach the surface of the organ, the hematomas as areas of more or less marked intraparenchymal or subcapsular hypoechogenicity, and the infarctions as clear and well-defined avascular areas [16, 17]. However, compared with CT, the most important limit of CEUS imaging is the impossibility to detect single lesions out of the excretory ways. In conclusion, it is reasonable that CEUS imaging will be in the future increasingly used in the follow-up of the non-surgical renal traumatisms especially in the young patients [18], but not in the first evaluation of the traumatised patient.

14.4.7 Phlogistic Pathology

CEUS imaging can have a role in patients with phlogosis. In agreement with the guidelines of the European Society of Urology for the diagnosis of pyelonephritis, the use of imaging techniques is indicated principally in patients non-responsive to medical therapy within the first 72 h or in the suspicion of complications. Since the ultrasound appearance is often variable and aspecific, the recourse to second-level imaging techniques is frequently required. CEUS imaging can detect the presence of acute pyelonephritis as parenchymal areas of hypoperfusion, generally of triangular morphology [19]. Small abscesses are visible as round lesions without contrast enhancement, at times with perilesional enhancement rim (Fig. 14.5) [19, 20]. The diagnostic accuracy of CEUS seems to be inferior in case of diffuse pyelonephritis because it is not possible to compare contemporaneously the kidneys for the focal and multifocal forms. Mitterberger et al.

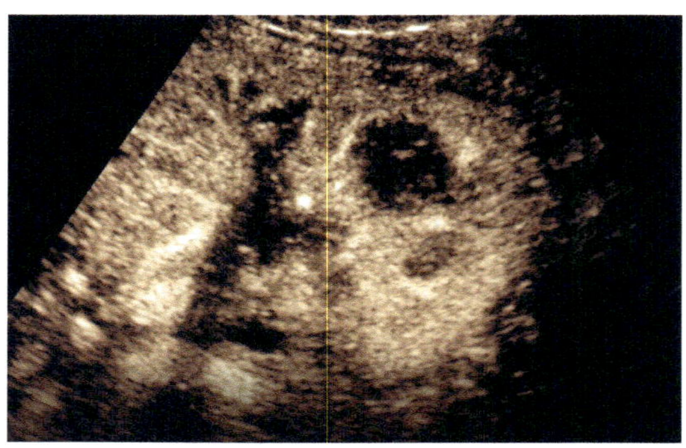

Fig. 14.5 Usefulness of the echo-contrastography in the renal phlogosis. Febrile patient, hypovascularised area at the III median of the right kidney. No signs of colliquation are visible in B-mode. At the echo-contrastography, in the mesorenal region a lesion is visible with peripheral enhancement and central colliquated area, compatible with an abscess collection (diagnosis confirmed for the disappearance of the lesion after medical therapy)

reported in selected subjects a sensibility of 98% and a specificity of 100% of CEUS imaging to detect diffuse pyelonephritis, with positive and negative predictive values of 100% and 89%, respectively [20].

14.4.8 Study of Patients Submitted to Ablative Therapies

Percutaneous or intraoperative (radiofrequency, thermo-ablation, laser, cryotherapy, etc.) ablative therapies are valid therapeutic options for the treatment of renal malignancies <4–5 cm in diameter [21], and it is reasonable that the indications will increase in the near future. Imaging techniques play a fundamental role not only in the identification of the lesions, but also in the evaluation of the therapeutic result of the treatment [22] and in the follow-up. Ultrasound imaging without contrast does not provide information on the therapeutic efficacy of the ablation performed. This limitation can easily be overcome by CEUS imaging. The echo-contrastographic test should be performed 5–10 min after the ablation, the time necessary to have the disappearance of the artefacts linked to procedure. The persistence of areas of contrast enhancement in the context of the lesion is considered the expression of residual neoplastic activity while the absence of enhancement excludes the residue or the recovery of the disease [16]. Because the diagnostic accuracy in evaluating the treatment results with CEUS imaging is quite similar to CT with contrast, CEUS is an effective alternative in the post-treatment control.

14.4.9 Renal Ischemia

In the case of clinical suspicion of renal infarction, colour and power Doppler are the first investigations useful for the identification of focal or diffusive perfusion defects. However, the diagnostic accuracy is reduced by the relative insensitivity of the Doppler techniques in the evaluation of the slow flows. Also, the unfavourable angle of insonation of the renal poles considerably limits the study of the flows [7]. CEUS imaging goes beyond both limits and allows the evaluation of the perfusion of the parenchyma in almost all clinical situations.

After the administration of the contrast medium the renal infarcts appear as regions with a wedge-like morphology and base turned towards the capsule, without enhancement. The excellent spatial resolution of CEUS allows to differentiate between renal infarcts and cortical ischemia (Fig. 14.6), in which it is possible to recognise the enhancement of segmentary, interlobar, and arciform vessels, and the absence of enhancement of the interlobular vessels of the renal cortex. The diagnostic sensibility of CEUS imaging is quite similar to angiography and CT [7]. However, unlike CT and MR with contrast medium, CEUS imaging does not present counter-indications in patients affected by renal insufficiency and has a specific indication in the clinical suspicion of acute cortical necrosis.

14.4.10 Renal Artery Stenosis

Colour Doppler is widely considered as the first-line technique of choice for the diagnosis of stenosis/obstruction of the renal artery. This technique presents evident advantages in patients with chronic renal insufficiency because it does not require the use of radiological contrast medium or gadolinium. The use of echo amplifiers, which increase around 30-fold the intensity of the arterial Doppler signal, allows a better visualisation of the renal arteries, reduces the duration of the test (and thus increases the productivity of the ultrasound surgeries), and reduces the number of undiagnostic tests. The main indication of CEUS imaging is in subjects in which the velocity/time curve is hard to obtain in basal conditions (calcifications, obesity, etc.). However, the capacity of CEUS imaging to improve the diagnostic accuracy is still debated [23]. In the near future, the application of new parametric software will reasonably permit a quantitative analysis of the CEUS curves and a more accurate definition of the renal perfusion and will probably add important elements in the diagnostics of

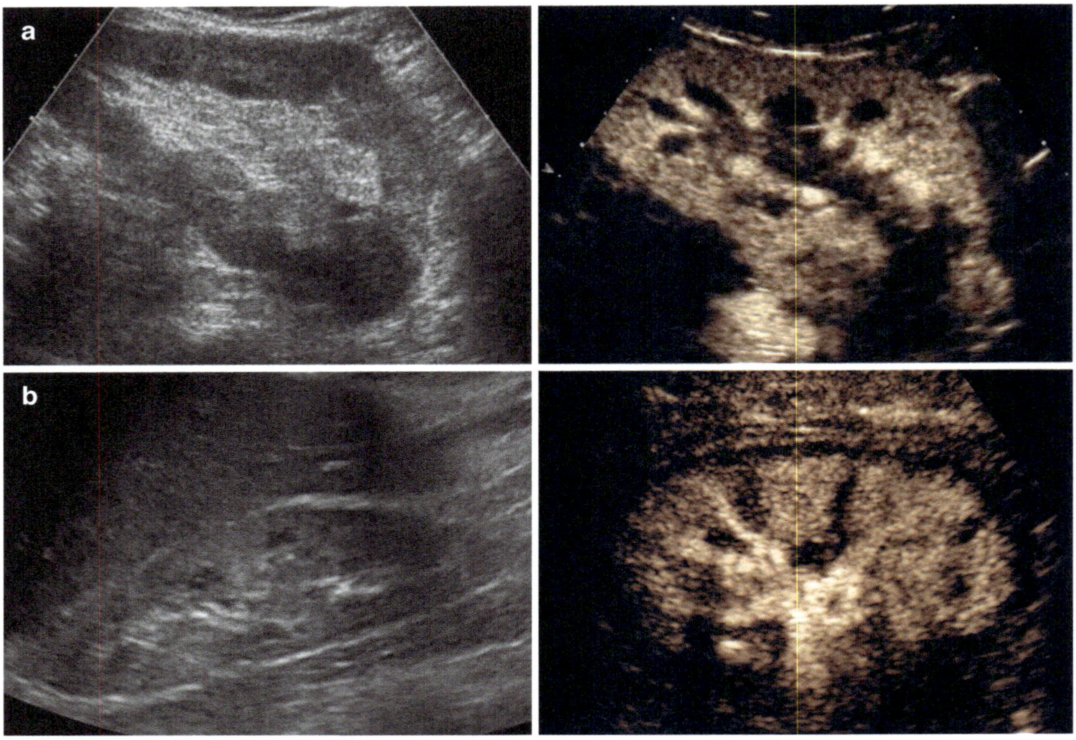

Fig. 14.6 Echo-contrastographic appearance of the renal ischemic lesions. (**a**) Acute renal infarct visible as a triangular shaped area at the third median of the kidney without enhancement. (**b**) Acute renal cortex, identifiable by the presence of flows in the segmentary, interlobar, and arciform vessels, and by the absence of enhancement in ample portion of the renal cortex

renal artery stenosis and in predicting the response to a possible PTA.

14.4.11 Vesicoureteral Reflux

The diagnosis of vesicoureteral reflex (VUR) is traditionally done with the conventional minctional cystography which represents the gold standard technique for the diagnosis, follow-up, and verification of the results after medical, surgical, or endoscopic treatment. However, the elevated radiant dose, aggravated by the prolonged radioscopic observation necessary in the phases of bladder filling and in the minctional phase and the inevitable irradiation of the gonads and the vertebral hematopoietic marrow, represents the main limitation of this technique in subjects often in paediatric age. Bladder CEUS imaging for the research of VUR had already been used in last decades. The only echocontrast means authorised by the AIFA was Levovist, at present no longer in production.

The most recent research refers to the SonoVue with diagnostic results that overlap with those of the Levovist and are clinically very satisfactory. As previously reported, CEUS imaging is without radiogenic risk but, as well as the classical retrograde cystography, it requires bladder catheterisation or direct puncture of the bladder, both invasive and not risk free. The test consists of the transurethral application of a catheter or the direct puncture of the bladder by the suprapubic way. 0.1–0.5 mL of SonoVue should be diluted in 500 mL of tepid physiological solution and slowly injected into the bladder. The progressive distension of the bladder is thus followed in real time by the suprapubic probe, demonstrating

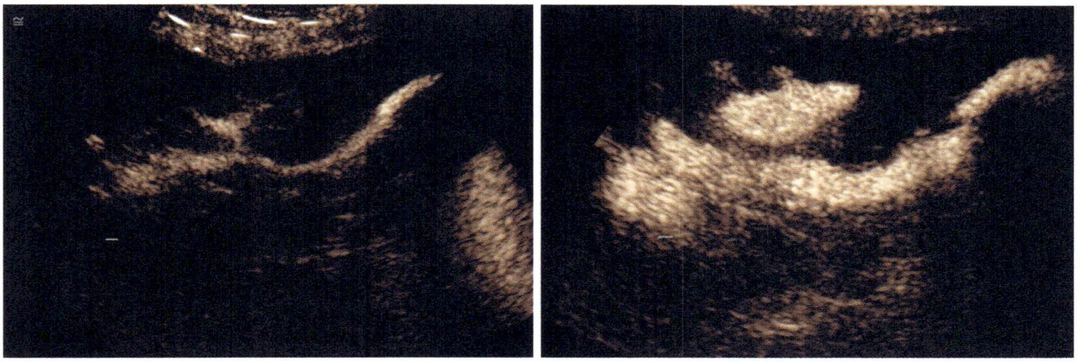

Fig. 14.7 Vesicoureteral reflux. It is visible that after the filling of the bladder with the contrast medium there is a progressive reflux of this in the ureter and in the renal calices of the transplanted kidney

mobile hyperechogenous spots referable to microbubbles, which progressively occupy all of the bladder lumen. After that the filling of the viscera has been obtained, and the reflux must be searched at the level of the ureters and pyelocaliceal system, slowly filling with hyperreflective bubbles. The scans of the kidneys and ureters are acquired in supine and prone decubitus before and after diuresis.

In the presence of RVU, echocystocontrastography provides images comparable with those obtained by traditional cystography, adopting the same classification criteria in 5 degree, according to the scheme proposed by the International Reflux Grading System on Voiding Cystourethrography (Fig. 14.7). The echocystocontrastography compensates the reduced angle of view, due to the relatively small size of the scanning surface obtained by the ultrasound probe, with the multiplanarity of the performable echotomograms and the possibility to record some clips where the whole excretory unit is wholly scanned allowing to represent the reflux dynamically. It also allows a prolonged observation and repeated fillings, increasing the likelihood of revealing an intermittent reflux.

Compared to minctional cystourethrography, the echocystocontrastography shows a sensibility of 57–100%, a specificity of 85–100%, a positive predictive value of 58–100%, and a negative predictive value of 87–100% for the search and quantification of vesicoureteral reflux [24]. The accuracy ranges from 78% to 96%, with the higher values obtained in the most recent works. We should also take into mind that the echocontrastographic test reported a 19% false negative at the minctional cystourethrography compared with 10% of false negatives reported by classical radiological technique. We have detected a concordance of the gravity of the reflux between the two techniques in 73.6% of the cases, while echocystography overestimated the reflux in 19.6%, in particular in the presence of grade I and II refluxes. In conclusion, echocystocontrastography is a highly reliable and reproducible technique, potentially capable of substituting the classical radiological cystourethrography, particularly in the follow-up of patients with RVU, in young girls with phlogosis of the lower urinary pathways and for the screening of children with severe vesicoureteral reflux.

14.4.12 Transplanted Kidney

The CEUS parametric study of the transplanted kidney allows us to effectively and objectively evaluate the entity of the parenchymal vascularisation of the graft. The few works reported in the literature with second-generation microbubbles suggest a great potential of CEUS imaging in the visualisation of the parenchymal perfusional deficits, from the alterations of the macro- to those of the microcirculation.

Perfusion, including the capillary microcirculation, is a universally recognised parameter of vitality and functionality of a tissue since pathological variations of the perfusion are detectable during acute and chronic rejection. The recent analytical applications of tracer kinetics, pixel by pixel, and the changes in the intensity of the signal induced by the administration of the microbubbles allow the definition of colour maps of the haemodynamic parameters (parametric maps) of the organ/structure/lesion investigated: i.e. regional blood volume, regional blood flow, and average transit time.

A delay in the cortical enhancement is frequent in patients affected by acute renal transplant rejection [25]. This finding is, however, unspecific since it is observed in the presence of each acute renal insufficiency and voluminous perirenal haematomas [25]. Another study has shown a reduction in the ratio between cortical and medullar blood flow during acute tubular necrosis [23].

Other authors have compared parametric CEUS imaging to ECD for the early diagnosis of chronic allograft nephropathy reporting a sensibility of CEUS imaging of 91% (82% for ECD), a specificity of 82% (64% for ECD), and an accuracy of 85% (73% for ECD). Interestingly, the use of echocontrast not only improves the diagnostic capacity of the ECD for the diagnosis of CAN but also provides quantitative information on the microvascular and perfusional integrity of the graft [26]. Moreover, CEUS imaging has a possible use also in the diagnosis of acute pyelonephritis in transplanted kidney, showing a diagnostic accuracy of 95% and a positive predictive value of 100% when compared to the gold standard, the gadolinium-enhanced MRI. However, the extremely high negative predictive value (75%) suggests that in case of negative CEUS we cannot exclude the disease. In this regard, a possible explanation could be the small sample size of the study.

References

1. Granata A, Zanoli L, Clementi S, Fatuzzo P, Di Nicolò P, Fiorini F. Resistive intrarenal index: myth or reality? Br J Radiol. 2014;87(1038):20140004.
2. Granata A, Zanoli L, Insalaco M, Valentino M, Pavlica P, Di Nicolò PP, Scuderi M, Fiorini F, Fatuzzo P, Bertolotto M. Contrast-enhanced ultrasound (CEUS) in nephrology: has the time come for its widespread use? Clin Exp Nephrol. 2015;19(4):606–15.
3. Bertolotto M, Catalano O. Contrast-enhanced ultrasound: past, present, and future. Ultrasound Clinics. 2009;4:339–67.
4. Claudon M, Cosgrove D, Albrecht T, et al. Guidelines and good clinical practice recommendations for contrast enhanced ultrasound (CEUS)—update 2008. Ultraschall Med. 2008;29:28–44.
5. Piscaglia F, Nolsøe C, Dietrich CF, Cosgrove DO, Gilja OH, Bachmann Nielsen M, Albrecht T, Barozzi L, Bertolotto M, Catalano O, Claudon M, Clevert DA, Correas JM, D'Onofrio M, Drudi FM, Eyding J, Giovannini M, Hocke M, Ignee A, Jung EM, Klauser AS, Lassau N, Leen E, Mathis G, Saftoiu A, Seidel G, Sidhu PS, ter Haar G, Timmerman D, Weskott HP. The EFSUMB guidelines and recommendations on the clinical practice of contrast enhanced ultrasound (CEUS): update 2011 on non-hepatic applications. Ultraschall Med. 2012;33(1):33–59.
6. Hoeffel C, Mulé S, Huwart L, Frouin F, Jais JP, Helenon O, Correas JM. Renal blood flow quantification in pigs using contrast-enhanced ultrasound: an ex vivo study. Ultraschall Med. 2010;31(4):363–9.
7. Piscaglia F, Bolondi L. The safety of Sonovue in abdominal applications: retrospective analysis of 23,188 investigations. Ultrasound Med Biol. 2006;32:1369–75.
8. Hoeffel C, Mule S, Huwart L, Frouin F, Jais JP, Helenon O, Correas JM. Renal blood flow quantification in pigs using contrast-enhanced ultrasound: an ex vivo study. Ultraschall Med. 2010;31(4):363–9.
9. Miller DL, Quddus J. Lysis and sonoporation of epidermoid and phagocytic monolayer cells by diagnostic ultrasound activation of contrast agent gas bodies. Ultrasound Med Biol. 2001;27(8):1107–13.
10. Miller DL, Dou C, Wiggins RC. Glomerular capillary hemorrhage induced in rats by diagnostic ultrasound with gas-body contrast agent produces intratubular obstruction. Ultrasound Med Biol. 2009;35(5):869–77.
11. Williams AR, Wiggins RC, Wharram BL, Goyal M, Dou C, Johnson KJ, Miller DL. Nephron injury induced by diagnostic ultrasound imaging at high mechanical index with gas body contrast agent. Ultrasound Med Biol. 2007;33(8):1336–44.
12. Ascenti G, Mazziotti S, Zimbaro G, et al. Complex cystic renal masses: characterization with contrast-enhanced US. Radiology. 2007;243:158–65.
13. Israel GM, Bosniak MA. How I do it: evaluating renal masses. Radiology. 2005;236:441–50.
14. Tamai H, Takiguchi Y, Oka M, et al. Contrast-enhanced ultrasonography in the diagnosis of solid renal tumors. J Ultrasound Med. 2005;24:1635–40.
15. Xu ZF, Xu HX, Xie XY, Liu GJ, Zheng YL, Lu MD. Renal cell carcinoma and renal angiomyolipoma: differential diagnosis with real-time contrast-

enhanced ultrasonography. J Ultrasound Med. 2010;29(5):709–17.

16. Meloni MF, Bertolotto M, Alberzoni C, et al. Follow-up after percutaneous radiofrequency ablation of renal cell carcinoma: contrast-enhanced sonography versus contrast-enhanced CT or MRI. AJR Am J Roentgenol. 2008;191:1233–8.
17. Catalano O, Aiani L, Barozzi L, et al. CEUS in abdominal trauma: multi-center study. Abdom Imaging. 2009;34:225–34.
18. Valentino M, Serra C, Zironi G, De Luca C, Pavlica P, Barozzi L. Blunt abdominal trauma: emergency contrast-enhanced sonography for detection of solid organ injuries. AJR Am J Roentgenol. 2008;191:1233–8.
19. Valentino M, Ansaloni L, Catena F, Pavlica P, Pinna AD, Barozzi L. Contrast-enhanced ultrasonography in blunt abdominal trauma: considerations after 5 years of experience. Radiol Med. 2009;114:1080–93.
20. Mitterberger M, Pinggera GM, Colleselli D, et al. Acute pyelonephritis: comparison of diagnosis with computed tomography and contrast-enhanced ultrasonography. BJU Int. 2008;101:341–4.
21. Gervais DA, McGovern FJ, Arellano RS, McDougal WS, Mueller PR. Renal cell carcinoma: clinical experience and technical success with radiofrequency ablation of 42 tumors. Radiology. 2003;226:417–24.
22. Goldberg SN, Gazelle GS, Mueller PR. Thermal ablation therapy for focal malignancy: a unified approach to underlying principles, techniques, and diagnostic imaging guidance. AJR Am J Roentgenol. 2000;174:323.
23. Ciccone MM, Cortese F, Fiorella A, Scicchitano P, Cito F, Quistelli G, Pertosa G, D'Agostino R, Guida P, Favale S. The clinical role of contrast-enhanced ultrasound in the evaluation of renal artery stenosis and diagnostic superiority as compared to traditional echo-color-Doppler flow imaging. Int Angiol. 2011;30(2):135–9.
24. McCarville MB. Contrast-enhanced sonography in pediatrics. Pediatr Radiol. 2011;41(Suppl 1):S238–42.
25. Fischer T, Dieckhofer J, Muhler M, et al. The use of contrast-enhanced US in renal transplant: first results and potential clinical benefit. Eur Radiol. 2005;15(Suppl 5):E109–16.
26. Schwenger V, Hinkel UP, Nahm AM, Morath C, Zeier M. Real-time contrast-enhanced sonography in renal transplant recipients. Clin Transpl. 2006;20(Suppl 17):51–4.

Functional MR Imaging in Native Kidney Dysfunction

15

Elena L. Indino, Alessandro Di Gaeta,
Riccardo Campa, and Valeria Panebianco

15.1 Functional MRI Tools

Since the function of the kidney centers on fluid regulation, magnetic resonance imaging (MRI) is naturally suited for in vivo measurement of various aspects of renal function, such as perfusion, filtration, diffusion, and oxygenation (Table 15.1). Because of its noninvasive nature and provision of quantitative measures of a wide variety of physiological parameters MRI represents an essential research and potentially diagnostic tool [1–3].

Table 15.1 MRI technique for in vivo measurement of renal function

Physiologic parameters	MRI tools
Perfusion	ASL, DCE, DWI, IVIM
Glomerular filtrations	DCE
Interstitial diffusion	DWI
Tissue oxygenation	BOLD
Tubular transit and sodium concentration	Na-MRI

15.2 Dynamic Contrast-Enhanced MRI (DCE-MRI)

DCE-MRI, or MR-renography, is used to characterize renal perfusion and vascular properties. Hemodynamic measurements rely on exogenous tracers that affect the blood MR characteristics. An intravenous injection of contrast agent (CA) alters two independent MR time constants and consequently creates dynamic contrast that can be detected using T1- and T2-weighted perfusion measurements (Fig. 15.1). By considering a set of images acquired before, during, and after a CA infusion (generally 3–5 min after CA injection), a region of interest (ROI) or individual voxel will display a characteristic signal intensity time course, which can be related to CA concentration. By fitting the DCE-MRI data to an appropriate pharmacokinetic model, physiological parameters can be extracted that relate to extraction fraction (EF), glomerular filtration rate (GFR), and renal blood flow. Determination of GFR by MRI data is feasible because the standard CA, Gd-DTPA, is freely filtered at the glomerulus and is not excreted and not reabsorbed. MR signal intensity can be translated to contrast media concentration in order to generate a concentration-time curve for any region of interest that depicts vascular, proximal, and distal phase in the cortex, as primary sources of data for perfusion models to calculate hemodynamic parameters. Various models have been proposed: deconvolution, two-compartment separable compartment model, three-compartment models, and a seven-compartment model. The potential to

E. L. Indino · A. Di Gaeta · R. Campa
V. Panebianco (✉)
Department of Radiological Sciences, Oncology and Pathology, Policlinico Umberto I, Sapienza University of Rome, Rome, Italy

A. Granata, M. Bertolotto (eds.), *Imaging in Nephrology*,
https://doi.org/10.1007/978-3-030-60794-4_15

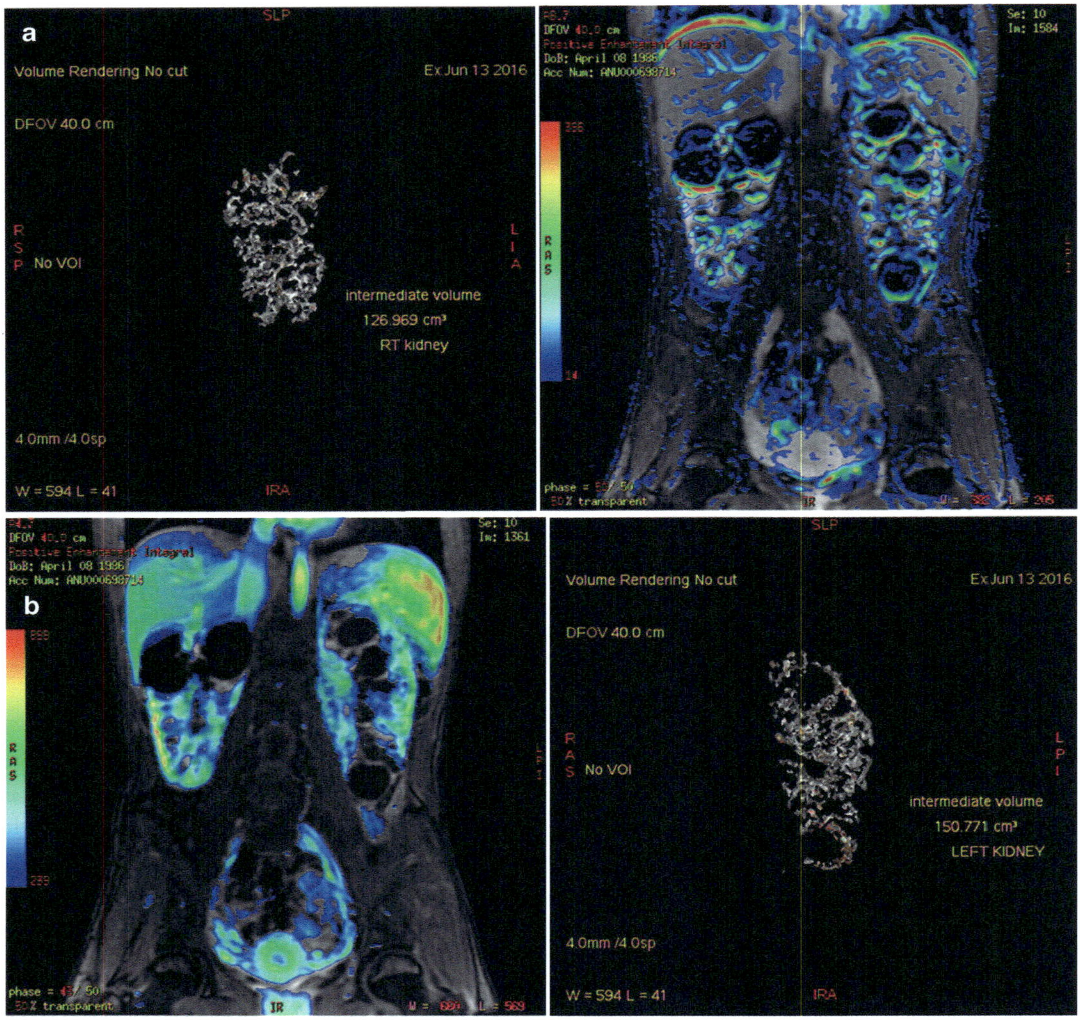

Fig. 15.1 (**a**) Coronal, axial, and sagittal T2W of a 36-year-old man with polycystic disease. (**b**) Qualitative approach with colorimetric maps of arterial enhancement and "functional" parenchyma

reap greater specificity from using higher order models depends on the available signal-to-noise (SNR) and the ability to obtain a high temporal resolution arterial input function (AIF) [4, 5].

15.2.1 Clinical Applications

Quantitative evaluation of renal function, most importantly, perfusion and filtration, is often required for diagnosis and monitoring of vascular diseases, renovascular hypertension, renal damage due to diabetes, renal transplantation, and functional urinary obstruction. In research settings, MR-renography has been shown to provide excellent anatomical detail and functional information in a single examination [6, 7].

15.3 Arterial Spin Labeling (ASL)

An emerging alternative to MR renography is ASL, which utilizes endogenous blood water as a contrast agent, not involving contrast injection to eliminate the risk of nephrogenic systemic fibrosis (NSF) in patients with compromised kidney function.

Perfusion is measured by acquiring a set of labeled (tagged) and nonlabeled (control) images. Spin labeling involves inversion of the magnetization of arterial blood using radiofrequency pulse. There are three types of spin labeling applicable to the method: flow-in, flow-out, and subtraction tag-on/off. All can be combined with HASTE sequence TrueFISP or with 2D or 3D acquisition with ECG trigger and/or respiratory gating. The technique to tag-on/off subtraction is the form of spin labeling that is more standard. The general concept of this method is to acquire two data sets, one with active tags on arterial flow and another with a set of untagged control. The subtraction between the two eliminates the signal stationary tissues keeping only the spins labeled getting angiographic image. It can perform angiographic examinations of the renal arteries with the possibility, also, to increase the temporal resolution of getting time-resolved magnetic resonance angiography (MRA) images.

15.3.1 Clinical Applications

Though, in patients with advanced RCC, ASL can evaluate outcomes of therapy, taking advantage of the high perfusion in tumors and in transplanted patients perfusion might indicate the stability of renal allograft function; ASL technical complexity has restricted its application primarily to research [8]. Moreover, a recent study showed that ASL is also promising for assessing renal perfusion in patients with metabolic syndrome and detecting hemodynamic responses to pharmacologic therapy.

15.4 Diffusion-Weighted MRI (DW-MRI)

Diffusion-weighted MRI (DW-MRI) is a noninvasive modality to characterize tissues based on Brownian motion of water molecules within them. Apparent diffusion coefficient (ADC) is a quantitative parameter calculated from DWI that combines the effects of capillary perfusion and water diffusion. The method requires no exogenous contrast agent and is therefore clinically applicable; the acquisition times (<1 min) are usually short enough to collect several slices within few breath-holds. The apparent diffusion constant (ADC), the DWI quantitative index, describes the average diffusivity of water molecules in all three directions, and is determined by fitting the curve of DWI-MR signal intensity versus b-values, a parameter that determines the diffusion weighting, to an exponentially decaying curve.

DWI-MRI in kidneys makes sense because of the organ's high blood flow and role in water filtration. DW-MRI in renal diseases is an evolving field and previous investigators have attempted to evaluate its utility in the characterization of renal parenchymal disease, renal infections, focal renal lesions, and allografts [9, 10].

15.4.1 Clinical Applications

Most pathologic conditions, including acute and chronic failure, chronic ureteral obstruction, and pyelonephritis, reduce ADC in the cortex and medulla compared with healthy kidneys. DWI differentiates stable from deteriorating allograft function in transplant patients, whereas ADC correlates with GFR in patients with renal artery stenosis. Decreases in ADC have been reported in RCC, although inflammatory lesions impose similar diffusion restrictions. A lower ADC might be consequent to increased cellularity that imposes barriers to free diffusion of water or to accumulation of fibroblasts.

15.5 Blood Oxygen Level-Dependent (BOLD)

BOLD MRI is a unique tool available for renal imaging research due to its sensitivity to the blood concentration of deoxyhemoglobin which acts as a MR contrast agent. The acquisition time is short (1–5 min). The presence of deoxyhemoglobin generates a susceptibility difference that locally perturbs the magnetic field and increases the spin-spin relaxation rate $R2^*$ of surrounding water. High R2* estimate corresponds to low tissue oxygenation or hypoxia, based on the assumption that blood and tissue oxygenation are at tight equilibrium.

15.5.1 Clinical Applications

There is increasing evidence that BOLD is sensitive to subtle intrarenal change induced by renal artery stenosis (RAS), enabling the prediction of possible renal failure at an earlier stage. Another important current application focuses on the differentiation between acute rejection and acute tubular necrosis as the cause for delayed graft function in transplanted kidney.

Several studies also support the use of BOLD to monitor changes in renal hemodynamics in diabetic patients.

15.6 Limitations and Future Directions

Despite the mentioned high potentials of these MRI tools, numerous critical points must still be recognized for each. Regarding DCE, determination of physiological parameters from MRR data requires several steps, including acquisition, image analysis, signal-to-concentration conversion, and tracer kinetic modeling. Each of these steps may contribute errors to the final results. Currently, for example, there is no agreement regarding the best acquisition scheme.

Technical complexity of ASL studies has restricted its application primarily to research, but more research is needed to validate ASL in human subjects.

Also the application of DWI has been limited to research. Lack of a standard protocol and ADC complexity of result interpretation are some of the issues restricting the renal application of this technique.

3T-MRI induces strong BOLD contrast but may also cause severe bulk susceptibility artifact due to the presence of bowel gas; moreover BOLD should be separated to other variables related to oxygenation such as perfusion, vascular volume fraction, and intrinsic spin relaxation.

Many other approaches are also in the exploratory phase, including diffusion tensor imaging (DTI) to study the directionality of water diffusion, Na-MRI to study corticomedullary sodium gradient, MR elastography to evaluate tissue mechanical property, and IVIM as a biomarker for renal perfusion.

References

1. Ebrahimi B, Textor SC, Lerman LO. Renal relevant radiology: renal functional magnetic resonance imaging. Clin J Am Soc Nephrol. 2014;9(2):395–405. https://doi.org/10.2215/CJN.02900313.
2. Takahashi T, Wang F, Quarles CC. Current MRI techniques for the assessment of renal disease. Curr Opin Nephrol Hypertens. 2015;24(3):217–23.
3. Zhang JL, Rusinek H, Chandarana H, Lee VS. Functional MRI of the kidneys. J Magn Reson Imaging. 2013;37(2):282–93. https://doi.org/10.1002/jmri.23717.
4. Schoenberg SO, Aumann S, Just A, Bock M, Knopp MV, Johansson LO, Ahlstrom H. Quantification of renal perfusion abnormalities using an intravascular contrast agent (part 2): results in animals and humans with renal artery stenosis. Magn Reson Med. 2003;49(2):288–98.
5. Bane O, Wagner M, Zhang JL, Dyvorne HA, Orton M, Rusinek H, Taouli B. Assessment of renal function using intravoxel incoherent motion diffusion-weighted imaging and dynamic contrast-enhanced MRI. J Magn Reson Imaging. 2016;44(2):317–26.
6. Montet X, Ivancevic MK, Belenger J, Jorge-Costa M, Pochon S, Pechère A, Terrier F, Vallée JP. Noninvasive measurement of absolute renal perfusion by contrast medium-enhanced magnetic resonance imaging. Investig Radiol. 2003;38(9):584–92.
7. Prowle JR, Molan MP, Hornsey E, Bellomo R. Measurement of renal blood flow by phase-contrast magnetic resonance imaging during septic acute kidney injury: a pilot investigation. Crit Care Med. 2012;40(6):1768–76. https://doi.org/10.1097/CCM.0b013e318246bd85.
8. Panebianco V, Iacovelli R, Barchetti F, Altavilla A, Forte V, Sciarra A, Cortesi E, Catalano C. Dynamic contrast-enhanced magnetic resonance imaging in the early evaluation of anti-angiogenic therapy in metastatic renal cell carcinoma. Anticancer Res. 2013;33(12):5663–6.
9. Chandarana H, Lee VS. Renal functional MRI: Are we ready for clinical application? AJR Am J Roentgenol. 2009;192(6):1550–7. https://doi.org/10.2214/AJR.09.2390.
10. Thoeny HC, De Keyzer F. Diffusion-weighted MR imaging of native and transplanted kidneys. Radiology. 2011;259(1):25–38. https://doi.org/10.1148/radiol.10092419.

Part III

Transplanted Kidney

Transplanted Kidney 16

Mauro Dugo, Rosario Maccarrone, Irene Campo, Francesco Pesce, Luca Di Lullo, and Antonio Granata

16.1 Introduction

Kidney transplantation, providing a better quality of life and long-term outcome compared to maintenance dialysis, represents an essential option for the replacement of kidney function, although the burden of graft loss remains very high [1].

Careful clinical monitoring and appropriate imaging diagnosis can play an important role in renal transplant patients. Different imaging tools are now available in routine clinical practice. Ultrasonography, both in B-mode and with Doppler ultrasound, is the most frequent first-line imaging approach in the posttransplant period [2].

However, its role and usefulness in case of parenchymal complications of the graft are not fully clarified [3]. Some patients still develop several complications, which might cause the loss of the graft or its dysfunction, as reported in Table 16.1. In Table 16.2 the list of common indications for kidney transplant imaging is reported.

In this chapter, we analyze the use and clinical relevance of imaging techniques in most common parenchymal graft complications, including:

(a) Acute or immediate complications, such as acute tubular necrosis, drug toxicity, acute graft pyelonephritis, and hyper-acute rejection
(b) Early complications, such as acute rejection, calcineurin inhibitor toxicity, and infectious acute graft pyelonephritis
(c) Chronic complications, such as chronic allograft nephropathy [4]

16.2 Methods for the Study of Renal Transplant

The ultrasonographic study of the v kidney is easy to perform given the superficial position of the graft. Convex probes with frequencies ranging from 3.5 to 5.0 MHz allow obtaining longitudinal, transversal, and oblique scans. In some cases, a linear probe with frequencies ranging from 6.0 to 10 MHz can be used (Fig. 16.1). To minimize technical failures, it is worthwhile standardizing the working methodology, starting the test in

M. Dugo (✉)
Nephrology and Dialysis Unit –AULSS2, Treviso, Italy

R. Maccarrone · A. Granata
Nephrology and Dialysis Unit, "Cannizzaro" Hospital, Catania, Italy

I. Campo
Department of Radiology, Civile Hospital, Conegliano, Italy

F. Pesce
Nephrology and Dialysis Unit - Department Nephrology, Dialysis and Transplant, Aldo Moro University, Bari, Italy

L. Di Lullo
Nephrology and Dialysis Unit - Colleferro Hospital, Rome, Italy

A. Granata, M. Bertolotto (eds.), *Imaging in Nephrology*, https://doi.org/10.1007/978-3-030-60794-4_16

Table 16.1 Post-transplant complications based on most likely occurrence periods

Early complications	**30–40%**
Acute rejection	20–40%
Acute tubular necrosis	10–30%
Urinary hemorrhage and/or leak	6%
Infections	
Fluid collection (abscess, hematoma, lymphocele, urinoma)	
Renal artery and/or vein thrombosis (rare)	Rare
Urinary obstruction	
Cyclosporine and tacrolimus toxicity	
Disease relapse	
Late complications	**60–70%**
Transplanted renal artery stenosis	10–12%
Renal infarction	
Cyclosporine and tacrolimus toxicity	
Infections	
Arteriovenous fistula	10%
Obstruction	
Transplanted renal vein stenosis	
Chronic allograft nephropathy	
Long-term complications	**1–2%**
De novo glomerulonephritis	
Recurrent disease	
Other complications	1%

Table 16.2 Imaging in kidney transplantation

Common indications for kidney transplant imaging
Routine surveillance imaging
Immediate postoperative evaluation
Fevers and chills
Follow peritransplant collections
Hypertension and/or unexplained graft dysfunction
Elevated or rising creatinine
Pain in region of transplant
Severe hypertension refractory to medical therapy
Decreased urine output

B-mode and identifying the site, form, and position of the graft. The morphological and echo-structural parameters observed at the scale of Gray's test (rapid volumetric increase over 20%, parenchymal hypoechogenicity, presence of a hyperechogenous shade between the echoes of the renal sinus and the walls of the renal pelvis, reduction in volume, and thinning of the parenchyma) might provide a large amount of information concerning a possible damage of the organ. Once the B-mode test is com-

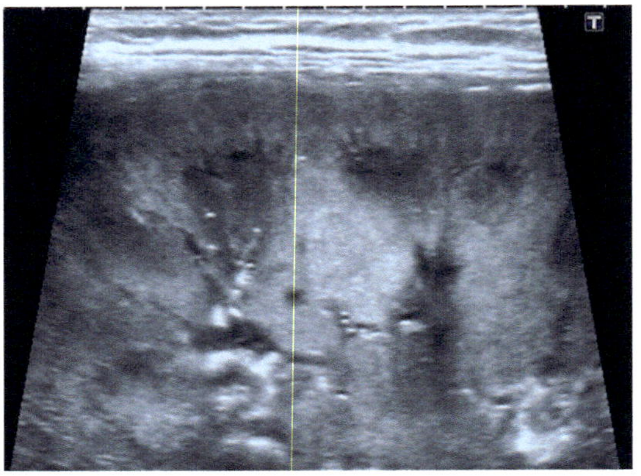

Fig. 16.1 B-mode ultrasonography with linear probe: healthy graft, detail of the parenchyma

pleted, B-flow, color Doppler imaging is fundamental for a rapid and clear assessment of arterial and venous perfusion of the organ. The extension of the box color must be limited, to improve the Doppler analysis capacity and the frame rate (FR). Pulse repetition frequency (PRF) should be set at values of 1.0–1.5 kHz and wall filter at values of 100 Hz and the color gain should be regulated as well, to optimize the image without aliasing and to avoid color diffusion to the perivascular tissues (color bleeding). Finally, the spectral analysis module should be activated with the positioning of the "sample volume" in the lumen of the interlobular artery and the recording of the velocity/time curve (V/t), which will allow obtaining the resistance index (RI) and the pulsatility index (PI).

16.2.1 Computed Tomography

CT may be complementary in the evaluation of renal transplant complications. If the patient's renal function allows, intravenous contrast-enhanced CT angiography (CTA) may be performed to noninvasively confirm a diagnosis of renal artery stenosis if, for example, PSVs are elevated at ultrasound.

Contrast-enhanced imaging can also be used to characterize indeterminate focal lesions detected at ultrasound as cystic or solid. Additionally, intravenous contrast-enhanced CT with excretory phase imaging (acquired 5–20 min after intravenous contrast material administration) can be used to confirm a urine leak or urinoma. Administration of intravenous contrast material should be avoided in individuals with impaired renal function because of the risk of developing contrast-induced nephropathy. Noncontrast CT is helpful to evaluate the full extent of a perinephric fluid collection and its relationship to surrounding structures if portions of the collection are obscured by bowel gas at ultrasound. Also, noncontrast CT is more accurate than ultrasound for the diagnosis of renal and ureteral stones, especially for small stones.

16.2.2 MR Imaging

MR imaging also plays a complementary role in the evaluation of renal transplant complications. Magnetic resonance angiography (MRA) can be used to noninvasively confirm renal artery stenosis.

Contrast-enhanced MR imaging can also characterize focal renal lesions as cystic or solid. Additionally, excretory phase imaging can be performed to diagnose a urine leak or urinoma.

Administration of gadolinium-based contrast agents in individuals with impaired renal function has been associated with the development of nephrogenic systemic fibrosis, a potentially fatal fibrosing condition. Contrast agents associated with the greatest number of nephrogenic systemic fibrosis cases are gadodiamide (Omniscan™), gadopentetate dimeglumine (Magnevist™), and gadoversetamide (OptiMARK™) and should not be administered to individuals with impaired renal function. Other gadolinium-based contrast agents are associated with few if any unconfounded cases of nephrogenic systemic fibrosis, and understanding of their potential role in the evaluation of individuals with impaired renal function is evolving.

16.2.3 Nuclear Medicine

Nuclear medicine studies may be used to evaluate transplant perfusion or to collect system injury following renal transplantation. Technetium-99 m (99mTc)-labeled pharmaceuticals are typically used, either 99mTc-mercaptoacetyl triglycine or 99mTc-diethylene triamine. The radiopharmaceutical is injected intravenously and sequential images are acquired to evaluate the vascular phase (flow phase), parenchymal phase (functional phase), and washout phase (excretory phase). Nuclear medicine studies are an option for patients with contraindications to iodinated and gadolinium-based intravenous contrast agents.

16.3 Ultrasound Evaluation of Normal Renal Transplant

The healthy transplanted kidney has ultrasound features comparable to the healthy native one; however, a more detailed two-dimensional image is apparent as the transplant is usually located more superficially, and thus higher frequency transducers can be utilized. The reniform outline and central echo complex, resulting from the collecting system and the renal vasculature together with any sinus fat, are well depicted, while the distinction between the renal cortex and the relative echo-poor medulla is usually apparent (Fig. 16.2). The size is similar to native kidneys, but after 2 months, the normal transplant kidney usually becomes hypertrophic and can elongate by 2–3 cm [5]. The collecting system of a well-functioning transplant is often slightly dilated, presumably because of a combination of an increased production of urine (since it is working as the sole kidney) and the loss of ureter's tonicity from denervation. However, in the unobstructed transplant, the filling should be minor and confined to the renal pelvis, while filling of the infundibula or the calyces is suspicious of significant outflow obstruction. In color Doppler imaging, arterial and venous flow should extend to within a few millimeters of the capsule throughout all renal segments, although this depends on the depth of the transplant kidney, the transducer frequency, and the sensitivity of the color Doppler settings. Occasionally flow will appear to be decreased or absent in deeper

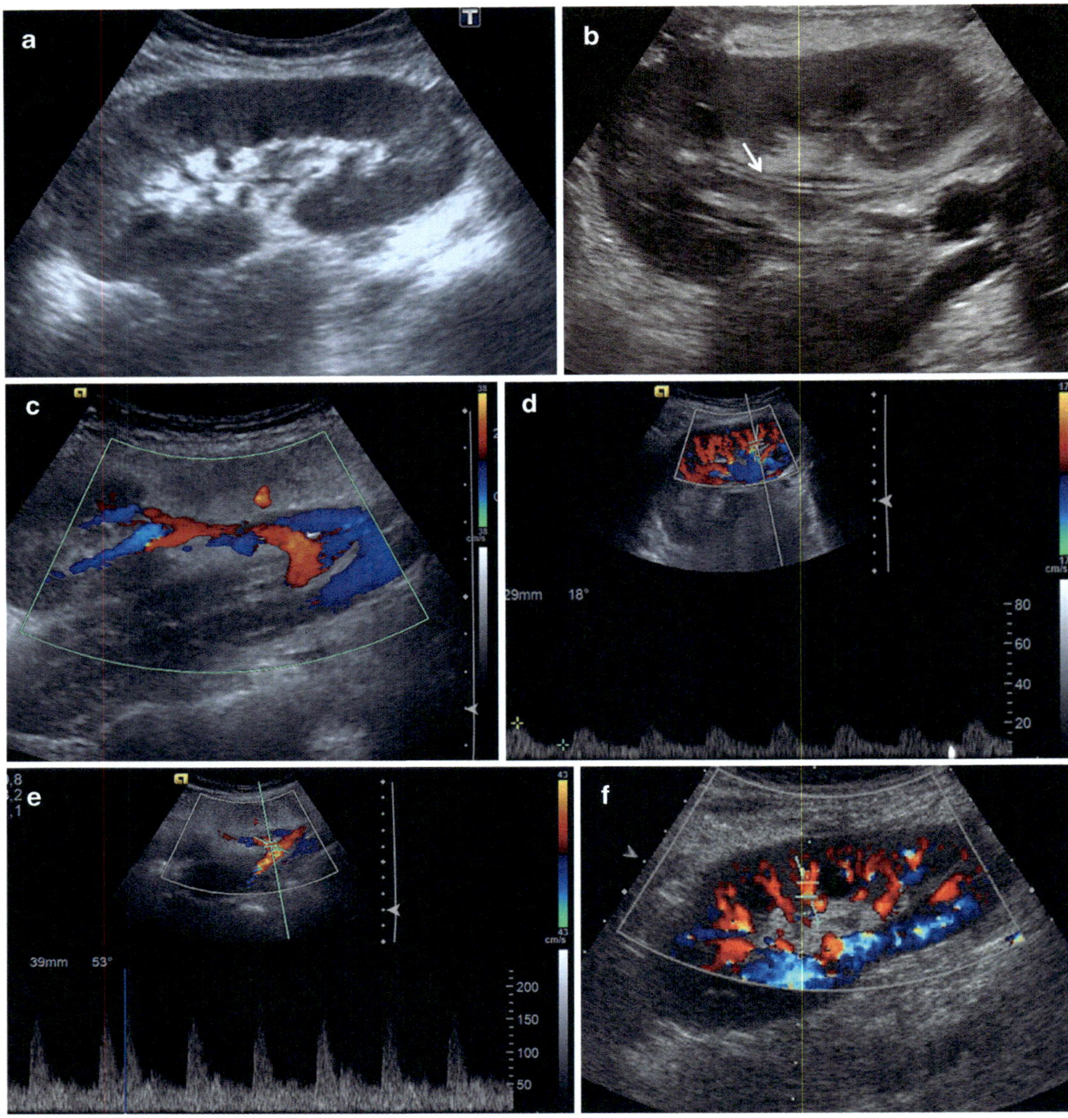

Fig. 16.2 (**a**) Normal transplant kidney on grayscale ultrasound demonstrates good contrast resolution between cortex and medulla. (**b**) Slight dilatation of the collecting system and pigtail catheter (arrow) is noted. (**c**) Normal renal artery and vein of the transplant kidney on color Doppler ultrasound. (**d**) Normal homogeneous blood flow throughout the transplant kidney on color Doppler ultrasound. Interlobar, arcuate, and peripheral cortical branches are illustrated. (**e**) Normal intrarenal artery waveform on spectral Doppler ultrasound shows a brisk systolic upstroke and high diastolic flow. Resistive index is normal (RI = 0.55). (**f**) Normal waveform of the renal artery on spectral Doppler ultrasound

portions of the kidney, which should prompt evaluation with B-flow or power Doppler, as it is more sensitive than color Doppler (Fig. 16.3). Spectral Doppler interrogation from the segmental and interlobar vessels shows the normal fast systolic upstroke with a subsequent slow decay in diastole, with forward flow being maintained until the next cardiac cycle. Thus, RI values of 0.8 or lower are expected, although the clinical context should be evaluated as well. The main renal artery is usually readily demonstrated but is often much more tortuous than that of the native

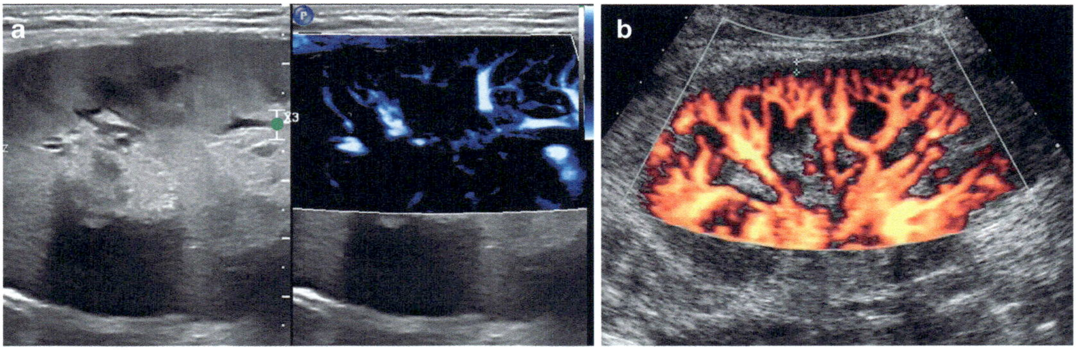

Fig. 16.3 Transplanted kidney: (**a**) b-flow; (**b**) power Doppler

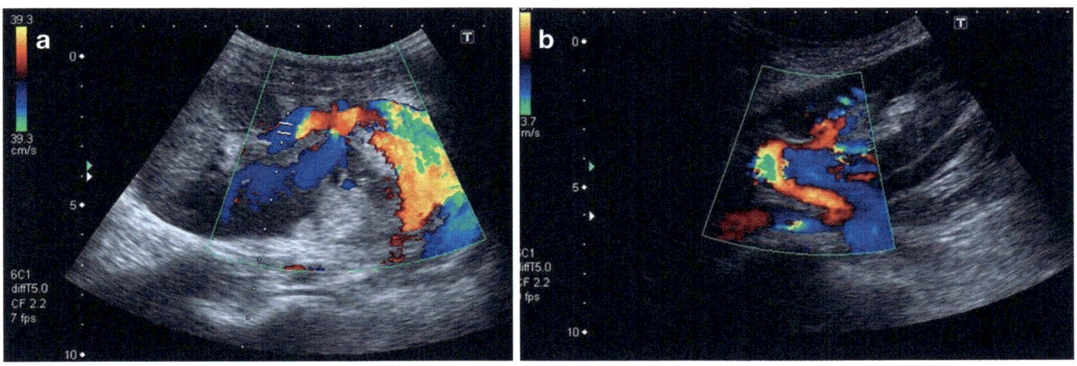

Fig. 16.4 The vascular pedicle can have different orientations that depend on the patient's characteristics and the size of the graft: (**a**) lateralized hilum and (**b**) medialized hilum

kidneys because of the way the transplant is relocated into the iliac fossa after the anastomoses have been performed (Fig. 16.4). Therefore, the straight portions of the artery as optimum locations for Doppler measurements are those that tend to lie parallel to the skin and thus subtend the worst beam-to-vessel angles. The branch and main renal veins are easily accessed for Doppler studies.

16.4 Parenchymal Complications

16.4.1 Immediate Graft Parenchymal Complications

"Immediate" graft parenchymal complications are all the adverse events occurring within the first week since the surgical procedure.

Immediate parenchymal complications are often responsible for delayed graft function and are associated with a higher rate of hospitalization and a worse graft survival both in the short and in the long period. These complications are mostly represented by hyper-acute rejection, acute tubular necrosis (ATN), calcineurin inhibitor toxicity, and acute pyelonephritis.

16.4.1.1 Hyper-Acute Rejection

Hyper-acute rejection has become a very rare event caused by the presence of preformed antibodies against HLA, ABO, or other alloantibody-to-donor endothelial surface antigens in the recipient, responsible for an immediate graft loss [6].

The diagnosis is made very early, within minutes or hours of transplantation in a recipient, often even in the theater, during the surgical intervention. The kidney usually stops functioning within minutes after transplantation and appears flaccid and blue-cyanotic, due to the thrombotic and inflammatory processes, with a graft loss rate above 60%.

Therefore, B-mode US in hyper-acute rejection management has a very limited usefulness due to the extremely quick necrosis process which involves the graft. Anyway, the sonographic features are nonspecific and like those observed in case of acute rejection and ATN; CDUS evaluation may show the complete absence of intrarenal blood flow [7].

16.4.1.2 Acute Tubular Necrosis (ATN)

ATN is one of the most frequent causes of delayed graft function (DGF) and is detected with different levels of severity in 20–60% of deceased donor renal transplantation biopsies.

It is the most common cause of early graft dysfunction observed during the first 48 h post-transplantation and is related to the reversible ischemic injury involving tubular renal cells in the pretransplant period. The main risk factors for acute tubular necrosis include deceased (vs. living) donor renal transplantation, donor hypotension, and prolonged warm and cold ischemia period.

The grayscale imaging feature of ATN is extremely variable and aspecific. Besides size variations, such as graft enlargement, decreased echogenicity and/or scattered heterogeneous areas of variable echogenicity with a loss of corticomedullary differentiation can be observed. Parenchymal edema and sometimes a complete compression of the renal sinus may also be seen. However, graft swelling or enlargement can also be caused by other conditions, including a normal early postoperative state, as well as delayed graft function, cellular or humoral rejection, acute CNI toxicity, and obstruction. Moreover, these findings may be observed to be totally normal as well or totally indistinguishable from an acute rejection. CDUS evaluation shows that a renal resistive index (RRI) is always greater than 0.80 (Fig. 16.5).

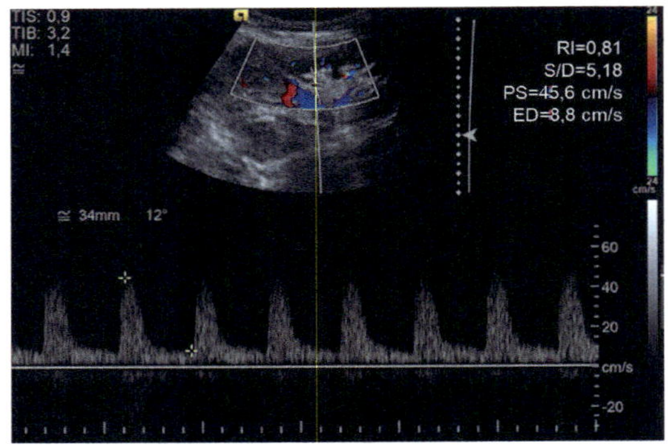

Fig. 16.5 Acute tubular necrosis: increase of the RI. The increase in RI has poor diagnostic accuracy

16.4.2 Early Graft Parenchymal Complications

16.4.2.1 Acute Rejection

Acute rejection is a major cause of graft dysfunction affecting more than 30% of transplanted kidneys. Most episodes of acute rejection occur between 48 h and 6 months after surgery. Despite a dramatic reduction in the incidence and severity of acute rejection due to the introduction of new immunosuppressive protocols in the past three decades, some kidneys do not regain function and even among patients who recover, acute rejection can have a negative impact on long-term graft survival. Clinical manifestations are unspecific and may include malaise and oliguria. The traditional symptoms, such as graft pain and tenderness, and fever occasionally, are now often absent, so that the clinical onset can also be completely silent. Laboratory findings mostly include increased serum creatinine, proteinuria, and sometimes pyuria.

US B-mode may be helpful mainly for excluding other causes of acute kidney injury, because in most cases the findings are similar to those observable in other acute parenchymal nephropathies (Fig. 16.6):

- Increased volume of the graft due to inflammatory edema (very frequent but nonspecific)
- Enlarged and hypoechogenous pyramids, due to medullary edema (early but nonspecific)

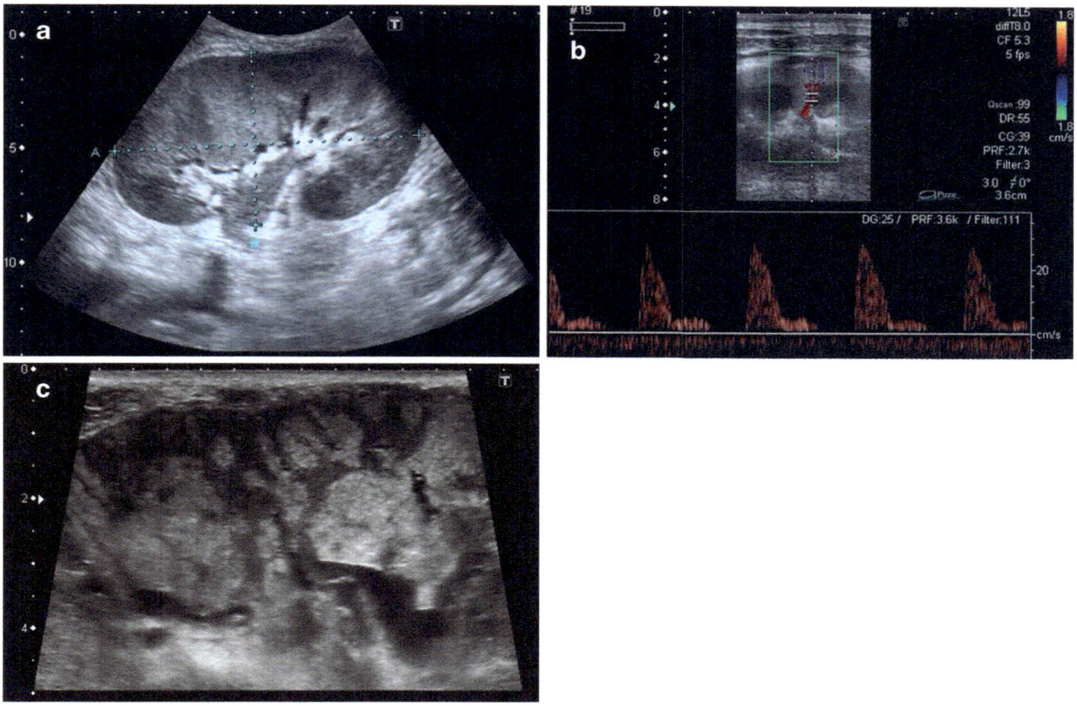

Fig. 16.6 Acute rejection: (**a**) sagittal ultrasonography shows an enlarged, globular shaped allograft with loss of renal sinus fat; (**b**) the study of the renal parenchyma, at the color Doppler with a linear probe, shows significant increase, poor vascularization, and RI = 1.00. The v/t curves show absence of the diastolic phase. (**c**) Acute rejection: B-mode linear probe shows inhomogeneity of the renal parenchyma. Kidney biopsy shows acute cell rejection

- Thickened and hyperechogenous cortex (rarely hypoechogenous cortex and increased medullar thickness, with consequent loss of the corticomedullary differentiation)
- Edema of the collecting system and focal parenchymal hypoechogenicity, due to focal infarctions
- Perigraft anechogenous collections due to necrosis and/or hemorrhages
- Increased parenchymal thickness with obliteration of the hyperechogenous pyelic sinus

With the color Doppler study it is possible to find out elevated RRI, an unspecific feature detectable also in ureteral obstruction, ATN, renal vein occlusion, pyelonephritis, and calcineurin inhibitor toxicity [8].

In patients receiving a kidney transplant, graft RRI is poorly correlated with the donor parameters such as age or allograft function while it is strictly connected with host-related factors such as pulse pressure (PP), intima-media thickness (IMT), and ankle brachial index (ABI).

In a study involving 321 renal allograft recipients, Naesens et al. confirmed that RRI was not related to graft function or intrarenal histologic disease pattern, while, being strictly connected with the recipient age, it could represent a survival indicator [9, 10].

In conclusion, there are no specific ultrasonographic signs of acute rejection of the graft, even though the presence of these patterns associated with a rapid worsening of renal function may help in the initial differential diagnosis of acute graft dysfunction.

Unfortunately, a definitive discrimination of ATN and AR by Doppler ultrasound is not possible [11].

Recently, contrast-enhanced ultrasound (CEUS) has been indicated as a new promising noninvasive imaging tool that may also be helpful in the early diagnosis of kidney transplant complications, such as delayed graft function (DGF) and acute allograft rejection.

Differently from conventional US techniques, CEUS allows a more precise study of graft microvascularization providing also quantitative information about transplant perfusion [12].

Schwenger et al. in 2006 tested the efficacy of real-time quantitative determination of arterial arrival of a US contrast medium in kidney transplantation demonstrating a higher accuracy of CEUS compared to CDUS in the estimation of graft perfusion [12].

Recently, Grzelak et al. showed that CEUS was a better tool in the identification of acute rejection than conventional techniques. Authors demonstrated, in patients with normal graft function, the regular inflow of contrast medium in all graft regions. Conversely, subjects with DGF showed delayed inflow of the contrast medium; moreover the time of inflow to the regions of interest significantly differed between ATN and acute rejection [13].

Therefore, this led to the suggestion that with the help of CEUS-derived parameters of the quantitative assessment, it could be possible to distinguish ATN from AR [14]. However, the ability of CEUS in differentiating between ATN, AR, and calcineurin inhibitor toxicity has not been investigated. Consequently, in the context of acute graft dysfunctions, performing a biopsy remains mandatory to obtain a definitive diagnosis.

16.4.2.2 Drug Toxicity

CNIs, such as tacrolimus and cyclosporine, are used as maintenance immunosuppressive therapy in almost all renal transplant recipients. Unfortunately, these compounds are also potentially nephrotoxic and a frequent cause of acute and chronic graft dysfunction.

Typically, CNI toxicity occurs during the first 3 months after transplantation when the therapeutic target is higher and may induce an impairment of renal function, which is mostly reversible after reducing the dose. However, when the CNI toxicity is severe and/or persisting, a chronic, progressive, and irreversible renal disease can result. Rarely, thrombotic microangiopathy leading to acute graft loss may be induced by CNI treatment in susceptible patients.

The standard US exam in CNI injury does not disclose specific features. Graft swelling, increased or decreased renal echogenicity, and loss of corticomedullary differentiation are usually observed at the common B-mode examination. At CDUS only a nonspecific RRI increase can be revealed. Long-term CNI toxicity is not generally differentiable from chronic allograft rejection, in which US may show small-sized graft with thinner cortical layer or normal findings, according to the degree of renal insufficiency.

Consequently, a biopsy may be required for the differential diagnosis with other acute or chronic causes of graft dysfunction.

16.4.2.3 Acute Graft Pyelonephritis (AGPN)

Acute graft pyelonephritis (AGPN) can complicate any phase of posttransplantation period. A recent analysis demonstrates that transplant recipients have a 72-fold higher risk of first-time hospitalization for pyelonephritis compared to matched population controls [15].

According to the literature [16], the diagnosis of AGPN should include (1) positive microbiology or imaging (urinary dipstick positive for nitrite and/or leukocyte esterase and/or a positive urine culture and/or ultrasound marks indicating pyelonephritis) and/or (2) positive laboratory test results (leukocyte count $\geq$12x 10^9 cells/L and/or C-reactive protein (CRP) $\geq$80 mg/L and/or temperature >37.8 °C) and/or (3) positive clinical signs (one or more of the following: graft-pain/flank pain, chills, clinical symptoms consistent with cystitis (dysuria, urge, suprapubic pain)). The variable incidence is around 20%. Important risk factors for this complication include immunosuppressive regimens, invasive urological procedures such as bladder catheterism or ureteral stenting (Fig. 16.7), and posttransplantation urethral bladder reflux (Fig. 16.8).

The early differential diagnosis is essential, because AGPN episodes increase the risk of scarring, acute rejection, and worsening of renal function. Imaging is necessary in AGPN both to

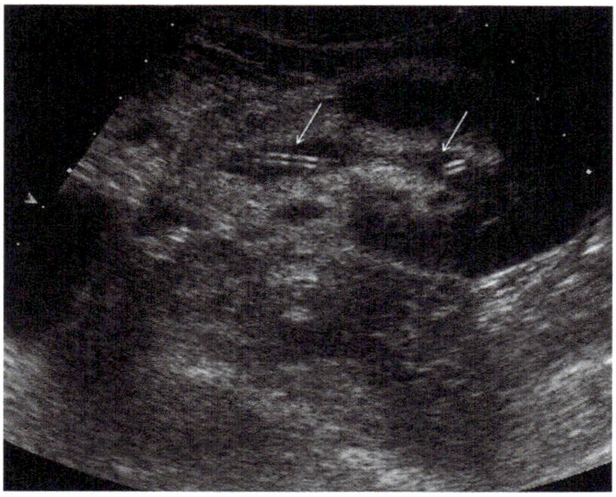

Fig. 16.7 Kidney transplanted into left iliac fossa. Presence of ureteral stent (arrows)

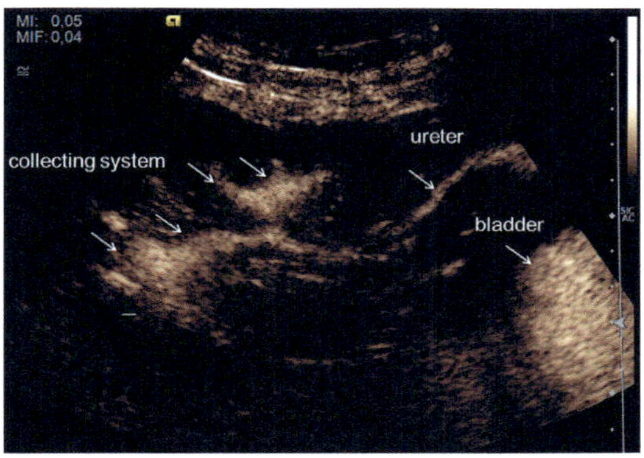

Fig. 16.8 Kidney transplanted into right iliac fossa. Acute relapsing pyelonephritis. Contrast-enhanced voiding urosonography with the intravesical administration of the ultrasound contrast agent SonoVue™ for vesicoureteral reflux detection

evaluate the presence and extent of complications such as renal and perirenal lesions and to detect potentially treatable causes [17].

The basal B-mode evaluation does not allow high accuracy (11–40% sensitivity and 50% specificity) in detecting renal parenchymal lesions. Standard US is more helpful in the presence of renal abscess or hydronephrosis, since these changes are usually characterized by inflammation-induced graft swelling, thickener sinus, and reduced corticomedullary differentiation.

Occasionally, parenchymal infections may display as focal acute pyelonephritis, which are characterized by hypo- or anechogenous and poorly defined areas with faded borders at US.

Posterior parietal reinforcement might be present as an expression of nonsuppurative paracellular inflammation related to interstitial edema and/or hemorrhages. CDUS has a higher sensitivity (38–63%) in detecting parenchymal abnormalities in case of AGPN. Power Doppler has been shown to have a higher sensitivity (41%) and specificity (89%), when compared with CDUS (Fig. 16.9).

Computed tomography (CT) is the gold standard for the diagnosis of AGPN, with an excellent performance in recognizing underlying obstructive causes such as calculi or anatomic alterations due to perirenal collections. On the other hand, CT imaging is highly expensive and implies a high-dose radiation and contrast media nephrotoxicity risk. Magnetic resonance imaging (MRI-DWI) is increasingly used in patients with posttransplant creatinine increase and may overcome CT limits.

The advent of newer US contrast agents helps to better detect areas of poor renal parenchymal perfusion. Contrast-enhanced US (CEUS) is a toxic-free, quick, and feasible procedure that can improve the detection of low flow by improving the signal-to-noise ratio, and can improve the sensitivity of US for AGPN (Fig. 16.10). For example, the presence at CEUS test of a triangular hypoechoic, hypoperfused area in the medulla indicates ischemic parenchymal lesions and is helpful for distinguishing between APN and a simple pyelitis. Acute rejection-induced hypoperfusion areas show a "diffuse pattern," easily distinguishable by the "triangular shape" of the focal hypoperfused areas characteristic of AGPN.

In a recent analysis Granata et al. demonstrated the utility of CEUS examination in the diagnosis of AGPN. CEUS resulted to be an excellent tool in the workup of complicated acute pyelonephritis, so that it might be considered as the imaging technique of choice in the evaluation and follow-up for these patients [18–21].

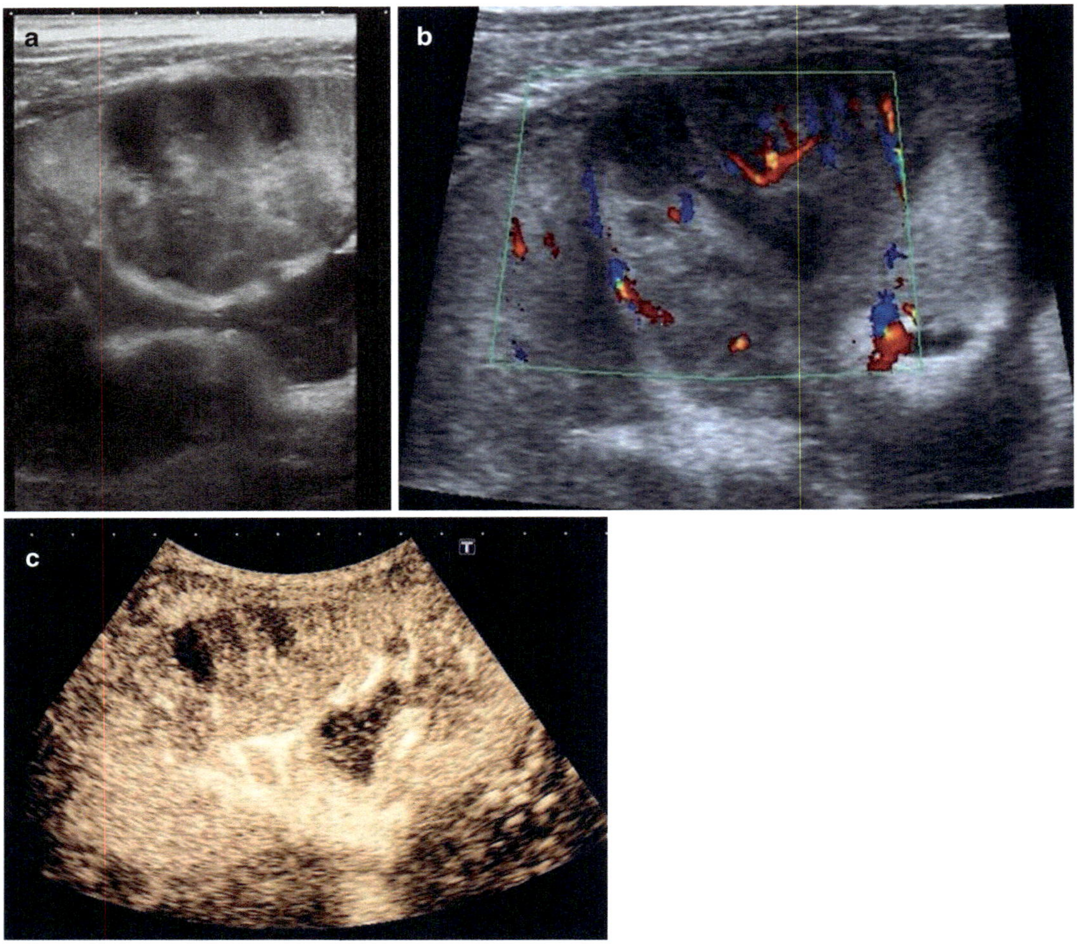

Fig. 16.9 Fever and chills in kidney-transplant patient. (**a**) B-mode ultrasound shows multiple hypo-anechoic areas; (**b**) color Doppler shows poor vascularization; and (**c**) contrast-enhanced ultrasound shows absence of vascularization. Diagnosis: sepsis secondary to abscess graft

16.4.2.4 Viral Infections: BK and Cytomegalovirus Nephropathy

BK (polyomavirus) and cytomegalovirus are viral infections that can lead to allograft dysfunction due to interstitial nephritis, glomerulopathy, or cytokine release. Additionally, adenoviral infections of the renal allograft are a rare cause of allograft dysfunction.

BK virus nephropathy occurs in up to 5–10% of kidney transplants, usually within the first 12–18 months of transplantation. The confirmatory diagnosis of BKV-associated nephropathy (BKVAN) is made by the discovery of viruria, viremia by PCR analysis, and tubule-interstitial changes at graft histology [22].

Information from diagnostic imaging is mostly not specific and of limited utility in the diagnosis of BKVAN. An uncommon exception is represented by the renal obstruction caused by the ureteral involvement of the virus. Moreover, other authors have described as specific some other findings using CT and ultrasound in transplanted patients affected by BKVAN [23].

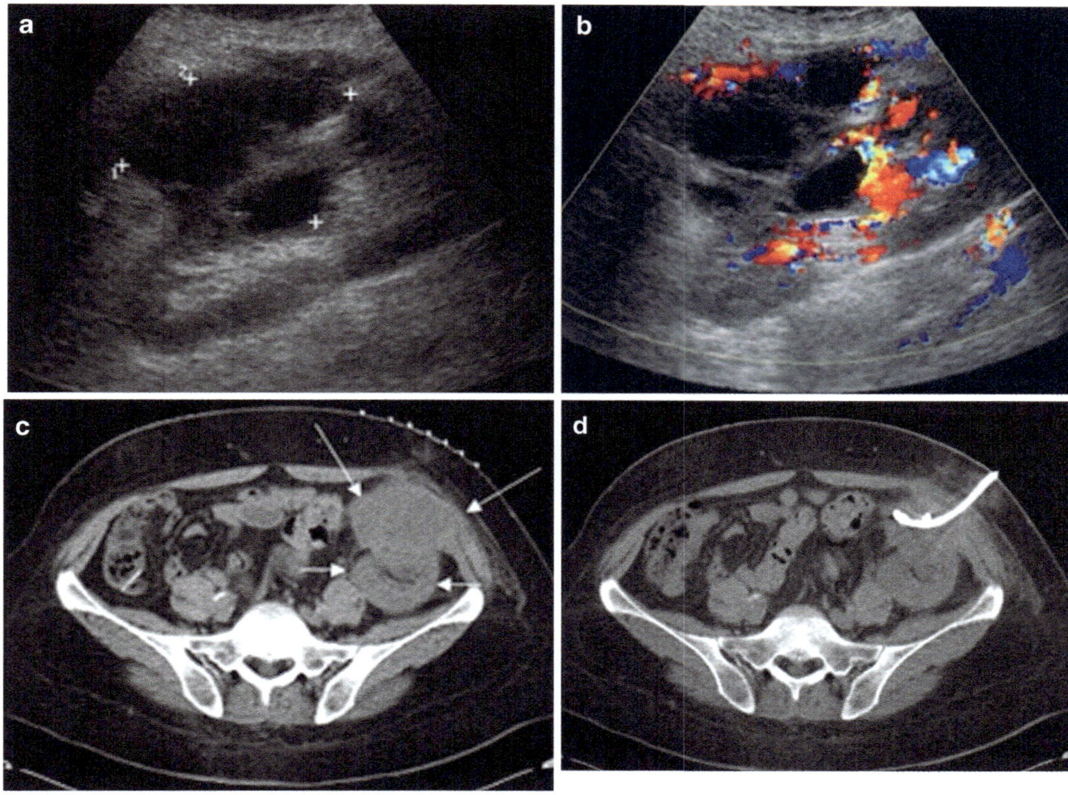

Fig. 16.10 Renal abscess. (**a**) Image A is a grayscale sagittal image through the transplant kidney that shows an exophytic multi-septated abscess (calipers). (**b**) A color Doppler image of the same area shows peripheral vascularity without any significant internal flow. (**c**) An axial CT scan image through the pelvis shows transplant kidney (short arrows) with the abscess protruding anteriorly (long arrows). (**d**) Image D shows a drain placed in the abscess (courtesy of Prof. Ishrad)

More recently, Dugo et al. have described typical CDUS patterns (Fig. 16.11) observed in 17 consecutive patients affected by BKVAN [24].

They used high-frequency sonography with a linear array transducer (56 mm linear probe, bandwidth 5–12 MHz) and reported the presence of characteristic localized hypoechoic areas from the papilla to the renal cortex alternating with normal echoic areas (zebralike pattern), without any vascular abnormality. Should these findings be confirmed in a larger population, CDUS could be proposed as a more specific imaging technique for the diagnosis of BKVAN (Fig. 16.12).

16.4.3 Late Graft Parenchymal Complications

16.4.3.1 Recurrent Primary Disease and "De Novo" Renal Disease

Primary glomerular disease recurrence must be considered as a possible and unpredictable cause of graft function impairment. Recurrence risk depends upon the specific glomerular disease. Glomerular diseases with the higher recurrence rate include primary focal segmental glomerulosclerosis (FSGS), primary membranous nephropathy, membranoproliferative glomerulonephritis, complement-mediated HUS, and C3 glomeru-

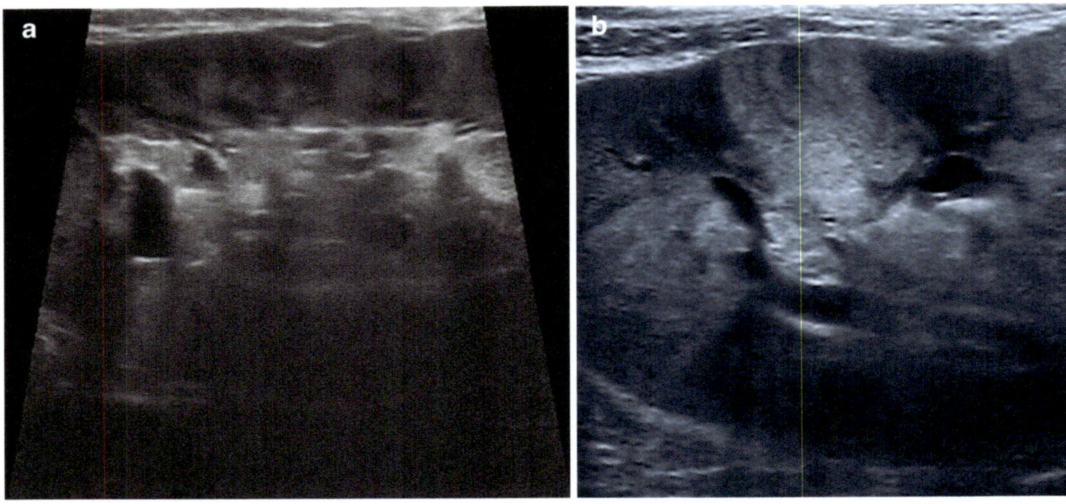

Fig. 16.11 The study with a linear probe highlights multiple hypoechoic parenchymal areas alternating with normoechoic areas (zebralike aspect); (**a**) and (**b**) show different zebralike aspects

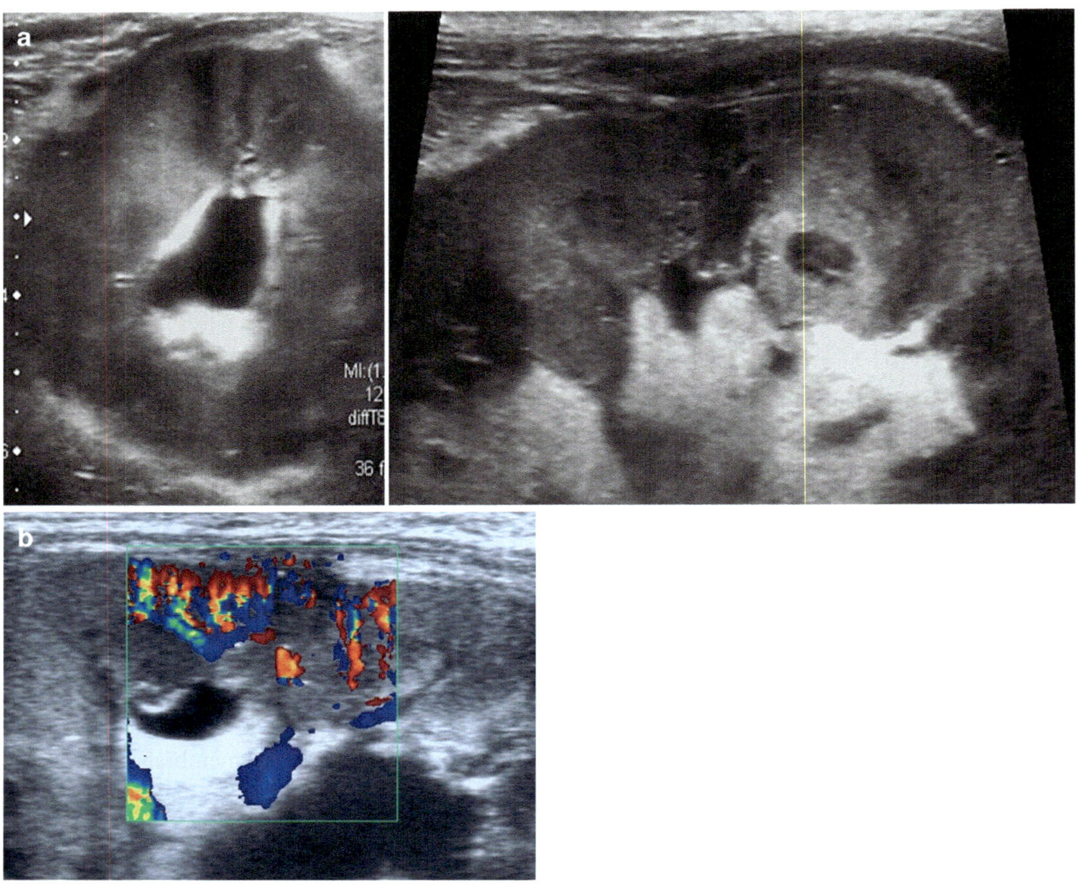

Fig. 16.12 Early BKVAN. (**a**) B-mode shows zebralike aspect and (**b**) persistence normal vascularization to color Doppler in hypo-anechoic areas

lopathy. Late recurrence (i.e., after more than 1 year posttransplant) has been described for many diseases, including FSGS, membranoproliferative glomerulonephritis, immunoglobulin A (IgA) nephropathy, and diabetic nephropathy. In all these conditions, imaging alone has a limited diagnostic role and graft biopsy remains mandatory for the precise diagnosis [25].

16.4.3.2 Chronic Renal Rejection

The most common cause of graft failure after the first year is the so-called chronic renal allograft nephropathy (CAN). CAN is a clinicopathological entity that the new revised Banff 2005 classification system redefined as "interstitial fibrosis and tubular atrophy (IF/TA), without evidence of any specific etiology."

CAN is characterized by a progressive decline of the renal function, often accompanied by arterial hypertension and proteinuria without manifestations of nephrotoxicity or acute rejection.

The diagnosis of CAN is not easily made, since the only alteration is represented by a progressive and slow increase of serum creatinine.

The differential diagnosis of CAN implies distinguishing among the many underlying conditions that cause progressive allograft dysfunction and/or are associated with similar histologic findings such as primary disease recurrence, transplanted renal artery stenosis, calcineurin inhibitor nephrotoxicity, BKVAN, rejection relapses, and occasionally obstructive nephropathies.

CDUS usefulness is limited to differentiate parenchymal chronic complications from vascular, surgical, and/or urological causes of graft dysfunction. Moreover, it guides the decision to perform graft histological examination. However, allograft biopsy remains the gold standard and is necessary in most cases to exclude potentially treatable causes of chronic rejection, such as chronic CIN.

In chronic rejection biopsies, glomerulosclerosis, tubular atrophy, interstitial fibrosis, and severe vascular involvement are usually observed. These changes are similar to those seen in native renal biopsies from patients with chronic kidney disease (CKD) and the US appearance is not different, showing:

- Reduced graft length/volume
- Reduced graft cortical thickness
- Increased graft cortical echogenicity
- Poor visibility of the renal pyramids and the renal sinus
- Marginal irregularities
- Papillary calcifications

On occasion, the chronic process can lead to the formation of lymphatic accumulation under renal capsular surface (subcapsular lymphocele) due to the occlusion of the intrarenal lymphatic collectors. US will show a thin subcapsular hypoechogenous band/strip.

At the color Doppler examination, reduced graft vascularity and interlobar RRI increase can be observed in most patients (Fig. 16.13).

A role for high RRI was described in the early 2000s as an early, strong negative predictor of long-term graft survival [26].

However, more recent data from Naesens et al. did not support such a relation between RRI and graft function or intrarenal histologic disease pattern. In fact, these authors showed in a 321 transplanted patients' cohort that RRI was strictly connected with the recipient and not to the donor age, reflecting the characteristics of the host and representing a recipient survival indicator [10–27].

A method to quantify the pixels of color of the power Doppler in the region of interest (ROI) has been recently described by Nankivell et al. [28].

According to this technique, parenchymal vascularization can be quantified in relation to the maximum fractional area (MFA) at the color Doppler and the distance between the most peripheral color pixels and the renal capsule.

This method has a proven excellent reproducibility and diagnostic accuracy. The distance between the peripheral color pixels and the renal capsule showed a 91% sensitivity in the diagnosis of CAN and reached 94% when combined with MFA. Scholbach et al. have suggested the use of tissue Doppler for the diagnosis of CAN to detect the tissue pulsatility index (PI: calculated as the ratio between the differences between systolic mean and diastolic mean in the ROI and the mean velocity), to quantify graft perfusion [29].

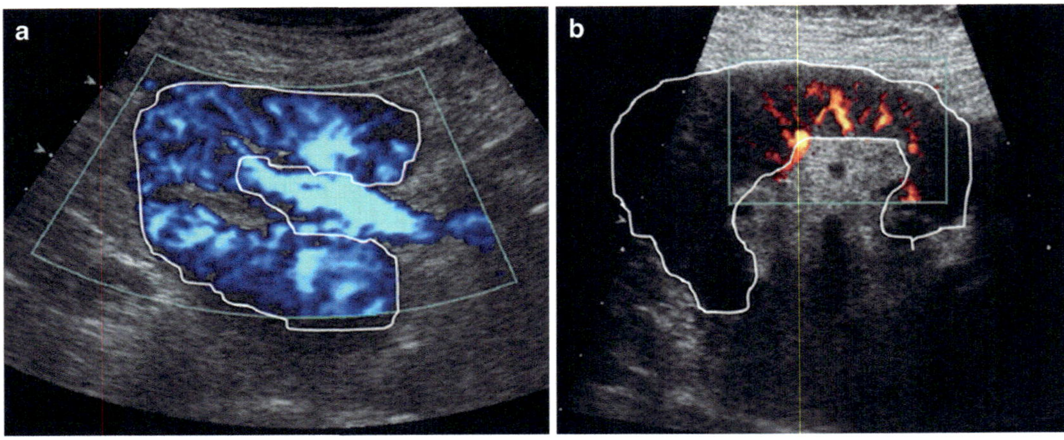

Fig. 16.13 Chronic allograft nephropathy. (**a**) Normal kidney vascularization; (**b**) significant reduced renal perfusion. At renal biopsy CAN diagnosis

Recently, novel ultrasonic technologies have been applied in the evaluation and diagnosis of kidney allograft status, such as contrast-enhanced ultrasonography (CEUS) and tissue elasticity quantification using acoustic radiation force impulse (ARFI) technology.

The quantitative information about microvascular perfusion of the renal allograft can be evaluated by CEUS, which can offer an improved diagnostic accuracy compared with CDUS for the detection of CAN. Moreover, the measure of graft perfusion parameters such as US RRI, pulsatility index, and renal blood flow estimated by CEUS is significantly more accurate compared to conventional CDUS [12]. Schwenger et al., in a small cohort of 26 transplanted subjects, demonstrated that quantitative determination of renal blood flow provided by CEUS has a significantly higher diagnostic power for the detection of graft dysfunction due to CAN compared with conventional color Doppler resistance indices. Nevertheless, those data should be confirmed in larger trials. In addition, the CEUS accuracy in the differential diagnosis between different causes of late graft dysfunctions has not yet been investigated [30].

Another novel tool in the evaluation of CAN is US-based elastography (elasticity) by the acoustic radiation force impulse method (ARFI). Parenchymal stiffness can be measured by this transient elastography technique and seems to correlate with histologic measures of interstitial fibrosis (Fig. 16.14).

Initially, encouraging results of ARFI efficacy in the quantification of liver fibrosis have led to the hypothesis of its potential effectiveness in detecting parenchymal fibrosis in kidney transplant as well. Accordingly, tissue elasticity measured by ARFI has been explored by Stock et al. as a new promising noninvasive technique for the assessment of renal allograft fibrosis. A moderate correlation between mean ARFI values and the grade of fibrosis and the BANFF category was found.

More recently, Lee et al. showed that there was no significant correlation between shear wave velocity (SWV) measured by ARFI and IF/TA or renal dysfunction. Tissue elasticity parameters were related to the time after transplantation and were influenced by graft hemodynamics.

Further long-term longitudinal assessments are necessary to confirm these results [31].

16.4.3.3 Neoplasm (Posttransplant Lymphoproliferative Disorder)

Renal transplant patients have a generally increased risk of neoplasm related primarily to chronic immunosuppression. Most neoplasms are skin cancers and lymphomas. Patients are also at increased risk for renal cell carcinoma,

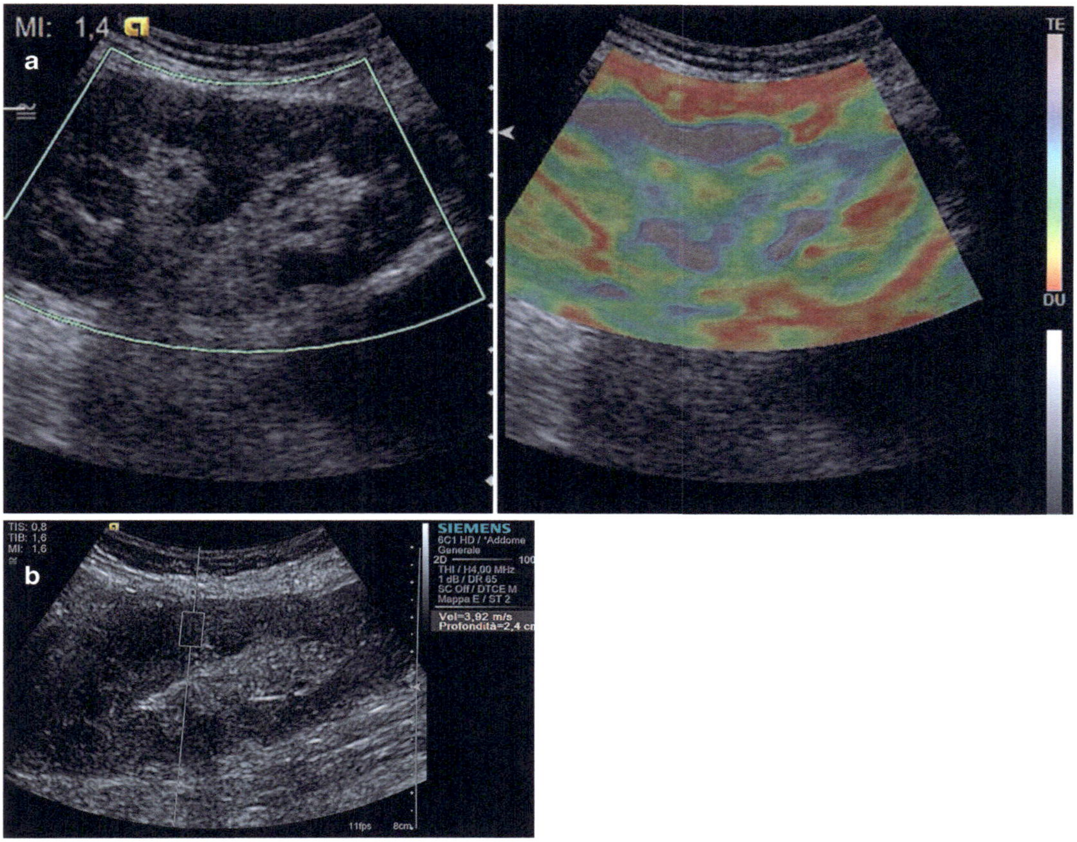

Fig. 16.14 Acoustic radiation force impulse method (ARFI) of transplanted renal shows elevated velocity (3.92 m/s) compatible for interstitial fibrosis

although most of these are in the native kidneys in patients with acquired cystic disease from hemodialysis. Ultrasonography may be used to screen for renal neoplasms in both the transplant and native kidneys, although marked atrophy and increased echogenicity in the native kidneys may decrease the ability to detect small tumors with ultrasonography [32].

Posttransplantation lymphoproliferative disorder (PTLD) is a general term for a variety of lymphoid disorders ranging from lymphoid hyperplasia to frank lymphoma. Most cases of PTLD are B-cell lymphocyte proliferations related to Epstein-Barr virus, although the heterogeneity of these disorders suggests a variety of mechanisms that predispose to lymphoproliferation.

PTLD after solid organ transplantation usually occurs within the first year; however, the median time of presentation for renal transplant patients is 5 years, as a result of less aggressive immunosuppressive therapy. The most common site for PTLD in renal transplant patients is the allograft, followed by extranodal involvement, with particular predilection for the gastrointestinal tract and liver. Typical patterns of kidney involvement include a heterogeneous hilar mass and multiple parenchymal masses. Although one may suspect PTLD based on sonographically detected renal or gastrointestinal abnormalities, the high frequency of multisystem involvement makes positron-emission tomography combined with CT the preferred imaging modality.

16.5 Vascular Complications

Recently, the improvement of immunosuppressive regimens has led to a progressive reduction in both early and long-term graft loss due to acute or chronic rejection. Accordingly, the relevance of other causes of premature kidney failure such as drug toxicity and metabolic consequences, infections, primary disease recurrence, and vascular complications has progressively increased [33].

Vascular complications after renal transplantation usually include renal artery stenosis and thrombosis, transplant renal vein thrombosis, biopsy-induced vascular injuries such as pseudoaneurysm, and intrarenal arteriovenous fistula formation [34] (Table 16.3).

Kidney transplant vascular complications are a life-threatening, relatively rare, event, accounting for approximately 10% of all posttransplant abnormalities. However, their diagnosis is extremely important because of the potential for rapid graft loss and poor prognosis. On the other hand, repair of vascular defects is mostly possible by angioplasty or surgical procedures, making graft conservation achievable [35].

Reducing the incidence of vascular complications depends to a great extent on a prompt and precise diagnosis. Ultrasound and color Doppler exam (CDUS) is frequently the first-line investigation for both suspected native renal tract and renal transplant vascular complications. It is a noninvasive, inexpensive, rapid, and safe tool with a high diagnostic performance when performed by an experienced operator [36, 37].

Other imaging techniques, such as computed tomography (CT) or magnetic resonance imaging (MRI), may be complementary and are often used as solving tools when US results are doubtful. Finally, angiographic methods remain the gold standard in the diagnosis and treatment of graft vascular abnormalities, even though its indication must be strictly based on a favorable risk/benefit ratio assessed by the nephrologist.

New promising ultrasound-based technologies have been developed such as contrast-enhanced sonography (CEUS). CEUS is a radiation and toxin-free, reproducible, and very rapid US imaging modality that showed to enhance the diagnostic performance of CDUS in many different settings avoiding the limitation and potentially dangerous effect of other radiological techniques. Therefore, it is reasonable to suppose a future widespread application also in transplant medicine [38, 39].

Table 16.3 Vascular complications of kidney transplant

Most common vascular renal transplantation complications
Renal artery stenosis
Renal artery thrombosis
Renal vein thrombosis
Pseudoaneurysm
Arteriovenous fistula

16.6 Transplanted Renal Artery Stenosis (TRAS)

16.6.1 Epidemiology

Renal artery stenosis (TRAS) is the most frequent vascular complication in renal transplant, accounting for 75% of all graft vascular defects. It is important to detect this process because it represents a potentially reversible cause of refractory hypertension and graft loss. The reported incidence ranges between 1 and 23%, even though its epidemiology substantially differs depending on the diagnostic approach and the time elapsed from the transplant. An incidence of 12.4% has been registered when transplanted patients undergo a planned Doppler examination during the first year of follow-up [40]. However in more recent and powered trials the incidence did not exceed 1–3% [41]. TRAS is more frequently diagnosed between 3 months and 2 years from the surgical procedure; however it can equally occur anytime. Discrepancies in the reported prevalence might also be explained by a not-well-established criterion for defining a hemodynamically significant TRAS. Factors associated with an increased risk of TRAS are the following: cadaveric kidney transplant, atherosclerosis in donor vessels, cytomegalovirus infection, younger donor age, and extended criteria donors [42].

16.6.2 Clinical Manifestations and Pathogenesis

Based on the anatomic localization of the stenosis we can distinguish three main types of TRAS: proximal due to recipient atherosclerotic arterial disease, anastomotic, and distal in the donor renal artery. However, considering the extension of the stenosis it can be differentiated into localized, diffuse, and multiple. In about half of all TRAS cases, the stenosis is localized and anastomotic and iatrogenic, being mainly caused by scarring related to the surgical procedure during explantation, clamping, and/or anastomosis of the vessel with the iliac artery axis [43]. Less commonly, multiple segments of the artery (or even the entire vessel) are stenotic. In these cases, the stenosis is generally the result of catheter-related trauma to the intima during the phase of cold ischemia, but it may also be caused by torsion and/or kinking occurred after surgical implantation [44]. Both anastomotic and distal donor stenosis may also be caused by rejection. An immunological mechanism has also been proposed, particularly in diffuse and multiple stenoses. In most cases, TRAS is asymptomatic, but in some patients it can result in resistant hypertension and/or graft dysfunction in the absence of rejection, ureteric obstruction, or infection, because of severe renal hypoperfusion. TRAS is the underlying cause of 5% of all posttransplant hypertension [45].

The pathophysiology of hypertension occurring in the setting of TRAS is comparable to the renovascular hypertension in the "one-kidney, one-clip" experimental models. However, since, differently from Goldblatt's models, the transplanted kidney is denervated, in this case the stenosis-induced kidney ischemia does not directly trigger the sympathetic response.

Nevertheless, as in non-transplanted patients with bilateral RAS or solitary kidney stenosis, the renin-angiotensin-aldosterone system (RAAS) is activated in TRAS. This leads to sodium and fluid retention and, in rare cases, patients may develop edema, congestive heart failure, or recurrent bouts of pulmonary edema. Moreover, in transplanted patients, a sudden, not-justified kidney function reduction after the administration of antiangiotensin drugs should be considered as suggestive of TRAS. An association with erythrocytosis has also been reported. Physical examination is mostly silent and a vascular bruit in the iliac fossa can often be present, but is not specific for significant stenosis [46]. Limited evidence regarding the progression showed that in most patients TRAS remains stable over time and can be treated medically. Occasionally a spontaneous regression has also been observed. There are reports of favorable long-term follow-up of hemodynamically significant stenosis treated by percutaneous angioplasty (PTA) [47]. On the other hand, the USRDS registry reported an adjusted hazard ratio for death and graft loss of 2.84 (95% CI 1.70–4.72) in transplant recipients with TRAS compared with those without TRAS [41].

16.6.3 Diagnosis

Although angiography remains the gold standard for the final diagnosis of TRAS, color Doppler examination, as performed by an experienced operator, plays an essential role in the screening, diagnosis, and follow-up. Other imaging techniques, such as computed tomography (CT) or magnetic resonance imaging (MRI), have a complementary role. New ultrasound-based techniques as contrast-enhanced ultrasound (CEUS) have already demonstrated to improve the diagnostic performance of color Doppler ultrasound examination (CDUS) examination, but are still under evaluation in transplanted kidney [39, 48].

16.6.4 Color Doppler Ultrasound (CDUS)

The CDUS examination, being performed at the bedside, is a noninvasive, highly sensible, specific, and inexpensive tool in the management of TRAS [49] (Fig. 16.15). It has progressively replaced renal scintigraphy because of its superior performance (87–94% sensitivity; 86–100% specificity) [50].

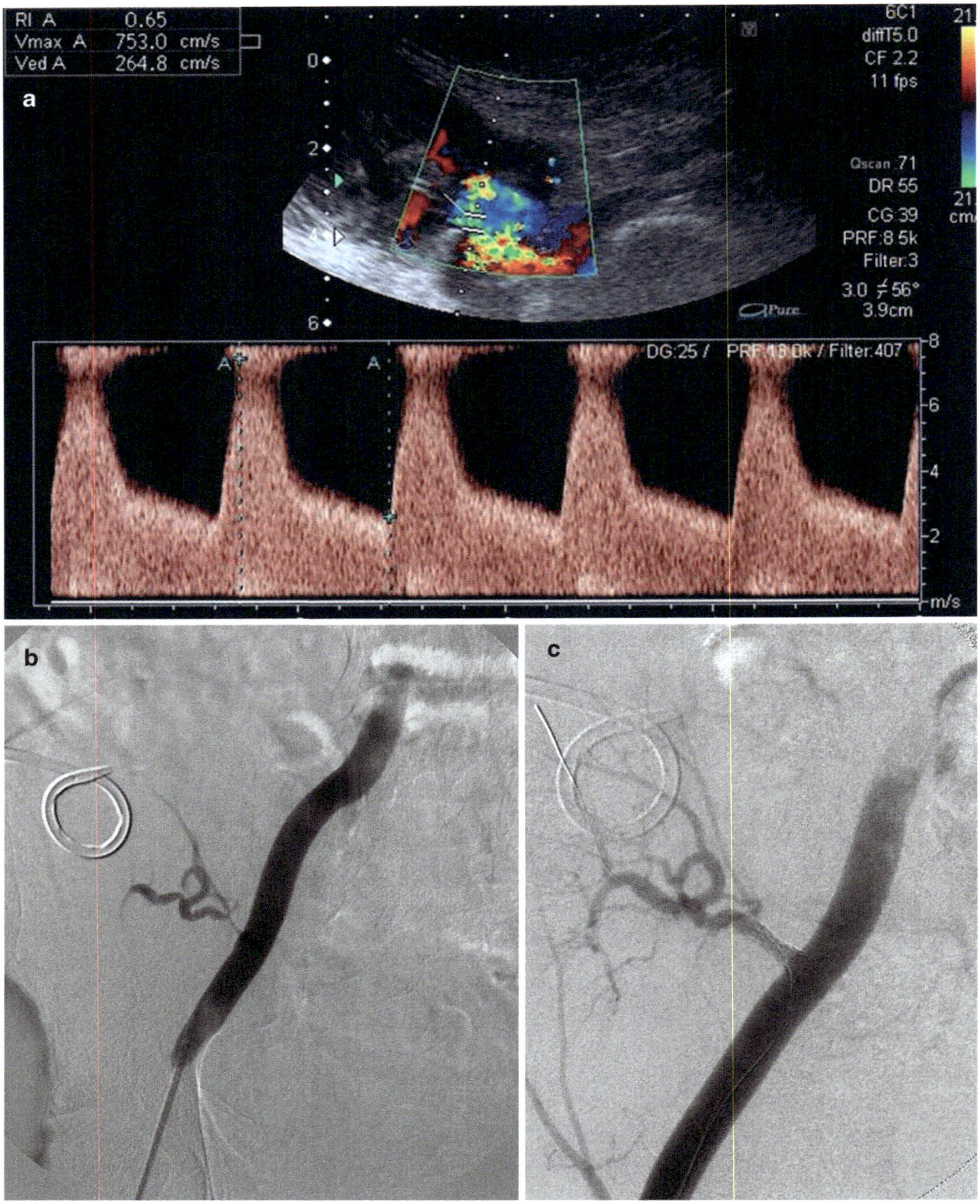

Fig. 16.15 Transplanted renal artery stenosis. Arterial hypertension and failure of the graft on 28th day. (**a**) CDUS finding of anastomotic aliasing of renal artery with high VPS (753 cm/s); (**b**) arteriography confirms anastomotic TRAS tightened; (**c**) PTA and stenting in the first part of the renal artery

CDUS allows assessing both the localization and hemodynamic significance of TRAS. Moreover, Doppler study is ideal to estimate the result of revascularization and helps in grading the stenosis during a long-term follow-up. The main disadvantages are that this investigation is operator dependent and time consuming [39]. As in the native kidney, CDUS evaluation criteria of RAS are based on direct findings at the level of the stenosis (proximal criteria), or on flow changes induced in the renal vasculature induced by the stenosis (distal criteria).

Differently from native kidney, in TRAS it is more difficult to set a peak systolic velocity (PSV) cutoff as a direct diagnostic criterion. Furthermore, the more frequent presence of transplant renal artery tortuosity and/or multiple renal arteries leads to incorrect insonation angles and reduces the accuracy of PSV assessment, thus representing a significant source of technical errors in CDUS evaluation. For the same reason, the direct visualization of color artifacts, such as aliasing at the site of the stenosis and presence of turbulence at color evaluation, may not be a sign of significant TRAS [49]. If possible, the operator should consult the surgery report to know whether multiple artery or anastomosis problems had been observed.

Elevated PSV of the RA is not necessarily indicative of TRAS. In fact, PSV as measured in a hypertrophic, well-functioning transplanted kidney may rise beyond 250–300 cm/s longwise the artery even in the absence of TRAS (Fig. 16.16). On the other hand, in case of chronic graft dysfunction with reduced organ volume, a focal PSV of 180–200 cm/s may be suggestive of significant stenosis, particularly when the other segments of the artery show markedly lower PSVs (40–50 cm/s) [51].

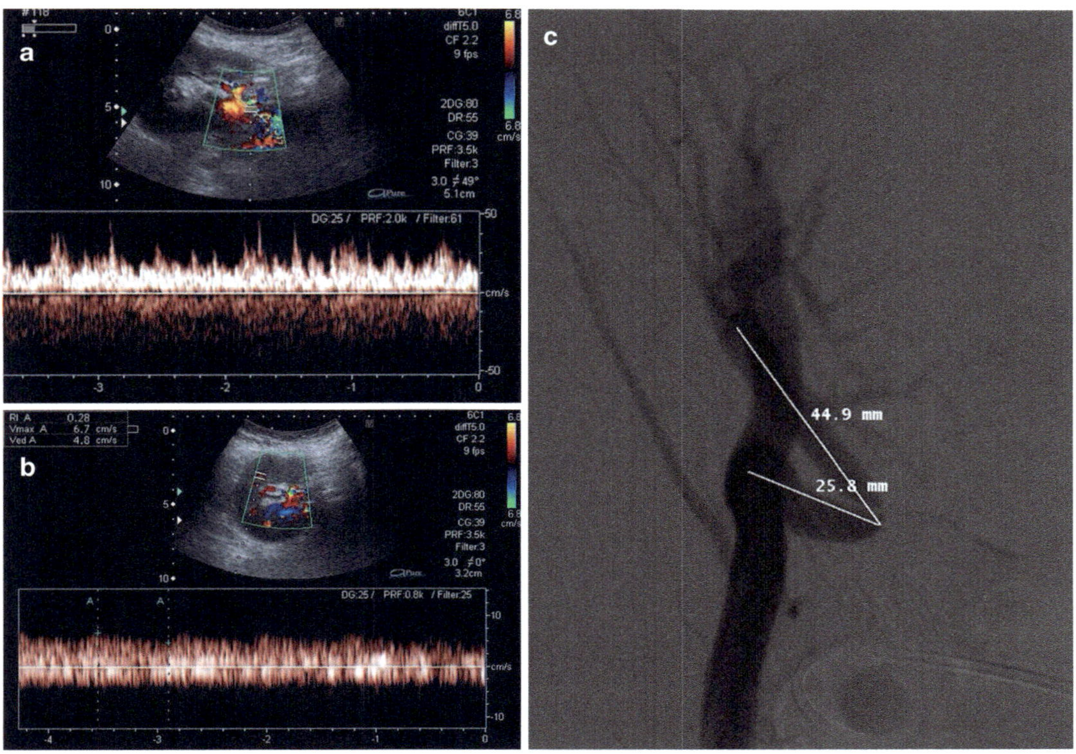

Fig. 16.16 Transplanted kidney renal artery stenosis (TRAS). (**a**) Renal artery with narrow angle determined by length greater than the vein; (**b**) tardus pardus phenomenon; (**c**) renal artery with narrow angulation determined by length greater than the vein (angiography)

Table 16.4 Detection of transplant artery stenosis

PSV	≥2.0 m/s	≥2.5 m/s	≥3.0 m/s
Specificity	67% (55–77%)	79% (65–82%)	93% (77–96%)
Sensitivity accuracy	100% (46–100%)	100% (46–100%)	80% (29–98%)
	68%	92%	81%

Therefore, an isolated acceleration of the flow that is 2.5 times higher than the pre- or post-stenotic velocity (e.g., PSV 250–270 vs. 80–120 cm/s) might represent a direct criterion for the diagnosis of TRAS. Concerns about a specific PVS limit have been deepened by a recent retrospective analysis of 844 transplanted kidneys performed by Robinson K. et al., in which almost 30% of renal transplants showed a PVS over 250 cm/s within the first 9 months and 19% had velocities over 250 cm/s also after the first-year posttransplant without any sign of graft dysfunction [51] (Table 16.4).

Eventually, some authors have pointed out that the PSV threshold for stenosis may also depend on the type of anastomosis, differing between end-to-side and end-to-end graft anastomosis, but this observation has not been confirmed in all studies [52]. Anyhow, in transplanted patients, when a high PSV is not associated with other clinical findings, a closer CDUS follow-up is advisable before immediate invasive intervention [53]. A recently proposed direct TRAS criterium is the ratio of PSV in the renal artery to the adjacent external iliac artery (RAA-to-EIA) with a threshold of 1.8 or greater, but its diagnostic and prognostic value is still poorly defined [54]. Looking at distal criteria, while the evaluation of the resistive index (RI) at CDUS may be very useful for the diagnosis (or recognizing) of RAS in native kidneys and predicting of the response to revascularization, in TRAS it has a less confirmed value. Initially, a high RI (<0.80 or higher) measured at least 3 months after transplantation had been found associated with both allograft failure and death with a functioning graft [55]. More recently, it has been demonstrated that RI reflects the recipient vascular status, but not the vasculature integrity of the graft [10, 27]. In addition, the waveform and resistive indexes of the transplanted kidney cannot be compared with the contralateral kidney, making more uncertain the interpretation of the results. A class of other distal parameters has been evaluated in RAS studies. The intrarenal parameters are measured from the intraparenchymal arteries which are often easier to evaluate than the main arteries [27, 53].

In native kidneys with significant renal artery stenosis, waveforms from the intraparenchymal arteries have been reported to be dampened [27].

This dampening has been evaluated quantitatively by measuring the prolonged rise time in early systole or qualitatively by assessing waveform shapes. Acceleration time (AT) alone is a validated high-sensitivity indirect index in the diagnosis of TRAS. In a small study performed by Gottlieb et al. a 0.10-s cutoff or a subjective assessment of dampening of the waveforms had a 95% accuracy in the detection of a hemodynamically significant TRAS, compared to a 62% obtained using the standard PVS threshold of 2.0 re/s as the sole criterion (Table 16.3).

CDUS is also particularly useful in the assessment of the effectiveness of perfusion restoration after revascularization procedures. When RI increases to the normal range, it invariably indicates restored kidney perfusion achieved by effective revascularization [56]. Doppler examination is essential for monitoring the TRAS during the posttreatment follow-up, allowing early diagnosis of recurrence, while MRA and spiral CTA are less suitable for assessing restenosis because of artifacts caused by the stent material [56]. Accordingly, CDUS follow-up to assess for restenosis may be warranted in patients after stent placement for TRAS, even in the absence of clinical signs of restenosis. Finally, because the number of patients affected by peripheral artery disease (older age and diabetes) that undergo kidney transplant is increasing, the possibility of a concomitant iliac artery disease that mimics TRAS (pseudo-TRAS) should always be considered [57].

Lesions upstream to the transplant anastomosis, reducing blood flow, may cause transplant hypoperfusion with signs and symptoms resembling TRAS. Also, these lesions may be detected by CDUS examination [57].

In summary, there is a reasonable level of consensus on a PVS above 250–300 cm/s as the limit to predict significant TRAS, in clinically suspicious patients, with an acceptable grade of sensitivity and specificity. In contrast to RAS in the native kidneys, indirect signs are less sensible and less accepted as valid diagnostic criteria in TRAS. In fact, an AT below 0.10 s is the only accepted distal criterion in this setting.

16.6.4.1 New Renal Ultrasound-Based Imaging: Contrast-Enhanced Ultrasound (CEUS)

In the evaluation of TRAS, contrast-enhanced ultrasound may be complementary to the standard CDUS examination. To date, few papers have tested the use of CEUS in TRAS, so that the role of this technique is still ill defined. Quantitative and qualitative CEUS examination seems to be a promising, quick, and noninvasive assay of graft perfusion, providing a real-time imaging of renal vasculature and perfusion [14, 40].

Longer time of contrast agent inflow indicates the presence of stenosis, and the rate of contrast agent inflow positively correlates with the severity of arterial stenosis on cross-sectional imaging.

Since PSV measurements require an angle of interrogation parallel to the vessel, which is not always obtainable by Doppler ultrasound, CEUS does not require identification of the renal artery, nor is it angle dependent. Furthermore, ultrasound examination during microbubble infusion can be used to quantify total organ and regional nutrient blood flow to the kidney [15, 58].

16.6.5 Nuclear Medicine Imaging (NMI)

NMI or isotope renography imaging of the allograft is a less invasive, non-nephrotoxic tool to evaluate graft function and perfusion, particularly in the early postoperative period. It may represent a complementary procedure for TRAS assessment when performed both at basal and after renin-angiotensin system inhibition [16]. The optimal radiopharmaceutical agent in individuals with normal renal function is still undefined. However, 99mTc-mercaptoacetyltriglycine (MAG-3) and 99mTc-diethylenetriaminepentriacetic acid (DTPA) are the most commonly used in clinical practice. Given its higher extraction rate, 99mTc-MAG3 is to be preferred over 99mTc-DTPA in patients with impaired kidney function [59].

Nevertheless, though in the past NMI was considered in the diagnostic algorithms of TRAS, it is now less applied because of its low specificity (almost 67%) compared to CDUS and MRI. For years, isotope renography (basal or after renin-angiotensin system stimulation) has been the most popular noninvasive screening procedure for TRAS. However, despite relatively good sensitivity (75%), the procedure is seriously limited by its poor specificity (67%).

16.6.6 CT and MRI Angiography

Computed tomography can provide excellent imaging by a three-dimensional reconstruction of graft vessels; however, it still requires the administration of nephrotoxic contrast agents, as in subtraction angiography [60]. Therefore, when clinical and less invasive instrumental features are strongly suggestive of hemodynamically significant stenosis, it is preferable to directly perform angiography that, in the case a TRAS is detected, allows to treat the stenotic vessel by angioplasty with or without stent placing (PTCA). Magnetic resonance imaging (MRI) can be safely used to diagnose or confirm TRAS and can be considered as a noninvasive alternative to CT angiography.

Gadolinium-based contrast agents are not nephrotoxic; nevertheless, they are not indicated when eGFR is below 30 mL/min due to the debated risk of nephrogenic systemic fibrosis.

Moreover, the opinions about MRI application in TRAS are contrasting, because some of them have reported that MRI angiography well correlates with digital subtraction angiography results, while others reported that, as compared with CDUS and digital subtraction angiography, MRI angiography may cause a conspicuous number of false positives (75%) due to artifacts. Other limitations may be related to the presence of clips on the anastomosis [52, 61].

16.6.7 Arteriography

Selective arteriography provides the precise diagnosis of RAS both in native and transplanted kidneys. Although its execution needs some relatively large amounts of potentially nephrotoxic radiocontrast medium, it is invasive and burdened by various complications such as thromboembolism, pseudoaneurysms, traumatic arteriovenous fistulas, and groin hematomas occurring in 10% of cases. Moreover, it can induce graft function loss with a reported incidence of 9% [62]. Therefore, angiographic techniques are not used as a screening tool, but are recommended in patients in whom a strong suspect TRAS has been previously elicited by other noninvasive screening tests or in patients particularly in those with a good expectancy of successful revascularization. Indeed, arteriography allows an immediate correction by transluminal angioplasty followed by balloon angioplasty and stent placement. Carbon dioxide images produce contrast columns like those with iodinated contrast media, giving images of the inflow iliac artery, artery anastomosis, and transplant renal artery with a resolution comparable to that of classical arteriography [62].

16.7 Renal Artery Thrombosis (RAT)

16.7.1 Epidemiology

The complete occlusion of the renal transplant artery is a rare and poor-prognosis vascular complication. Mainly, it occurs in the early postoperative period, even though very few papers reported cases detected after the first month, especially in rejected kidney or in a kidney with high-grade TRAS39. The incidence peak is observed in the first 48 h after surgery [63]. In the literature, the reported incidence of thrombotic complications in case series is about 0.5–6% and is more frequent in recipients of cadaveric donor kidneys and in pediatric age which may occur in 35% of transplanted kidneys, as reported by the North American Pediatric Renal Transplant Cooperative Study (NAPRTCS) [64]. Recognized risk factors are the following: hypovolemia, atherosclerosis of the donor vessels, technical errors, administration of the monoclonal antibody such as OKT3 (plus high-dose methylprednisolone), antiphospholipid antibodies, high-dose steroids especially as premedication, a too long cold ischemia time, and delayed graft function recovery. A clinical history of renal or extrarenal venous thrombosis, diabetic nephropathy, and peri- and early postoperative poor hemodynamic status is significantly associated with an increased risk of RAT and renal vein occlusions.

Transplant centers should consider prevention strategies in at-risk population such as patients with thrombophilic states or coagulation abnormalities, children, patients with a previous history of vascular thrombosis, and patients who lost a first kidney transplant because of graft thrombosis if not related to technical errors.

16.7.2 Clinical Manifestations and Pathogenesis

Usually, graft arterial thrombosis is characterized by sudden anuria and graft tenderness and/or severe pain over the graft region. Thrombocytopenia can be caused by platelet accumulation and consumption after thrombus formation. In the suspicion of RAT an urgent investigation is mandatory because it may result in immediate graft loss without a prompt correction. On occasion, segmental infarctions may be completely silent.

16.7.3 Diagnosis

CDUS has a 100% sensitivity and specificity in the detection of RAT and it typically leads to the complete absence of arterial flow within the kidney, from the point of occlusion along the vessel to distal arterial branches and with the complete absence of venous flow [65]. An occlusion that involves a segmental artery producing a segmental infarction occurs with the absence of arteriovenous flow only in the affected segment. Power Doppler imaging can be an excellent tool in these cases, because of its capacity to identify low-flow vessels, even though sometimes an arteriography proof is required [65]. Renal vascular thrombosis may be confirmed by supplementary imaging modalities including angiography, scintigraphy, CT, and MRI. As in TRAS, CEUS may be applied in the detection of RAT. It may provide an immediate diagnosis, without recourse to other potentially nephrotoxic agents. In addition, with CEUS clinicians can directly obtain additional information not available from other modalities about the microcirculation [38].

16.8 Renal Vein Thrombosis (TTRV)

16.8.1 Epidemiology, Clinical Manifestations, and Pathogenesis

Transplanted renal vein thrombosis (TTRV), affecting between 0.4% and 6% of all renal allografts, is an infrequent vascular complication, but it commonly causes early graft loss [66].

Even though in most cases the pathogenesis is undefined, TTRV is frequently the consequence of a technical problem with the vein or the extension of a lower-limb venous occlusion [66]. Similarly, to deep vein thrombosis (TVP), TTRV risk factors are coagulation disorders such as factor V Leiden mutation, metabolic diseases, high hematocrit, renal impairment, nephrotic syndrome, rejection, infections, and calcineurin inhibitor treatment. In this regard, USRDS data reported in transplanted subjects an increased incidence of TVP episodes (2.9 episodes/1000 person-years) compared to normal population [67]. The clinical presentation is comparable to RAT displaying as a sudden drop in urine output combined with graft tenderness and enlargement, swelling, and proteinuria, resulting in an immediate graft dysfunction. It may represent a life-threatening condition leading to a dramatic graft rupture and hemorrhage [68]. Moreover, only a small number of reported cases were successfully treated by surgical procedure or by less invasive intra-arterial injections of antifibrinolytic agents, such as recombinant tissue plasminogen activator or urokinase.

16.8.2 Diagnosis

16.8.2.1 Ultrasound-Based Diagnosis (CDUS and CEUS)

CDUS is an easy and accurate technique in TTVR diagnosis. The most common CDUS feature in the presence of complete TTRV is the absence of the venous color signal associated with a scarce or absent vessel's compressibility. Less frequently, the occlusion may be incomplete [67]. In case of total graft's vein occlusion, the Doppler trace shows a typical "reverse" diastolic flow, with the wave flow below the baseline and a peculiar bidirectional flow in the parenchymal arteries (Fig. 16.17). The intrarenal arteries' reverse flow is a 100% specific evidence of TTRV and an immediate indication for sudden surgical transplanted kidney revision regardless of any further diagnostic confirmation.

In addition, the color imaging of the hilar region may display a complete lack in venous flow.

Other B-mode combined, but less specific, signs are graft enlargement with augmented parenchymal thickening, decreased echogenicity, and reduced or absent corticomedullary differentiation [67]. An incomplete occlusion and/or graft renal vein stenosis is a very uncommon event. External factors such as perinephric fluid collection (hematomas, lymphocele, urinomas) and perivascular fibrosis may cause renal vein narrowing by compression (Fig. 16.18). The CDUS and B-mode findings are less suggestive in the context of incomplete vein occlusions. Usually, the most accepted diagnostic criterion for a partial TTRV is a 3–4-fold rise in the PSV between the stenotic and prestenotic segments [69, 70]. CEUS has been demonstrated to be an excellent tool in assessing venous patency in renal trans-

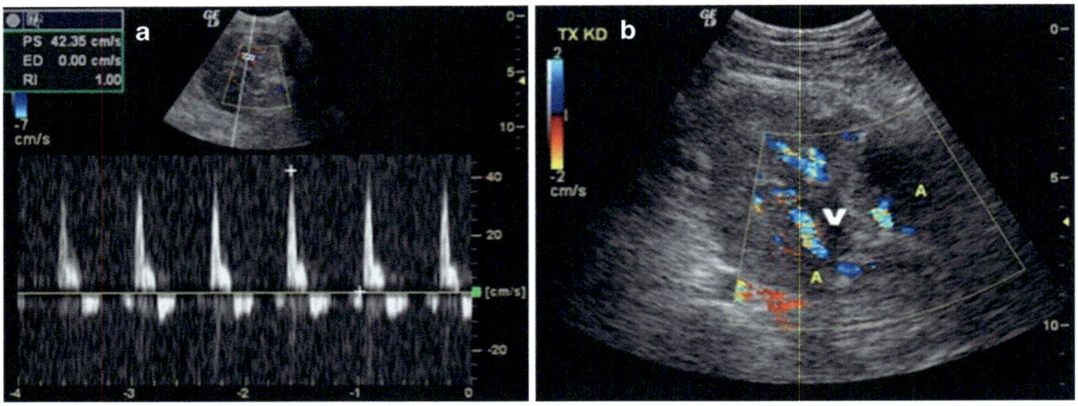

Fig. 16.17 Renal vein thrombosis. (**a**) Doppler US of an intrarenal arcuate artery shows reversal of the diastolic flow below the baseline; (**b**) color Doppler image through the renal hilum shows two renal arteries (A) with no flow in the central renal vein (V) consistent with renal vein thrombosis (courtesy of Prof. Ishrad)

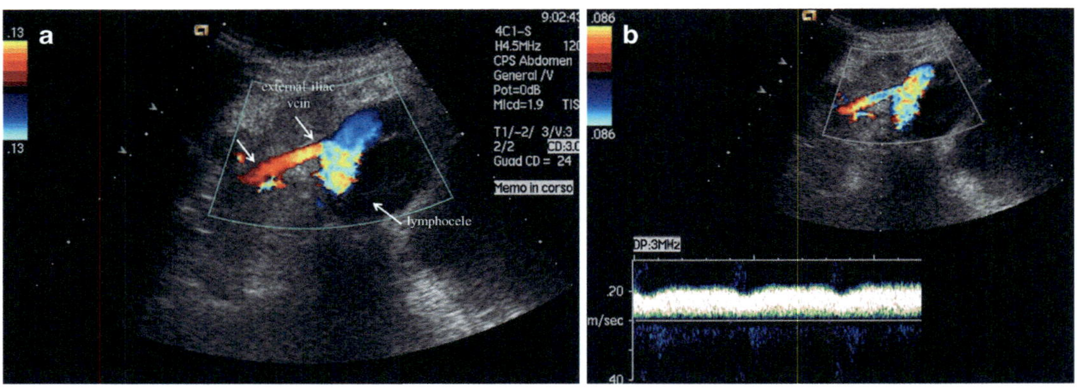

Fig. 16.18 Stenosis of the transplanted renal vein. (**a**) Color Doppler ultrasound shows external compression of the homolateral external iliac vein and (**b**) significantly increased PSV (200 cm/s)

plants. It allows quantifying cortical perfusion and microcirculation. Recently, more specific thrombus-targeting microbubble media have also been tested in animal models aiming at improving the efficiency and precision in the detection of thrombi.

16.8.2.2 Arteriography

Eventually, an angiographic (or other investigations) confirmation may be needed if CDUS findings are highly suggestive of partial and treatable TTRV or when clinical evidences are strongly suspicious of stenosis, despite ambiguous imaging results.

16.9 Arteriovenous Fistulas and Pseudoaneurysms

16.9.1 Epidemiology, Clinical Manifestations, and Pathogenesis

AVFs are unusual both native and transplanted kidney vascular complications, accounting for 1–2% of all vascular lesions [71]. They are a well-known kidney biopsy consequence and, for this reason, a certain incidence is inevitable, especially in per-protocol transplanted kidney biopsies. In animal studies, the incidence after biopsy is close to 50%; however, in human angiographic studies the incidence in native kidneys is almost 15–16%. Isolated case of post-ureterorenoscopy lithotripsy and congenital AVFs and infection-related pseudoaneurysms have been described in literature.

During kidney biopsy, the concurrent puncture and damage of an artery and vein walls, producing a vessel junction, may result in an AVF. On the other hand, pseudoaneurysms can develop when the damage is limited to the arterial wall. Both lesions are generally small, asymptomatic, and likely to resolve spontaneously. Even though sometimes AVFs may be more extended, inducing a renal perfusion reduction and leading to graft ischemia, indeed they may be a concerning source of intragraft hemorrhages. Therefore, only large AVFs deserve to be invasively treated.

Pseudoaneurysms are always clinically silent; nevertheless they are at high risk of bleeding; consequently, the treatment is mandatory and not related to the lesion's size [72]. Selective embolization is the treatment of choice with an 80% rate of good outcome.

16.9.2 Diagnosis

16.9.2.1 Ultrasound-Based Diagnosis (CDUS and CEUS)

We can appreciate AVFs at the B-mode examination only when they display a huge extension. On the other hand, they can be steadily visualized at color mode as localized areas with both arterial and venous flow with the characteristic appearance of a color mosaic pattern. Moreover, this feature allows to discriminate high-flow AVFs, presenting an accelerate flow even though increasing the PRF until only the anomalous focus. This maneuver usually produces diagnostic results. Spectral analysis may show increased systo-diastolic flow around the interest area with normal or reduced resistive and pulsatility indexes compared to nearby vessels, whereas Doppler waveform from draining vein shows higher flow velocities and an arterialized pattern occurs in around 30% of all cases (Fig. 16.19).

Pseudoaneurysms display at B-mode as anechoic circular areas, similarly to cystic lesions, while at the color Doppler analysis, they exhibit a turbulence and "to-and-fro" flow comparable to that seen in pseudoaneurysms involving the arterial anastomosis and distal tract (Figs. 16.20 and 16.21). Even in the suspect of AVFs and pseudoaneurysms, echocontrast exam may be one of the best suitable diagnostic investigations. As previously mentioned, CEUS provides a 30-fold more accurate renal circulation. Furthermore, it may be very useful to detect parenchymal perfusion impairment that leads to kidney function decline in large AVFs. This may help to identify and discriminate AVFs that urgently need to be treated [73]. CEUS seems

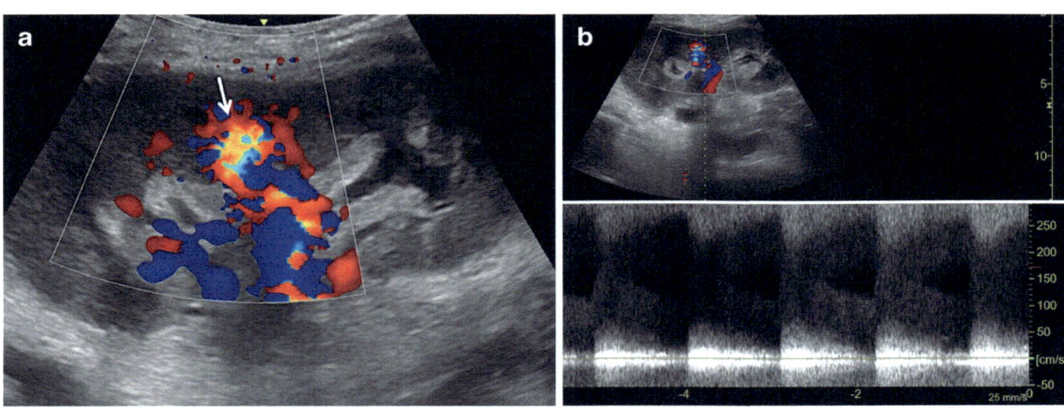

Fig. 16.19 (**a**) Color Doppler ultrasound shows large-caliber interlobar artery and vein. The resistance index of the nutrient artery is 0.50 (vs. approximately 0.80 in other regions of the graft). The venous spectrum reflects markedly pulsatile flow that cannot be found in other interlobar veins. Post-biopsy arteriovenous fistula (arrow); (**b**) Doppler shows alternating flow

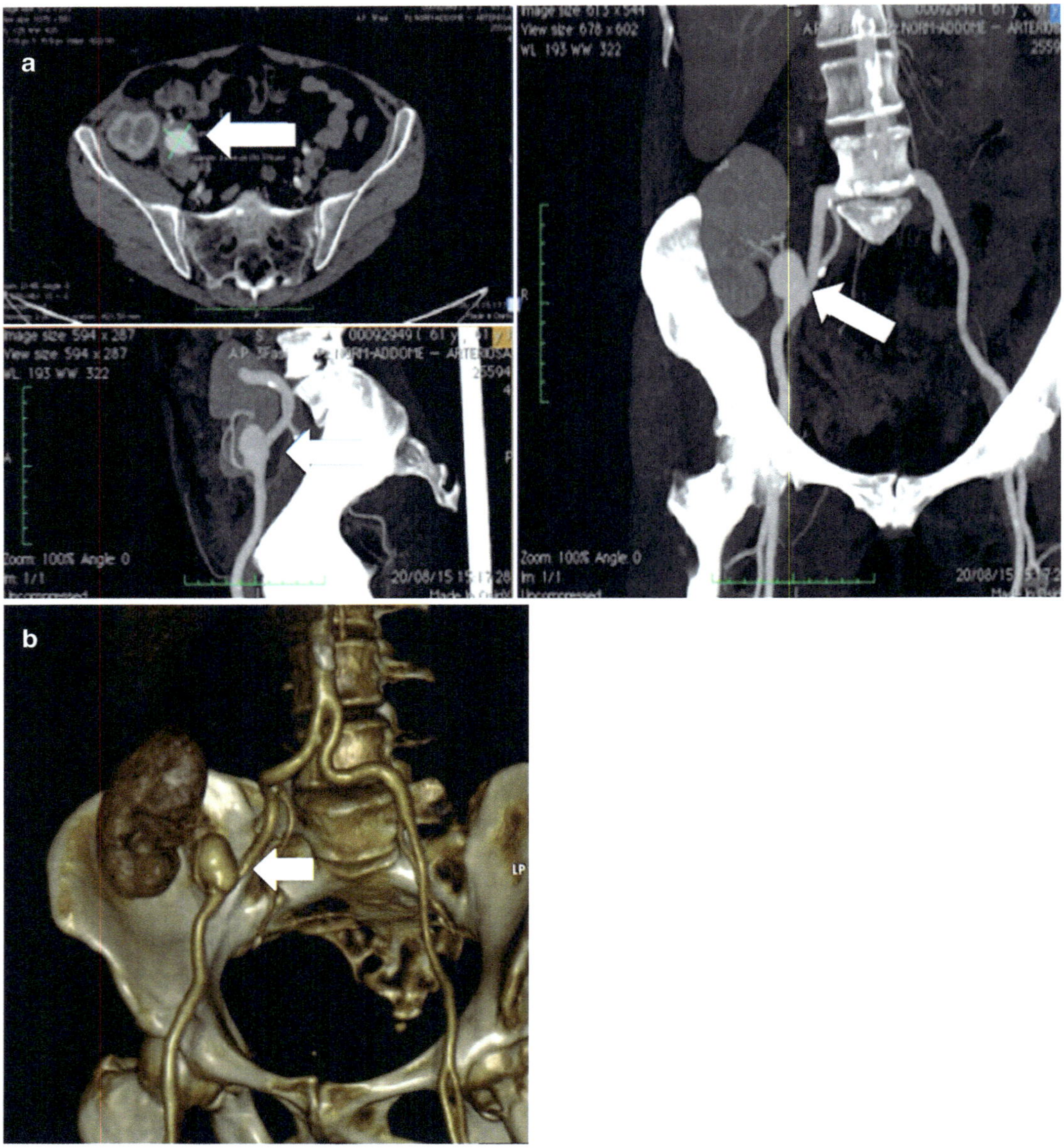

Fig. 16.20 (**a**) Abdominal computed tomography scan angiography demonstrates the presence of a pseudoaneurysm at the level of the arterial anastomosis of the renal graft (arrow). (**b**) Volume rendering demonstrates the anastomotic pseudoaneurysm (arrow)

to be a viable diagnostic option even in pseudoaneurysm characterization and follow-up with high sensibility and specificity [74]. It would appear in few described cases that echocontrast exam improved the identification of the lesion's margins and, consequently, a more accurate size estimation [75]. Accordingly, CEUS might be used in the monitoring of coil embolization effectiveness; indeed contrast sonography has been demonstrated to be helpful in the study of small bleeding focus, refining the diagnosis of kidney parenchyma hemorrhages.

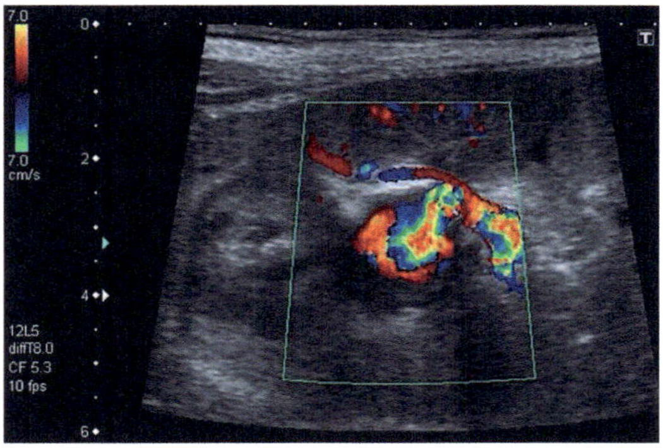

Fig. 16.21 Renal pseudoaneurysm. Color Doppler ultrasonography shows the typical swirling signal called "yin-yang" sign

16.9.2.2 Arteriography

Arteriography is not justified when AVF is clearly asymptomatic and a prompt treatment is not required. However, when necessary, arteriography transcatheter embolization is a safe and effective minimally invasive technique to treat biopsy-related vascular injuries in renal transplants.

16.10 Rare Vascular Complications

Torsion of the vascular pedicle of the transplanted kidney is extremely rare. It is caused by intraperitoneal placement of the graft (which occurs during combined renal-pancreatic transplants). Because of its increased mobility, the kidney may rotate around the vascular pedicle, causing vascular occlusion that will lead to parenchymal necrosis and graft loss if not identified promptly. The clinical presentation varies: it may resemble acute rejection or renal vein thrombosis. Ultrasonography can facilitate the diagnosis by documenting a change in the orientation of the kidney, so that the hilum is anterior rather than posterior. Color Doppler ultrasound findings are variable with low diagnostic accuracy. Dissection of the iliac artery and the renal artery are extremely rare events, which are caused by dissection of the aorta and present the same features on CDUS.

Torsion is determined by the rotation of the allograft around its vascular pedicle. This may completely compromise kidney transplant vascular perfusion leading to immediate graft loss if not timely recognized. Data in literature are very scarce and this complication has been described in only 24 cases. It is more frequent in intraperitoneal graft placement, which usually occurs during combined renal-pancreatic transplants [76].

Grafts that are intraperitoneally located are more likely to rotate around the vascular pedicle due to their increased mobility [77].

Similarly, to TTRV the clinical presentation is not specific and symptoms may include nausea, vomiting, abdominal pain, and signs of acute kidney injury such as decreased urine output with sudden kidney function impairment [77]. Renal allograft torsion requires a rapid surgical detorsion to avoid allograft loss. For these reasons, imaging diagnosis plays an essential role in the detection of these events.

16.10.1 Diagnosis

16.10.1.1 Ultrasound-Based Diagnosis (CDUS and CEUS)

As the first step, US B-mode evaluation can document a different orientation of the kidney compared to previous exams (the hilum may exhibit an anterior rather than posterior position). CDUS findings are inconsistent and in this setting the diagnostic value is very low. Main features are the following: augmented renal resistive index and high PVS at the main renal artery anastomosis. At the beginning, when the torsion is not complete, it may only result in venous involvement [78].

Then, as the twisting progresses, the arterial implication evolves from a decreased resistive index until the complete lack of blood flow on color Doppler, eventually showing also a reverse diastolic flow. Afterwards, the torsion may include the ureter; consequently the graft may also display enlargement and hydronephrosis at standard B-mode [78].

CEUS, providing a better vascular visualization, may allow to better appreciate the vascular kinking and/or torsion [78]. As in RAT, the presence of ischemia or impending necrosis may be demonstrated by a delayed or absent enhancement of the corticomedullary area and nephrographic phases of contrast [78].

16.10.1.2 CT and MRI Angiography

The change in axis of the allograft can be more precisely documented on cross-sectional imaging such as CT and MRI, even though obtaining more accurate imaging should not delay surgical treatment, and since patients with pedicle torsion have a severe renal impairment the use of iodinate contrast agents or gadolinium is not recommendable. Recently, iron-based contrast agents have been investigated in transplanted patients [79].

16.11 Conclusions

Both grayscale B-mode and color Doppler ultrasound are portable inexpensive first-step tools in the management of graft parenchymal and vascular complications. These methods provide a quick differential diagnosis with other causes of graft failure such as surgical complications, hydronephrosis, and early large perinephric collections. CDUS and calculation of the RI (the peak systolic velocity minus the end diastolic velocity divided by the peak systolic velocity) can confirm suspicions of allograft dysfunction and might be a useful tool in biopsy indication and subsequent transplant follow-up.

New advanced techniques such as CEUS might overcome standard CDUS limitations in the next future providing unique functional data in grafts, with promising results in terms of monitoring graft function, optimizing antirejection therapy, and thus minimizing the risk of nephrotoxicity. Additional, well-designed studies are needed to further validate their role in these settings.

References

1. Meier-Kriesche HU, Schold JD, Srinivas TR, Kaplan B. Lack of improvement in renal allograft survival despite a marked decrease in acute rejection rates over the most recent era. Am J Transplant. 2004;4(3):378–83.
2. O'Neill WC, Baumgarten DA. Ultrasonography in renal transplantation. Am J Kidney Dis. 2002;39:663–78.
3. Granata A, Di Nicolò PP, Scarfia VR, Insalaco M, Lentini P, Veroux M, Fatuzzo P, Fiorini F. Renal transplantation parenchymal complications: what Doppler ultrasound can and cannot do. J Ultrasound. 2015;18(2):109–16.
4. Granata A, Clementi S, Clementi A, Di Pietro F, Scarfia VR, Insalaco M, Aucella F, Prencipe M, Figuera M, Fiorini F, Sicurezza E. Parenchymal complications of the transplanted kidney: the role of color-Doppler imaging. G Ital Nefrol. 2012;29(S57):S90–8.
5. Lockhart ME, Wells CG, Morgan DE, Fineberg NS, Robbin ML. Reversed diastolic flow in the renal transplant: perioperative implications versus transplants older than 1 month. AJR Am J Roentgenol. 2008;190(3):650–5.
6. Colvin RB. Antibody-mediated renal allograft rejection: diagnosis and pathogenesis. J Am Soc Nephrol. 2007;18(4):1046–56.
7. Sharfuddin A. Renal relevant radiology: imaging in kidney transplantation. CJASN. 2014;9(2):416–29.
8. Fischer T, Mehrsai A, Salem S, Ahmadi H, Baradaran N, Tahe-rimahmoudi M, Nikoobakht MR, Rezaeidanesh M, Mansoori D, Pourmand G. Role of resistive index measurement in diagnosis of acute rejection episodes following successful kidney transplantation. Transplant Proc. 2009;41(7):2805–7.
9. Heine GH, Gerhart MK, Ulrich C, Kohler H, Girndt M. Renal Doppler resistance indices are associated with systemic atherosclerosis in kidney transplant recipients. Kidney Int. 2005;68:878–85.
10. Naesens M, Heylen L, Lerut E, Claes K, De Wever L, Claus F, et al. Intrarenal resistive index after renal transplantation. N Engl J Med. 2013;369:1797–806.
11. Dupont PJ, Dooldeniya M, Cook T, Warrens AN. Role of duplex Doppler sonography in diagnosis of acute allograft dysfunction-time to stop measuring the resistive index? Transpl Int. 2003;16:648–52.
12. Schwenger V, Hinkel UP, Nahm AM, Morath C, Zeier M. Real-time contrast-enhanced sonography in renal transplant recipients. Clin Transplant. 2006;20(Suppl 17):51–4.
13. Grzelak P, Szymczyk K, Strzelczyk J, Kurnatowska I, Sapieha M, Nowicki M, Stefanczyk L. Perfusion of kidney graft pyramids and cortex in contrast-enhanced ultrasonography in the determination of the cause of delayed graft function. Ann Transplant. 2011;16:48–53.
14. Girometti R, Stocca T, Serena E, Granata A, Bertolotto M. Impact of contrast-enhanced ultrasound in patients with renal function impairment. World J Radiol. 2017;9(1):10–6.
15. Graversen ME, Dalgaard LS, Jensen-Fangel S, Jespersen B, Østergaard L, Søgaard OS. Risk and outcome of pyelonephritis among renal transplant recipients. BMC Infect Dis. 2016;16:264.
16. Brown ED, Chen MYM, Wolfman NT, et al. Complications of renal transplantation: evaluation with US and radionuclide imaging. Radiographics. 2000;20:607–22.

17. Pelle G, Vimont S, Levy PP, Hertig A, Ouali N, Chassin C, Arlet G, Rondeau E, Vandewalle A. Acute pyelonephritis represents a risk factor impairing long-term kidney graft function. Am J Transplant. 2007;7:899–907.
18. Granata A, Andrulli S, Fiorini F, Basile A, Logias F, Figuera M, Sicurezza E, Gallieni M, Fiore CE. Diagnosis of acute pyelonephritis by contrast-enhanced ultrasonography in kidney transplant patients. Nephrol Dial Transplant. 2011;26(2):715–20.
19. Granata A, Floccari F, Insalaco M, Clementi A, Di Lullo L, D'Amelio A, Zamboli P, Logias F, Romano M, Fiorini F. Ultrasound assessment in renal infections. G Ital Nefrol. 2012;29(Suppl 57):S47–57.
20. McArthur C, Baxter GM. Current and potential renal applications of contrast-enhanced ultrasound. Clin Radiol. 2012;67(9):909–22.
21. Fontanilla T, Minaya J, Cortés C, Hernando CG, Arangüena RP, Arriaga J, Carmona MS, Alcolado A. Acute complicated pyelonephritis: contrast-enhanced ultrasound. Abdom Imaging. 2012;37(4):639–46.
22. Chang CY, Gangji A, Chorneyko K, Kapoor A. Urological manifestations of BK polyomavirus in renal transplant recipients. Can J Urol. 2005;12:2829–36.
23. Tourret J, Mercadal L, Penna RR, Brocheriou I, Barrou B. Visualizing BK virus nephropathy. NDT Plus. 2010;3(2):185–6.
24. Dugo M, Mangino M, Meola M, Petrucci I, Valente ML, Laurino L, Stella M, Mastrosimone S, Brunello A, Virgilio B, Rizzolo M, Maresca MC. Ultrasound findings of BK polyomavirus-associated nephropathy in renal transplant patients. J Nephrol. 2017;30(3):449–53.
25. Allen PJ, Chadban SJ, Craig JC, Lim WH, Allen RDM, Clayton PA, Teixeira-Pinto A, Wong G. Recurrent glomerulonephritis after kidney transplantation: risk factors and allograft outcomes. Kidney Int. 2017;92(2):461–9.
26. Radermarcher J, Mengel M, Ellis S, Stuht S, Hiss M, et al. The renal arterial resistance index and renal allograft survival. N Engl J Med. 2003;349:115–24.
27. Di Nicolò P, Granata A. Renal resistive index: not only kidney. Clin Exp Nephrol. 2017;21(3):359–66.
28. Nankivell BJ, Chapman JR, Gruenewald SM. Detection of chronic allograft nephropathy by quantitative Doppler imaging. Transplantation. 2002;74(1):90–6.
29. Scholbach T, Girelli E, Scholbach J. Tissue pulsatility index: a new parameter to evaluate renal transplant perfusion. Transplantation. 2006;81:751–5.
30. Harvey CJ, Sidhu PS. Bachmann Nielsen M contrast-enhanced ultrasound in renal transplants: applications and future directions. Ultraschall Med. 2013;34(4):319–21.
31. Lee J, Oh YT, Joo DJ, Ma BG, Lee AL, Lee JG, Song SH, Kim SU, Jung DC, Chung YE, Kim YS. Acoustic radiation force impulse measurement in renal transplantation: a prospective, longitudinal study with protocol biopsies. Medicine (Baltimore). 2015;94(39):e1590.
32. Lentini P, Granata A, Ciancio A, Gallieni M. Regular ultrasound examination of transplanted kidneys allows early diagnosis of renal cell carcinoma and conservative nephron sparing surgery. Arch Ital Urol Androl. 2011;83(4):195–9.
33. Ghazanfar A, Tavakoli A, Augustine N. Management of transplant artery stenosis and its impact on long-term allograft survival: a single-centre experience. Nephrol Dial Transpl. 2011;26:336–43.
34. Osman Y, Shokeir A, Ali-el-Dein B, Tantawy M, Wafa EW, et al. Vascular complications after live donor renal transplantation: study of risk factors and effects on graft and patients survival. J Urol. 2003;169:859–62.
35. Estrada CC, Musani M, Darras F, Suh H, Abate MT, Mani A, Nord EP. 5 years experience with drug eluting and bare metal stents as primary intervention in transplant renal artery stenosis. Transplant Direct. 2017;3(2):e128.
36. Rodgers SK, Sereni CP, Horrow MM. Ultrasonographic evaluation of the renal transplant. Radiol Clin N Am. 2014;52(6):1307–24.
37. Granata A, Floccari F, Lentini P, Vittoria S, Di Pietro F, Zamboli P, et al. Vascular complications following kidney transplant: the role of color-Doppler imaging. G Ital Nefrol. 2012;29(S57):S99–S105.
38. Granata A, Zanoli L, Insalaco M, Valentino M, Pavlica P, Di Nicolò PP, Scuderi M, Fiorini F, Fatuzzo P, Bertolotto M. Contrast-enhanced ultrasound (CEUS) in nephrology: has the time come for its widespread use? Clin Exp Nephrol. 2015;19(4):606–15.
39. Granata A, Floccari F, Logias F, Insalaco M, Di Lullo L, Andrulli S, Zamboli P, Ricciardi B, Fiorini F. Contrast enhanced ultrasound in renal diseases. G Ital Nefrol. 2012;29(Suppl 57):S25–35.
40. Weir MR, Salzberg DJ. Management of hypertension in the transplant patient. J Am Soc Hypertens. 2011;5:425–32.
41. Hurst FP, Abbott KC, Neff RT, et al. Incidence, predictors and outcomes of transplant renal artery stenosis after kidney transplantation: analysis of USRDS. Am J Nephrol. 2009;30(5):459–67.
42. Pararajasingam R, Riad H, Chalmers, Etemadi J, Rahbar K, Haghighi AN, Bagheri N, Falaknazi K, Ardalan MR, Ghabili K, Shoja MM. Renal artery stenosis in kidney transplants: assessment of the risk factors. Vasc Health Risk Manag. 2011;7:503–7.
43. Chen W, Kayler LK, Zand MS, Muttana R, Chernyak V, DeBoccardo GO. Transplant renal artery stenosis: clinical manifestations, diagnosis and therapy. Clin Kidney J. 2015;8(1):71–8.
44. Willicombe M, Sandhu B, Brookes P, Gedroyc W, Hakim N, Hamady M, Hill P, McLean AG, Moser S, Papalois V, Tait P, Wilcock M, Taube D. Postanastomotic transplant renal artery stenosis: association with de novo class II donor-specific antibodies. Am J Transplant. 2014;14(1):133–43.
45. Weir MR, Burgess ED, Cooper JE, Fenves AZ, Goldsmith D, McKay D, Mehrotra A, Mitsnefes

MM, Sica DA, Taler SJ. Assessment and management of hypertension in transplant patients. J Am Soc Nephrol. 2015;26(6):1248–60.
46. Roberts JP, Ascher NL, Fryd DS, et al. Transplant renal artery stenosis. Transplantation. 1989;48:580–3.
47. Ngo AT, Markar SR, De Lijster MS, Duncan N, Taube D, Hamady MS. A systematic review of outcomes following percutaneous Transluminal angioplasty and stenting in the treatment of transplant renal artery stenosis. Cardiovasc Intervent Radiol. 2015;38(6):1573–88.
48. Zhang X, Wang H, Liu S, Yan J, Liu X, Xu D, Tian C. Three-Dimensional Computed Tomography Reconstruction in Transplant Renal Artery Stenosis. Exp Clin Transplant. 2017;
49. Granata A, Fiorini F, Andrulli S, Logias F, Gallieni M, Romano G, Sicurezza E, Fiore CE. Doppler ultrasound and renal artery stenosis: an overview. J Ultrasound. 2009;12(4):133–43.
50. Erley CM, Duda SH, Wakat JP, et al. Noninvasive procedures for diagnosis of renovascular hypertension in renal transplant recipients—a prospective analysis. Transplantation. 1992;54:863–7.
51. Robinson KA, Kriegshauser JS, Dahiya N, Young SW, Czaplicki CD, Patel MD. Detection of transplant renal artery stenosis: determining normal velocities at the renal artery anastomosis. Abdom Radiol (NY). 2017;42(1):254–9.
52. Gao J, Li JC, Xiao MS, Ng A, Trost D, Goldstein M, et al. Color duplex sonography in severe transplant renal artery ste- nosis: a comparison of end-to-end and end-to-side arterial anastomoses. Clin Imaging. 2009;33:116–22.
53. Siskind E, Lombardi P, Blum M, Tyrell R, Villa M, Kuncewitch M, Olsen EM, Alex A, Lumermann L, Bhaskaran MC, Jhaveri KD, Sachdeva M, Calderon K, Greben C, Putterman D, Gandras E, Caplin D, D'Agostino C, Pellerito J, Coppa G, Molmenti EP. Significance of elevated transplant renal artery velocities in the postoperative renal transplant patient. Clin Transplant. 2013;27:E157–60.
54. de Morais RH, Muglia VF, Mamere AE, et al. Duplex Doppler sonography of transplant renal artery stenosis. J Clin Ultrasound. 2003;31(3):135–41.
55. Radermacher J, Mengel M, Ellis S, Stuht S, Hiss M, Schwarz A, Eisenberger U, Burg M, Luft FC, Gwinner W, Haller H. The renal arterial resistance index and renal allograft survival. N Engl J Med. 2003;349:115–24.
56. Bruno S, Ferrari S, Remuzzi G, Ruggenenti P. Doppler ultrasonography in posttransplant renal artery stenosis: a reliable tool for assessing effectiveness of revascularization? Transplantation. 2003;76(1):147–53.
57. Aslam S, Salifu MO, Ghali H, Markell MS, Friedman EA. Common iliac artery stenosis presenting as renal allograft dysfunction in two diabetic recipients. Transplantation. 2001;71:814–7.
58. Wei K, Le E, Bin JP, Coggins M, Thorpe J, Kaul S. Quantification of renal blood flow with contrast-enhanced ultrasound. J Am Coll Cardiol. 2001;37:1135–40.
59. Fananapazir G, Bashir MR, Corwin MT, Lamba R, Vu CT, Troppmann C. Comparison of ferumoxytol-enhanced MRA with conventional angiography for assessment of severity of transplant renal artery stenosis. J Magn Reson Imaging. 2017;45(3):779–85.
60. Sun IO, Hong YA, Kim HG, Park HS, Choi SR, Chung BH, Chun HJ, Choi BS, Park CW, Kim YS, Yang CW. Clinical usefulness of 3-dimensional computerized tomographic renal angiography to detect transplant renal artery stenosis. Transplant Proc. 2012;44(3):691–3.
61. Gaddikeri S, Mitsumori L, Vaidya S, Hippe DS, Bhargava P, Dighe MK. Comparing the diagnostic accuracy of contrast-enhanced computed tomographic angiography and gadolinium-enhanced magnetic resonance angiography for the assessment of hemodynamically significant transplant renal artery stenosis. Curr Probl Diagn Radiol. 2014;43(4):162–8.
62. Spinosa DJ, Isaacs RB, Matsumoto AH, Angle JF, Hagspiel KD, Leung DA. Angiographic evaluation and treatment of transplant renal artery stenosis. Curr Opin Urol. 2001;11:197–205.
63. Wu CK, Leu JG, Wei CC, Hsieh SC. Acute thrombosis of a transplanted renal artery after gastric ulcer bleeding in a patient with a long-term well-functioning renal allograft: a case report and literature review. Medicine (Baltimore). 2016;95(30):e4301.
64. McDonald RA, Smith JM, Stablein D, Harmon WE. Pretransplant peritoneal dialysis and graft thrombosis following pediatric kidney transplantation: a NAPRTCS report. Pediatr Transplant. 2003;7:204.
65. Cosgrove DO, Chan KE. Renal transplants: what ultrasound can and cannot do. Ultrasound Q. 2008;24(2):77–87.
66. Ponticelli C, Moia M, Montagnino G. Renal allograft thrombosis. Nephrol Dial Transplant. 2009;24(5):1388–93.
67. Drudi FM, Cascone F, Pretagostini R, Ricci P, Trippa F, Righi A, et al. Role of color Doppler US in the evaluation of renal transplant. Radiol Med. 2001;101:243–50.
68. Giustacchini P, Pisanti F, Citterio F, et al. Renal vein thrombosis after renal transplantation: an important cause of graft loss. Transplant Proc. 2002;34:2126–7.
69. Schwenger V, Hinkel UP, Nahm AM, et al. Color doppler ultrasonography in the diagnostic evaluation of renal allografts. Nephron Clin Pract. 2006;104:c107–12.
70. Gao J, Ng A, Shih G, et al. Intrarenal color duplex ultrasonography: a window to vascular complications of renal transplants, J Ultrasound Med , 2007, 26 (pg. 1403–1418).
71. Middleton WD, Kellman GM, Melson GL, Madrazo BL. Postbiopsy renal transplant arteriovenous fistulas: color Doppler US characteristics. Radiology. 1989;171(1):253–7.
72. Antonopoulos IM, Yamacake KG, Tiseo BC, Carnevale FC, Z E Jr, Nahas WC. Renal pseudoaneu-

rysm after core-needle biopsy of renal allograft successfully managed with superselective embolization. Int Braz J Urol. 2016;42(1):165–7.
73. Siracusano S, Bertolotto M, Ciciliato S, Valentino M, Liguori G, Visalli F. The current role of contrast-enhanced ultrasound (CEUS) imaging in the evaluation of renal pathology. World J Urol. 2011;29(5):633–8.
74. Durkin N, Deganello A, Sellars ME, Sidhu PS, Davenport M, Makin E. Post-traumatic liver and splenic pseudoaneurysms in children: diagnosis, management, and follow-up screening using contrast enhanced ultrasound (CEUS). J Pediatr Surg. 2016;51(2):289–92.
75. Helck A, Hoffmann RT, Sommer WH, Notohamiprodjo M, Albyaa H, Reiser M, Clevert DA. Diagnosis, therapy monitoring and follow up of renal artery pseudoaneurysm with contrast-enhanced ultrasound in three cases. Clin Hemorheol Microcirc. 2010;46(2–3):127–37.
76. Ozmen M, Bilgic I, Ziraman I, Koc M. Torsion of extraperitoneally transplanted kidney: an unusual complication. Exp Clin Transplant. 2013;11(2):186–90.
77. Sofue K, Vikraman DS, Jaffe TA, Chaubal GN, Bashir MR. Graft kidney torsion after simultaneous kidney-pancreas transplant: report of 2 cases and literature review. J Comput Assist Tomogr. 2015;39(4):506–9.
78. Dewan R, Dasyam AK, Tan H, Furlan A. Renal Allograft Torsion: US and CT Imaging Findings of a Rare Posttransplant Complication. Case Rep Radiol. 2016;2016:4273780.
79. Sebastià C, Quiroga S, Boyé R, Cantarell C, Fernandez-Planas M, Alvarez A. Helical CT in renal transplantation: normal findings and early and late complications. Radiographics. 2001;21(5):1103–17.

17 Sonographic Evaluation of Surgical Complications of Kidney Transplantation

Massimiliano Veroux, Domenico Zerbo, Daniela Corona, Nunziata Sinagra, and Pierfrancesco Veroux

17.1 Introduction

The use of renal transplantation has significantly increased in developed and developing countries for treatment of chronic renal failure and is nowadays considered the best replacement therapy for patients with end-stage renal disease. Kidney transplantation has been offered to an increased number of patients and this has led to an increased use of marginal deceased donor, which may increase the risk of surgical complications after transplantation. Consequently, the understanding of the normal and abnormal imaging features of the transplanted kidney has become even more important for the radiologists and technologists around the world [1, 2]. Many healthcare providers who do not deal with these patients on a regular basis will not have enough experience in this regard. Hence it is important to evaluate a renal graft at various stages and to identify the imaging findings, which suggest an abnormality of the renal graft. Early detection and management of the anatomic and vascular abnormalities in the early and late posttransplant period could be extremely useful to improve the graft survival.

M. Veroux (✉) · D. Zerbo · D. Corona
N. Sinagra · P. Veroux
Vascular Surgery and Organ Transplant Unit, Department of Surgical and Medical Sciences and Advanced Technologies, University Hospital of Catania, Catania, Italy
e-mail: veroux@unict.it

In the early postoperative period, ultrasound (US) is the most frequently used imaging modality for evaluating renal transplant, because of its portability and rapid technique, without the need for intravenous contrast or ionizing radiation [1, 3–6]. Typically, a baseline examination may be obtained within the first 24–48 h using both grayscale and Doppler imaging. These baseline images establish the renal size and echogenicity, the status of the collecting system and ureter, and the size and location of any postoperative perinephric fluid collections. Additionally, any preexisting renal parenchymal lesions can be noted on this baseline scan. US is also helpful in the management of postoperative complications, such as draining perinephric fluid collections or placing a percutaneous nephrostomy tube [1, 3, 4, 6].

The healthy kidney graft has the same appearance of the native kidney, but its evaluation is usually simpler due to the superficial position of the transplanted kidney in the iliac fossa. The renal artery normally shows a low-resistance waveform with a resistance index (RI) of less than 0.7 [1, 3, 4]. The resistance index depends on graft vessels, but it could be influenced more by the recipient's vessels and their elasticity [7]. An elevated RI (>0.9) may be found in cases of renal vein obstruction, urethral obstruction, and pyelonephritis [6], and RI should be a useful tool for monitoring graft function and should be determined in every graft exploration [8, 9].

A. Granata, M. Bertolotto (eds.), *Imaging in Nephrology*, https://doi.org/10.1007/978-3-030-60794-4_17

Real-time US guidance is helpful in directing the renal biopsy; not only does US guidance aid in avoiding the main vessels, but it also affects preferable sampling of the glomeruli through angling of the needle tangentially toward the renal cortex [1].

In recent years, contrast-enhanced sonography has been used more frequently for a better evaluation of cortical arteries that could not be explored satisfactorily with color Doppler or power Doppler. Ultrasonography contrast agents are composed of a shell of biocompatible materials, including proteins, lipids, or biopolymers [6]. These agents are safe and not nephrotoxic. Contrast-enhanced sonography may permit a complete exploration of the cortical region of the kidney and can explore even the renal artery and vein: it can be used to differentiate renal artery stenosis from kinking and may help to identify kidney-transplant recipients with vascular rejection [10]. Contrast-enhanced ultrasound allows for quick and noninvasive assessment of parenchymal kidney graft perfusion. It enables confirmation of transplant artery stenosis diagnosis in the early postoperative period and helps assess the degree of stenosis [11]. Moreover, Stenberg et al. [12] demonstrated that contrast-enhanced sonography is able to detect perfusion defects more accurately than DTPA.

17.2 Sonographic Evaluation of Surgical Complications of Kidney Transplantation

These complications can be classified as parenchymal complications, perinephric fluid collections, vascular complications, and urologic complications.

17.2.1 Focal Renal Parenchymal Lesions

Focal lesions are a less common occurrence in the transplanted kidney. Hematoma, focal contusion, or scar may occur as a result of surgery or biopsy.

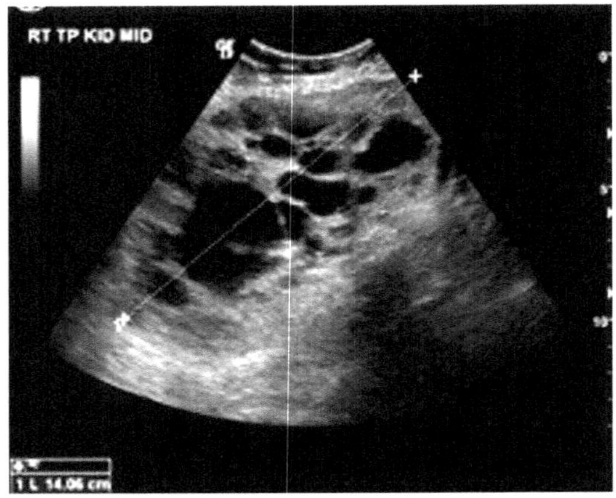

Fig. 17.1 Acquired cystic disease of the transplant kidney. US image through the transplant kidney shows slightly enlarged kidney with numerous cystic changes

Additionally, stones or small tumors may incidentally be carried from a donor kidney during the transplant process. Long-term dialysis may lead to acquired cystic changes (Fig. 17.1). Other parenchymal lesions that may develop in the graft include renal carcinoma, transitional cell cancer, lymphoproliferative disorders, simple or complex cysts, and infective lesions [1, 2].

17.2.2 Perinephric Fluid Collections

Perinephric fluid collections occur during the early posttransplant period of up to 50% of renal transplants [1, 2, 13, 14], and include hematomas, lymphoceles, urinomas, and abscesses. Differential diagnosis between the various types of perinephric fluid collection with US may be difficult, and the clinical signs and postoperative time may suggest the correct etiology. Hematomas and urinomas are usually seen in the early postoperative period, whereas lymphoceles typically are not present until 4–8 weeks after transplantation.

17.2.2.1 Urinoma or Urinary Leak

Urinomas occur in 1–5% [1, 15] of transplant cases, most commonly in the first 2 weeks. Usually it is due to ureteral necrosis for acute rejection or anastomotic leaks. Leaks are most often found at the distal ureter or at the site of ureterocystostomy; they are caused by ureteric ischemia or surgical technique. In such cases, urinomas are seen in the early posttransplant period, usually after removal of the urinary catheter (V–VI postoperative day). Urine leaks may present also later, within the first 30 days, with reduced urine output, deteriorating renal function and pain at the site of transplant surgery. Urinomas are extraperitoneal collections that are typically seen between the bladder and kidney and may occasionally rupture intraperitoneally. Urinomas typically present with a fluid collection adjacent to pelvis but separate from the bladder. Ultrasound demonstrates anechoic fluid collections (urinary ascites) [1, 2, 5, 16]. Diagnosis is often confirmed with ultrasound-guided aspiration to detect elevated creatinine that may help to differentiate urinomas from lymphocele, the latter having a creatinine in the fluid comparable to serum.

17.2.2.2 Hematoma

Hematomas are a common complication of the early postoperative period; the incidence of significant posttransplant hematomas is 4–8% [2, 17]. Perinephric hematomas complicate up to 7% of renal biopsies and can be subcapsular with an increase in size collection [18]. They frequently appear on US as complex crescentic collections around the kidney, and it is typically heterogeneous and avascular on color Doppler. In early phases, hematomas are usually anechoic, and with a decreasing echogenicity when lysis of the clot occurs (Fig. 17.2). Measurement of hematomas on baseline scans is important, as they normally will gradually decrease in size over time. A hematoma that increases in size should raise suspicion of an active or repeat bleed [1, 2].

17.2.2.3 Lymphoceles

Lymphocele is a common complication after kidney transplantation, with a reported incidence ranging from 0.6% to 33.9% [1, 3–6, 14]. The lymphocele may be a consequence of lymphatic disruption during preparation of the recipient iliac vessels or alternatively may derive from the graft itself due to an incomplete lymphatic vessel ligation during bench surgery. They usually occur 4–8 weeks after transplant [2, 3] and they are located in a medial position between the graft and the bladder. While lymphoceles are usually asymptomatic, larger ones may cause a mass effect and compression of the ureter or adjacent structures, wound infection, and deep vein thrombosis due to compression of external iliac vein. At clinical examination, lymphoceles are usually not detectable except in larger lymphocele, which may present with a soft mass in the iliac fossa. Many recent studies highlighted the relation between immunosuppression and occurrence of lymphocele, particularly in patients treated with everolimus or sirolimus. US typically shows lymphoceles as anechoic collections and may have septations [1, 3–6, 14].

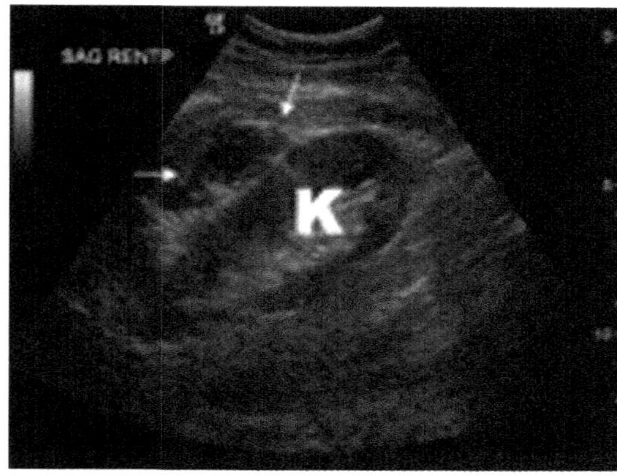

Fig. 17.2 Postsurgical hematomas. Dual image shows a hematoma (arrows) seen as complex fluid collection anterior to the kidney (K)

17.2.2.4 Perinephric Abscesses

Infection is not altogether unusual after transplant, but the formation of a perinephric abscess is relatively uncommon. The abscess may develop by either infection of a perinephric collection or extension of renal abscess into perinephric space. Pain and fever are typical of the clinical presentation. In a febrile patient, any collection near the graft should be considered potentially infected. US is nonspecific in differentiating the abscess from other collections; however, presence of air (seen as echogenic interface with ring-down artifacts) is suggestive of an abscess. Typically, a perinephric collection is an avascular collection with septation and debris [16].

17.2.3 Vascular Complications

Vascular complications may affect less than 10% of patients but they are associated with significant morbidity and may even lead to graft loss. Early identification and intervention in cases of vascular complication may save the graft. Color Doppler US and duplex waveform are the preferred methods of initial evaluation of early vascular complications [19].

17.2.3.1 Renal Artery Stenosis (RAS)

RAS is the most commonly encountered vascular complication in renal transplants [20, 21], and it occurs in up to 10% of cases and is responsible for roughly 1–5% of cases of posttransplant hypertension [1, 2, 20–22]. There is a wide variability in the reported incidence of RAS, mainly for the lack of a clear definition of hemodynamically significant RAS. Most of the definitions reported in the literature vary from 50% to 80% incidence of RAS, although in most cases a definitive angiographic documentation is lacking [23].

Most commonly, it presents within the first 3 months following transplant, but it may develop early or late. In more than 50% of patients, RAS presents at the site of anastomosis, and it has been shown that end-to-end anastomosis has a threefold risk of RAS than end-to-side anastomoses [21]. Pre-anastomosis stenosis usually occurs as a result of preexisting recipient atherosclerotic disease or in the donor vessel. Anastomotic stenosis usually is the result of vessel perfusion injury or incorrect suture technique. RAS may also be a consequence of acute rejection episodes of polyoma virus infection. With the increasing age of deceased donor, the incidence of RAS is increasing, due to the higher rate of atherosclerotic disease in donor renal artery. Moreover, RAS is more common in transplants from deceased donors than living donors, suggesting that some immunological factors and prolonged cold ischemia time may play a role [4].

RAS may present with refractory hypertension or with hypertension associated with graft dysfunction. Color Doppler ultrasound has been used for many years in screening for transplant renal artery stenosis [24]. Its noninvasive nature, portability, low cost, and lack of iodine contrast make it very useful for detecting RAS and monitoring recurrence after interventional or surgical correction [25]. Characteristic US findings in cases of RAS include focal areas of color aliasing, turbulence, and spectral broadening. A peak systolic velocity of >200 cm/s or a Doppler frequency shift of greater than 7.5 kHz when a 3 MHz transducer is used is an expected finding [1, 3, 4, 26] (Fig. 17.3), but they can be visualized

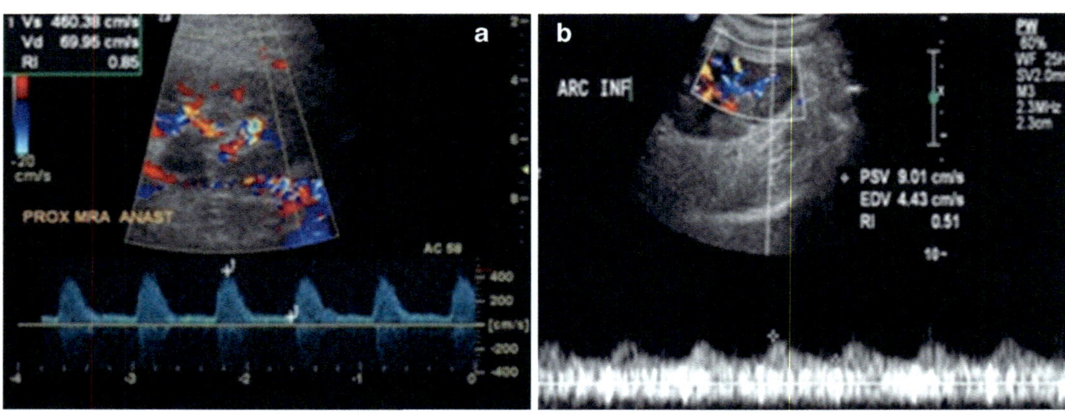

Fig. 17.3 (**a**, **b**) Renal artery stenosis. Image A, a color Doppler and spectral waveform image through the anastomotic region of the transplant renal artery, shows increased velocity (460 cm/s) through the anastomotic area. Image B, a color Doppler and waveform through the intrarenal arcuate artery, shows a delayed and slow upstroke with a "tardus parvus" waveform

only when the degree of stenosis exceeds 80% [27]. A velocity ratio of stenotic to prestenotic segment greater than 2:1 is another supportive finding. An additional helpful finding is a tardus parvus waveform (delayed systolic upstroke) distal to the stenosis and in the intrarenal arcuate arteries [1, 3, 4] (Fig. 17.3). Again, a pathologically low RI within the graft (0.6 or less) may be highly specific for stenosis >50% [5]. Numerous twists and turns of the transplant renal artery may contribute to defective Doppler angle correction on color flow imaging: in such cases, power Doppler may be useful in providing a better delineation of transplant renal artery [9]. The examination of the transplant renal artery may be difficult due to the tortuosity of the vessel leading to erroneous insonation angles; other sources of error are renal artery stretching and/or kinking, which can cause false acceleration [4].

The iliac arteries should also be examined to evaluate the preanastomotic peak systolic velocity max, because iliac stenosis can lead to reduced renal function similar to that observed in the presence of RAS [19].

17.2.3.2 Renal Artery Thrombosis

Renal artery thrombosis is a less common complication of transplant, occurring in less than 0.5–2% of cases [1, 3, 5]. Surgical technique leading to kinking or torsion of the artery or dissection of the arterial wall is often the cause, so that arterial thrombosis usually occurs very early in the posttransplant period. Other precipitating factors include acute or hyperacute rejection, acute tubular necrosis, and hypercoagulable states. Often, it results in transplant loss [1, 3, 19]. Clinical manifestations include absent urinary output and tenderness and swelling in the graft area. Moreover, although the graft lacks innervation, the inflammatory process within the transplanted graft may lead to an intense inflammatory response in the adjacent visceral peritoneum leading to severe localized pain over the graft [4].

The most common US finding is the absence of arterial and venous flow distal to the thrombus and in the intrarenal vessels. Segmental infarction appears as poorly marginated, hypoechoic masses, or a hypoechoic mass with a well-defined echogenic wall. Global infarction appears as a diffusely enlarged kidney [28].

The absence of flow on US is a rare finding in severe cases of acute rejection [1–3]. It is important to adjust technical parameters to avoid a false-positive result. Power Doppler US may help to demonstrate flow in a technically difficult patient [1, 3].

17.2.3.3 Renal Vein Thrombosis

Thrombosis of the renal vein is a rare cause of transplant dysfunction, occurring in 4–5% of cases [1, 3–5]. When caused by surgical complications, such as an extrinsic compression of the graft or a kinking, it occurs in the early posttransplant period [29, 30]. Clinically, it presents with abrupt onset of graft tenderness accompanied by swelling and oliguria. In most cases patients present with acute pain in the iliac fossa with hematuria and deteriorating hemodynamic parameters, due to the graft rupture [30]. On grayscale US, echogenic material may be seen within the renal vein. Duplex US studies demonstrate findings of absent venous flow in the main renal vein and diastolic reversal of the arterial flow in the main artery and/or intrarenal arteries [1, 3–5] (Figs. 17.4 and 17.5). The high resistance caused by renal vein thrombosis results in typical bidirectional flow in the intrarenal arteries (the arterial waveform will be positive during systole and negative during diastole) [31].

A high resistive index may accompany partial venous thrombosis. In some cases, an increase in segmental venous velocity may be seen in partial thrombus, kinking of the vein, or extrinsic pressure by a fluid collection. The kidney may be enlarged and hypoechoic on grayscale imaging and may demonstrate effacement of the renal sinus.

17.2.3.4 Arteriovenous Fistulas and Pseudoaneurysms

Percutaneous biopsy of renal transplants is crucial in determining the cause of transplant dysfunction and making the correct treatment decisions. However, renal biopsy may lead to vascular complications such as arteriovenous fis-

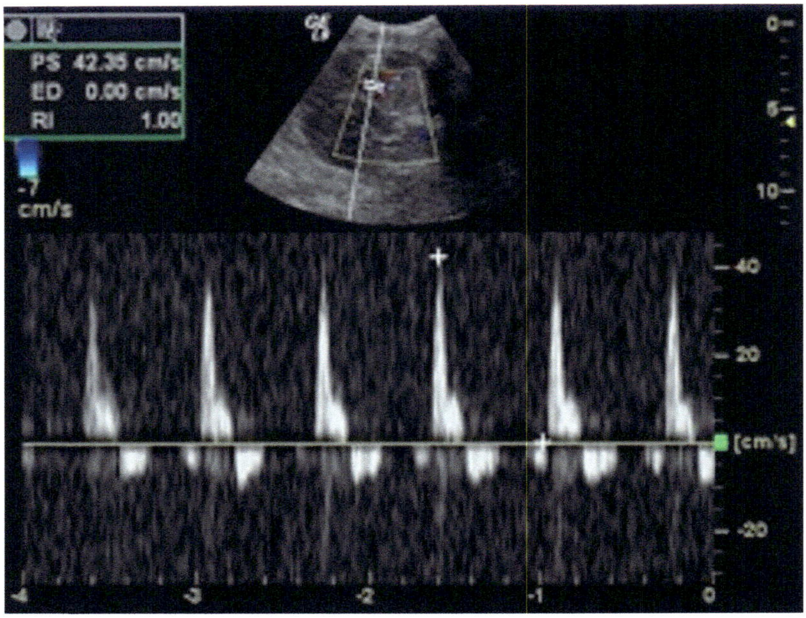

Fig. 17.4 Renal vein thrombosis. Doppler US of an intrarenal arcuate artery shows reversal of the diastolic flow below the baseline

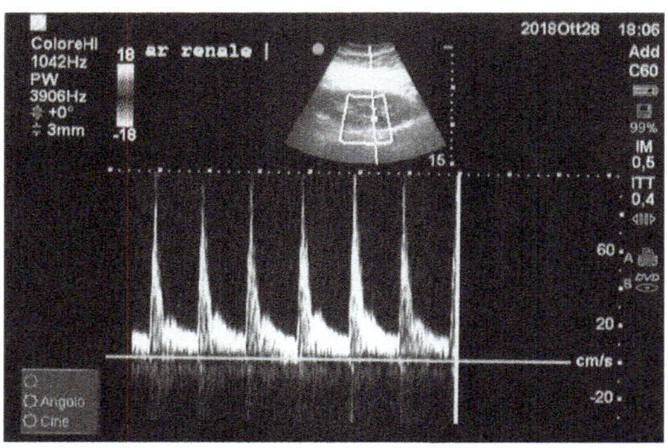

Fig. 17.5 Partial renal vein thrombosis. Doppler ultrasound showed increased resistance with an initial diastoli flow reversal

tula (AVF) or pseudoaneurysm formation in 1–18% of cases [1, 3–5, 26, 33–35]. An arteriovenous fistula occurs as a result of simultaneous laceration of a renal artery branch and an adjacent renal vein during a graft biopsy.

Usually, AVF and pseudoaneurysm are self-limiting and resolve spontaneously. Predisposing factors include arterial hypertension, renal medullary disease, central renal biopsies, and multiple needle passes [26, 32, 33]. Grayscale US imaging usually cannot identify small AVF which can be easily visualized at color Doppler sonography as a focal area of turbulent flow and aliasing that extends outside the confines of normal vessels in the renal parenchyma. This appearance is caused by the fistula vibration and the vibration interfaces in the perivascular tissues produce phase shifts in the reflected sound wave and result in random color assignment [4].

AVF appears as abnormal high velocity in an isolated renal artery with aliasing in the paired vein [1, 3, 4]. The feeding artery shows a high-velocity, low-resistance waveform, while the draining vein shows arterialization (Fig. 17.6). Approximately 70% of AVFs will resolve spontaneously within 2 years, whereas the remaining can be symptomatic or persist [36]. Large AVFs may cause renal ischemia through the "steal phenomenon" [1, 3].

Pseudoaneurysm (PA) after a biopsy is usually intrarenal, while extrarenal PA is very uncommon and is often a consequence of incorrect surgical anastomosis or peri-anastomotic infections. PA appears as a simple or minimally complex cystic structure on grayscale US [1, 3]. Color Doppler imaging shows turbulent, swirling flow pattern within the PA. Pseudoaneurysms with a narrow neck without venous communication show a classic machinelike alternating to-and-fro Doppler

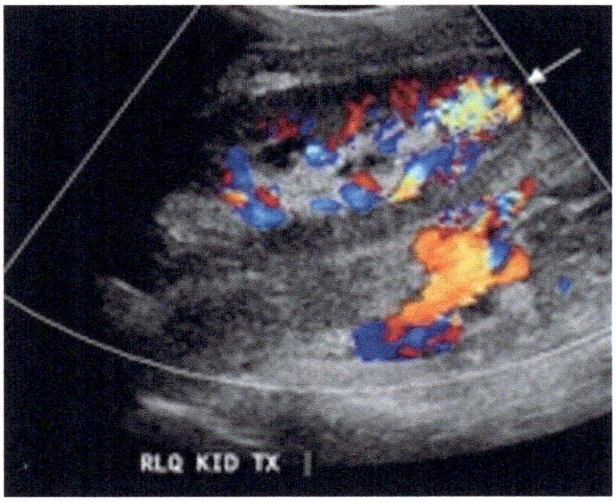

Fig. 17.6 Arteriovenous fistula at the lower pole in the area of previous biopsy. Color Doppler image through the transplant kidney that shows color aliasing and turbulence at the lower pole suggestive of high velocity (arrow)

spectrum at their necks. When associated with AVF, PA shows a high-velocity, low-resistance spectrum at their necks, with minimally pulsatile high-velocity flow in the draining vein [4, 37]. PAs are usually self-limiting and resolve spontaneously, but larger PAs (>2 cm in diameter) may require intervention, due to the higher risk of rupture.

17.2.4 Complications of the Collecting System and Ureter

Urological complications are less frequent thanks to the improved surgical techniques, and most urological complications occur during the first month posttransplant. Currently, rates vary from 3% to 10% [38, 39]. Ureteric obstruction and urine leak are the most common of these, and the transplant ureter tends to be commonly involved because of its delicate limited blood supply that originates from the renal hilum. The surgical techniques of vesicoureteral anastomosis adopted in kidney transplantation are associated with a low incidence of postoperative urinary leaks of obstruction, and the use of indwelling stents for 4–6 weeks reduced significantly the incidence of such complications. The upper part of prophylactic ureteral stent can be visualized as echogenic parallel lines in the pelvis, whereas the lower end can be similarly seen in the fundus of the bladder.

17.2.4.1 Ureteral Obstruction

While mild fullness of the collecting system and ureter is a common finding on US due to loss of tonicity secondary to denervation, true ureteral obstruction occurs in about 2–5% of cases [40–43]. The site of obstruction most commonly involved is the anastomosis into the bladder and roughly 90% of stenosis occurs in the distal third of the ureter [4]. Ureteral obstruction is caused by ureteral ischemia, infection, ureteral kinking, edema at the anastomosis, and extrinsic compression of the ureters by fluid collections. Most commonly, the distal third of the ureter is affected [1, 3]. Other causes include acute rejection, BK virus-induced ureteral stenosis, and nephrolithiasis as a consequence of prolonged stay of ureteral stent.

Commonly, immediately after the transplantation a mild hydronephrosis is seen because of edema at the ureteroneocystostomy site: quite often, this is a self-limited sonographic finding and usually completely resolves within a few days after transplantation. Because the transplanted kidney is denervated, most patients will not complain of the typical renal colic when obstruction occurs: moreover, when there has been a prior obstruction in the past, clinical and sonographic evaluation of the caliceal or ureteral obstruction may be difficult, because once the urothelium has been stretched it may never collapse again, making the distinction between functional obstruction and residual dilatation very difficult.

Grayscale US shows dilation of the renal pelvis and calyces (Fig. 17.7). The transplant ureter is actually easier to evaluate compared to the native ureters because of its relatively anterior position, allowing for visualization of the site of obstruction on US examination (Fig. 17.8).

In cases of dilated collecting systems, urinary obstruction may be differentiated from non-obstruction by scintigraphy. Obstruction may also be ruled out by delayed radionuclide imaging or diuretic administration. Antegrade urography is helpful for identifying the site of

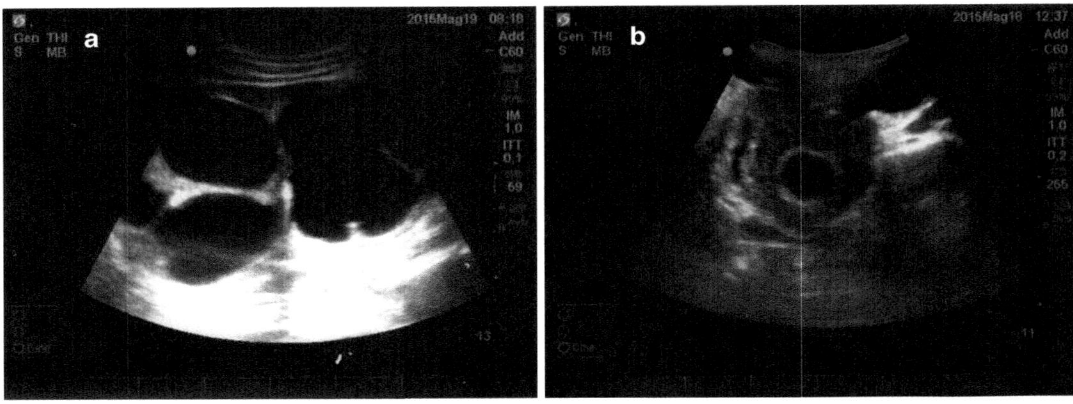

Fig. 17.7 (**a**, **b**) Hydronephrosis. Image A shows a transplant kidney with severe hydronephrosis and proximal hydroureter with reduction of the parenchymal thickness. Image B shows a severe increase in the wall of bladder due to urethral stenosis, responsible for the hydronephrosis

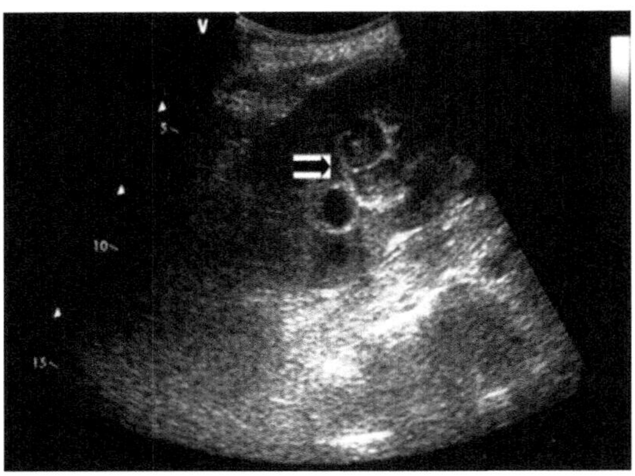

Fig. 17.8 Fungus balls. Graft sonography demonstrates a mild hydronephrosis with the presence of an isoechogenic mass in the calyceal system (arrow)

obstruction prior to therapy, which is often by percutaneous nephrostomy, ureteral stenting, or balloon dilatation [1, 3].

US may also detect pyelonephritis, clots, fungus, tumors, and stones. Pyelonephritis appears as a thickening of the urothelium, a finding that may also be seen in chronic rejection [1, 4].

References

1. Herman H, Irshad A, Ackerman S, Shazly M. Diagnostic challenges in kidney transplantation. In: Veroux M, Veroux P, editors. Kidney Transplantation: Challenging the future. UAE: Bentham Science Editor; 2012. p. 168–85.
2. Veroux M, Corona D, Veroux P. Kidney transplantation: future challenges. Minerva Chir. 2009;64:75–100.
3. Irshad A, Ackerman SJ, Campbell AS, Aris M. An overview of renal transplantation: current practice and use of ultrasound. Semin Ultrasound. 2009;30:298–314.
4. Sharfuddin A. Imaging evaluation of kidney transplant recipients. Semin Nephrol. 2011;31:259–71.
5. Martino P, Lucarelli G, Palazzo S, Teceschi M, Impedovo SV, Di Lorenzo V, Ditonno P, Battaglia M, Selvaggi FP. Surgical complications of renal transplantation: ultrasound diagnosis. Arch Ital Urol Androl. 2010:221–5.
6. Jimenez C, Lopez MO, Gonzales E, Selgas R. Ultrasonography in kidney transplantation: values and new developments. Transplant Rev. 2009;23:209–13.
7. Heine Gh GMK, Ulrich C, Kohler H, Girndt M. Renal Doppler resistance indices are associated with systemic atherosclerosis in kidney transplant recipients. Kidney Int. 2005;68:878–85.
8. Radermacher J, Mengel M, Ellis S, et al. The renal arterial resistance index and renal allograft survival. N Engl J Med. 2003;349:115–24.
9. Singh AK, Sahani DV. Imaging of the renal donor and transplant recipient. Radiol Clin N Am. 2008;46:79–93.
10. Fischer T, Filimonow S, Dieckhöfer J, et al. Improved diagnosis of early kidney allograft dysfunction by ultrasound with echo enhancer: a new method for the diagnosis of renal perfusion. Nephrol Dial Transplant. 2006;2:2921–9.
11. Grzelak P, Kurnatowska I, Nowicki M, Muras K, Podgórski M, Strzelczyk J, Stefańczyk L. Detection of transplant renal artery stenosis in the early postoperative period with analysis of parenchymal perfusion with ultrasound contrast agent. Ann Transplant. 2013;18:187–94.
12. Stenberg B, Chandler C, Wyrley-Birch H, Elliott ST. Post-operative 3-dimensional contrast-enhanced ultrasound (CEUS) versus Tc99m-DTPA in the detection of post-surgical perfusion defects in kidney transplants - preliminary findings. Ultraschall Med. 2014;35:273–8.

13. Tublin ME, Dodd GDIII. Sonography of renal transplantation. Radiol Clin N Am. 1995;33:447–59.
14. Pozniak MA, Dodd GD, Kelcz F. Ultrasonographic evaluation of renal transplantation. Radiol Clin N Am. 1992;30:1053–66.
15. Noorbala MH, Gholamrezaie HR. Study of surgical complications between primary and secondary renal transplants. Transplant Proc. 2005;37:2154–6.
16. Sutherland T, Temple F, Chang S, Hennessy O, Lee W-K. Sonographic evaluation of renal transplant complications. J Med Imag Radiat Oncol. 2010;54:211–8.
17. Borrego J, Burgos FJ, Galmes I, et al. Surgical complications in 479 renal transplantations. Actas Urol Esp. 1994;18:253–7.
18. Preda A, Van Dijk LC, Van Oostaijen JA, Pattynama PMT. Complication rate and diagnostic yield of 515 consecutive ultrasound guided biopsies of renal allografts and native kidneys using a 14-gauge Biopty gun. Eur Radiol. 2003;13:527–30.
19. Granata A, Clementi S, Londrino F, Romano G, Veroux M, Florini F, Fatuzzo P. Renal transplant vascular complications: the role of Doppler ultrasound. J Ultrasound. 2015;18:101–7.
20. Hurst Fp AKC, Neff RT, et al. Incidence, predictors and outcomes of transplant renal artery stenosis after kidney transplantation: analysis of USRDS. Am J Nephrol. 2009;30:459–67.
21. Henning BF, Kuchlbauer S, Boger CA, et al. Percutaneous transluminal angioplasty as first-line treatment of transplant renal artery stenosis. Clin Nephrol. 2009;71:543–9.
22. Mangray M, Vella JP. Hypertension after kidney transplantation. Am J Kidney Dis. 2011;57:331–41.
23. Weir MR, Salzberg DJ. Management of hypertension in the transplanted patient. J Am Soc Hypertens. 2011;5:425–32.
24. De Morais RH, Muglia VF, Mamere AE. Duplex Doppler sonography in transplant renal artery stenosis. J Clin Ultrasound. 2003;31:135–41.
25. Gao J, Li J, Meng-Su X, et al. Color duplex sonography in severe transplant renal artery stenosis: a comparison of end-to-end and end-to-side arterial anastomoses. Clin Imaging. 2009;33:116–22.
26. Grenier N, Claudon M, Trillaud H, et al. Noninvasive radiology of vascular complications in renal transplantation. Eur Radiol. 1997;7:385–91.
27. Brown ED, Chen MY, Wolfman NT, Ott DJ, Watson NE Jr. Complications of renal transplantation: evaluation with US and radionuclide imaging. Radiographics. 2000;20:607–22.
28. Akbar SA, Jafri SZ, Amendola MA, Madrazo BL, Salem R, Bis KG. Complications of renal transplantation. Radiographics. 2005;25:1335–56.
29. Veroux M, Corona D, Giuffrida G, Gagliano M, Giaquinta A, Tallarita T, Zerbo D, Cappellani A, Sorbello M, Veroux P. A rare cause of iliocaval thrombosis in kidney transplantation. Transplant Proc. 2009;41(4):1405–6.
30. Veroux M, Veroux P, Puliatti C, Fiamingo P, Macarone M, Cappello D. Renal allograft rupture caused by acute tubular necrosis. Chir Ital. 2003;55(5):753–5.
31. Elsayes KM, Menias CO, Willat J, Azar S, Harvin HJ, Platt JF. Imaging of renal transplant: utility and spectrum of diagnostic findings. Curr Probl Diagn Radiol. 2011;40:127–39.
32. Martinez T, Palomares M, Bravo JA, et al. Biopsy-induced arteriovenous fistula and venous aneurysm in a renal transplant. Nephrol Dial Transplant. 1998;13:2937–9.
33. Barley FL, Kessel D, Nicholson T, et al. Selective embolization of large symptomatic iatrogenic renal transplant arteriovenous fistula. Cardiovasc Interv Radiol. 2006;29:1084–7.
34. Yablon Z, Recupero P, McKenna J, Vella J, Parker MG. Kidney allograft biopsy: timing to complications. Clin Nephrol. 2010;74:39–45.
35. Gainza FJ, Minguela I, Lopez-Vidaur I, Ruiz LM, Lampreade I. Evaluation of complications due to percutaneous renal biopsy in allografts and native kidneys with color-coded Doppler sonography. Clin Nephrol. 1995;45:303–8.
36. Nakatani T, Uchida J, Han YS, et al. Renal allograft arterio-venous fistula and large pseudoaneurysm. Clin Transpl. 2003;17:9–12.
37. Pearl AL. Diagnostic imaging in kidney transplantation. In: Danovitch GM, editor. Handbook of kidney transplantation. Philadelphia: Lippincot Williams Wilkins; 2007. p. 291–310.
38. Gogus C, Yaman O, Soygur T, Beduk Y, Gogus O. Urological complications in renal transplantation: long-term follow-up of the Woodruff ureteroneocystostomy procedure in 433 patients. Urol Int. 2002;69:99–101.
39. Kocak B, Baker TB, Koffron AJ, Leventhal JR. Ureteral complications in the era of laparoscopic living donor nephrectomy: do we need to preserve the gonadal vein with the specimen? J Endourol. 2010;24:247–51.
40. Nankivell BJ, Chapman JR. Chronic allograft nephropathy: current concepts and future directions. Transplantation. 2006;81:643–54.
41. Granata A, Di Nicolò P, Scarfia VR, Insalaco M, Lentini P, Veroux M, Fatuzzo P, Fiorini F. Renal transplantation parenchymal complications: what Doppler ultrasound can and cannot do. J Ultrasound. 2014;18:109–16.
42. Veroux M, Corona D, Giuffrida G, Gagliano M, Tallarita T, Giaquinta A, Zerbo D, Cappellani A, Veroux PF. Acute renal failure due to ureteral obstruction in a kidney transplant recipient with Candida albicans contamination of preservation fluid. Transplant Infect Dis. 2009;11:266–8.
43. Granata A, Clementi S, Londrino F, Romano G, Veroux M, Fiorini F, Fatuzzo P. Renal transplant vascular complications: the role of Doppler ultrasound. Ultrasound. 2014;18(2):101–7. https://doi.org/10.1007/s40477-014-0085-6.

Functional MR Imaging in Transplanted Kidney Dysfunction

18

Alessandro Di Gaeta, Elena L. Indino, Maurizio Del Monte, and Valeria Panebianco

18.1 Blood-Oxygen Level-Dependent MRI

In blood-oxygen level-dependent (BOLD) MRI deoxyhemoglobin is the endogenous contrast agent for noninvasive assessment of tissue oxygen availability. BOLD MRI has been used to measure intrarenal medullary oxygenation in pathologic conditions early after allograft period [3, 6]. In literature, most studies use multiple gradient-recoiled echo sequences, which results in a parameter of R2* related to deoxyhemoglobin's concentration [6, 7, 17]. The measure of the rate of signal loss in a specific region is measured using regions of interest (ROIs) tool. The R2* levels negatively correlate with oxygen bioavailability in tissues. Usually R2* levels can be impaired in acute and chronic graft rejection, ureteral obstruction, acute ischemic injury, and hypertension.

During acute ischemic injury [7, 17] R2* levels in ROIs placed in both renal cortex and medulla (respectively, CR2* and MR2*) are increased. However, in inflammatory and immune-mediated kidney injury, MR2* levels are decreased; this effect can be related to changes in hemodynamics and/or toe of reduction of oxygen consumption in medulla, probably related to decreased tubular function [3, 6]. For example, R2* values in the medulla are lower in both acute tubular necrosis (ATN) and acute rejection (AR), if compared to normal kidney. However these two etiologies can be differentiated using certain threshold R2* values (AR patients usually have lower MR2* values than ATN) [3, 7].

Chronic allograft nephropathies are a state of chronic inflammation which results in decreased R2* values in both cortex and medulla (CR2* and MR2*). This effect is due to increased oxygen levels related to either an increased oxygen delivery or a reduced oxygen extraction in the kidney [16, 17].

18.2 Arterial Spin Labeling (ASL)

ASL is a noninvasive technique, based on the use of magnetically labeled protons in arteries. Therefore protons in arterial blood are endogenous tracers, and there is no need for contrast agent injection. Its application in renal evaluation has been validated by several studies [12, 15]. The most common sequences used are FAIR (flow-sensitive alternating inversion recovery) for perfusion preparation and True-FISP (true fast imaging with steady precession) for data acquisition; however several repetitions and high-field magnets are needed, due to low signal-to-noise ratio (SNR), and high time resolution sequences, because of blood T1 decay [12].

A. Di Gaeta · E. L. Indino · M. Del Monte
V. Panebianco (✉)
Department of Radiological Sciences, Oncology and Pathology, Policlinico Umberto I, Sapienza University of Rome, Rome, Italy

A. Granata, M. Bertolotto (eds.), *Imaging in Nephrology*,
https://doi.org/10.1007/978-3-030-60794-4_18

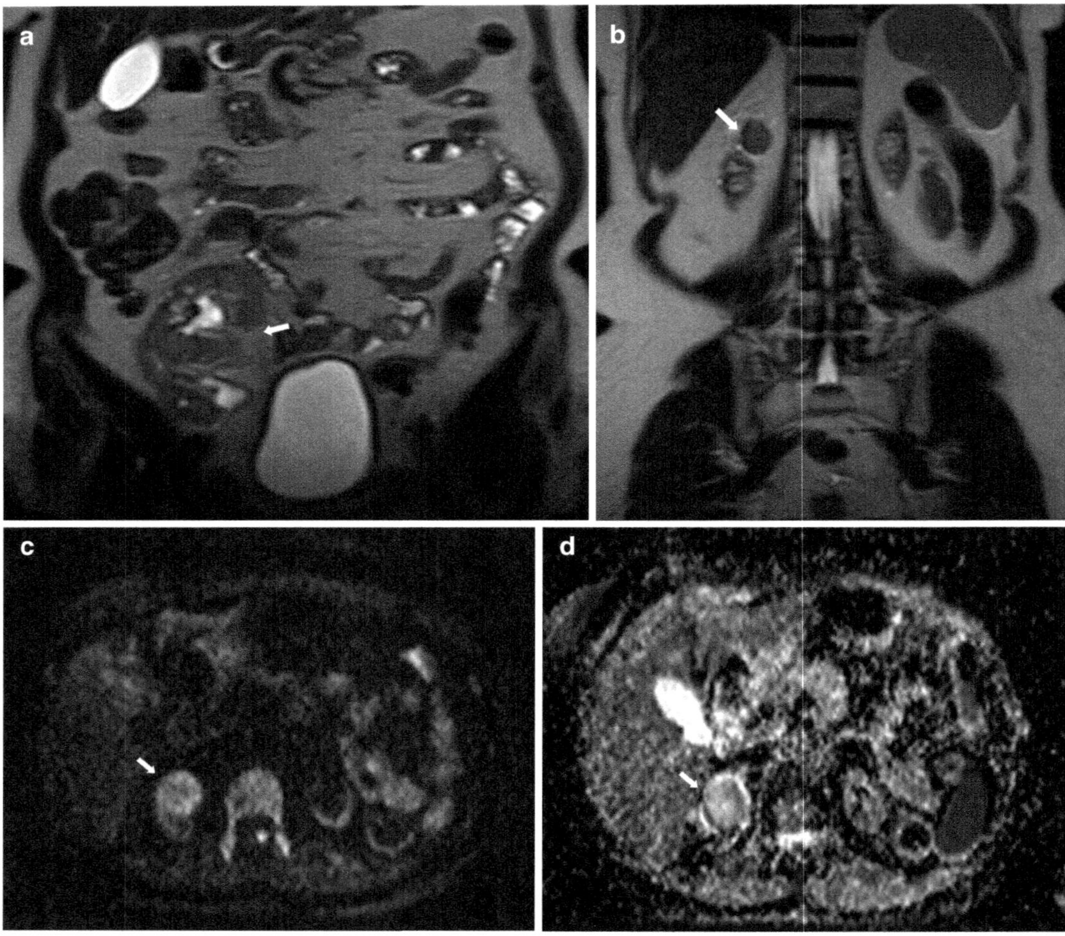

Fig. 18.1 Coronal T2W images in a 57-year-old patient who underwent kidney transplantation 10 years earlier. During follow-up for mild calyceal dilatation (**a**) in the graft, a well-rounded solid formation was discovered on her native right kidney at the superior pole (**b**) that showed signal restriction at DWI (**c–d**). The lesion was biopsied and was diagnosed a primitive renal neoplasm

ASL plays a prevalent role in the evaluation of delayed graft function (DGF) [15]. In the early postoperative period after kidney transplantation, DGF occurs in 20–25% of patients who have undergone transplantation from deceased donor and is a significant diagnostic and clinical challenge [9, 13]. This condition is defined as nonreduction of serum creatinine (S-creatinine) or need for dialysis in the first week after transplantation. Main risk factors are cold ischemia and advanced donor, and can result in acute allograft rejection, impaired allograft function, and graft loss [13, 14]. The importance of early detection of DGF is evident in order to limit irreversible allograft damage. Usually renal perfusion in allografts from DGF patients is significantly lower than in allografts with initial renal function, which present higher perfusional values [15]. In clinical practice DGF renal perfusion well correlates with renal function, and early perfusion impairment predicts the development of DGF and the need for dialysis early after transplantation. Moreover renal perfusion measurement may help to risk stratify the patients and to evaluate the cause of renal dysfunction early after transplantation (Figs. 18.1 and 18.2).

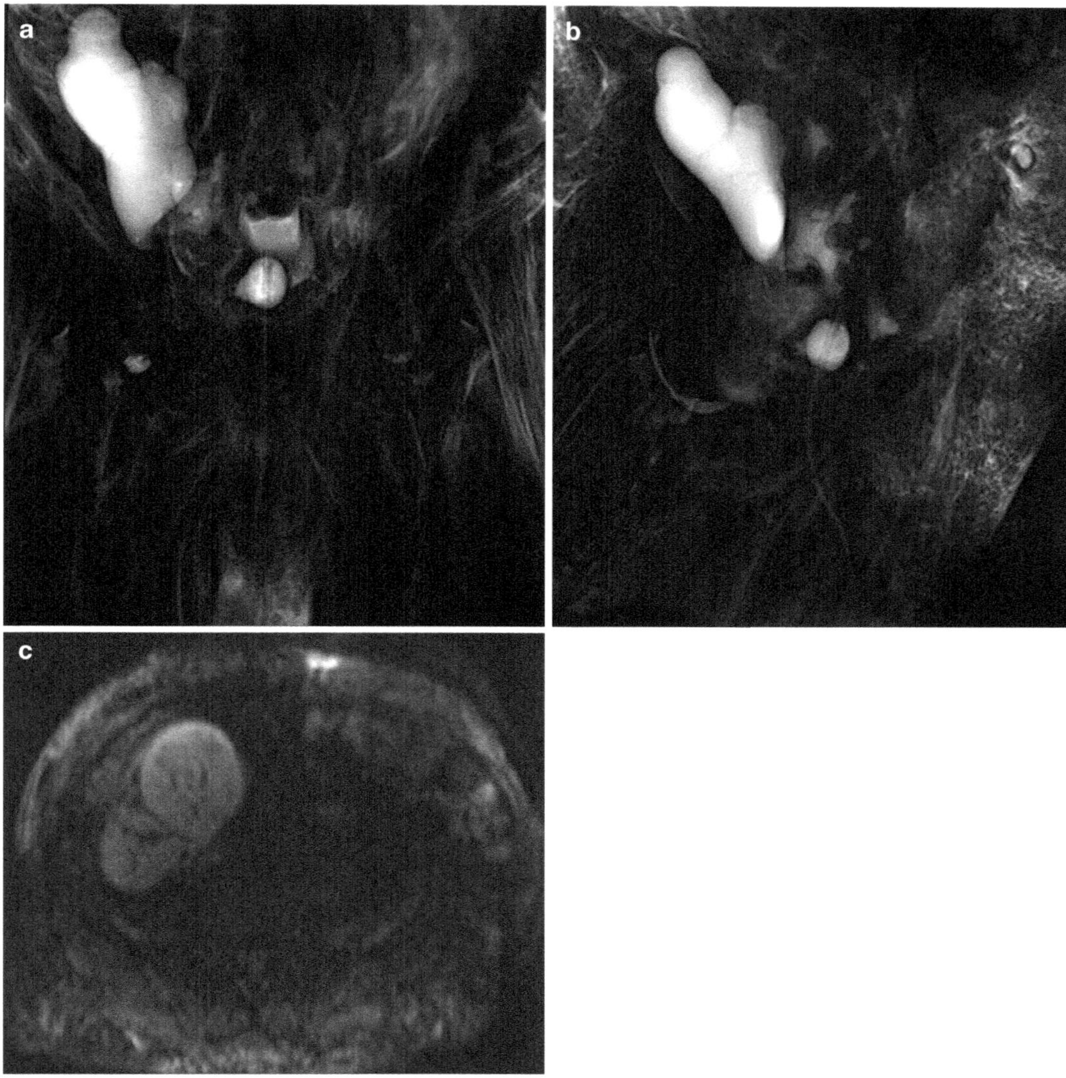

Fig. 18.2 Perirenal fluid collection in a patient who underwent renal transplantation after 15 days. In MRI images a perirenal fluid collection is seen with mild ureteral compression. Heavily T2W images on coronal and parasagittal planes (oriented on the major axis of the grafted kidney) did not show communication with urinary pathway (in order to exclude anastomosis dehiscence and urinomas). The collection was suddenly drained placing a percutaneous drainage

18.3 Diffusion-Weighted and Diffusion Tensor Imaging

Diffusion-weighted MR imaging (DW-MRI) is a noninvasive MRI tool to obtain functional information about the renal allograft. Its application is essential in monitoring patients early after kidney transplantation [2, 5]. DW-MRI yields a total "apparent diffusion coefficient" (ADCT) that provides simultaneous information on diffusion and perfusion properties. ADC values of medulla and cortex have to be analyzed separately due to their intrinsic characteristic. However DW-MRI may in addition provide information on microcirculation, quantified with the "perfusion fraction" (FP), and "perfusion-free" diffusion (ADCD) [2, 5, 19]. The former represents the microcirculation of blood and/or movement of fluids in predefined structures such as tubules and glomeruli. In kidneys, diffusion properties may be anisotropic because the main anatomic structures, like vessels and tubules, exhibit a radial orientation.

The fractional anisotropy (FA) of tissues is a measure of the directionality of diffusion, especially evident in medulla. It is assessed by using diffusion tensor imaging (DTI) [4].

In normal kidney FP and ADCT values are slightly higher in the cortex than in medulla, while ADCD does not change. In renal allograft a lack of corticomedullary difference is seen in diffusion parameters, probably related to either denervation or effects of immunosuppressive drugs [2, 5]. In acute rejection (AR) and acute tubular necrosis (ATN), the values of ADCT and FP are reduced, while ADCD is usually similar in both cortex and medulla [5, 14, 19]. The most accurate indicator for allograft function is FP that correlates with estimated glomerular filtration rate (eGFR) and is an important indicator for assessment immediately after transplant.

In abnormal function of allograft reduction of ADC values is seen in cortex and medulla; in such cases, where recovery occurs from dysfunction, an increasing of ADC value is seen, suggesting the importance of DWI in monitoring graft rejection episodes [18, 19].

DTI may be more sensitive than DWI detecting pathological changes in renal microstructure. In fact, at a lower rate of renal function impairment, FA value reduction in medullary is more pronounced than the reduction in ADC values [14, 18, 19].

In contrast to its high sensitivity, DTI does not have high specificity and is not able to differentiate between different pathological conditions in allograft dysfunction (e.g., acute rejection, acute tubular necrosis), requiring further investigation [4, 18].

18.4 MR Angiography

Vascular complication most commonly seen in renal transplantation includes renal artery or vein thrombosis and renal artery stenosis [9–11]. Gadolinium-enhanced 3D magnetic resonance angiography (MRA) is an accurate reproducible technique for evaluating renal artery and vein complications [1].

Dynamic contrast-enhanced perfusional MRI (DCE-MRI) during i.v. injection of contrast agent is a useful instrument in the evaluation of vascular kidney pedicle patients. In the arterial phase, it is possible to evaluate arterial vessel, vascular anastomosis, and vessel patients. In case of arterial stenosis, narrowing of the vessel is seen and, occasionally, a slight dilatation of pre-stenotic segment [8, 10, 14].

Usually arterial thrombosis is seen as a filling defect in the arterial lumen, which is frequently associated to perfusional cortical defects. It is important to depict small anomalous renal arteries (e.g., polar and accessory arteries) as possible thrombosis location, in the absence of filling defects in principal renal vascular pedicle and parenchymal intensity impairment. Cortical defects in arterial phase are seen when the disease involves also small vessels [8].

Intraparenchymal small arterioles can be affected by other pathological processes such as rejection, cyclosporine toxicity, acute tubular necrosis, infection, and transplantation-related malignancies [10].

Loss of renal corticomedullary differentiation (CMD) on T1W images is finding in renal allografts undergoing rejection. MRI evidence of loss of CMD has a sensitivity of 97%; however, this finding is nonspecific and observed also in cyclosporine toxicity and other infiltrative or diffuse renal parenchymal diseases [1, 11]. Chronic rejection results in loss of CMD on T1-weighted images. The degree of loss of CMD on DCE-MRI may correlate with the severity of rejection [14].

At last, the necessity of MRA to rule out transplant-related malignancies should not be forgotten. Transplant recipients are at higher risk of developing neoplastic disease than general population, as a result of the following:

- Chronic immunosuppression and antigenic stimulation
- Increased susceptibility to oncogenic viral infections
- Direct neoplastic action of immunosuppressants

Particularly, the most common entities are infection-related malignancies, lymphoproliferative disease (non-Hodgkin and Hodgkin lymphomas), and Kaposi sarcoma, as well as cancers of the liver, stomach, oropharynx, anus, vulva, and penis [10].

18.5 MR Nephro/Urography

In the assessment of renal allograft functional and structural data, nephro/urography MRI (MRNU) plays an essential role. In fact, this study can provide either excellent anatomical information through T2-weighted sequences or functional and parenchymal data through post-contrast T1-weighted sequences [1, 10].

Heavily T2-weighted pulse sequences result in high signal intensity in stationary fluids (bile, urine, cerebrospinal fluid, and bowel fluid) and low signal intensity in solid organs and moving fluids. Commonly, T2W sequences are post-processed in maximum intensity projection (MIP) reconstruction that enables rotational view for a better analysis of suspected areas of disease without overlapping of structures. This approach shows the morphologic appearance of the collecting system, such as the detection of the level and type of ureteral obstruction and stenosis, but does not provide information about renal function, localization of eventual urinary leakage, and differential diagnosis of perirenal collection after transplant (urinomas, hematomas, and lymphoceles). In this case, post-gadolinium-enhanced T1-weighted sequence is the exam of choice.

Through dynamic contrast-enhanced imaging (DCE-MRI) and placing region of interest (ROI) at the level of evaluating structures, a semiquantitative evaluation of kidney function is possible supported by computing intensity/time curves, giving information on the eGFR and gadolinium renal excretion in the collecting system [8, 11]. If any impairment of the curve is shown, the underlying cause must be searched (prerenal, intrarenal, postrenal). Renal and ureteral urine leaks result from disruption of the calyces, infundibula, renal pelvis, or ureters; generally, T2W sequences' hyperintense and T1W hypointense collection is seen in the perirenal and periureteral space that can be challenging in differentiating from a lymphocele (other common complications after transplantation). Delayed post-gad images (obtained 5–20 min after contrast material injection) are the key for demonstrating a urine leak because gadolinium in urine increases the attenuation of the urinoma over time, differentiating lymphoceles which do not show progressive enhancement [10].

One study reported renography to be an encouraging tool in the differentiation of intrinsic causes of renal dysfunction, like ATN and AR. Yamamoto et al. [20] calculated GFR and mean transit time of the tracer in the kidney (MTTK) and in each vascular (MTTA) and tubular (MTTT) compartment. As a result, the GFR and MTTK were significantly lower in patients with allograft dysfunction; in particular the fractional MTT of the tracer in tubular compartment (MTTT/K) was high in ATN than AR. However fractional MTT of the tracer for vascular compartment (MTTA/K) was higher in AR than ATN. These results are encouraging for the implementation of these techniques in the clinical practice of graft evaluation.

References

1. Hwang JK, Moon IS, et al. Contrast enhanced magnetic resonance angiography in the early period after kidney transplantation. Transplant Proc. 2013;45:2925–30. https://doi.org/10.1016/j.transproceed.2013.08.039.
2. Thoeny HC, De Keyzer F. Diffusion-weighted MR imaging of native and transplanted kidneys. Radiology. 2011;259:25–38. https://doi.org/10.1148/radiol.10092419.
3. Thoeny HC, Zumstein D, Vermathen P, et al. Functional evaluation of transplanted kidneys with diffusion-weighted and BOLD MR imaging: initial experience. Radiology. 2006;241:812–21. https://doi.org/10.1148/radiol.2413060103.
4. Lanzman RS, Ljimani A, Wittsack HJ, et al. Kidney transplant: functional assessment with diffusion-tensor MR imaging at 3T. Radiology. 2013;266:218–25. https://doi.org/10.1148/radiol.12112522.
5. Kaul A, Sharma RK, Gupta A, et al. Assessment of allograft function using diffusion-weighted magnetic resonance imaging in kidney transplant patients. Saudi J Kidney Dis Transpl. 2014;25:1143–7.

6. Sadowski EA, Fain SB, Grist TM, et al. Assessment of acute renal transplant rejection with blood oxygen level-dependent MR imaging: initial experience. Radiology. 2005;236:911–9. https://doi.org/10.1148/radiol.2363041080.
7. Han F, Xiao W, Chen J, et al. The significance of BOLD MRI in differentiation between renal transplant rejection and acute tubular necrosis. Nephrol Dial Transplant. 2008;23:2666–72. https://doi.org/10.1093/ndt/gfn064.
8. Martin DR, Sharma P, Votaw JR, et al. Individual kidney blood flow measured with contrast-enhanced first-pass perfusion MR imaging. Radiology. 2008;246:241–8. https://doi.org/10.1148/radiol.2461062129.
9. Dimitroulis D, Bokos J, Kostakis A, et al. Vascular complications in renal transplantation: a single-center experience in 1367 renal transplantations and review of the literature. Transplant Proc. 2009;41:1609–14. https://doi.org/10.1016/j.transproceed.2009.02.077.
10. Huber A, Heuck A, Reiser M, et al. Contrast-enhanced MR angiography in patients after kidney transplantation. Eur Radiol. 2001;11:2488–95. https://doi.org/10.1007/s003300100992.
11. Gufler H, Rau WS, et al. Contrast enhanced MR angiography with parallel imaging in the early period after renal transplantation. J Magn Reson Imaging. 2009;29:909–16. https://doi.org/10.1002/jmri.21726.
12. Artz NS, Sadowski EA, Fain SB, et al. Reproducibility of renal perfusion MR imaging in native and transplanted kidneys using non-contrast arterial spin labeling. J Magn Reson Imaging. 2011;33:1414–21. https://doi.org/10.1002/jmri.22552.
13. Cavaille-Coll M, Bala S, Velidedeoglu E, Hernandez A, Archdeacon P, Gonzalez G, Neuland C, Meyer J, Albrecht R. Summary of FDA workshop on ischemia reperfusion injury in kidney transplantation. Am J Transplant. 2013;13:1134–48.
14. Katja Hueper, Faikah Gueler, Dagmar Hartung et al. Functional MRI detects perfusion impairment in renal allografts with delayed graft function. Am J Physiol Renal Physiol 308: F1444 –F1451, 2015, https://doi.org/10.1152/ajprenal.00064.2015.
15. Heusch P, Wittsack H-J, Lanzman RS, et al. Functional evaluation of transplanted kidneys using arterial spin labeling MRI. JMRI. 2014;40:84–9. https://doi.org/10.1002/jmri.24336.
16. Djamali A, Sadowski EA, Becker BN, et al. BOLD-MRI assessment of intrarenal oxygenation and oxidative stress in patients with chronic kidney allograft dysfunction. Am J Physiol Renal Physiol. 2007;292:F513–22. https://doi.org/10.1152/ajprenal.00222.2006.
17. Fei Han, Wenbo Xiao, Jianghua Chen et al. The significance of BOLD MRI in differentiation between renal transplant rejection and acute tubular necrosis. Nephrol Dial Transplant (2008) 23: 2666–2672 doi: https://doi.org/10.1093/ndt/gfn064.
18. Katja H, Abedalrazag A, Hartung D, et al. Diffusion-Weighted Imaging and Diffusion Tensor Imaging Detect Delayed Graft Function and Correlate With Allograft Fibrosis in Patients Early After Kidney Transplantation. JMRI. 2016;44:112–21.
19. Eisenberger U, Thoeny H, Vermathen P, et al. Evaluation of renal allograft function early after transplantation with diffusion-weighted MR imaging. Eur Radiol. 2010;20:1374–83. https://doi.org/10.1007/s00330-009-1679-9.
20. Yamamoto A, Zhang JL, Lee VS, et al. Quantitative evaluation of acute renal transplant dysfunction with low-dose three-dimensional MR renography. Radiology. 2011;260:781–9. https://doi.org/10.1148/radiol.11101664.

Part IV

Inteventional Procedures and New Trends

Elastography of the Kidney

19

Nicolas Grenier, Jean-Luc Gennisson, Clément Marcelin, Yann Le Bras, and Lionel Couzi

19.1 Introduction

Non-invasive characterization of renal parenchymal diseases is a challenge for nephrologists. Imaging could play a major role in the future for that purpose but our techniques still require more validation in terms of diagnosis or prognosis. To now, imaging of the kidney has been mainly based on morphological evaluation of the parenchyma and intrarenal vasculature by using ultrasound (US) sonography and Doppler, computed tomography (CT) or magnetic resonance imaging (MRI). Besides these morphological aspects, functional and structural parameters become more and more accessible using US and MRI. Whereas functional parameters are essentially provided by MRI, as perfusion, filtration, oxygenation and diffusion, structural parameters can be provided by both, as elastography.

Elastography is an attractive technique, which was already demonstrated in the liver [1–3], but the technique is still not specific enough to be considered as a marker of fibrosis by itself and is often used in addition to biopsy or blood marker analysis. Whereas US elastography has gained experience and validation in clinical practice, MR elastography (MRE) is developing rapidly, also mainly in the field of liver diseases. Within the kidney, much more validation is required to define a potential role for characterization of diffuse tissue changes.

As in the liver, the main factor of chronic renal function alteration is related to progressive changes of extracellular matrix leading to progression of fibrosis. This process, called chronic kidney disease (CKD), shows an increased incidence and prevalence in developed countries, particularly in the context of diabetes and hypertension-related nephropathies [4]. It causes end-stage renal failure, with its extensive morbidity and mortality and increases health costs. In

N. Grenier (✉)
Service d'Imagerie Diagnostique et Interventionnelle de l'Adulte, Groupe Hospitalier Pellegrin, CHU de Bordeaux, Place Amélie Raba-Léon, Bordeaux Cedex, France

Université Bordeaux Segalen, Bordeaux, France
e-mail: nicolas.grenier@chu-bordeaux.fr

J.-L. Gennisson
Imagerie par Résonance Magnétique Médicale et Multi-Modalités, CNRS UMR8081, Université Paris Sud, CEA Service Hospitalier Frédéric Joliot, Orsay, France

C. Marcelin · Y. Le Bras
Service d'Imagerie Diagnostique et Interventionnelle de l'Adulte, Groupe Hospitalier Pellegrin, CHU de Bordeaux, Place Amélie Raba-Léon, Bordeaux Cedex, France

L. Couzi
Université Bordeaux Segalen, Bordeaux, France

Place du Gal Leclerc 91401, Orsay, France

Service de Néphrologie, Groupe Hospitalier Pellegrin, CHU de Bordeaux, Place Amélie Raba-Léon, Bordeaux Cedex, France

A. Granata, M. Bertolotto (eds.), *Imaging in Nephrology*, https://doi.org/10.1007/978-3-030-60794-4_19

most types of kidney diseases, CKD progression is characterized by progressive fibrotic processes that may involve first either glomeruli (glomerulosclerosis) or interstitial space (interstitial fibrosis) depending on the initial nephropathy [5, 6]. Similarly, in renal transplantation, the development of interstitial fibrosis and tubular atrophy (IF/TA), previously called chronic allograft nephropathy (CAN) [7, 8], is the major determinant of renal allograft failure.

Therefore, development of new non-invasive methods for identification and quantification of fibrosis would be worthwhile. Because it is a progressive process, CKD justifies developing more efficient diagnostic strategies by using non-invasive methods. These new approaches require defining and validating adequate imaging biomarkers, with their intrinsic variability and inter-operator reproducibility before to be used in clinical practice. Diffusion-weighted MRI (DW-MRI) was recently proposed in experimental interstitial renal fibrosis [9] but no clinical validation has been reported yet. Application of US elastography to the kidney has been shown to be possible and the first results are encouraging. However, the kidney is a much more complex organ than the liver, with two anatomical compartments, cortex and medulla, a high vascularity and a urinary excretion function. Therefore, all these parameters have to be taken into account to better understand the intrinsic and extrinsic factors of variation on elasticity measurements before extending this method to large clinical trials.

19.2 Elastography Techniques

19.2.1 US Elastography

Several techniques have been proposed, classified into two main categories: quasi-static techniques and dynamic techniques which do not provide the same information on mechanical parameters. With quasi-static elastography, a qualitative strain map of the investigated organ is obtained, whereas with dynamic elastography, a quantitative map or a quantitative value of elasticity is provided.

Quasi-static elastography, also called by manufacturers "real-time elastography", was the first elastography technique, developed by Ophir et al. [10]. This technique is based on a quasi-static deformation, or strain (ε) of the medium which is related to elasticity, defined by the Young's modulus (E), through the Hooke's law (Eq. 19.1):

$$E = \sigma / \varepsilon \tag{19.1}$$

where σ is the stress applied to the medium. As σ is never known, E cannot be quantified with this technique.

In order to obtain calculated strain maps, images before and after compression of the tissue are extracted (Fig. 19.1). The main limits of this technique are the absence of quantification and the impossibility to apply that strain to deep organs as native kidneys.

Conversely, dynamic elastography is a quantitative technique based on the propagation of mechanical or elastic waves, so-called shear waves, in the body which is considered as quasi-incompressible. Here, the Young's modulus is directly related to the shear wave speed (V_S), $E = 3\rho V_S^2$, where ρ is the tissue density of about 1000 kg.m^{-3}. By generating a shear wave within the tissues using an external source (a low-frequency vibrator or an US radiation force) and by using 1D or 2D US to follow their propagation, dynamic elastography can extract a quantitative value of the speed of shear waves. Three main dynamic elastography methods have been proposed: FibroScan®-transient elastography, acoustic radiation force impulse (ARFI) and supersonic shear wave imaging (SSI):

- FibroScan®-transient elastography was the first quantitative elastography method proposed by Sandrin et al. [11]. It is a 1D US technique based on the use of a low-frequency vibrator (50 Hz), which transmits transient mechanical wave in the medium and one single US transducer (5 MHz) that catches the propagating shear wave (Fig. 19.2). The generated tissue displacement is estimated by an ultrafast 1D US speckle tracking method. By calculating the

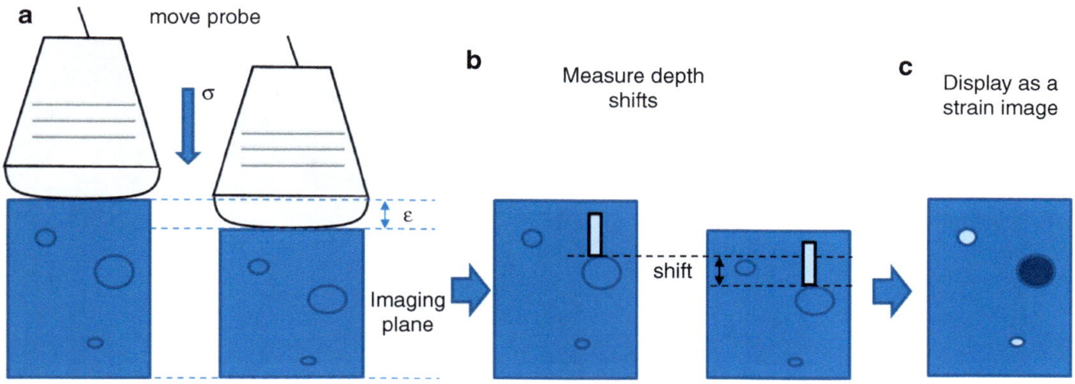

Fig. 19.1 Quasi-static elastography. Principle of quasi-static elastography. (**a**) The probe is placed at the surface of the investigated organ and a small compression is applied. Images are acquired before and after compression. (**b**) By taking small windows within the image of raw ultrasound signals, a displacement shift in depth is recovered. (**c**) Then by calculating the derivative of the displacement the final strain image is obtained and displayed (published with permission from Grenier et al., US Clinics 2013;8:551)

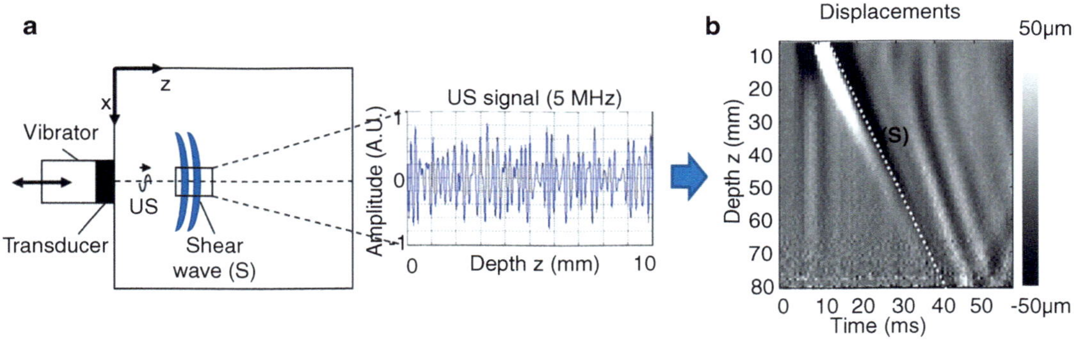

Fig. 19.2 FibroScan®-transient elastography. (**a**) Principle: a slight low-frequency pulse (typically 50 Hz) is given at the surface of the investigated medium with the front face of the transducer working in emission-reception at a high frame rate (some kHz). This pulse induces the propagation of shear waves which induces movement within the raw frequency ultrasound signal recorded. (**b**) By cross-correlating the acquired signals, a displacement map showing shear wave propagation in depth as a function of time is calculated. The shear wave speed is then recovered by estimating the slope of the shear wave (published with permission from Grenier et al., US Clinics 2013;8:551)

shear wave phase as a function of depth, the phase velocity of the shear wave at the central frequency is then estimated in a given window of depth (from 20 to 60 mm).

- The quantitative ARFI technique is based on the use of an US radiation pressure which acts as a shear wave source. This radiation pressure field is generated at the focal spot by focusing US during a long period of time (hundreds of µs versus 1–10 µs for classical US B-mode). The resulting shear waves are locally followed using 1D US with a high frame rate (several kHz) closely to the source. At last a time-of-flight algorithm is used to obtain shear wave velocity values (Fig. 19.3a). Even if US is used in a 1D mode for elasticity measurement, a 2D B-mode image is also provided at the same time to position the elasticity region of interest at the desired location within the organ (Fig. 19.3b). New developments make it now possible to provide 2D maps with superficial probes (Fig. 19.3c).
- The SSI technique is based on the association of production of an acoustic radiation force to

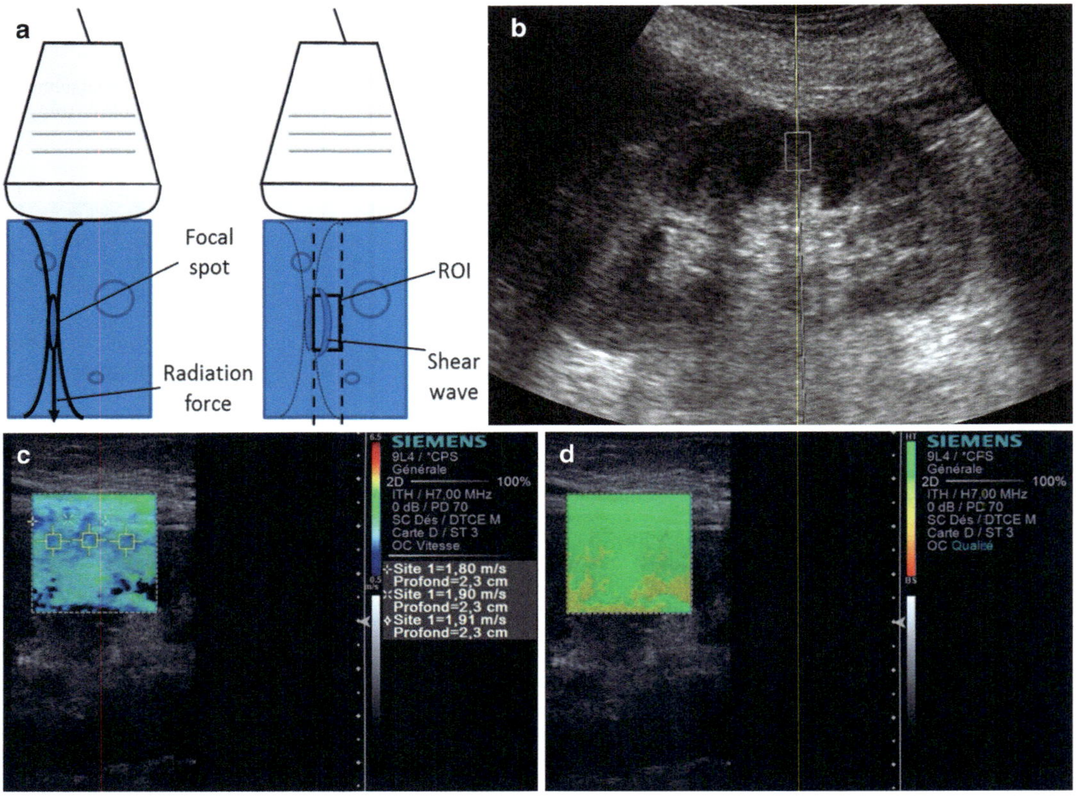

Fig. 19.3 Acoustic radiation force imaging (ARFI). (**a**) Principle: a radiation force is created from a focal spot within the organ by focusing ultrasound (left). This creates a local shear wave source that is propagated perpendicularly to the ultrasound axis. On few transducers close to the focal spot, the displacements of the shear wave are recovered allowing a 1D measurement of shear elasticity in the ROI (right) (published with permission from Grenier et al., US Clinics 2013;8:551). (**b**) Example of intrarenal shear wave velocity measurement with the ARFI technique. (**c**) Using high-frequency probes, it is now possible to obtain 2D maps, but not in real time (here in a transplant). (**d**) To verify the reliability (or variability) of measurements, a "quality map" can also be displayed: green meaning low variability and red high variability

generate a Mach cone and an US ultrafast imaging sequence [12]. The Mach cone is generated by several successive focalized US spots at 4–5 different depths producing 4–5 interfering spherical shear waves. This creates a quasi-plane shear wave front in the imaging plane (Fig. 19.4a) illuminating almost all the medium. Then, the entire plane is imaged with an ultrafast US technique (until 20,000 images/s). At last from the resulting movie of the propagating shear wave, by using a time-of-flight algorithm, a real-time quantitative map is calculated (Fig. 19.4b).

19.2.2 MR Elastography

MRE is also able to obtain information about the stiffness of tissue by assessing the propagation of mechanical waves through the tissue with a special MRI technique. The technique essentially involves three steps: (1) generating shear waves in the tissue by applying vibrations with frequencies ranging from 50 to 500 Hz using an external driver as a source of motion, (2) imaging induced waves inside the body using dynamic phase-contrast MRE where propagating shear waves in tissue are encoded into the phase of the MR images

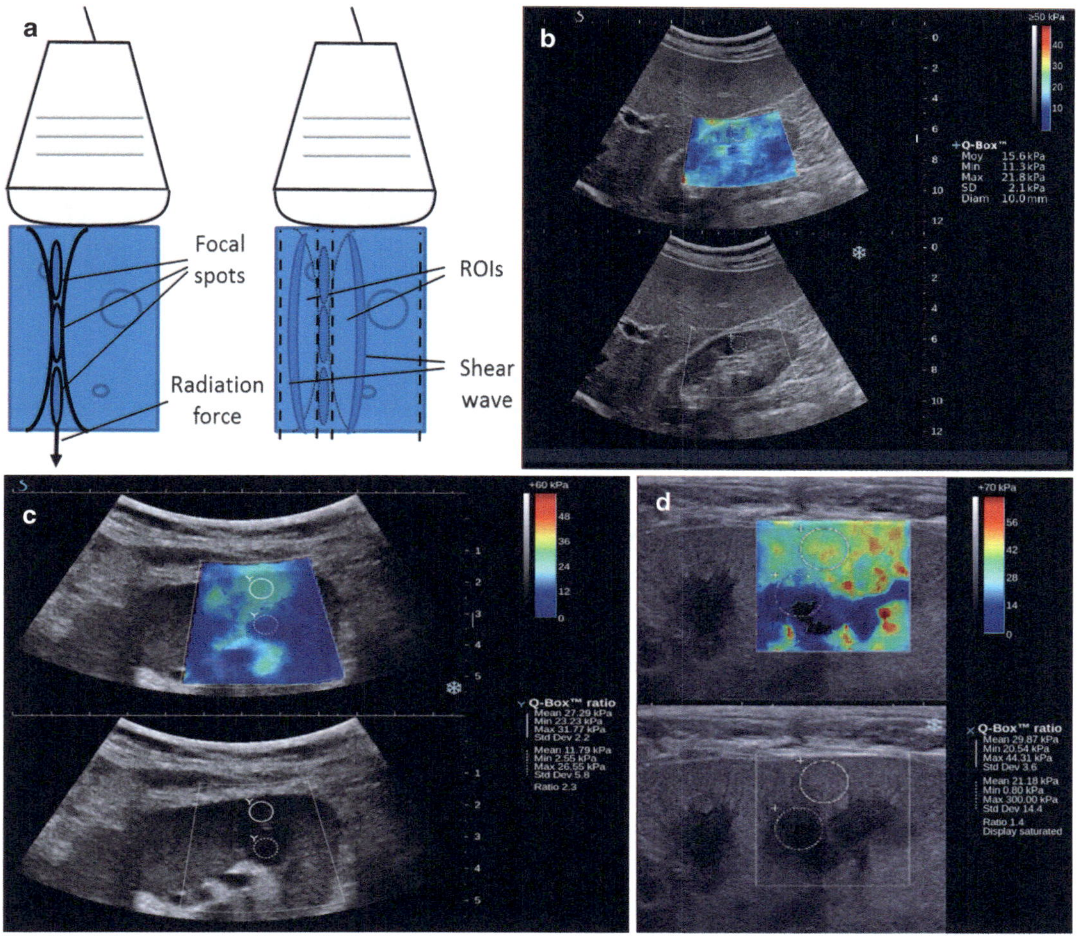

Fig. 19.4 Supersonic shear wave imaging (SSI). (**a**) Principle: Multiple focal spots are created in depth along the same axis, generating a Mach cone acting as a shear wave source (left). By using an ultrafast imaging mode, the propagating shear wave is caught in the entire field of imaging allowing the reconstruction of a 2D elasticity map (right) (published with permission from Grenier et al., US Clinics 2013;8:551). (**b–d**) Examples of elasticity mapping in a native kidney using a low-frequency probe (**b**) and in a transplanted kidney using either a low-frequency probe (**c**) or a high-frequency probe (**d**)

with the help of motion-encoding gradients, and (3) processing the images of the shear waves to generate quantitative maps of tissue stiffness, called elastograms by using mathematical inversion algorithms based on equations of motion, with simplifying assumptions (isotropy, homogeneity and incompressibility) [13].

MRE is already being used clinically for the assessment of patients with chronic liver, heart and brain diseases, and the technology is becoming available as an upgrade on conventional MRI scanners. The experience in renal diseases is still limited.

19.3 Technical Impact on Renal Sampling

The quasi-static elastography technique is inadequate for renal purposes because the kidneys are deep and because they do not provide quantitative data [14, 15]. Dynamic elastography techniques based on shear wave propagation are more appropriate.

Among these techniques, the FibroScan® elastography system is, to our sense, also inappropriate for the kidney for several reasons: (1) First, there is no B-mode control and, as the sample volume is fixed in depth and size, it is extremely difficult and hazardous to position adequately the sample volume on the renal parenchyma which is located at a variable depth and, moreover, to focus sampling on the cortex versus medulla. A manual adjustment could be considered in transplanted kidneys, because it is more superficially located, but it stays hazardous without real-time sonographic control; moreover, such adjustment would require to modify the pressure put on the probe which would change elasticity values; (2) second, the mechanical wave has to be applied on a rigid surface, such as the rib cage, to avoid compression effects by the probe, which is impossible for the kidney. Despite these limitations, FibroScan® transient elastography was used in two recent series of transplanted kidneys [16–18]. The latter reported that body mass index, skin allograft distance and peri- or intrarenal fluid accumulation were important confounders of successful KS measurements. The same authors mentioned that the heterogeneous renal morphology and several technical confounding factors negatively affect the measurability of elasticity by this technique. Further technical modifications were called to improve its applicability for kidney assessment.

The ARFI system is more appropriate because it is US guided, allowing to position a sample volume in depth and to selectively sample cortex and medulla [19]. It provides a monodimensional (1D) real-time sampling (Fig. 19.3b) or a fixed bi-dimensional (2D) quantitative mapping.

The SSI technique provides a real-time bidimensional quantitative mapping and is implemented on low-frequency curved arrays, for native and deep-transplanted kidneys (Fig. 19.4b,c), and on high-frequency linear arrays, for superficial transplanted kidneys (Fig. 19.4d).

19.4 Normal Values and Reproducibility

Table 19.1 summarizes the normal cortical values obtained with US techniques in the literature. Using ARFI, four studies reported mean normal renal elasticity values in healthy volunteers [20]; normal values were between 2.15 m/s and 2.49 m/s, corresponding approximately to 13.9 and 18.6 kPa in terms of Young's modulus (Table 19.1); and similar values were always obtained between right and left kidneys [21, 22, 25]. Using SSI, normal cortical elasticity values measured within native renal kidneys of 127 healthy volunteers, age ranging between 17 and 63 years old, appeared quite low, with a large distribution: 5.2 ± 2.9 (1–13) kPa and 4.9 ± 2.9 (1–26) kPa in men and women, respectively [24]. The reasons of such discrepancies remain unclear and call for a large comparative study of normal native kidneys.

Table 19.1 Normal cortical values with shear wave techniques

Study	Technique	SWV value (m/s)	Elasticity (kPa)
Guo et al. [20]	ARFI	2.15 ± 0.51	13.9
Bob et al. [21]	ARFI	2.42 ± 0.70	17.6
Bota et al. [22]	ARFI	2.49 ± 0.81	18.6
Goya et al. [23]	ARFI	2.35 ± 0.39	16.6
Arda et al. [24]	SSI	–	5.0 ± 2.9
	SSI	–	4.40 (3.68, 5.70)

Changes in renal cortical stiffness with age have been reported in both children and adults. In children, SWV values increased between year 1 and year 5 [25]. Conversely, in adults, these values showed a tendency to decrease with age (18–30y = 2.94 ± 0.60 m/s; 31–50y = 2.26 ± 0.82 m/s; 51–65y = 2.48 ± 0.8 m/s). In a cohort of 281 healthy subjects, a negative statistically significant correlation between age and SWV was also reported [23]. A decrease of renal blood flow could explain the fact that kidneys would become softer with age.

Several studies evaluated reproducibility of ARFI measurements in native kidneys (Table 19.2). In the largest series, a strong agreement was obtained between measurements in right and left kidneys obtained by two operators (ICC = 0.71 for right kidney and 0.69 for left kidney) [21]. Smaller ICCs were obtained in healthy subjects as compared to patients with kidney diseases (0.68 vs. 0.75) and in women as compared with men (0.59 vs. 0.78). ICC also decreased in subjects over

Table 19.2 Reproducibility of shear wave measurements

Study	Technique	No. of patients	Kidney	Intra-observer ICC	Inter-observer ICC
Guo et al. [20]	ARFI	40	Native	0.6 (95% CI: 0.31–0.81, $p = 0.001$)	0.64 (95% CI: 0.13–0.82, $p = 0.011$)
Hu et al. [26]	ARFI	32	Native	0.71 (95% CI: 0.39–0.86, $p = 0.001$)	0.63 (95% CI: 0.23–0.82, $p = 0.004$)
Bob et al. [21]	ARFI	107	Native	0.71 (95% CI: 0.53–0.83)	
Syversveen et al. [19]	ARFI	30	Transplanted		0.31 (95% CI: −0.03 to 0.60)
Grenier et al., [27]	SSI	43	Transplanted		0.60 (95% CI: 0.34–0.76, $p = 0.3 \times 10^{-4}$)

50 years, in over-weighted and obese subjects (0.66 and 0.36, respectively), and with a sampling depth under 4 cm and over 6 cm (0.32 and 0.60, respectively) compared to the window of 4–6 cm (0.81). In the two other series, ICCs between 0.60 and 0.71, and between 0.63 and 0.64, were obtained for intra- and inter-observer reproducibility, respectively. In renal transplants, the mean intra-observer coefficient of variation (CV) was 22% for observer 1 and 24% for observer 2 [19]. Inter-observer agreement, expressed as ICC, was only 0.31 (95% CI: −0.03 to 0.60).

Using SSI in renal transplants, intra- and inter-observer variation coefficients of cortical elasticity were 20% and 12%, respectively [27]. According to the distribution CVs in this cohort, a CV <27% was obtained for each observer in 75% of cases.

These results confirm the moderate-to-low reproducibility of all these techniques requiring several samplings for each measurement, at least five.

19.5 Elastography and Renal Function

Considering the relationship between renal stiffness and level of renal function, several studies found either no correlation [27] or only a weak correlation between elastography parameters and GFR values either in native kidneys for three different types of nephropathies as glomerulonephritis, diabetic nephropathy or nephrosclerosis [23, 28, 29] or in transplants. However, whereas this relationship was noted as positive in two of the three studies on native kidneys, with renal stiffness decreasing with GFR drop [28, 29], it was reported as negative in a large cohort of diabetic nephropathy (renal stiffness being lower for healthy volunteers than for diseased patients) [23] and in transplanted kidneys. These discrepancies also remain unexplained.

Considering the relationship between renal stiffness and stage of dysfunction, elastography has been unable to predict accurately CKD stages. No relation was found between SWV values and CKD stage by Wang et al. [30]. Two other studies showed a statistically significant correlation only when SWVs were compared between stage 0 and stages 4 and 5 [29] or between stages 1–4 and stage 5 [20], again with a decrease of SWV values when stages increase.

The same threshold value was found by Goya et al. [23] with an 84.1% sensitivity and a 67.3% specificity.

19.6 Elastography and Histopathological Changes

An increase in the extracellular matrix synthesis, with excessive fibrillary collagens, characterizes the development of chronic lesions in the glomerular, interstitial and vascular compartments, leading progressively to end-stage renal failure [5]. Mechanisms participating in these processes are increasingly identified and various therapeutic interventions have been shown to prevent or to favour regression of fibrosis in several experimental models [31].

19.6.1 Preclinical Studies

To our knowledge, only one study attempted to evaluate US elastography in an experimental model [32]: it was a rat model of glomerulosclerosis induced by L-NAME administration, and the objective was to use SSI to detect kidney cortex elasticity changes and predict histopathological development of fibrosis. This study showed that cortical elasticity values increase with the development of intrarenal disease. When followed longitudinally, these values increased to approximately 76% of their baseline values 4 weeks after the onset of the model and remained stable 3 weeks later. A high degree of positive correlation between the enhanced renal stiffness and the degree of renal dysfunction, measured by the proteinuria/creatininuria ratio, was very encouraging, but no correlation could be found between the semi-quantitative scoring system (addition of several graded items evaluated qualitatively) and SSI. Preclinical studies on more fibrotic animal models would be worthwhile.

19.6.2 Clinical Studies on Native Kidneys

The studies on correlation between SWV values and pathologic alterations in native kidneys provided very discordant results.

One study of 163 patients [26] showed a moderate negative correlation with pathologic parameters ($r = -0.422$ to -0.511) with significantly lower mean SWV values in kidneys with severe histologic impairment than in kidneys with mild or moderate histologic impairment and healthy controls.

A second study of 76 patients [33] showed a positive linear correlation with fibrosis with higher mean SWV values in subcapsular parenchyma of kidneys with various percentages of renal fibrosis (<25%, 25%–50%, >50%) than in non-fibrotic kidneys.

A third study of 45 patients [30] did not show any significant correlations with renal fibrosis.

19.6.3 Clinical Studies on Transplanted Kidneys

The natural history of IF/TA in transplanted kidneys has been well studied through protocol biopsies. The early phase, which generally occurs during the first years post-transplantation, is characterized by fibrogenesis and emergence of tubulo-interstitial damage due to immunologic phenomena; the late phase is characterized by the worsening of parenchymal lesions (irreversible interstitial fibrosis, tubular atrophy, arteriolar hyalinosis) and the occurrence of glomerular sclerosis leading to graft lost [7, 8]. Non-invasive markers of these pathological changes are lacking and protocol biopsies are still the only reliable tool for the diagnosis of IF/TA.

Several studies have been performed on renal transplants because it is more superficially located allowing more accurate measurements. Most of them were performed with low-frequency probes (Fig. 19.4b) but high-frequency probes can also be used in very superficial kidneys (Fig. 19.4c, b). The correlation between renal elasticity quantification and intra-renal pathological changes is also controversial in the literature but the number of enrolled patients for biopsy is quite limited.

Using the FibroScan®, a study performed on 52 biopsied transplants [18] obtained significantly higher stiffness in allografts with histologically confirmed advanced fibrosis. The sensitivity and specificity to detect renal allograft fibrosis with a cut-off of 40 kPa were 54% and 73%, respectively. Two other groups [16, 17] found a positive correlation between renal stiffness and degree of interstitial fibrosis.

With ARFI, Syversveen et al. [19], in 30 patients scheduled for biopsy, did not found any correlation between shear wave velocity values and grade of fibrosis. The median values were 2.8 m/s (range: 1.6–3.6), 2.6 m/s (range: 1.8–3.5) and 2.5 m/s (range: 1.6–3) for grades 0 (n = 12), 1 (n = 10) and 2/3 (n = 8) fibrosis, respectively. These values did not differ significantly in transplants without and with fibrosis (grade 0 vs. grade 1, P = 0.53, and grade 0 vs. grades 2/3, P = 0.11). However, SWV was increasing with the time after transplantation.

Using SSI in 49 consecutive kidney-transplant recipients scheduled for renal biopsy [27] none of each individual score of the semi-quantitative Banff classification, including interstitial fibrosis (ci), was correlated with the measurement of cortical stiffness. Moreover, cortical stiffness was correlated with neither the level of interstitial fibrosis measured by quantitative image analysis nor the scoring and grading of IF/TA. However, renal cortical stiffness did correlate with the sum of the scores of chronic lesions and the sum of the scores of all individual lesions (r = 0.34, p = 0.05, and r = 0.41, p = 0.03, respectively).

One possible explanation for such discrepancies is the non-specificity of stiffness changes related to interstitial fibrosis. These results suggest that the degree of renal cortical stiffness does not reflect any specific intra-renal change, such as fibrosis, but rather the association of several renal microlesions, especially chronic lesions and haemodynamic changes.

19.7 Factors of Variation Influencing Elasticity Measurement in the Kidney

Factors of variation influencing elasticity measurements in the kidney are numerous, and probably responsible for the lower reproducibility and lower performances in assessing renal parenchymal diseases than liver parenchymal diseases, and also for the discrepancies observed in the literature. Measuring SWV within the kidney with any of these systems must be cautious because it is sensitive to many mechanical parameters. A clear assessment of these factors of variation is essential to decrease the intrinsic variability of in vivo measurements, and to increase the reproducibility of the method. These factors are compressibility of renal transplants, anisotropy of renal architecture, high degree of renal vascularity and possible increase of urinary pressure.

Whereas native kidneys are quite deep within the abdomen and hardly compressible, renal transplants are more superficially located in the iliac fossa. This is why a manual compression of renal parenchyma by the US probe is possible during scanning. The same phenomenon is observed on the liver parenchyma with higher elasticity values on the left lobe, using a compliant epigastric window, than on the right lobe, using a rigid intercostal window. This is why Syversveen et al. [19] evaluated, quantitatively, the effect of probe compression on elasticity values, using a mechanical device and calibrated compression forces with ARFI on the renal cortex of 31 kidney transplants. Comparison showed highly significant differences of mean shear wave velocity between the five different compression weights.

In the kidney, the intrinsic architecture of the parenchyma is highly oriented, or anisotropic: Henle loops and vasa recta within the medulla and collecting ducts within the cortex and medulla are parallel and oriented from the capsule to the papilla within each renal segment. Using MRI, the degree of anisotropy has been estimated to be around 15% in the cortex and 30% in the medulla [34]. An in vivo evaluation of the effect of intrarenal anisotropy on elasticity values was performed in pig kidneys, scanned preoperatively [35]. Acquisitions were performed in a renal segment with a pyramid axis parallel to US beam, and then in a renal segment with a pyramid axis perpendicular to US beam. When emission of the ultrasound beam is sent parallel to renal microstructures, the shear wave propagates perpendicular to these, creating multiple vascular and tubular interfaces, thus decreasing its speed of propagation and resulting in lower elasticity values. Conversely, when emission of the ultrasound beam is sent perpendicular to these structures, the shear wave propagates at a higher speed, without interfaces, resulting in higher elasticity values. The mean variation of the shear modulus due to anisotropy was 10.5% in the outer cortex, 29.7% in the inner cortex and 31.8% in the medulla in normal conditions. Therefore, when performing renal US elastography, a clear identification of sampled renal segments and their orientation according to the US beam is mandatory. This is of prime importance for inter-patient comparisons and longitudinal follow-up.

The kidney is highly vascularized, mainly the cortex, with an eighth of the cardiac blood flow being distributed into each kidney. The degree of vascular pressure also influences elasticity values. In the same pig study, a significant decrease of elasticity was noted after ligation of the renal artery (Fig. 9). A decrease of elasticity was also observed using MR elastography during ischaemia, with cortical and medullary stiffness changing by ~30% and ~20%, respectively [36]. Conversely, in our pig study, a huge increase of renal elasticity was observed after ligation of the renal vein.

Asano et al. [28] evaluated the impact of vascular factors influencing SWV values by measuring the brachial-ankle pulse wave velocity, as an indicator of arteriosclerosis of large vessels, in 183 patients. They showed that a low SWV was obtained in patients with a high brachial-ankle pulse wave velocity, demonstrating that diminution of blood flow may affect SWV values in the kidneys more than the progression of tissue fibrosis.

Finally, urinary obstruction is known to increase intra-renal pressure, mostly when acute and complete. The same pig study confirmed that elasticity values were highly influenced by the degree of urinary obstruction in a linear fashion. As a consequence, urinary obstruction will have to be ruled out before to attribute an increased elasticity to tissue changes. Particular attention will have to be paid to the degree of bladder filling in kidney-transplant patients because, due to the shortness of the ureter and due to its denervation, a filled bladder may induce a dilatation of the pyelocaliceal system. Based on these observations, Dillman et al. [37] attempted to determine if SWV measurements obtained either before or after intravenous diuretic administration can be used to discriminate obstructive hydronephrosis from unobstructive hydronephrosis in children, with diuretic renal scintigraphy as the reference standard. Unfortunately, these measurements did not enable discrimination of obstructive hydronephrosis from unobstructive hydronephrosis in this context.

In summary, quantification of tissue stiffness using ultrasound is more complex within the kidney than within the liver. Due to compartmentalization and high tissue heterogeneities, 2D sonography-guided techniques seem more appropriate than transient elastography. Variability of measurements is higher than in the liver, probably explaining the discrepancies observed between cortical stiffness and age, renal function and histological changes. Therefore, more experience is needed in preclinical models and in patient cohorts with pathological correlation to better understand which are the physical factors of variation and the histopathological causes of elasticity changes. Non-invasive imaging could participate in this challenge in the near future using functional, structural or molecular approaches. MRE is still under development.

Disclosures of Potential Conflicts of Interest: N.G. is a member of the scientific advisory board of SuperSonic Imagine, and J.L.G. is a scientific consultant for SuperSonic Imagine.

References

1. Bavu E, Gennisson JL, Couade M, Bercoff J, Mallet V, Fink M, Badel A, Vallet-Pichard A, Nalpas B, Tanter M, Pol S. Non-invasive in vivo liver fibrosis staging using supersonic shear imaging: a clinical study. Ultrasound Med Biol. 2011;37:1365–73.
2. Castera L, Forns X, Alberti A. Non-invasive evaluation of liver fibrosis using transient elastography. J Hepatol. 2008;48:835–47.
3. Palmeri ML, Wang MH, Rouze NC, Abdelmalek MF, Guy CD, Moser B, Diehl AM, Nightingale KR. Noninvasive evaluation of hepatic fibrosis using acoustic radiation force-based shear stiffness in patients with nonalcoholic fatty liver disease. J Hepatol. 2011;55:666–72.

4. El Nahas M. The global challenge of chronic kidney disease. Kidney Intern. 2005;68:2918–29.
5. Chatziantoniou C, Boffa JJ, Tharaux PL, Flamant M, Ronco P, Dussaule JC. Progression and regression in renal vascular and glomerular fibrosis. Intern J Exp Pathol. 2004;85:1–11.
6. Ricardo SD, van Goor H, Eddy AA. Macrophage diversity in renal injury and repair. J Clin Invest. 2008;118:3522–30.
7. Nankivell BJ, Borrows RJ, Fung CL, O'Connell PJ, Allen RD, Chapman JR. The natural history of chronic allograft nephropathy. New Eng J Med. 2003;349:2326–33.
8. Stegall MD, Park WD, Larson TS, Gloor JM, Cornell LD, Sethi S, Dean PG, Prieto M, Amer H, Textor S, Schwab T, Cosio FG. The histology of solitary renal allografts at 1 and 5 years after transplantation. Am J Transplant. 2011;11:698–707.
9. Togao O, Doi S, Kuro-o M, Masaki T, Yorioka N, Takahashi M. Assessment of renal fibrosis with diffusion-weighted MR imaging: study with murine model of unilateral ureteral obstruction. Radiology. 2010;255:772–80.
10. Ophir J, Cespedes I, Ponnekanti H, Yazdi Y, Li X. Elastography: a quantitative method for imaging the elasticity of biological tissues. Ultrasonic Imaging. 1991;13:111–34.
11. Sandrin L, Fourquet B, Hasquenoph JM, et al. Transient elastography: a new noninvasive method for assessment of hepatic fibrosis. Ultrasound Med Biol. 2003;29:1705–13.
12. Bercoff J, Tanter M, Fink M. Supersonic shear imaging: a new technique for soft tissue elasticity mapping. IEEE Trans Ultrason Ferroelectr Freq Control. 2004;51:396–409.
13. Mariappan YK, Glaser KJ, Ehman RL. Magnetic resonance elastography: a review. Clin Anat. 2010;23:497–511.
14. Gao J, Min R, Hamilton J, Weitzel W, Chen J, Juluru K, Rubin JM. Corticomedullary strain ratio: a quantitative marker for assessment of renal allograft cortical fibrosis. J Ultrasound Med. 2013;32:1769–75.
15. Weitzel WF, Kim K, Rubin JM, Wiggins RC, Xie H, Chen X, Emelianov SY, O'Donnell M. Feasibility of applying ultrasound strain imaging to detect renal transplant chronic allograft nephropathy. Kidney Intern. 2004;65:733–6.
16. Arndt R, Schmidt S, Loddenkemper C, Grünbaum M, Zidek W, van der Giet M, Westhoff TH. Noninvasive evaluation of renal allograft fibrosis by transient elastographyDOUBLEHYPHENa pilot study. Transpl Int. 2010;23:871–7.
17. Lukenda V, Mikolasevic I, Racki S, Jelic I, Stimac D, Orlic L. Transient elastography: a new noninvasive diagnostic tool for assessment of chronic allograft nephropathy. Int Urol Nephrol. 2014;46:1435–40.
18. Sommerer C, Scharf M, Seitz C, Millonig G, Seitz HK, Zeier M, Mueller S. Assessment of renal allograft fibrosis by transient elastography. Transpl Int. 2013;26:545–51.
19. Syversveen T, Brabrand K, Midtvedt K, Strøm EH, Hartmann A, Jakobsen JA, Berstad AE. Assessment of renal allograft fibrosis by acoustic radiation force impulse quantification-a pilot study. Transpl Int. 2011;24:100–5.
20. Guo LH, Xu HX, Fu HJ, Peng A, Zhang YF, Liu LN. Acoustic radiation force impulse imaging for noninvasive evaluation of renal parenchyma elasticity: preliminary findings. PLoS One. 2013;11(8):e68925.
21. Bob F, Bota S, Sporea I, Sirli R, Petrica L, Schiller A. Kidney shear wave speed values in subjects with and without renal pathology and inter-operator reproducibility of acoustic radiation force impulse elastography (ARFI)DOUBLEHYPHENpreliminary results. PLoS One. 2014;26(9):e113761.
22. Bota S, Bob F, Sporea I, Şirli R, Popescu A. Factors that influence kidney shear wave speed assessed by acoustic radiation force impulse elastography in patients without kidney pathology. Ultrasound Med Biol. 2015;41:1–6.
23. Goya C, Kilinc F, Hamidi C, Yavuz A, Yildirim Y, Cetincakmak MG, Hattapoglu S. Acoustic radiation force impulse imaging for evaluation of renal parenchyma elasticity in diabetic nephropathy. Am J Roentgenol. 2015;204:324–9.
24. Arda K, Ciledag N, Aktas E, Aribas BK, Kose K. Quantitative assessment of normal soft-tissue elasticity using shear-wave ultrasound elastography. Am J Roentgenol. 2011;197:532–6.
25. Lee MJ, Kim MJ, Han KH, Yoon CS. Age-related changes in liver, kidney, and spleen stiffness in healthy children measured with acoustic radiation force impulse imaging. Eur J Radiol. 2013;82:e290–4.
26. Hu Q, Wang XY, He HG, Wei HM, Kang LK, Qin GC. Acoustic radiation force impulse imaging for noninvasive assessment of renal histopathology in chronic kidney disease. PLoS One. 2014;29(9):e115051.
27. Grenier N, Poulain S, Lepreux S, et al. Quantitative elastography of renal transplants using supersonic shear imaging: a pilot study. Eur Radiol. 2012;22(10):2138–46. https://doi.org/10.1007/s00330-012-2471-9.
28. Asano K, Ogata A, Tanaka K, Ide Y, Sankoda A, Kawakita C, Nishikawa M, Ohmori K, Kinomura M, Shimada N, Fukushima M. Acoustic radiation force impulse elastography of the kidneys: is shear wave velocity affected by tissue fibrosis or renal blood flow? J Ultrasound Med. 2014;33:793–801.
29. Bob F, Bota S, Sporea I, Sirli R, Popescu A, Schiller A. Relationship between the estimated glomerular filtration rate and kidney shear wave speed values assessed by acoustic radiation force impulse elastography: a pilot study. J Ultrasound Med. 2015;34:649–5.
30. Wang L, Xia P, Lv K, Han J, Dai Q, Li XM, Chen LM, Jiang YX. Assessment of renal tissue elasticity by acoustic radiation force impulse quantification with histopathological correlation: preliminary experience in chronic kidney disease. Eur Radiol. 2014;24:1694–9.

31. Boffa JJ, Lu Y, Placier S, Stefanski A, Dussaule JC, Chatziantoniou C. Regression of renal vascular and glomerular fibrosis: role of angiotensin II receptor antagonism and matrix metalloproteinases. J Am Soc Nephrol. 2003;14:1132–44.
32. Derieppe M, Delmas Y, Gennisson JL, Deminière C, Placier S, Tanter M, Combe C, Grenier N. Detection of intrarenal microstructural changes with supersonic shear wave elastography in rats. Eur Radiol. 2012;22:243–50.
33. Cui G, Yang Z, Zhang W, Li B, Sun F, Xu C, Wang K. Evaluation of acoustic radiation force impulse imaging for the clinicopathological typing of renal fibrosis. Exp Ther Med. 2014;7:233–5.
34. Ries M, Jones RA, Basseau F, Moonen CT, Grenier N. Diffusion tensor MRI of the human kidney. J Magn Reson Imaging. 2001;14:42–9.
35. Gennisson JL, Grenier N, Combe C, Tanter M. Supersonic shear wave elastography of in vivo pig kidney: influence of blood pressure, urinary pressure and tissue anisotropy. Ultrasound Med Biol. 2012;38:1559–67.
36. Warner L, Yin M, Glaser KJ, Woollard JA, Carrascal CA, Korsmo MJ, Crane JA, Ehman RL, Lerman LO. Noninvasive in vivo assessment of renal tissue elasticity during graded renal ischemia using MR elastography. Investig Radiol. 2011;46:509–14.
37. Dillman JR, Smith EA, Davenport MS, DiPietro MA, Sanchez R, Kraft KH, Brown RK, Rubin JM. Can shear-save elastography be used to discriminate obstructive hydronephrosis from nonobstructive hydronephrosis in children? Radiology. 2015;277:259–67.

20 Renal Biopsy

Antonio Granata, Francesco Pesce, Paola Suavo-Bulzis, Rosario Maccarrone, Campo Irene, Carlo Manno, Giorgio Battaglia, and Loreto Gesualdo

20.1 Introduction

The development of renal biopsy is tightly bound to the birth of nephrology. This specialty did not stem from internal medicine and the study of kidney diseases was mainly an interest of physiologists. The performance and interpretation of renal biopsy were, along with the introduction of dialysis and transplantation, major drivers in determining the emergence of nephrology as a specialty in the 1960s.

The history of the renal biopsy is very interesting. It is difficult to identify who actually performed the first biopsy, as this depends on the definition of biopsy (e.g., open, closed) and/or on the indication (e.g., as part of another procedure or as a goal in itself). The importance of renal pathology in nephrology, taking advantage of renal biopsy, was underlined in 1951 by Iversen and Brun in Copenhagen in a study of 42 patients dialyzed for acute renal failure as the underpinning cause (amyloidosis, diabetic nephropathy, hypercalcemia, and chronic glomerulonephritis) was identified and treated while awaiting the recovery of diuresis [1]. In this study, the biopsy was performed with patients in sitting position; intravenous pyelography was performed to visualize the lower right pole and the needle used (length 180 mm, diameter 1.9 mm) was connected to a syringe that was taking off a core piece of kidney by vacuum section, but the adequate tissue was obtained only in 53% of biopsies. A minimum of bleeding complication of transient gross hematuria was reported. In 1954, Kark and Muehrcke in Chicago modified the procedure by placing the patient in the prone rather than in the upright position with a pillow under the abdomen to lift up the right kidney to avoid the spleen [2]. They used an exploring needle to localize the kidney prior to the insertion in blind approach of a biopsy needle, the Franklin modified Vim-Silverman needle, a precursor of the needle used today. The renal tissue was trapped in the needle and then sheared off obtaining a success rate in 96% of biopsies and no major complication was reported. The anatomical landmarks of percutaneous renal biopsy were the XII rib, the ilium (iliocostalis angle), and the spinous apophysis of lumbar vertebra. Intravenous pyelography was

A. Granata (✉)
Department of Nephrology and Dialysis, "Cannizzaro" Emergency Hospital, Catania, Italy

F. Pesce · P. Suavo-Bulzis · C. Manno · L. Gesualdo
Department of Nephrology Dialysis and Transplant, Aldo Moro University, Bari, Italy

R. Maccarrone
Nephrology and Dialysis Unit, San Giovanni di Dio Hospital Agrigento, Agrigento, Italy

C. Irene
Department of Radiology, Civile Hospital, Conegliano, Italy

G. Battaglia
Nephrology and Dialysis Unit, Santa Marta e Santa Venera Hospital, Acireale, Italy

A. Granata, M. Bertolotto (eds.), *Imaging in Nephrology*, https://doi.org/10.1007/978-3-030-60794-4_20

used to detect the lower pole of the kidney and the measurements were transferred back to the patient. Furthermore, a magnifying glass was used to observe the presence of glomeruli and to increase the efficiency of the technique.

In 1957, in Italy Dr. Bonomini faced several difficulties in introducing renal biopsy into clinical practice because it was still considered too risky for the patient, and yielding unreliable results. Indeed, the judging committee stated that percutaneous renal biopsy was too dangerous and ethically unacceptable when the book "*La biopsia renale percutan*ea" by Leonardi and Ruol was presented for a prestigious Italian medical award [3].

In 1960, at the first meeting of the International Society of Nephrology in Evian and Geneva, several papers discussed about renal biopsy. In March 1961, in the United Kingdom, an influential CIBA Foundation Symposium on "Renal Biopsy, Clinical and Pathological Significance" marked the advent of this technique.

In the following years, ultrasound, the imaging technique with the lowest associated risk, was used to localize the lower pole of the kidney, and it has been since then widely adopted and improved. Recently, the application of molecular biology techniques in the analysis of renal biopsy has allowed a better definition of the pathogenesis of renal diseases and has opened new avenues to identify targeted therapies. On the other hand, renal biopsy is a "*conditio sine qua non*" for the correct diagnosis of acute and chronic renal diseases which key aspects can be summarized as follows. The procedure provides diagnosis and modifies the clinical diagnosis in 25–50% of cases. The histological diagnosis guides treatment by describing the reversibility and activity of lesions and may change the therapy in 30–40% of patients. Furthermore, the renal biopsy predicts prognosis by assessing specific pathologic features and the extent of changes and also validates outcomes when used as an endpoint in clinical trials.

20.2 Indications for Renal Biopsy

In clinical practice there are numerous indications for renal biopsy. In the presence of acute kidney injury and increased serum creatinine, renal biopsy may be indicated if the ultrasound imaging does not show a reduced kidney volume or there are no other contraindications. The presence of proteinuria at urine analysis is an indication for renal biopsy since it is usually a sign of increased permeability of glomerulus or of failure of tubular reabsorption (usually, it leads to low-level proteinuria). Proteinuria of 1–3 g/day is usually asymptomatic, while higher levels lead to nephrotic syndrome and edema. Nephrotic syndrome defined as proteinuria >3.5 g/day, hypoalbuminemia, edema, hyperlipidemia, and lipiduria is due to increased glomerular permeability to albumin and other plasma proteins and is a mandatory indication to biopsy in adults and in children with atypical features. The presence of hematuria, asymptomatic or symptomatic (gross hematuria), isolated or associated with subnephrotic proteinuria, is an indication to perform a renal biopsy, since it is usually a sign of glomerular inflammation and disruption of the glomerular basal membrane, especially when red blood cell casts are found in urine analysis. When hematuria is combined with acute renal failure and red cell casts, the term nephritic syndrome should be used.

Nephritic syndrome is characterized by hematuria, proteinuria, elevated serum creatinine, and loss of function due to decreased glomerular blood flow, hypertension, and edema for salt retention. Finally, renal biopsy should be performed when there is a renal involvement during systemic diseases (Table 20.1).

In case of transplanted kidney, any cause of allograft dysfunction that is not readily explained by pre-renal or post-renal causes will usually prompt a biopsy.

20.3 Contraindications for Renal Biopsy

In advanced chronic kidney disease, renal biopsy is generally contraindicated, whereas in case of potentially reversible moderate dysfunction a renal biopsy can be taken into account. The absolute contraindication to perform a renal biopsy is generally the following: uncontrolled bleeding diathesis, uncontrolled severe arterial hyperten-

Table 20.1 Common indications for biopsy of native and transplanted kidneys

Native	Nephrotic syndrome
	Proteinuria >1 g/day (unless likely diabetic nephropathy)
	Hematuria of likely renal origin with additional evidence of glomerular disease
	Suspected multisystem disease (e.g., ANCA vasculitis, SLE, cryoglobulinemia)
	Suspicion of "intrinsic" renal disease: renal impairment or active urinary sediment (e.g., glomerulonephritis or tubulointerstitial nephritis with urine dipstick abnormalities)
	Assessment of response to therapy (e.g., following immunosuppression for glomerulonephritis)
Transplant	Unexplained allograft dysfunction
	Assessment of therapy response (e.g., following treatment of rejection)
	"Protocol" biopsy in patients at high risk of rejection

Table 20.2 Contraindications

Absolute	Anticoagulant therapy or coagulopathy (unless supported by clotting factor transfusion)
	Hypertension >160/90 mmHg
	Morbid obesity
	Platelet count <50 × 10^9/L (unless supported by platelet transfusion)
	Polycystic kidney disease
	Acute kidney infection
	Hydronephrosis
Relative	Other bleeding diathesis (including uremia)
	Antiplatelet therapy within 7 days
	Single functioning native kidney
	Small, scarred kidneys (typically <9 cm in bipolar length)
	Uncooperative patient

sion, solitary kidney, multiple renal cysts, renal mass or renal neoplasm, acute pyelonephritis and perinephric abscess, end-stage or near-end-stage kidney disease with small kidneys, patients unable to cooperate, obese patients, or patients with respiratory difficulties (Table 20.2).

However, the list of contraindications needs to be evaluated in each case. Indeed, the approach in high-risk patients has changed rapidly, as new techniques develop and a consensus statement is necessary. The same contraindications reported for the native kidney are valid for the transplanted kidney.

20.4 Equipment

Equipment includes drapes, disinfectant sponges, gauze pads, blade scalpel 11, anesthetic syringe, 10 mL of 1–2% lidocaine anesthetic solution, and automatic spring-loaded biopsy gun (with 14/16 gauge [4] and 15/19 cm long needle with a penetration depth of 22 mm and sample notch of 18 mm) but some (although not all) studies indicate lower yield with smaller (18-gauge) needles [5, 6]. Other factors, such as patient characteristics (e.g., kidney size) and operator experience, may also affect diagnostic yield. Sterile gloves, eye protection, gown, surgical cap, mask, spinal anesthesia needle (22 G × 120 mm), needle guide sterile kit, and full-size sterile drape are also required (Fig. 20.1). Ultrasound machines with convex array, high resolution, and Doppler schedule are preferred for this procedure. Additional equipment needed is the following: sterile transduction gel, acoustically transparent sterile transducer sheath, software with marks of guide with an inclination of 20–30°, and sterile rubber bands or clips to secure the sheath around the transducer.

20.5 Preparation of the Patient

The evening before the procedure the patient should have a light meal and an enema should be administered. On the morning of the biopsy, the patient must be fasting. Any antihypertensive drugs should be regularly given. A peripheral vein must be cannulated and blood pressure should be measured. The bladder must be emptied. Although kidney biopsy is very important for diagnosis, prognosis, and appropriate therapy, the risk/benefit ratio must always be assessed, especially for bleeding complications.

A successful procedure depends on patient-related factors, such as a thorough preparation of the patient, clinical, laboratory, and instrumental monitoring post-procedure and procedure-related

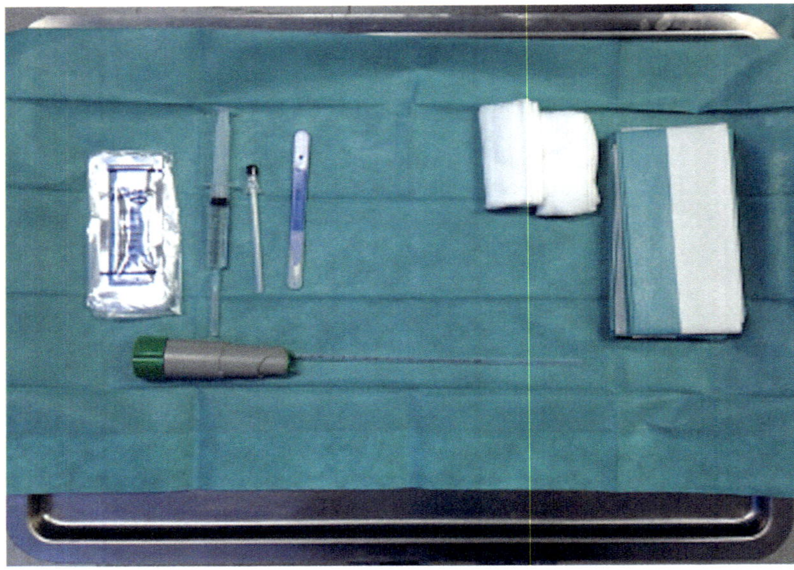

Fig. 20.1 Complete kit to perform renal biopsy: sterile gloves, gown, surgical cap, spinal anesthesia needle, needle guide sterile kit

factors, for example adequacy of specimen-handling techniques, consensus approach on clinical indications, and experience of the operator.

A first question in clinical practice is about choosing whether to perform the renal biopsy on inpatients or outpatients.

Shortening the after-biopsy observation period (e.g., outpatient management or 6–8-h monitoring) may reduce the safety of procedure.

However, a study has shown that complications occur in 89% of patients within a 24-h period. Therefore, after biopsy, an observation up to 24 h remains optimal, but since 11% of major complications occur after 24 h, some patients may require a longer period of hospitalization [7].

The prerequisites of procedure are focusing on medical history and examination of the patient, ultrasound evaluation of the kidneys (form, size, and cortical thickness), bleeding time, and laboratory data such as hemoglobin, platelets, prothrombin time, partial thromboplastin time, blood group, and sometimes dosage of von Willebrand factor and lupus anticoagulant. A specific test has not been established that can select patients with a major risk of post-biopsy bleeding and the impact of bleeding time on the complication rate is controversial [8]. In the future, evaluating some measure of platelet function, through a platelet function analyzer (PFA-100), may have a role in predicting risk.

The alterations of coagulation parameters should be corrected prior to the renal biopsy depending on the cause: erythrocyte transfusion in case of anemia, infusion of coagulation factors (e.g., factor VIII) if plasma levels are reduced, or administration of desmopressin acetate (DDAVP, dosage of 0.4 μg/kg/intravenous or 0.3 μg/kg/subcutaneous) if bleeding time is prolonged.

All antiplatelet or anticoagulant drugs should be stopped. Antiplatelet agents should be withdrawn from 5 to 10 days before the biopsy, for warfarin and dicoumarol drugs 5 days of interruption is needed, while for novel oral anticoagulant drugs (e.g., apixaban, rivaroxaban, dabigatran) 1–2 days is enough.

During the withdrawal period, sodic heparin or low-molecular-weight heparins should be administered and interrupted 12 h before the renal biopsy.

The management of patients who have an elevated thrombotic risk is different. Those taking two drugs (aspirin plus clopidogrel) for recent (<6–12 months) angioplasty and coronary stents should stop clopidogrel 5 days before the biopsy maintaining the administration of aspirin; tirofiban, an antiplatelet agent characterized by short plasmatic half-life, should be introduced 3 days before the biopsy and withdrawn 8 h before the biopsy. This approach presents an intermediate hemorrhagic risk but an elevated thrombotic risk; thus the patient should be monitored for 24 h after the renal biopsy in intensive cardiologic unit. A specific informed consent for cardiologic risk should be obtained.

As regards this crucial point attaining the risk management, an explicit informed consent, personally signed by a conscious patient and specific for the procedure of renal biopsy, should be obtained. The informed consent occurs in various steps; first, the physician who prescribed renal biopsy should inform the patient about the benefits deriving from a certain diagnosis and specific treatments. In the second step, the operator should describe the phases of the procedure, the possible complications, and the means to prevent and treat them.

Finally, the patient should confirm the consent or the refusal to procedure; for underage patient or the patient unable to understand, the physician should conform to the law of his/her country.

20.6 Position of the Patient

Kidney biopsy is usually performed in prone position (Fig. 20.2a). Lower pole of the left kidney is chosen to lower the risk of major hemorrhagic complications. If the patient is obese or has breathing difficulty, supine anterolateral position (SALP) may be more suitable (Fig. 20.2b). A recent study has shown that performing renal biopsy in SALP in obese patients ensures greater comfort and less breathing difficulties when compared to prone position, with no reduction in diagnostic yield or increase in complications [9].

20.7 Ultrasound Survey

A renal biopsy is typically performed by a suitably trained nephrologist or radiologist and ultrasounds are employed in both prebioptic and postbioptic phases.

20.7.1 Prebiopsy Ultrasound Study

Before performing the PRB, some recommendations are essential to reduce the risk of complications.

Prebioptic ultrasound study is essential to assess the presence of anatomical abnormalities of the kidney (e.g., presence of multiple cysts, hydronephrosis, solitary kidney) that may represent a risk factor for complications.

Prebiopsy renal study should be performed in the B-mode and with color Doppler (CD) in order

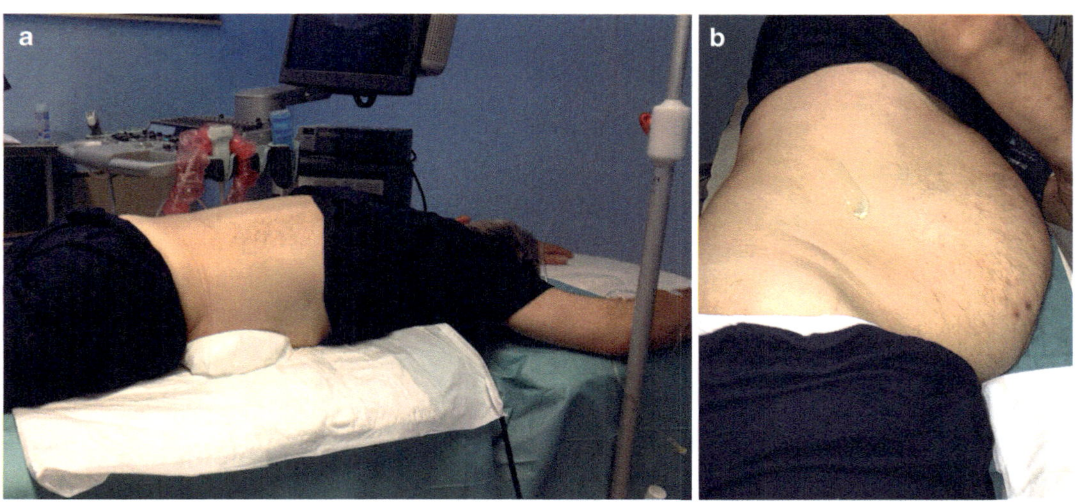

Fig. 20.2 Patient position. It is preferable to perform the biopsy with the patient in the prone position (**a**), if a patient is obese the supine anterolateral position is recommended (**b**)

to identify anomalous vessels that might be damaged by the needle during the procedure (Fig. 20.3), allowing the operator to choose the right kidney, when safer.

Anomalous vessels have been detected in about 10% of patients during the ultrasound study; complication rate appears to be reduced when color Doppler is performed [10].

Preparation of the patient needs an attentive medical history and examination, and renal ultrasound evaluation of form, size, and cortical thickness (Fig. 20.4). Furthermore, ultrasound guidance during the procedure allows the visualization of the biopsy needle and its path, with better performances than free-hand renal biopsy and a drastic reduction of the incidence of postbioptic complications, even in case of inexperienced operators [11].

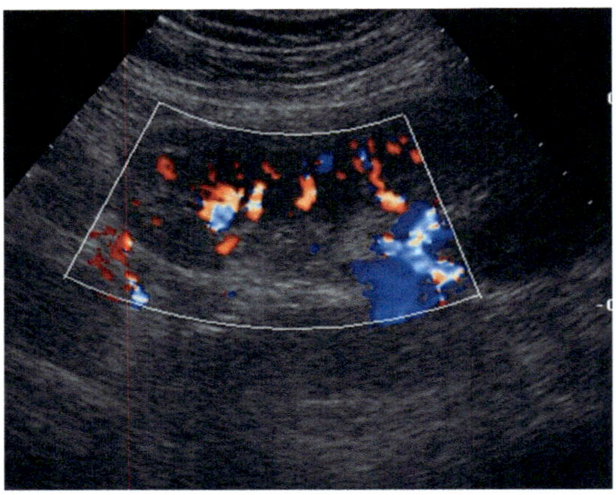

Fig. 20.3 Pre-biopsy evaluation. It is essential to evaluate renal vasculature with color Doppler to identify the presence of an abnormal vascularization

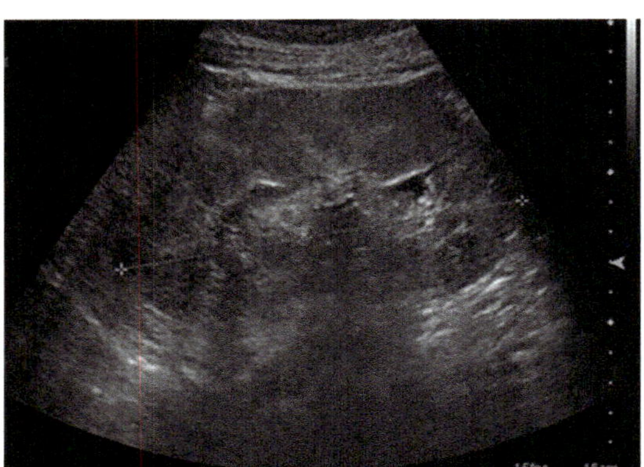

Fig. 20.4 Pre-biopsy evaluation. It is essential to evaluate the size of the parenchyma and the cortical thickness of the kidney

20.7.2 Procedure of Renal Biopsy

A rigorous algorithm describing the procedure step by step may increase the ratio of benefit/harm.

A meticulous preparation of the patient, including the informed consent, the biopsy technique, and the adequacy of management of the renal specimen, increases the benefits and provides diagnostic and therapeutic aspects. The reduction of risks depends on the operator's expertise and accurate clinical, laboratory, and instrumental postbioptic monitoring, even if the patient is asymptomatic.

In the clinical practice, renal biopsy may be performed on inpatients or outpatients. The most used is the eco-driven technique in prone position or, especially for obese patients, in anterior-lateral position (SALP).

The left kidney is preferred for the greater distance from the vena cava and the inferior pole for the greater and easier accessibility. The use of the lower pole compared to a mesorenal area, in addition to reducing the risk of damaging the vessels to the renal hilum, allows to sample more renal cortical tissue.

20.7.3 Performing the Biopsy in the Prone Position

The patient is placed in a prone position, possibly with a pillow under the abdomen in order to reduce the physiological dorsal lordosis and bring the kidney closer to the surface (Fig. 20.5).

The sterile field is prepared by disinfecting the skin region involved in the procedure and covering the remaining areas with sterile drapes. Operators must operate in sterile conditions. The ultrasound probe used during the biopsy procedure is usually a 3.5 MHz convex probe and it is covered with a suitable sterile probe cover; sterile gel is used. The preliminary ultrasound visualiza-

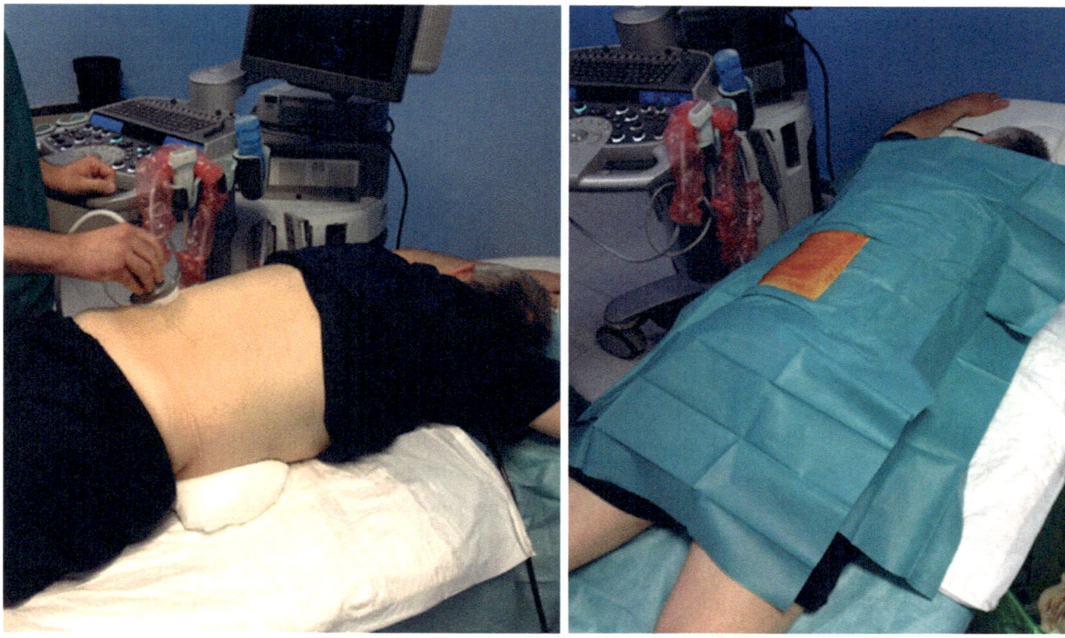

Fig. 20.5 To perform renal biopsy with prone patient, it is recommended to introduce a pillow under the abdomen to reduce the dorsal lordosis, thus bringing the kidney closer to the skin

tion of the lower pole of the left kidney is performed, assessing the most favorable trajectory for the introduction of the needle. The ultrasound device is programmed to highlight on the monitor the trajectory of the needle, and the probe is equipped with a needle guide.

We proceed to local anesthesia. Sometimes a skin incision may facilitate the entry of the needle to reach the kidney.

Under ultrasound guidance, the biopsy needle is introduced with an inclination of about 20° or 30° through the subcutaneous tissue, the muscular planes, and the fascia, until it stops immediately above the renal capsule (Fig. 20.6). A color box is placed to evaluate the presence of anomalous vessels. In the presence of abnormal vessels, the operator chooses whether to change trajectory to avoid them or to perform renal biopsy at the lower pole of the contralateral kidney.

Renal biopsy should be performed in B-mode.

In this phase, the collaboration of the patient is fundamental, who must maintain a short-time apnea in order to avoid displacement of the kidney simultaneous to the respiratory acts.

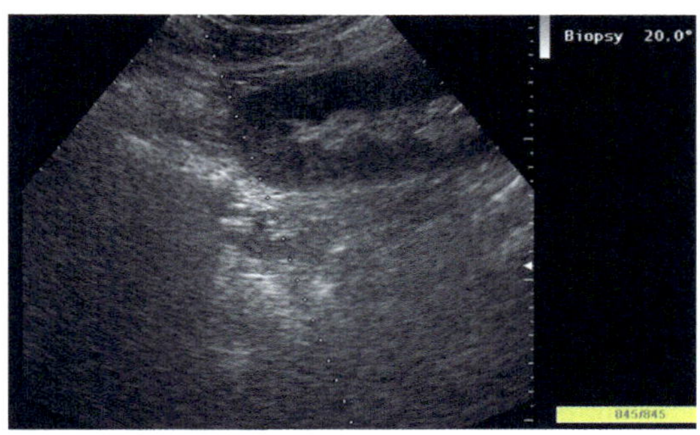

Fig. 20.6 The inclination of the biopsy needle must be about 20°–30°; it must cross the subcutis, the muscles, and the fascia and stop above the renal capsule

When the optimal position is reached, the needle is on the renal capsule, the patient is immobile, and the automatic needle is triggered, thus activating the descent of the mandrel at first and, then, of the shirt, imprisoning the sample.

The needle is extracted from the kidney and the biopsy sample is removed, and deposited on a gauze soaked in physiological solution or in a sterile container containing physiological solution.

Generally, two or three samples should be taken and evaluated by stereoscopic microscope to check the presence of cortical tissue and an adequate sampling of glomeruli.

Finally, a compression on the wound for 5–10 min and an ultrasonography check after 60 min should be done. In this phase, an early complication could be detected.

A further ultrasound and CD check are performed to exclude hemorrhagic complications and/or hemodynamic alterations (e.g., AVF) after the procedure.

The patient is transferred to the hospital bed, taking care to avoid sudden and supine movements. In this way the compressive and hemostatic effect of abdominal pressure is exploited.

During the post-procedure period, the patient is recommended bed rest in supine position for at least 24 h and blood pressure and arterial pulse are monitored; if necessary, hemoglobin and hematocrit are monitored every 4–6 h. The first postbioptic urine sample should be examined for macroscopic hematuria.

An ultrasound check should be done 24 h after the biopsy. Until that moment, the patient must rest in a supine position.

Good communication with the patient is essential for the entire duration of the procedure, since its collaboration is a necessary condition for the success of the biopsy and for the minimization of risks.

In developed countries numerous renal biopsies are performed in obese patients who have a high risk for bleeding complications, severe respiratory difficulties, and poorer ultrasound visualization of the kidney. Some technical precautions have been proposed in these high-risk patients, including computerized tomography guidance, laparoscopic renal biopsy, and trans-jugular biopsy.

However, computerized tomography guidance does not prevent the respiratory difficulties associated with the prone position, while laparoscopic renal biopsy, although safe and effective, requires general anesthesia and lengthy recovery times. Finally, trans-jugular renal biopsy is more invasive than percutaneous biopsy and yet is associated with a lower diagnostic yield due to the fact that the cortex is more distal.

20.7.4 Performing the Biopsy in the Supine Anterolateral Position (SALP)

This technique can be used in obese patients (BMI >30) to avoid some inconveniences, such as poor respiratory compliance for the prone position, deeper position of the inferior renal pole, and difficulty for some to maintain the same position for a long time. This technique has a significantly lower complication rate than the prone position and has excellent diagnostic power with a better compliance of the patient.

In the SALP position a towel is placed under the ipsilateral shoulder and gluteus to raise the hip by an angle of 30°. The ipsilateral arm is placed over the head of the patient while the contralateral is abducted and used for intravenous perfusion. The ipsilateral leg is slightly flexed over a pillow and the contralateral one is flexed and abducted. This position provides full exposure of Petit's triangle, thus providing enough space to perform ultrasound scanning and to easily orientate the ultrasound-guided puncture toward the inferior renal pole. After shaving and draping the chosen area, an ultrasound check of the kidney is performed to determine the ideal trajectory of the needle. The identification of the lower kidney pole with ultrasounds is easy and the quality of image resolution is high. After local anesthesia, an automatic needle is ultrasound guided to the capsule on the lower pole of the kidney and fired into the renal parenchyma.

20.8 Percutaneous Renal Transplant Biopsy

The biopsy of transplanted kidney is usually easier to perform, since the graft is more superficial and easier to reach.

The graft is located on the anterior part of the lower abdomen, in the pelvis. It lays over the iliopsoas muscle and it is retroperitoneal (in case of multiple transplants, its position may be intraperitoneal).

The patient is in supine position, and the biopsy is performed after B-mode and color Doppler ultrasound study.

About the preparation of the patient, there is no difference from the biopsy of native kidney. The chosen spot is usually the upper pole of the graft, to reduce major vascular complications (damaging principal vessels of the kidney, very close to the lower pole).

In case of suspect of rejection, biopsy of different spots of the kidney is necessary, since inflammatory lesions may have a heterogeneous distribution.

20.9 Monitoring

The observation time of the patient after renal biopsy must be at least 12 h (33% of complications occur after 8 h), although monitoring the patient for more than 24 h would be safer since the complication rate within 24 h is about 91% [7].

During this period, the patient must remain enticed. In case of low back pain, abdominal pain, or sudden pressure drop it is necessary to repeat immediately a blood count and, when possible, a Doppler ultrasound and a CT scan.

Hourly monitoring of blood pressure is needed during the 6-h period after the procedure.

A check of the hemoglobin value should be performed after 4–6 h and after 24 h the renal biopsy.

A color Doppler study must be performed on the following day. The patient should be resting at home for 7 days, averting car trips and physical activity for 2 weeks.

A study involving a remarkable number of patients found that 91% of major complications occurred within 12 h of PRB, with 7.4% occurring between 12 and 24 h and 1.85% occurring after 24 h [12].

Discharging uncomplicated outpatients after a 24-h observation period after renal biopsy would be the safest choice.

20.10 Complications

Few systematic data exist to estimate the complication rate of kidney biopsy, although recently many studies have been focusing on invasive procedures (e.g., thoracentesis, central venous catheter insertion, and liver biopsy).

When evaluating whether to perform a renal biopsy, benefit/risk ratio should be weighed out.

The standard procedure for kidney biopsy involves the use of ultrasounds and an automated spring-loaded biopsy device that may be associated with lower rates of procedural complications.

Bleeding complications include asymptomatic hematomas (Fig. 20.7a, b) detected only by

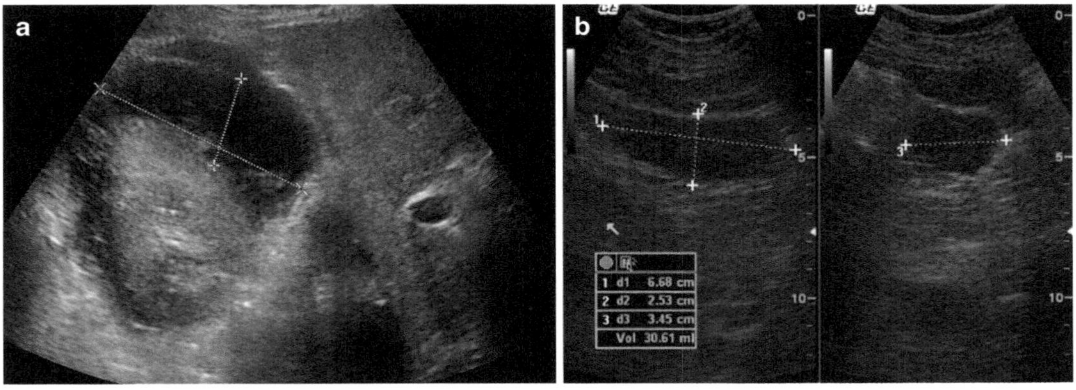

Fig. 20.7 Post-biopsy complications: hematomas could be symptomatic (**a**) or asymptomatic (**b**)

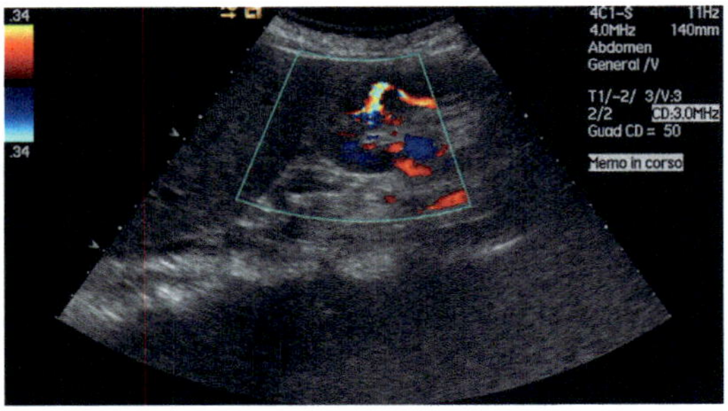

Fig. 20.8 Post-biopsy complications. FAV is often small and does not require angiographic intervention

post-biopsy ultrasound study, macroscopic hematuria, blood loss requiring erythrocyte transfusion, arteriovenous fistula (Fig. 20.8), and, rarely, complications that require angiographic intervention or nephrectomy.

A rare complication is the page kidney, caused by a large hematoma in the perinephric or subcapsular space resulting in extrinsic compression of the involved kidney, renal ischemia, activation of the renin-angiotensin-aldosterone system, and systemic hypertension [13].

Early ultrasonography performed immediately after the procedure and 1 h after the biopsy was clinically helpful in predicting the risk of major bleeding complications [14, 15].

On the other hand, a systematic use of color Doppler ultrasonography in monitoring patients after a renal biopsy is crucial for an early diagnosis of post-procedural arterio-venous fistula [16].

There is no consensus, among different studies, about the incidence of complications associated with kidney biopsy and their possible predictors, because of the presence of some biases (e.g., definition of complication, patient enrollment, procedural technique, and monitoring protocols) [7, 8].

The occurrence of post renal-biopsy bleeding complications has been systematically evaluated in a cohort of 471 patients who underwent real-time ultrasound-guided automated percutaneous renal biopsy in our single center [8].

The incidence of post renal-biopsy bleeding complications detected by systematic ultrasound and clinical examination was relatively high (34.1%), although bleeding complications were generally not relevant; only 1.2% required interventions for major complications (two cases of arterio-venous fistulas and four large hematomas). Two out of six patients required blood transfusions for relevant hemoglobin reduction and cardiovascular instability, hypotension, and tachycardia. Three patients underwent angiographic evaluation of the bleeding and Gelfoam trans-arterial catheter embolization of the lesion; one only patient underwent a surgical nephrectomy.

Clinical symptoms (discomfort or lumbar pain) were present in only a small part (2.5%) of the cohort. After evaluating several demographic, clinical, laboratory, and needle-related indicators, only gender, age, and baseline partial thromboplastin time were found to be significantly predictive of the risk of post-bioptic bleeding. This risk was greater in women and patients with higher baseline partial thromboplastin times, while, paradoxically, in older patients the risk of post-biopsy bleeding complications was significantly lower [8].

However, a phase IV randomized controlled trial on 162 patients has shown that treatment with desmopressin acetate decreases the risk of bleeding after a renal biopsy and reduces hematoma size in patients without coagulation defects [17]. Desmopressin is a synthetic derivative of vasopressin that exerts its hemostatic effects by increasing the levels of von Willebrand factor and factor VIII.

Post-biopsy bleeding was significantly less common in desmopressin-treated patients than in placebo-treated patients (13.7% vs. 30.5%, respectively). Among the 36 patients who experienced bleeding, the median hematoma size was 208 mm^2 versus 380 mm^2 in patients receiving desmopressin and placebo, respectively. Mean hospitalization duration was 1 day shorter in desmopressin-administered group than in the control one, which led to considerable cost savings. No other differences were found between the two groups in terms of secondary outcome results. The treatment caused no serious adverse events, and there were only mild side effects in three patients (a transient and nonrelevant tachycardia).

In a recent systematic review and meta-analysis, the authors aimed to evaluate the incidence of hemorrhagic complications (macroscopic hematuria and need for erythrocyte transfusion) after ultrasound-guided biopsy with automated spring-loaded biopsy device, in order to identify potential risk factors for bleeding complications [18]. Including 34 publications for the analysis was an important limitation of the review; only one of these was a randomized controlled trial, 13 studies were prospective, and 20 were retrospective. The rate of macroscopic hematuria was 3.5% and erythrocyte transfusion was 0.9%.

Significantly higher rates of transfusion were seen when using 14-gauge needles, serum creatinine level >2.0 mg/dL, female gender, acute kidney injury, mean age of 40 years or older, and mean systolic blood pressure greater than 130 mm Hg.

In conclusion, the risk of hemorrhagic complications is relatively low when the renal biopsy is ultrasound guided and performed with automated biopsy needles. However, in order to improve patient safety, the use of large-gauge needles (14 gauge) should be discouraged.

Since the prognostic value of potential risk factors is debatable, the search for more sensitive tests to assess coagulation disorders and better identify patient and procedural characteristics requires more studies in order to perform biopsy safely.

Finally, the use of desmopressin should be considered, since the only randomized controlled trial included in this review demonstrates the risk reduction of bleeding complication. This drug should be administered cautiously in patients with high thromboembolic risk.

20.11 Conclusion

The advent of ultrasound methods in interventional procedures has drastically reduced complications, especially when performing renal biopsy. This procedure, if performed by trained physicians, has a high success rate and few complications. Renal biopsy is essential for diagnosis and prognosis and nephrologists should train their fellows in order to perform renal biopsy safely.

References

1. Iversen P, Brun C. Aspiration biopsy of the kidney. Am J Med. 1951;11:324–30.
2. Kark RM, Muehrcke RC. Biopsy of kidney in prone position. Lancet. 1954;266:1047–9.
3. Fogazzi G, Cameron S. The early introduction of percutaneous renal biopsy in Italy. Kidney Int. 1999;56:1951–61.
4. Burstein DM, Korbet SM, Schwartz MM. The use of the automatic core biopsy system in percutaneous renal biopsies: a comparative study. Am J Kidney Dis. 1993;22:545–52.
5. Mai J, Yong J, Dixson H, Makris A, et al. Is bigger better? A retrospective analysis of native renal biopsies with 16 gauge versus 18 gauge automatic needles. Nephrology (Carlton). 2013;18:525–30.
6. Roth R, Parikh S, Makey D, et al. When size matters: diagnostic value of kidney biopsy according to the gauge of the biopsy needle. Am J Nephrol. 2013;37(3):249–54.
7. Whittier WL, Korbet SM. Timing of complications in percutaneous renal biopsy. J Am Soc Nephrol. 2004;15:142–7.
8. Manno C, Strippoli GFM, Arnesano L, et al. Predictors of bleeding complications in percutaneous ultrasound-guided renal biopsy. Kidney Int. 2004;66:1570–7.
9. Gesualdo L, Cormio L, Stallone G, et al. Percutaneous ultrasound-guided renal biopsy in supine antero-lateral position. Nephrol Dial Transplant. 2008;23:971–6.
10. Granata A, Floccari F, Ferrantelli A, et al. Does systematic preliminary colour Doppler study reduce kidney biopsy complication incidence? Int J Nephrol. 2011;2011:1. https://doi.org/10.4061/2011/419093.
11. Maya ID, Maddela P, Barker J, Allon M. Percutaneous renal biopsy: comparison of blind and real-time ultrasound-guided technique. Semin Dial. 2007;20:355–8.
12. Prasad N, Kumar S, Manjunath R, et al. Real-time ultrasound guided percutaneous renal biopsy with needle guide by nephrologists decreases post-biopsy complications. Clin Kidney J. 2015;8:151–6.
13. Dopson SJ, Jayakumar S, Velez JC. Page kidney as a rare cause of hypertension: case report and review of the literature. Am J Kidney Dis. 2009 Aug;54(2):334–9.
14. Waldo B, Korbet SM, Freimanis MG, et al. The value of post-biopsy ultrasound in predicting complications after percutaneous renal biopsy of native kidneys. Nephrol Dial Transplant. 2009;24:2433–9.
15. Ishikawa E, Nomura S, Hamaguchi T, et al. Ultrasonography as a predictor of overt bleeding after renal biopsy. Clin Exp Nephrol. 2009;13:325–31.
16. Rollino C, Garofalo G, Roccatello D, et al. Colour-coded Doppler sonography in monitoring native kidney biopsies. Nephrol Dial Transplant. 1994;9:1260–3.

17. Manno C, Bonifati C, Torres DD, Campobasso N, Schena FP. Desmopressin acetate in percutaneous ultrasound-guided kidney biopsy. A randomized controlled trial. Am J Kidney Dis. 2011;57:850–5.
18. Mackinnon B, Fraser E, Simpson K, Fox JG, Geddes C. Is it necessary to stop antiplatelet agents before a native renal biopsy? Nephrol Dial Transplant. 2008;23:3566–70.

21 Peritoneal Dialysis Catheter

Matthias Zeiler and Antonio Granata

Abbreviations

PD	Peritoneal dialysis
US	Ultrasound
CEUS	Contrast-enhanced ultrasound
CT	Computed tomography
MR	Magnetic resonance
EPS	Encapsulating peritoneal sclerosis

21.1 Introduction

Peritoneal dialysis (PD) is an established outpatient treatment method for end-stage renal disease. In contrast to hemodialysis PD offers more freedom and independence of therapy corresponding to higher quality of life, especially in younger and independent patients. In order to perform PD, a flexible silastic Teflon tube with up to two Dacron cuffs is inserted in a curved manner subcutaneously through the rectus muscle. The external cuff should be placed at least 2 cm from the exit site, whereas the inner cuff in the rectus muscle close to the internal muscular fascia and peritoneum. The cuffs fix the catheter to the surrounding tissue by a foreign body reaction, thus immobilizing the catheter and creating a barrier against the spreading of infection along the catheter. The catheter can be divided into three functional parts: the external part from the skin exit side to the external cuff, the subcutaneous tunnel between the external and internal cuff, and the intra-abdominal part. The intraperitoneal part of the catheter might be configured in a straight or curled manner, and has numerous side holes in order to facilitate a rapid dialysis fluid exchange. The distal end of the PD catheter is placed in the lower abdomen for optimal drainage of the dialysis fluid [1].

The use of ultrasound (US) in PD started in the late 1980s [2]. The catheter is visualized always in a transverse and longitudinal scan with linear or convex transducers of at least 5–7 MHz (Figs. 21.1 and 21.2). The Dacron cuff appears as a hyper-echoic tissue around the catheter with posterior acoustic shadow (Fig. 21.3). The catheter itself is represented as a double-binary structure in the longitudinal scan, thus representing the anterior outer surface, anterior inner surface, posterior inner surface, and posterior outer surface of the catheter (Fig. 21.4). The side holes of the catheter can be visualized as incisions or irregularities of the outer surface of the catheter in the case of a direction parallel to the transducer (Fig. 21.5), or as tagged hyper-echoic reflections in the case of oblique direction to the transducer (Fig. 21.6). The evaluation of complications in

M. Zeiler (✉)
Nephrology and Dialysis Unit, "Carlo Urbani" Hospital, Jesi, Italy

A. Granata
Department of Nephrology and Dialysis, "Cannizzaro" Emergency Hospital, Catania, Italy

A. Granata, M. Bertolotto (eds.), *Imaging in Nephrology*, https://doi.org/10.1007/978-3-030-60794-4_21

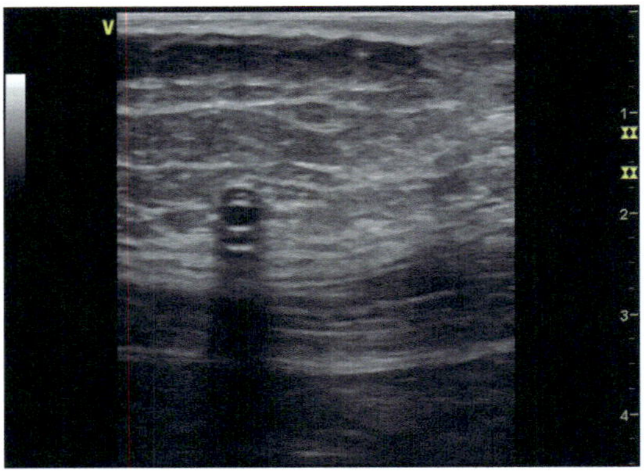

Fig. 21.1 Normal subcutaneous tunnel of the peritoneal catheter without hypo-echoic rim around the catheter in transverse view

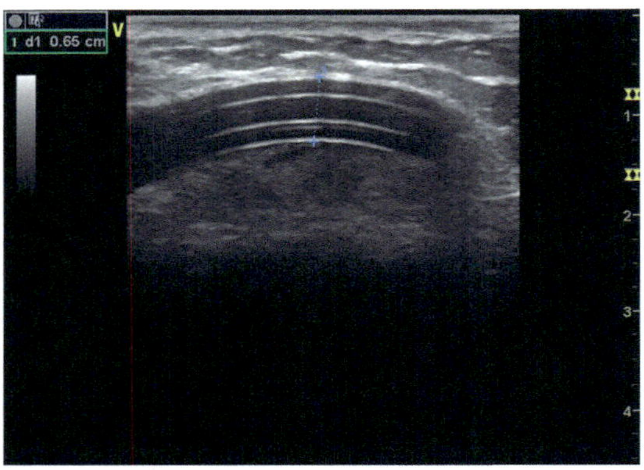

Fig. 21.2 Normal subcutaneous tunnel of the peritoneal catheter without hypo-echoic rim around the catheter in longitudinal view. The diameter of the catheter is indicated

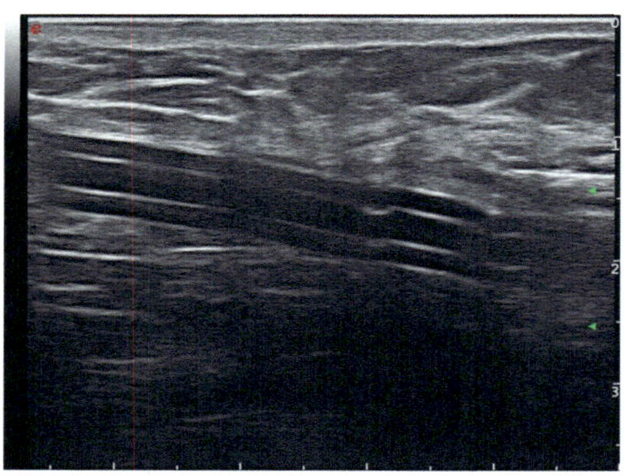

Fig. 21.3 Dacron cuff of the peritoneal catheter with posterior ultrasound shadow in longitudinal view

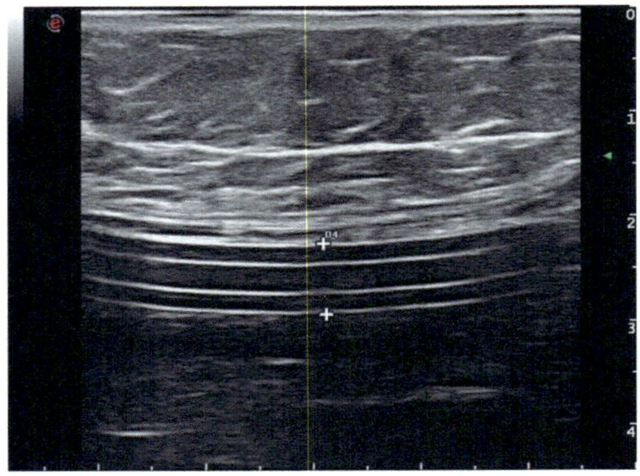

Fig. 21.4 Intraperitoneal tract of the peritoneal catheter in longitudinal view. The catheter follows the anterior abdominal wall

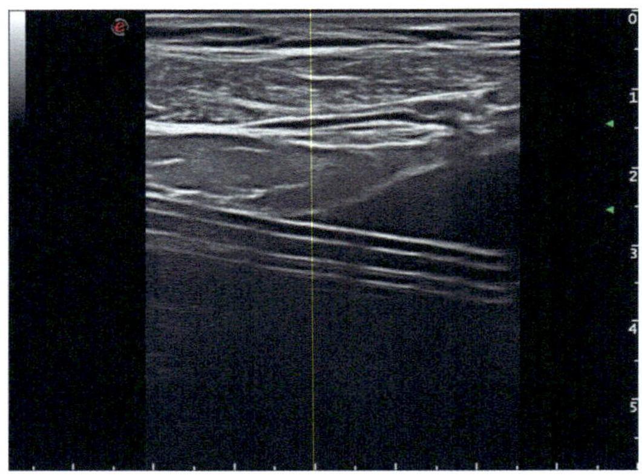

Fig. 21.5 Intraperitoneal tract of the peritoneal catheter. The irregularity of the catheter contour is caused by the catheter side holes

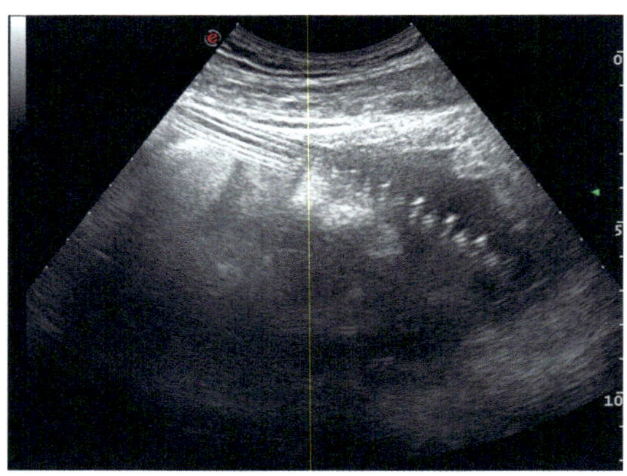

Fig. 21.6 Intraperitoneal tract of the peritoneal catheter with the tip in the lower abdomen. The irregularity of the catheter contour, as tagged hyper-echoic reflections, is caused by the catheter side holes

PD is mostly completed by catheterography or fluoroscopy [3], computed tomography (CT) with or without peritoneography [4–6], and magnetic resonance (MR) peritoneography [7–8].

21.2 Catheter-Related Infections

Scientific interest was focusing on the evaluation by US of the exit site and subcutaneous tunnel tract of the catheter in patients with catheter-related infection already in the late 1980s [2, 9–15]. An infection of the exit side presents as redness with or without secretion. Often, the mere clinical examination is inadequate to exclude an infection of the Dacron cuff or the subcutaneous tunnel in the early stage of infection [11]. Initially, US was utilized only in B-mode with linear transducers of at least 7 MHz. The aim of these studies was to correlate the outcome of the peritoneal catheter, with endpoints like catheter removal due to persistent infection or peritonitis, and due to US signs of inflammation at the subcutaneous tunnel. The US sign of inflammation taken into consideration was the thickness of the hypo-echoic rim around the peritoneal catheter or the cuff, respecting edema formation, of at least 1 mm thickness (Fig. 21.7) [12, 13]. By this way it is possible to differentiate between infection of the exit site without external cuff involvement, infection of the subcutaneous tunnel with involvement of the superficial cuff, and infection of abdominal wall abscesses or infection of the deep cuff embedded in the rectus muscle (Figs. 21.8 and 21.9). A frequency of every 2 weeks was proposed for follow-up measurement of the hypo-echoic rim thickness, beginning from clinical signs of infection or from start of antibiotic therapy [12]. The reduction of the hypo-echoic rim thickness is associated with technical catheter survival and reduction of peritonitis risk. Frequently, after healing of exit site, cuff, or tunnel infection, there will remain a hypo-echoic rim of less than 1 mm thickness around the catheter (Fig. 21.10). On the other

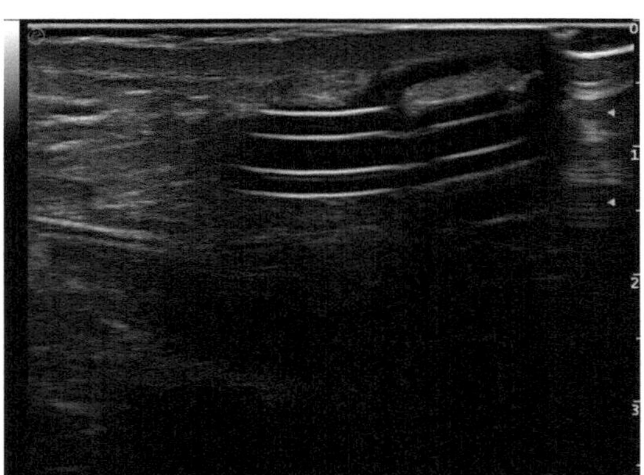

Fig. 21.7 Infection of the external Dacron cuff. Hypo-echoic rim around the cuff of the catheter in the subcutaneous tissue with thickness of more than 1 mm

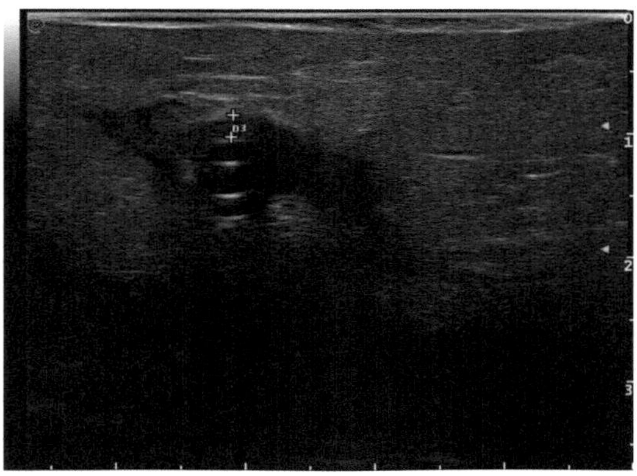

Fig. 21.8 Infection of the subcutaneous tunnel of the catheter. Hypo-echoic rim around the subcutaneous tunnel in the subcutaneous tissue with thickness of more than 1 mm and infiltration laterally to the catheter

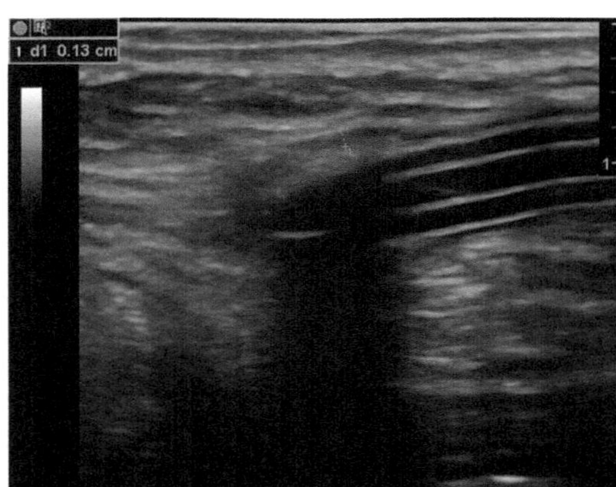

Fig. 21.9 Infection of the deep internal Dacron cuff of the catheter. Hypo-echoic rim around the cuff of the catheter with thickness of more than 1 mm. The Dacron cuff generates a posterior ultrasound shadow

hand, catheters which have never experienced an infection might not present a hypo-echoic rim around the catheter (Fig. 21.2). An additional US sign of inflammation in B-mode is the reduction of sharpness or blurring of the surrounding tissue (Fig. 21.11).

Hypervascularization associated to inflammation precedes hypo-echoic rim formation, thus having the potential of anticipating the diagnosis of catheter-related infections (Fig. 21.12). Nowadays, not only B-mode but also color Doppler US should be utilized for examination of the exit site, cuffs, and subcutaneous tunnel [16]. Power Doppler is more sensitive than color-flow

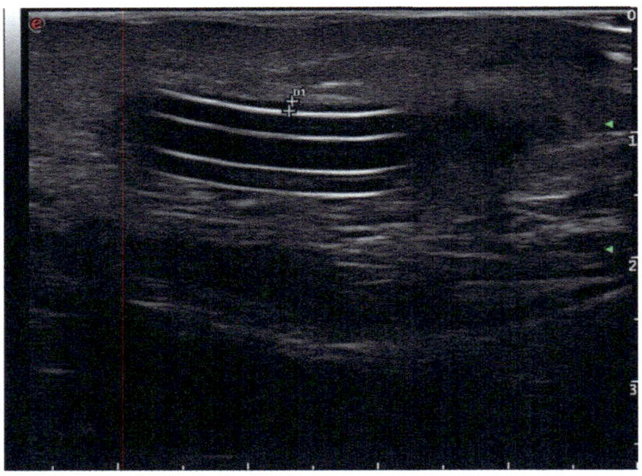

Fig. 21.10 Resolution of infection of the subcutaneous tunnel. The hypo-echoic rim at the anterior side of the catheter is reduced to less than 1 mm thickness after antibiotic treatment

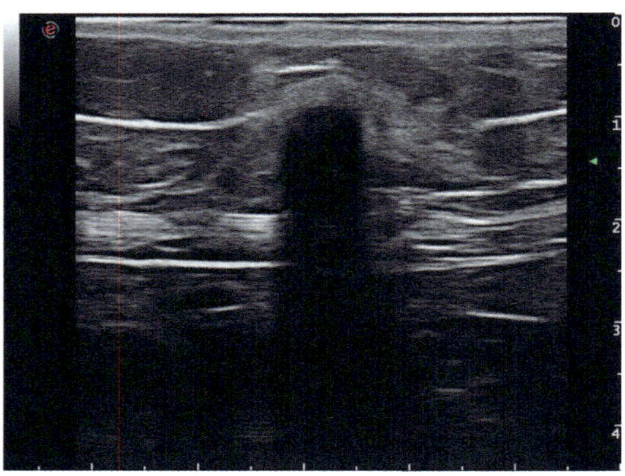

Fig. 21.11 Infection of the external Dacron cuff of the catheter. Blurring of the surrounding subcutaneous tissue in early stage of cuff infection

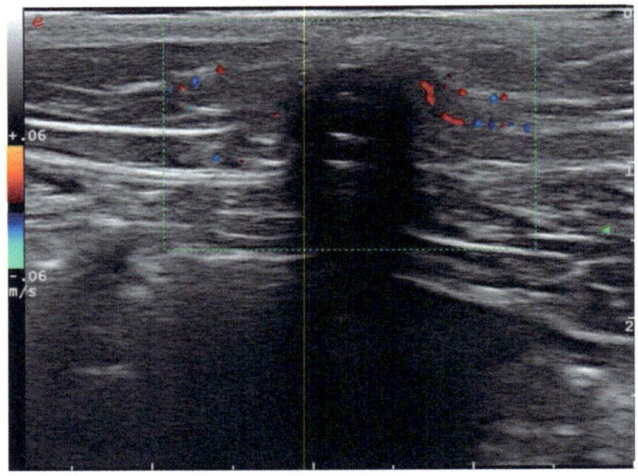

Fig. 21.12 Infection of the external Dacron cuff of the catheter. Blurring of the surrounding subcutaneous tissue in the absence of a hypo-echoic rim formation. Color Doppler evidences local hypervascularization

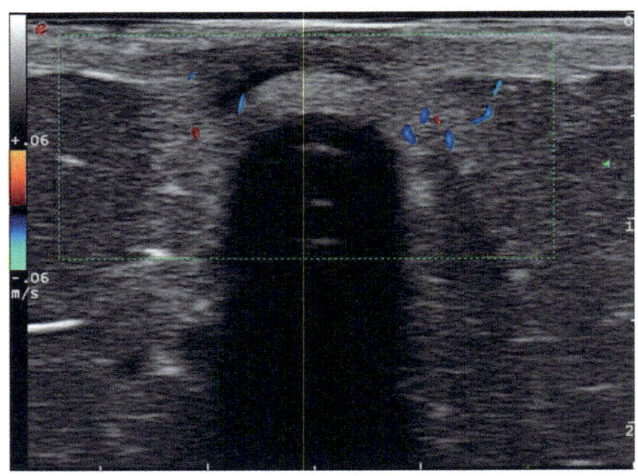

Fig. 21.13 Infection of the external Dacron cuff of the catheter. Hypo-echoic rim formation at the external Dacron cuff of the catheter. Color Doppler evidences local hypervascularization

Doppler in the evaluation of tissue hypervascularization associated to inflammation (Figs. 21.13 and 21.14). The quantification of the Doppler signal, in order to overcome the user dependence, remains a problem to be resolved in the future. In rheumatology, an image analysis counting the pixel quantity was proposed for follow-up examinations in arthritis [17]. Treatment success of catheter-related infections is reflected by the reduction of edema and Doppler signal quantity. Often, Doppler signals persist for longer time, even after the regression of the pericatheter hypo-echoic rim.

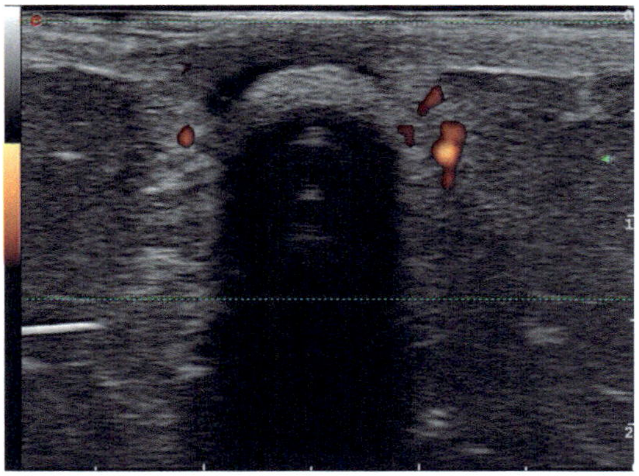

Fig. 21.14 Infection of the external Dacron cuff of the catheter. Hypo-echoic rim formation at the external Dacron cuff of the catheter (same patient as in Fig. 21.13). Power Doppler amplifies the perception of local hypervascularization

Table 21.1 Differential diagnosis of Doppler US and B-mode signs at the peritoneal catheter

	Doppler US positive	Doppler US negative
Hypo-echoic rim >1 mm Around the catheter	Ongoing infection Trauma (major entity) Recent catheter placement Leakage	
Hypo-echoic rim <1 mm Around the catheter	Subclinical infection Infection in regression Trauma (minor entity)	Normal condition Absence of infection or trauma

The possible combination of US signs (hypo-echoic rim and Doppler signals) and respective differential diagnoses is summarized in Table 21.1.

Main therapeutic strategies in PD catheter-related infections are [1]:

- Local antiseptic and antibiotic therapy for circumscribed exit-site infections.
- Systemic antibiotic therapy for tunnel and cuff infections.
- Surgical removal of the external cuff ("cuff shaving" procedure) under systemic antibiotic therapy in the case of persistence of infection at the external cuff, but absence of subcutaneous tunnel infection: This procedure can be combined with catheter splicing and partial replacement with configuration of a new tunnel and exit site.
- Surgical removal of the entire catheter including the Dacron cuffs under systemic antibiotic therapy in the case of persisting tunnel infection, deep cuff infection, peritonitis, or abdominal wall abscess.

Thus, US is helpful in the planning of a targeted therapeutic approach.

21.3 Peritoneal Catheter Malfunction

Peritoneal catheter malfunction, due to insufficient or absent dialysis fluid inflow or outflow, can be evaluated by several imaging methods utilizing classically abdomen X-ray, CT, and catheter fluoroscopy [3, 18–20]. Abdomen X-ray as well as computed tomography evidence intra-abdominal catheter position and distribution of gas and feces. Catheter fluoroscopy or catheterography has certain diagnostic importance as this technique can be combined directly with interventional procedures like flexible guidewire or stiff wire manipulations in the presence of catheter dislocation or omental wrapping [21–28]. Only recently US has been gaining application in the evaluation of catheter malfunction such as catheter localization, catheter occlusion by thrombus, adherences, omental wrapping, erroneous catheter placement, and catheter kinking in the subcutaneous tract [29–32].

In order to improve the distinction of the PD catheter from the surrounding tissue, the peritoneal cavity should be filled, if possible, with dialysis fluid of at least 1 L in adults. In pediatric patients evaluation of causes of catheter malfunction is facilitated by the limited profundity of structures, and thus the examination can be performed without filling of the abdominal space. Evaluation of the catheter position by US might replace abdomen X-ray. A good agreement between US and X-ray for the detection of the

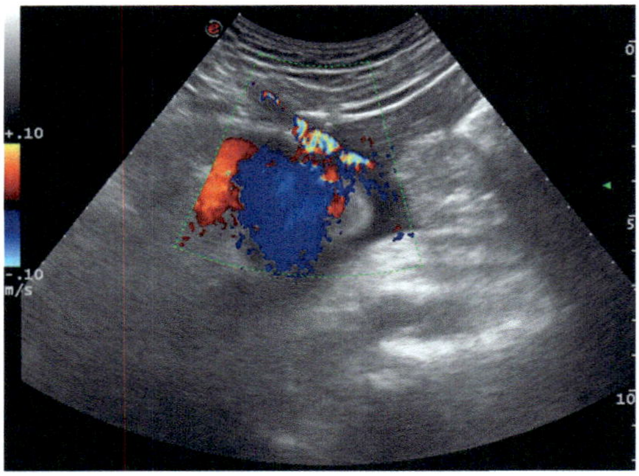

Fig. 21.15 Functional testing of the catheter by color Doppler. Color Doppler flow generated by forced injection of dialysis fluid through the catheter demonstrating absence of obstruction

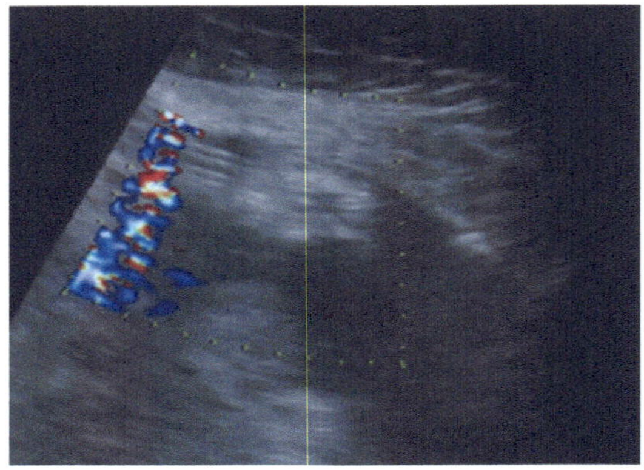

Fig. 21.16 Functional testing of a catheter by color Doppler. Malfunction by omental wrapping documented by the absence of Doppler flow signals at the distal part of the catheter and by the presence of adhesion of hyperechoic tissue around the catheter

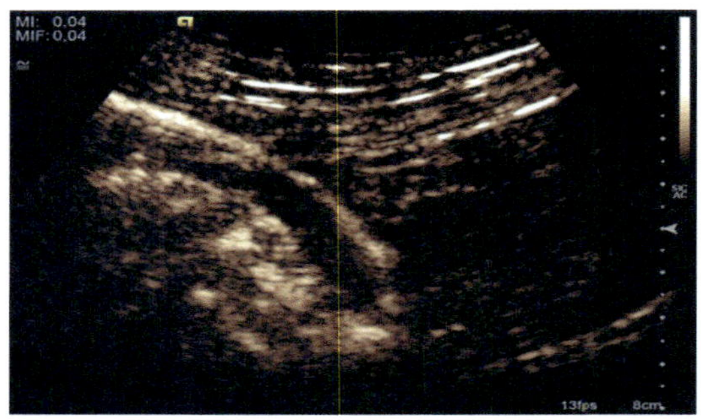

Fig. 21.17 Functional testing of a catheter by CEUS. Malfunction by omental wrapping documented by the absence of CEUS signals around the distal part of the catheter and normal inflow of contrast media quite up to the tip of the catheter

catheter in the inferior abdominopelvic regions has been reported in patients presenting catheter malfunction [30]. Radiographies could be reserved to patients in which the catheter cannot be well visualized by US, such as in the presence of severe obesity, meteorism, or missing patient collaboration, when a fecal impaction is suspected or in the presence of curled catheter.

Catheter function is evaluated classically by fluoroscopy. The inflow and the intraperitoneal distribution of the contrast agent are evidencing causes of catheter malfunction. Catheter function can also be evaluated dynamically by color Doppler [31] or contrast-enhanced ultrasound (CEUS) [30]. Color Doppler utilizes dialysis fluid or saline as a signal-generating agent. Therefore by gravity, compression on the dialysis bag, or injection with a syringe, dialysis fluid is forced inside the catheter (Fig. 21.15). A higher than normal flow rate is needed to increase the amount of signals to be acquired as the dialysis fluid does not contain Doppler effect-enhancing particles despite some microscopic air bubbles. Shaking of the dialysis fluid, thus generating microscopic air bubbles, increases the Doppler signal quantity. Absence of Doppler signals at the side holes of the peritoneal catheter corresponds to occlusion. In the case of adhesions or omental wrapping, fatlike tissue attached to the catheter is documented together with absence of Doppler signals in the affected zone (Fig. 21.16). CEUS bypasses the disadvantage of signal generation by the direct injection of ultrasound contrast agent [33–35] (Fig. 21.17). In contrast to color Doppler US utilizing dialysis fluid or saline, the intraperitoneal application of ultrasound contrast agent actually is classified as an off-label procedure.

21.4 Leakage and Defects of the Peritoneal Wall

Leakage of the peritoneal fluid into the subcutaneous tissue is a known complication in PD during the first month after catheter placement or other surgical interventions. Clinically, leakage can be suspected in the case of subcutaneous edema and inflammatory signs with orange peel skin or in the case of liquid discharge at the exit site during PD. US of the abdominal wall confirms the presence of subcutaneous edema by hypo-echoic bands in B-mode and local inflammation by hypervascularization in Doppler [36] (Figs. 21.18 and 21.19). Often it is possible to demonstrate the origin of leakage like small abdominal wall defects or incomplete surgical wound healing. Leakage along the catheter originating directly from the peritoneal entrance site is evidenced by a hypo-echoic rim around the subcutaneous tunnel (Fig. 21.20). CT peritoneography, with intraperitoneal ionic contrast media of 60–100 mL in 2 L of dialysate, evidences the leakage of contrast media into subcutaneous tissue in late scans or after an overnight dialysate rest [37, 38]. In the suspicion of a retroperitoneal leakage of dialysis fluid a CT peritoneography or a T2-weighted MR peritoneography, utilizing the presence of dialysate as contrast media, should be performed [39, 40].

Defects of the continuity of the abdominal wall, such as umbilical hernia, incisional hernia, and inguinal or scrotal hernia, can be diagnosed easily by US (Figs. 21.21 and 21.22). Due to the increased intra-abdominal pressure during PD

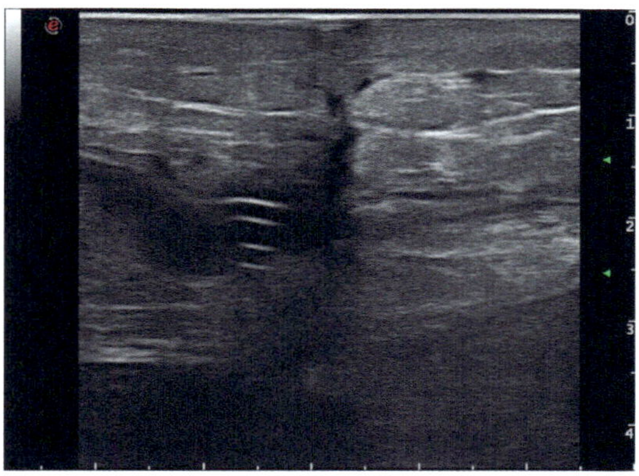

Fig. 21.18 Leakage of peritoneal dialysis fluid into the subcutaneous tissue. Dialysis fluid exits from the peritoneal cavity along the surgical incision, documented by the presence of hypo-echoic bands. The patient presents local pain

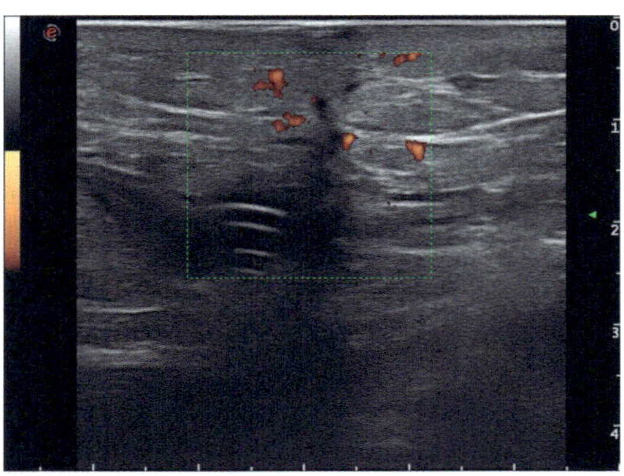

Fig. 21.19 Leakage of peritoneal dialysis fluid into the subcutaneous tissue. Power Doppler evidences local hypervascularization (same patient as in Fig. 21.18)

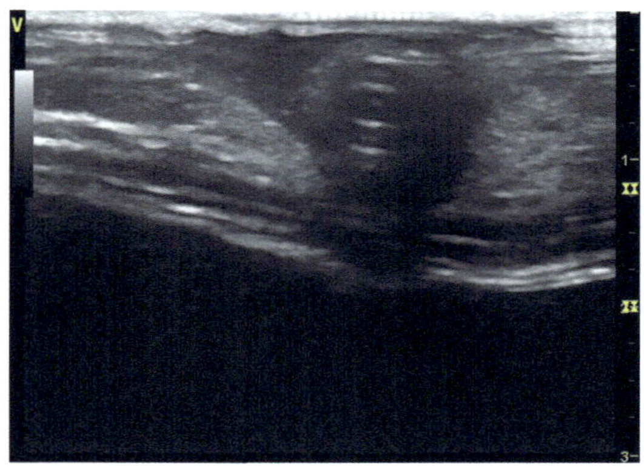

Fig. 21.20 Leakage of peritoneal dialysis fluid. Dialysis fluid exits around the deep internal Dacron cuff of the catheter, and thus the Dacron cuff "floats" in a hypo-echoic effusion

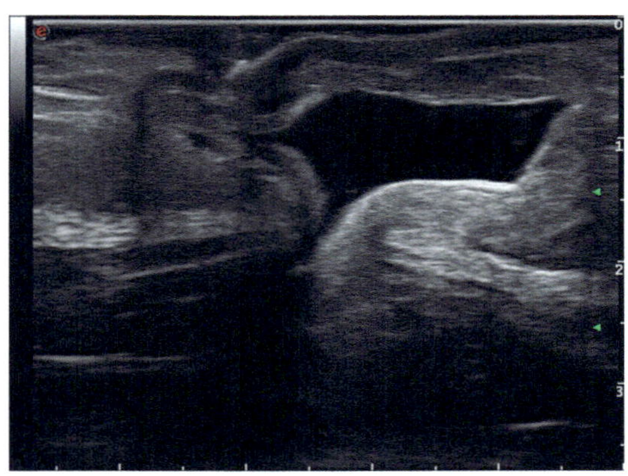

Fig. 21.21 Umbilical hernia. Hernia sac in the subcutaneous tissue filled with dialysis fluid

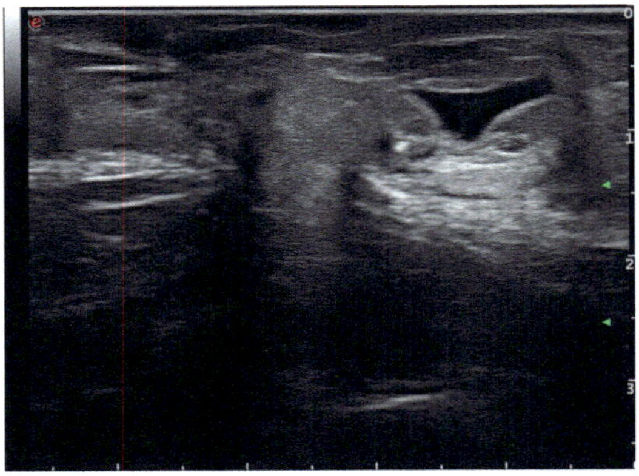

Fig. 21.22 Umbilical hernia. Herniation of omental tissue into the umbilical hernia sac provoked by augmented intra-abdominal pressure (same patient as in Fig. 21.21)

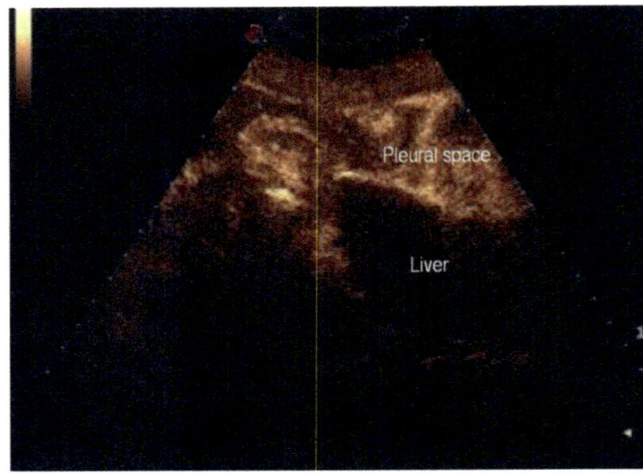

Fig. 21.23 Pleuroperitoneal defect resulting in pleural effusion in a peritoneal dialysis patient. CEUS evidences the migration of contrast agent from the peritoneal cavity to the pleural space (by courtesy of Michele Principe MD, San Giovanni Rotondo, Italy)

therapy these defects have a tendency to increase by time [41]. A feared complication is the irreversible incarceration of fat tissue or intestinal structures in the herniation sac. Reduction or absence of Doppler signals in the entrapped tissue indicates hypoperfusion or necrosis. In the preoperative management, US is more helpful in the case of smaller circumscribed defects, whereas CT in the case of larger defects.

Peritoneal-pleural defects cause symptomatic hydrothorax in PD patients. From a simple clinical point, a high glucose concentration (>500 mg/dl) of the pleural fluid already indicates the presence of glucose-containing PD fluid. Peritoneal scintigraphy with Tc-99 m DTPA or Tc-99 m sulfur colloid is useful in the evaluation of all kind of hernias including pleuroperitoneal communications in PD patients [42, 43]. Alternatively, CT or MR peritoneography can be performed, in the same manner as used for the evaluation of leakage [44–46]. Even CEUS can be used for peritoneal-pleural defects as this method evidences the migration of US contrast agent from the peritoneal cavity into the affected pleural space (Fig. 21.23) [47, 48].

21.5 Peritoneal Adherences

Screening for peritoneal adherences is useful in patients with preceding multiple abdominal interventions. The prevalence of adherences correlates to the number of previous interventions or peritonitis episodes. The risk of an intestinal lesion at surgical catheter placement, and at surgical revision for catheter malfunction, increases in the presence of intra-abdominal adhesions. Multiple extensive adherences are often associated to incomplete outflow of dialysis fluid or to catheter malfunction due to compartmentalization of the peritoneal cavity. US evaluates the "sliding viscera sign," defined as the movement of the viscera against the anterior abdominal wall during respiration of at least 1 cm extension [49–52]. This simple US sign excludes the presence of adherences. The importance of static examination techniques like computed tomography (CT) and magnetic resonance (MR) is restricted. They might evidence only extensive adherences in the presence of dialysate or ascites. The technique of motion signature analysis in dynamic cinematographic MR for abdominal adhesions is under development [53].

21.6 Prevention of Inferior Epigastric Artery Lesion

A lesion of the inferior epigastric artery is a feared complication during catheter percutaneous placement or removal [54]. The inferior epigastric artery originates from the external iliac artery forming by the superior epigastric artery

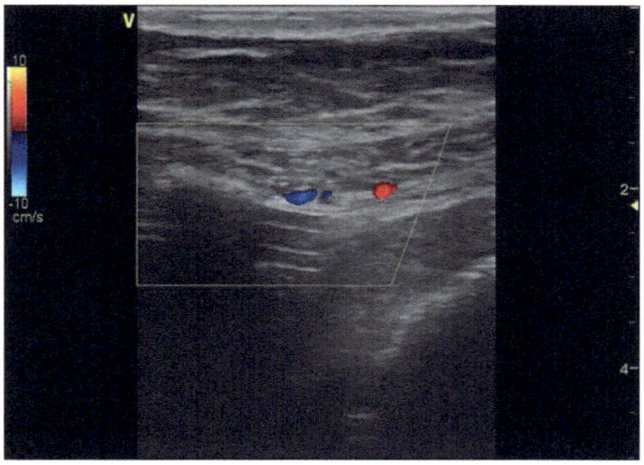

Fig. 21.24 Inferior epigastric artery. Course of the artery close to the deep internal Dacron cuff of the catheter evidenced by color Doppler

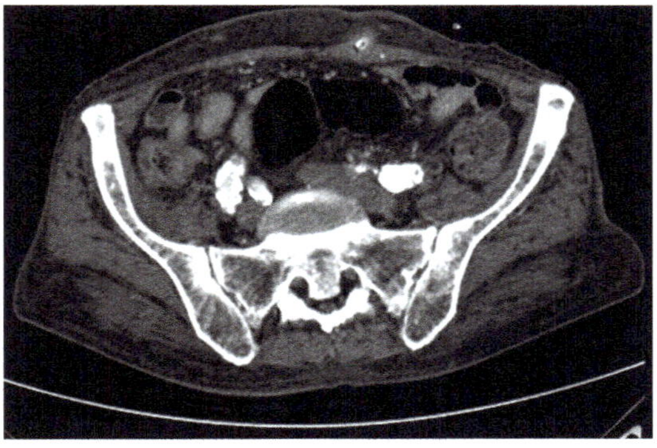

Fig. 21.25 Inferior epigastric artery. Course of the artery close to the deep internal Dacron cuff of the catheter in computed tomography. Presence of contrast enhancement around the catheter due to infection

an anastomosis with the internal thoracic artery [55]. This artery bypasses the periumbilical zone at the posterior side of the rectus muscle. This zone is usually used for the placement of the peritoneal catheter (Figs. 21.24 and 21.25). Especially at peritoneal catheter removal, in the presence of fibrotic scar tissue and local inflammation, a prior localization of the inferior epigastric artery by Doppler US is helpful to reduce the risk of inferior epigastric artery lesion. The course of the inferior epigastric artery is evidenced by color Doppler US and marked on the skin surface utilizing a colored pen.

21.7 Catheter Placement

The placement of the PD catheter across the abdominal wall can be performed by several techniques [1]: classic open surgery, video laparoscopic assisted procedure, and fluoroscopic or US-guided placement. US controls the subcutaneous and trans-muscular tunneling avoiding lesion of the inferior epigastric artery and erroneous placement of the deep catheter cuff. Under US control, a 21-gauge needle is inserted across the subcutaneous tissue and the rectus muscle into the abdominal space at an angulation of 45° with caudal direction. A guidewire is inserted through the needle into the peritoneal cavity followed by removal of the puncture needle. The guidewire serves as a guide for the introduction of tissue dilatators. To complete the procedure, the PD catheter is inserted across a peel-away sheath. US confirms the correct placement of the internal catheter cuff outside of the peritoneal cavity and the correct direction of the catheter to the lower abdominopelvic regions [56–59]. US-guided placement should be preferred to fluoroscopy alone, as it enables a direct view of the subcutaneous and trans-muscular structures during placement; furthermore it identifies vascular structures and local parietal adherences and avoids cuff malplacement [60]. Percutaneous catheter placement using a combination of ultrasound and fluoroscopy seems to be safe even in patients with prior abdominal surgeries [61].

21.8 Peritoneal Thickening

Peritoneal dialysis leads to a progressive thickening of the peritoneum [62, 63]. The thickness of the parietal peritoneum correlates with the transport status of the peritoneal membrane [64]. A thicker membrane reflects a faster peritoneal transport type classified by the quotient of dialysate versus plasma creatinine (D/P creatinine) during the 4-h peritoneal dialysis equilibration test. The maximal thickness of the parietal peritoneum is documented utilizing a linear transducer

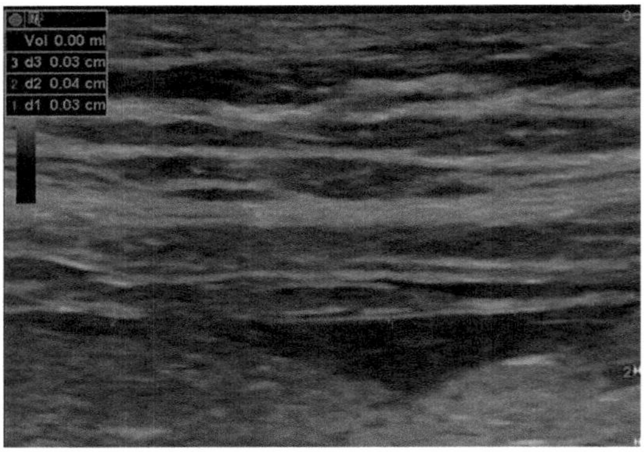

Fig. 21.26 Peritoneal thickness. Parietal peritoneum in a patient after 22 months of peritoneal dialysis

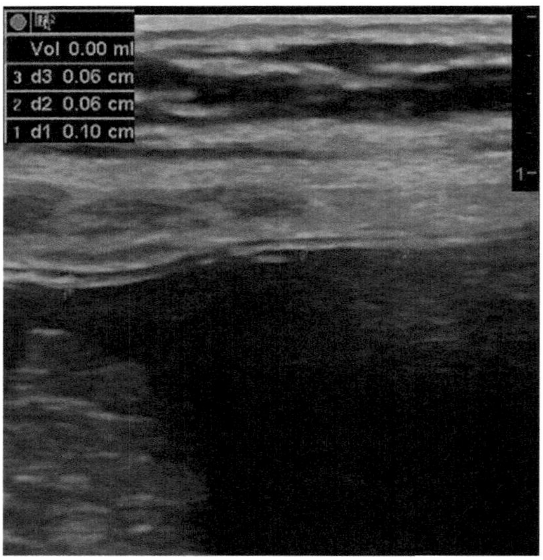

Fig. 21.27 Peritoneal thickness. Parietal peritoneum in a patient after 8 years of peritoneal dialysis. The subcutaneous tissue appears to be reduced and transformed in hypoechoic bands

of at least 10 MHz placed longitudinally in at least three different abdominal quadrants after having filled the abdominal cavity with dialysis fluid of at least 1 L (Figs. 21.26 and 21.27). The mean thickness of the peritoneum in adults performing PD for less than 2 years is between 0.44 and 0.65 mm, whereas in patients performing PD for more than 2 years mean peritoneal thickness is between 0.41 and 0.93 mm. In the inferior abdominopelvic regions there will be, on one side, a higher variability of thickness, but also a tendency of increased peritoneal thickening in contrast to upper umbilical regions. In children peritoneal thickness is correlated not only to the peritoneal transport status but also to body height, body mass index, duration of PD, and number of peritonitis episodes [65]. Thus, evaluation of peritoneal thickness by US cannot substitute a peritoneal equilibration test, but will evidence the tendency of progressive peritoneal-mesenchymal transformation for each patient.

21.9 Intraperitoneal Cyst or Abscess Formation

Frequent peritonitis episodes accelerate the thickening of the peritoneal membrane, but also favor the formation of intraperitoneal cysts like pseudocysts or mesenteric cysts [66–69]. The US aspect is variable between simple cyst and complicated cyst with a thick capsule and internal septa, in relation to the histopathological origin (Fig. 21.28). US is a complementary examination in contrast to CT (Fig. 21.29) and MR [70], but seems to be helpful in the follow-up of smaller cystic lesions [71].

Abdominal abscesses as a consequence of peritonitis might develop in about 1% of peritonitis episodes. Clinical symptoms like persisting

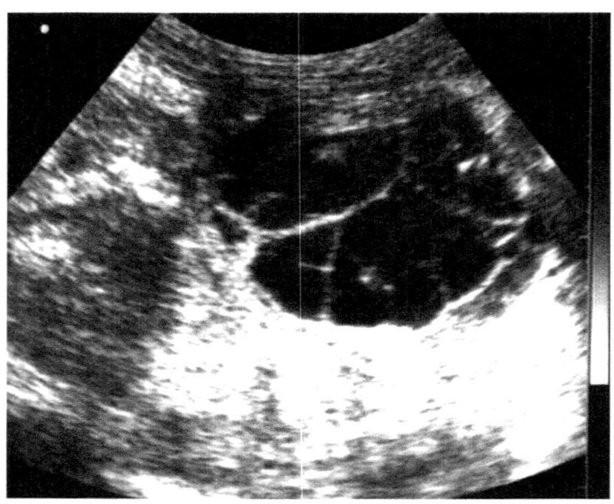

Fig. 21.28 Intraperitoneal cyst formation. Poly-septated cyst attached to the anterior abdominal wall in a patient with multiple peritonitis episodes. Histology confirmed a mesenteric cyst

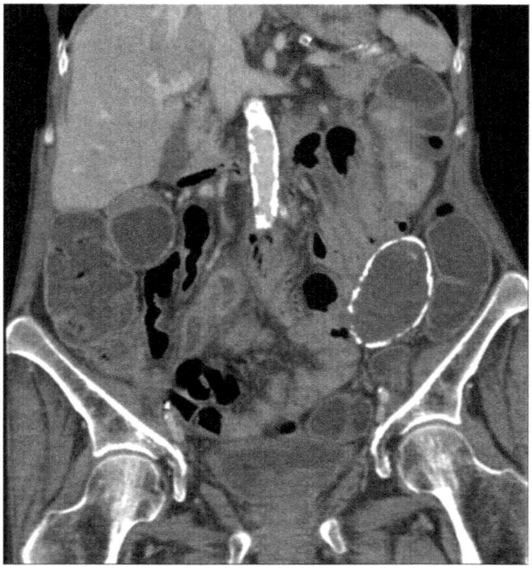

Fig. 21.29 Reconstruction in the coronal plane of a CT examination of the abdomen evidencing an intraperitoneal calcified cyst in the left lower abdomen in a patient with multiple peritonitis episodes. At CT examination the patient presented signs of intestinal occlusion

abdominal pain, fever, inappetence, and inflammatory signs despite appropriate antibiotic therapy might be indicative of abscess formation. Even in this case US is only a complementary examination to CT and MR [72].

21.10 Intestinal Perforation

Patients presenting with cloudy effluent and abdominal pain are presumed to have peritonitis. An intestinal perforation causing peritonitis is a feared complication in PD. Clinically, perforation can be suspected in patients who are presenting signs of severe infection and insufficient response to antibiotic therapy. Drainage of air during peritoneal dialysis confirms the clinical suspect. Perforation is mostly associated to diverticulitis in lesser part to catheter decubitus with bowel erosion. An upright abdomen or thorax X-ray might show air under the diaphragm (Figs. 21.30 and 21.31). In the lateral view of the abdomen in supine position the examiner should

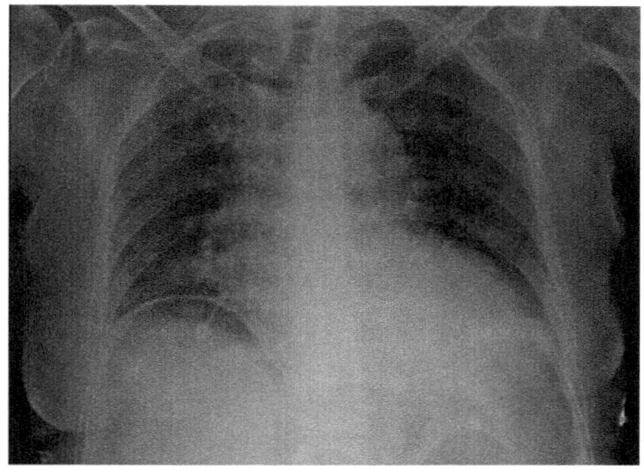

Fig. 21.30 Thorax radiography in a peritoneal dialysis patient with intestinal perforation. Air under the diaphragm on the right side

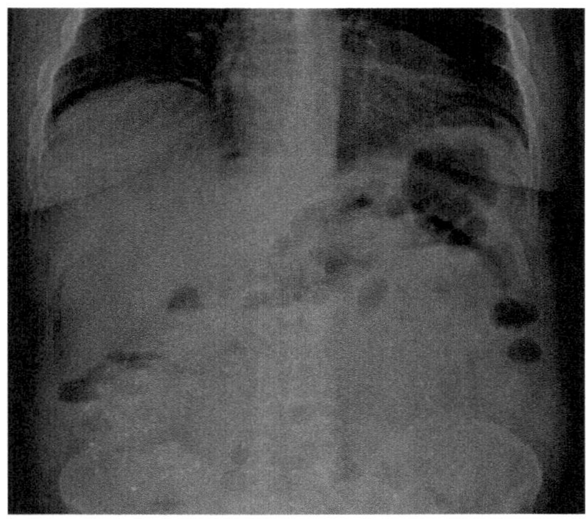

Fig. 21.31 Abdomen radiography in supine position in a peritoneal dialysis patient with intestinal perforation. Air under the diaphragm on both sides, intestinal air levels due to intestinal paralysis. Traces of lanthanum carbonate in the intestine

differentiate between intestinal air levels and free air bubbles. The accuracy of radiography depends mainly on the quantity of free air in the abdomen. CT is more sensitive than radiography and US [73, 74] (Figs. 21.32 and 21.33). Furthermore, CT examination is helpful in localizing the presumed origin of perforation (Fig. 21.34). On the other hand, air under the diaphragm in PD patients without peritonitis signs is mainly due to faulty bag exchange procedures [75].

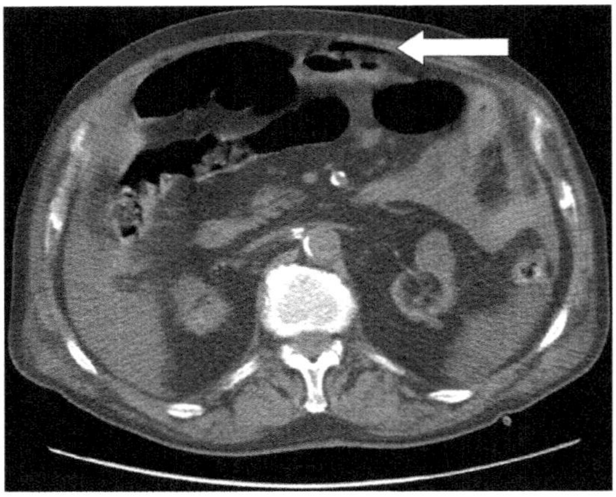

Fig. 21.32 CT examination of the abdomen in a peritoneal dialysis patient with intestinal perforation presenting free air under the anterior abdominal wall (white arrow), not visible in the lateral radiography of the abdomen

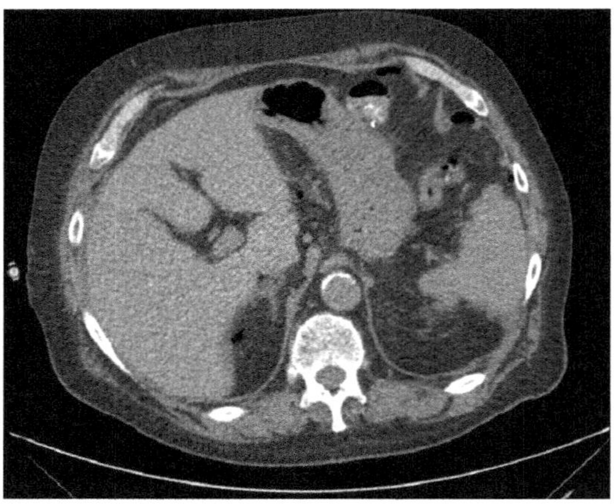

Fig. 21.33 CT examination of the abdomen in a peritoneal dialysis patient with intestinal perforation presenting multiple small free air accumulations. The abdominal radiography was negative

21.11 Encapsulating Peritoneal Sclerosis

Encapsulating peritoneal sclerosis (EPS) is a condition of progressive fibrotic peritoneal thickening, due to inflammatory peritoneal-mesenchymal transformation and vascular endothelial cell injury, which encapsulates intestinal loops causing initially unspecific clinical symptoms, such as inappetence, weight loss,

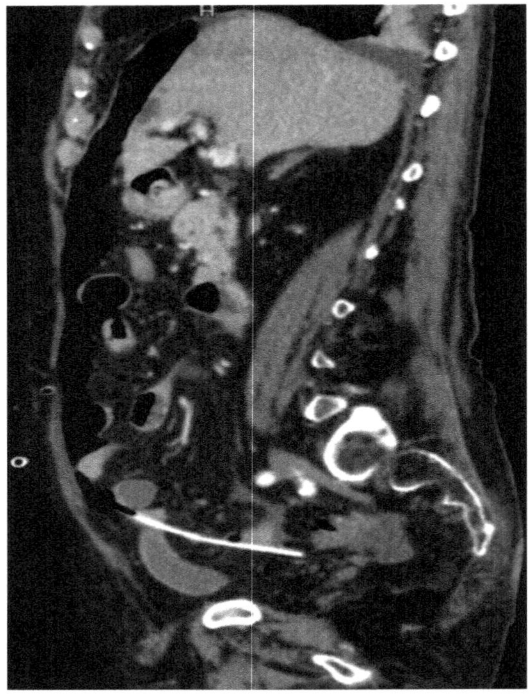

Fig. 21.34 Reconstruction in paramedian sagittal plane of a CT examination of the abdomen in a peritoneal dialysis patient with intestinal perforation. Extensive free air accumulation under the anterior abdominal wall. Air bubbles along the peritoneal dialysis catheter in the pelvic cavity indicating the origin of the perforation in the posterior region of the pelvis

altered bowel habit, and bloody dialysis fluid, up to symptomatic intestinal occlusion due to fibrous cocoon formation in advanced stages [76–78]. The ongoing inflammation results in corpusculated dialysate, intra-abdominal fibrin septa, adherences, intraperitoneal compartmentalization, and peritoneal calcifications. Long-term PD patients with frequent peritonitis episodes developing ultrafiltration failure are at high risk of EPS. Further risk factors developing EPS are acute cessation of PD, organ transplantation, high glucose concentration of dialysis fluid, and young patient age. US and CT are mainly applied when EPS is suspected [79–90] (Fig. 21.35). A normal US or CT does not exclude the development of EPS in the future; thus screening for EPS in asymptomatic patients without ultrafiltration failure is not recommended [83, 85, 88]. CT with endovenous contrast media and abdomen filled

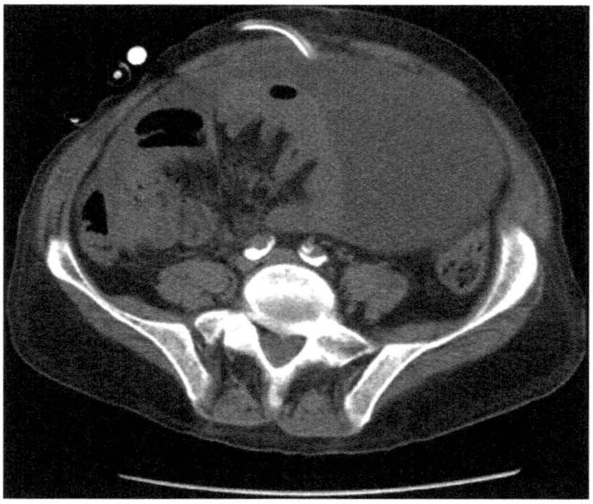

Fig. 21.35 Encapsulating peritoneal sclerosis. Presence of adherent bowel loops, bowel tethering, and air-fluid levels in bowel loops at CT examination

with dialysis fluid is the reference method when EPS is suspected and for disease monitoring. Nevertheless, the inter-observer agreement regarding CT findings of EPS is very variable [83, 84]. The signs of EPS detectable by the different radiological methods are summarized in Table 21.2. There are few studies regarding MR imaging in EPS [91]. The findings in MR are similar to CT (Fig. 21.36). A dynamic cinematographic MR coupled with advanced image analysis, which evaluates the propagation of abdominal motion, was proposed in EPS patients [92]. EPS-affected patients presented a normal movement only under the diaphragm, but no propagation into the lower abdomen. Up to now, the essential diagnostic elements in EPS are the combination of clinical and CT findings.

21.12 Conclusions and Outlook

Ultrasound is extremely useful in the ambulatory management of PD patients. The major part of complications in PD can be evaluated by US, Doppler US, or CEUS. The high spatial resolution and the capacity of analysis of complex three-dimensional structures by US are limited by a reduced accuracy in deep or extensive structures, or structures containing calcifications or gas. Doppler US is helpful in anticipating diag-

Table 21.2 Imaging techniques and findings in EPS

Imaging technique	Findings in EPS
Abdominal X-ray	Dilated small bowel loops Air-fluid levels Peritoneal calcifications
Follow-through contrast media studies of the intestine	Bowel motility disturbances Separated, rigid, dilated bowel loops Varying degrees of obstruction accompanied by hypermotility
US	Disturbed motility of bowel loops Dilated fixed loops matted together and tethered posteriorly Haustration of the ileum Intraperitoneal echogenic strands Echogenic "sandwich-appearance" membrane formation Thickened trilaminar appearance of the bowel wall
CT MR	Variable diameter of bowel segments Adherent, dilated bowel loops Bowel tethering Air-fluid level Loculated ascites Thickened intestinal wall Peritoneal thickening Increased density of mesenteric fat Entrapped fluid collections Peritoneal calcifications

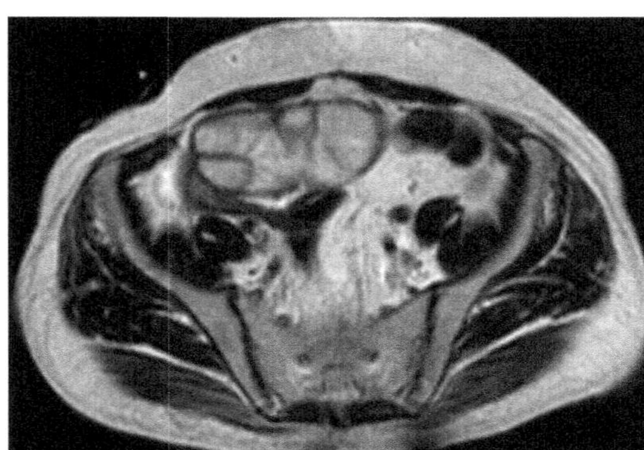

Fig. 21.36 Encapsulating peritoneal sclerosis. Adherent bowel loops surrounded by a thick capsule in MR examination at an early stage of disease

nosis of cuff and tunnel infections. CEUS finds its place together with Doppler US in the dynamic evaluation of catheter malfunction, thus reducing the necessity of fluoroscopy, CT, or MR peritoneography. CT remains a cornerstone for the diagnosis of EPS. The value of dynamic cinematographic MR in the clinical management of PD patients remains to be investigated.

References

1. Santarelli S, Amici G, Bernacconi T, Bonforte G, Ceraudo E, Dell'Aquila R, Galli E, Iadarola GM, Maffei S, Sardellini C, Zeiler M, La Milia V, Virga G, Brunori G, Garosi G, Cancarini G. The peritoneal dialysis catheter. J Nephrol. 2013;26(Suppl 21):4–75. https://doi.org/10.5301/JN.2013.11633.
2. Holley JL, Foulks CJ, Moss AH, Willard D. Ultrasound as a tool in the diagnosis and management of exit-site infections in patients undergoing continuous ambulatory peritoneal dialysis. Am J Kidey Dis. 1989;14:211–6.
3. Scabardi M, Ronco C, Chiaramonte S, Feriani M, Agostini F, La Greca G. Dynamic catheterography in the early diagnosis of peritoneal catheter malfunction. Int J Artif Organs. 1992;15:358–64.
4. Twardowski ZJ, Tully RJ, Ersoy FF, Dedhia NM. Computerized tomography with and without intraperitoneal contrast for determination of intraabdominal fluid distribution and diagnosis of complications in peritoneal dialysis patients. Trans Am Soc Artif Intern Organs. 1990;36:95–103.
5. Hollett MD, Marn CS, Ellis JH, Francis IR, Swartz RD. Complications of continuous ambulatory peritoneal dialysis: evaluation with CT peritoneography. AJR Am J Roentgenol. 1992;159:983–9. https://doi.org/10.2214/ajr.159.5.1344976.
6. Cochran ST, Do HM, Ronaghi A, Nissenson AR, Kadell BM. Complications of peritoneal dialysis: evaluation with CT peritoneography. Radiographics. 1997;17:869–78. https://doi.org/10.1148/radiographics.17.4.9225388.
7. Prokesch RW, Schima W, Schober E, Vychytil A, Fabrizii V, Bader TR. Complications of continuous ambulatory peritoneal dialysis: findings on MR peritoneography. AJR Am J Roentgenol. 2000;174:987–91. https://doi.org/10.2214/ajr.174.4.1740987.
8. Prischl FC, Muhr T, Seiringer EM, Funk S, Kronabethleitner G, Wallner M, Artmann W, Kramar R. Magnetic resonance imaging of the peritoneal cavity among peritoneal dialysis patients, using the dialysate as "contrast medium". J Am Soc Nephrol. 2002;13:197–203.
9. Domico J, Warman M, Jaykamur S, Sorkin MI. Is ultrasonography useful in predicting catheter loss? Adv Perit Dial. 1993;9:231–2.
10. Plum J, Sudkamp S, Grabensee B. Results of ultrasound assisted diagnosis of tunnel infections in continuous ambulatory peritoneal dialysis. Am J Kidney Dis. 1994;23:99–104.
11. Korzets Z, Erdberg A, Golan E, Ben-Chitrit S, Verner M, Rathaus V, Bernheim J. Frequent involvement of the internal cuff segment in CAPD peritonitis and exit-site infection - an ultrasound study. Nephrol Dial Int. 1996;11:336–9.
12. Vychytil A, Lorenz M, Schneider B, Hörl WH, Haag-Weber M. New criteria for management of catheter infections in peritoneal dialysis patients using ultrasonography. J Am Soc Nephrol. 1998;9:290–6.
13. Vychytil A, Lilaj T, Lorenz M, Hörl WH, Haag-Weber M. Ultrasonography of the catheter tunnel in peritoneal dialysis patients: what are the indications? Am J Kidney Dis. 1999;33:722–7.
14. Kwan TH, Tong MK, Siu YP, Leung KT, Luk SH, Cheung YK. Ultrasonography in the management of exit site infections in peritoneal dialysis patients. Nephrology (Carlton). 2004;9:348–52. https://doi.org/10.1111/j.1440-1797.2004.00331.x.
15. Karahan OI, Taskapan H, Yikilmaz A, Oymak O, Utas C. Ultrasound evaluation of peritoneal catheter tunnel in catheter related infections in CAPD. Int Urol Nephrol. 2005;37:363–6. https://doi.org/10.1007/s11255-004-0173-1.
16. Somma G, Trattelli G, Coppola C, Auricchio M. Studio pragmatico sul ruolo degli ultrasuoni nel management delle complicanze infettive del catetere peritoneale. Role of ultrasounds in the management infectious complications of peritoneal catheter. G Ital Nefrol. 2017;34:157–64.
17. Hau M, Kneitz C, Tony HP, Keberle M, Jahns R, Jenett M. High resolution ultrasound detects a decrease in pannus vascularisation of small finger joints in patients with rheumatoid arthritis receiving treatment with soluble tumour necrosis factor α receptor (etanercept). Ann Rheum Dis. 2002;61:55–8. https://doi.org/10.1136/ard.61.1.55.
18. Scanziani R, Pozzi M, Pisano L, Santagostino Barbone G, Dozio B, Rovere G, Gabella P, Magri F. Imaging work-up for peritoneal access care and peritoneal dialysis complications. Int J Artif Organs. 2006;29:142–52.
19. Stuart S, Booth TC, Cash CJ, Hameeduddin A, Goode JA, Harvey C, Malhotra A. Complications of continuous ambulatory peritoneal dialysis. Radiographics. 2009;29:441–60. https://doi.org/10.1148/rg.292085136.
20. Cakir B, Kirbaş I, Cevik B, Ulu EM, Bayrak A, Coşkun M. Complications of CAPD: evaluation with CT. Diagn Interv Radiol. 2008;14:212–20.
21. Kappel JE, Ferguson GM, Kudel RM, Kudel TA, Lawlor BJ, Pylypchuk GB. Stiff wire manipulation of peritoneal dialysis catheters. Adv Perit Dial. 1995;11:202–7.
22. Simons ME, Pron G, Voros M, Vanderburgh LC, Rao PS, Oreopoulos DG. Fluoroscopically-guided manipulation of malfunctioning peritoneal dialysis catheters. Perit Dial Int. 1999;19:544–9.

23. Savader SJ, Lund G, Scheel PJ, Prescott C, Feeley N, Singh H, Osterman FA Jr. Guide wire directed manipulation of malfunctioning peritoneal dialysis catheters: a critical analysis. J Vasc Interv Radiol. 1997;8:957–63.
24. Kim HJ, Lee TW, Ihm CG, Kim MJ. Use of fluoroscopy-guided wire manipulation and/or laparoscopic surgery in the repair of malfunctioning peritoneal dialysis catheters. Am J Nephrol. 2002;22:532–8.
25. Ozyer U, Harman A, Aytekin C, Boyvat F, Ozdemir N. Correction of displaced peritoneal dialysis catheters with an angular stiff rod. Acta Radiol. 2009;50:139–43. https://doi.org/10.1080/02841850802631983.
26. Xie JY, Ren H, Kiryluk K, Chen N. Peritoneal dialysis outflow failure from omental wrapping diagnosed by catheterography. Am J Kidney Dis. 2010;56:1006–11. https://doi.org/10.1053/j.ajkd.2010.03.034.
27. Miller M, McCormick B, Lavoie S, Biyani M, Zimmerman D. Fluoroscopic manipulation of peritoneal dialysis catheters: outcomes and factors associated with successful manipulation. Clin J Am Soc Nephrol. 2012;7:795–800. https://doi.org/10.2215/CJN.09850911.
28. Narayan R, Fried T, Chica G, Schaefer M, Daniel MD. Minimally invasive fluoroscopic percutaneous peritoneal dialysis catheter salvage. Clin Kidney J. 2014;7:264–8. https://doi.org/10.1093/ckj/sfu042.
29. Esposito F, Di Serafino M, Sgambati P, Erra P, Mercogliano C, Pecoraro C, Oresta P. Ultrasound in the diagnosis of peritoneal catheter obstruction in children. Kidney Int. 2012;82:499. https://doi.org/10.1038/ki.2012.132.
30. Zeiler M, Zanoli L, Scarfia RV, Santarelli S, Granata A. Peritoneal dialysis catheter position evaluated by ultrasound: can it replace abdomen X-ray in patients presenting catheter misplacement? Ultraschall Med. 2017;38:538–43. https://doi.org/10.1055/s-0043-103953.
31. Zeiler M, Lenci FF, Dellabella S, Santarelli S. Colour Doppler ultrasound for peritoneal catheter malfunction. Nephrol Dial Transplant. 2015;30(Suppl 3):iii537. https://doi.org/10.1093/ndt/gfv196.02.
32. Esposito F, Di Serafino M, Ambrosio C, Panico MR, Malacario F, Mercogliano C, Pecoraro C, Oresta P. Chronic peritoneal dialysis in children: the role of ultrasound in the diagnosis of peritoneal catheter obstruction. J Ultrasound. 2016;19(3):191–6. https://doi.org/10.1007/s40477-016-0209-2.
33. Heinzmann A, Müller T, Leitlein J, Braun B, Kubicka S, Blank W. Endocavitary contrast enhanced ultrasound (CEUS) – work in progress. Ultraschall Med. 2012;33:76–84. https://doi.org/10.1055/s-0031-1299056.
34. Müller T, Blank W, Leitlein K, Kubicka S, Heinzmann A. Endocavitary contrast-enhanced ultrasound: a technique whose time has come? J Clin Ultrasound. 2015;43:71–80. https://doi.org/10.1002/jcu.22250.
35. Granata A, Zanoli L, Insalaco M, Valentino M, Pavlica P, Di Nicolò PP, Scuderi M, Fiorini F, Fatuzzo P, Bertolotto M. Contrast-enhanced ultrasound (CEUS) in nephrology: has the time come for its widespread use? Clin Exp Nephrol. 2015;19:606–15. https://doi.org/10.1007/s10157-014-1040-8.
36. Portoles J, Coronel F, Ganado T. Abdominal wall leakage on CAPD: usefulness of ultrasonography. Nephron. 1995;69:348–9.
37. Maxwell AJ, Boggis CR, Sambrook P. Computed tomographic peritoneography in the investigation of abdominal wall and genital swelling in patients on continuous ambulatory peritoneal dialysis. Clin Radiol. 1990;41:100–4.
38. Litherland J, Lupton EW, Ackrill PA, Venning M, Sambrook P. Computed tomographic peritoneography: CT manifestations in the investigation of leaks and abnormal collections in patients on CAPD. Nephrol Dial Transplant. 1994;9:1449–52.
39. Lam MF, Lo WK, Chu FS, Li FK, Yip TP, Tse KC, Chan TM, Lai KN. Retroperitoneal leakage as a cause of ultrafiltration failure. Perit Dial Int. 2004;24:466–77.
40. Lam MF, Lo WK, Tse KC, Yip TP, Lui SL, Chan TM, Lai KN. Retroperitoneal leakage as a cause of acute ultrafiltration failure: its associated risk factors in peritoneal dialysis. Perit Dial Int. 2009;29:542–7.
41. Mahale AS, Katyal A, Khanna R. Complications of peritoneal dialysis related to increased intra-abdominal pressure. Adv Perit Dial. 2003;19:130–5.
42. Johnson J, Baum S, Smink RD. Radionuclide imaging in the diagnosis of hernias related to peritoneal dialysis. Arch Surg. 1987;122:952–4.
43. Juergensen PH, Rizvi H, Caride VJ, Kliger AS, Finkelstein FO. Value of scintigraphy in chronic peritoneal dialysis patients. Kidney Int. 1999;56:1111–9. https://doi.org/10.1046/j.1523-1755.1999.0550031111.x.
44. Fletcher S, Turney JH, Brownjohn AM. Increased incidence of hydrothorax complicating peritoneal dialysis in patients with adult polycystic kidney disease. Nephrol Dial Transplant. 1994;9:832–3.
45. Kang TW, Kim CK. Pleuroperitoneal communication of peritoneal dialysis demonstrated by multidetector-row CT peritoneography. Abdom Imaging. 2009;34:780–2. https://doi.org/10.1007/s00261-008-9468-5.
46. Xu T, Xie J, Wang W, Ren H, Chen N. Peritoneal-pleural leaks demonstrated by CT peritoneography. Case Rep Nephrol. 2015;5:135–9. https://doi.org/10.1159/000430806.
47. Matsumura M, Mizutani E, Suzuki T, Tsurumi H, Uni R, Higashihara T, Nakahara K, Takano H. Successful diagnosis and treatment of peritoneal dialysis-related pleuroperitoneal communication by contrast-enhanced ultrasonography and thoracoscopic surgery. Perit Dial Int. 2017;37:485–6. https://doi.org/10.3747/pdi.2016.00295.
48. Prencipe MA, Damiani F, Del Giudice A, Di Giorgio G, Aucella F. CEUS (contrast enhanced ultrasound) nella dialisi peritoneale complicata da idrotorace. G Ital Nefrol. 2017;34(S70):31.

49. Borzellino G, De Manzoni G, Ricci F. Detection of abdominal adhesions in laparoscopic surgery. A controlled study of 130 cases. Surg Laparosc Endosc. 1998;8:273–6.
50. Tu FF, Lamvu GM, Hartmann KE, Steege JF. Preoperative ultrasound to predict infraumbilical adhesions: a study of diagnostic accuracy. Am J Obstet Gynecol. 2005;192:74–9. https://doi.org/10.1016/j.ajog.2004.07.034.
51. Piccolboni D, Ciccone F, Settembre A. High resolution ultrasound for pre-operative detection of intraperitoneal adhesions: an invaluable diagnostic tool for the general and laparoscopic surgeon. J Ultrasound. 2009;12:148–50. https://doi.org/10.1016/j.jus.2009.09.001.
52. Larciprete G, Valli E, Meloni P, Malandrenis I, Romanini ME, Jarvis S, Rossi F, Barbati G, Cirese E. Ultrasound detection of the "sliding viscera" sign promotes safer laparoscopy. J Minim Invasive Gynecol. 2009;16:445–9. https://doi.org/10.1016/j.jmig.2009.03.023.
53. Fenner J, Wright B, Emberey J, Spencer P, Gillott R, Summers A, Hutchinson C, Lawford P, Brenchley P, Bardhan KD. Towards radiological diagnosis of abdominal adhesions based on motion signatures derived from sequences of cine-MRI images. Phys Med. 2014;30:437–47. https://doi.org/10.1016/j.ejmp.2013.12.002.
54. Messana JM, Block GA, Swartz RD. Injury to the inferior epigastric artery complicating percutaneous peritoneal dialysis catheter insertion. Perit Dial Int. 2001;21:313–5.
55. Wong C, Merkur H. Inferior epigastric artery: surface anatomy, prevention and management of injury. Aust N Z J Obstet Gynaecol. 2016;56:137–41. https://doi.org/10.1111/ajo.12426.
56. Maya ID. Ultrasound/fluoroscopy-assisted placement of peritoneal dialysis catheters. Semin Dial. 2007;20:611–5. https://doi.org/10.1111/j.1525-139X.2007.00371.x.
57. Abdel-Aal AK, Gaddikeri S, Saddekni S. Technique of peritoneal catheter placement under fluoroscopic guidance. Radiol Res Pract. 2011;2011:141707. https://doi.org/10.1155/2011/141707.
58. Golay V, Trivedi M, Roychowdhary A, Arora P, Sarkar D, Singh A, Dasgupta S, Pandey R. Ultrasound-guided CAPD catheter insertion. Perit Dial Int. 2013;33:454–8. https://doi.org/10.3747/pdi.2012.00206.
59. Abdel-Aal AK, Dybbro P, Hathaway P, Guest S, Neuwirth M, Krishnamurthy V. Best practice consensus protocol for peritoneal dialysis catheter placement by interventional radiologists. Perit Dial Int. 2014;34:481–93. https://doi.org/10.3747/pdi.2013.00029.
60. Shanmugalingam R, Makris A, Hassan HC, Li Y, DeGuzman I, Nandakoban H, Aravindan A, Narayanan G, Wong JKW. The utility of sonographic assessment in selecting patients for percutaneous insertion of peritoneal dialysis catheter. Perit Dial Int. 2017;37:434–42. https://doi.org/10.3747/pdi.2017.00006.
61. Jalandhara N, Balamuthusamy S, Shah B, Souraty P. Percutaneous peritoneal dialysis catheter placement in patients with complex abdomen. Semin Dial. 2015;28:680–6. https://doi.org/10.1111/sdi.12406.
62. Duman S, Ozbek SS, Gunay ES, Bozkurt D, Asci G, Sipahi S, Kircelli F, Ertilav M, Özkahya M, Ok E. What does peritoneal thickness in peritoneal dialysis patients tell us? Adv Perit Dial. 2007;23:28–33.
63. Temiz G, Sahin G, Mukerrem G, Ozkurt S, Degirmenci NA, Yalcin AU. Ultrasonographic evaluation of peritoneal membrane thickness and comparison with the effectiveness and duration of CAPD. Int Urol Nephrol. 2013;45:1761–6. https://doi.org/10.1007/s11255-013-0504-1.
64. Lee TS, Yang JY, Wang HP, Tsai TJ, Yang Y. Peritoneal thickening is not inevitable in long-term peritoneal dialysis and is associated with peritoneal transport characteristics: a two-centre sonographic study. Nephrol Dial Transplant. 2008;23:1005–10. https://doi.org/10.1093/ndt/gfm726.
65. Yavaşcan Ö, Aksu N, Alparslan C, Sarıtaş S, Elmas CH, Eraslan AN, Duman S, Mir S. The importance of ultrasonographic measurement of peritoneal wall thickness in pediatric chronic peritoneal dialysis patients. Ren Fail. 2015;37:381–6. https://doi.org/10.3109/0886022X.2014.1001280.
66. Namasivayam J. Intraperitoneal pseudocyst formation as a complication of continuous ambulatory peritoneal dialysis. Br J Radiol. 1991;64(761):463–4.
67. Sahpazova E, Ruso B, Kuzmanovska D. Intraperitoneal pseudocyst formation: complication of fungal peritonitis in continuous ambulatory peritoneal dialysis. Hippokratia. 2007;11:219–20.
68. Zeiler M, Santarelli S, Cangiotti AM, Agostinelli RM, Monteburini T, Marinelli R, Ceraudo E, Cutini G. Giant mesenteric cyst of mesothelial origin in a haemodialysis patient with previous peritoneal dialysis therapy. Nephrol Dial Transplant. 2010;25:1004–6. https://doi.org/10.1093/ndt/gfp680.
69. Baer G, Wagner A, Selbach J, Otto M, Weiner SM. Abdominal pseudocysts following peritoneal dialysis-associated peritonitis: a report of 3 cases. Am J Kidney Dis. 2010;55:e15–9. https://doi.org/10.1053/j.ajkd.2009.12.019.
70. Kurachi H, Murakami T, Nakamura H, Hori S, Miyake A, Kozuka T, Tanizawa O. Imaging of peritoneal pseudocysts: value of MR imaging compared with sonography and CT. Am J Roentgenol. 1993;161:589–91. https://doi.org/10.2214/ajr.161.3.8352112.
71. Ercan Z, Yildirim T, Merhametsiz O, Yayar O, Haspulat A, Ayli MD. Abdominal pseudocyst development in a peritoneal dialysis patient with a ventriculoperitoneal shunt: an indication for switch to hemodialysis? Perit Dial Int. 2014;34:470–1. https://doi.org/10.3747/pdi.2013.00069.
72. Boroujerdi-Rad H, Juergensen P, Mansourian V, Kliger AS, Finkelstein FO. Abdominal abscesses

complicating peritonitis in continuous ambulatory peritoneal dialysis patients. Am J Kidney Dis. 1994;23:717–21.

73. Lee FT Jr, Leahy-Gross KM, Hammond TG, Wakeen MJ, Zimmerman SW. Pneumoperitoneum in peritoneal dialysis patients: significance of diagnosis by CT. J Comput Assist Tomogr. 1994;18:439–42.
74. Okamoto T, Ikenoue T, Matsui K, Miyazaki M, Tsuzuku Y, Nishizawa Y, Kubota M. Free air on CT and the risk of peritonitis in peritoneal dialysis patients: a retrospective study. Ren Fail. 2014;36:1492–6. https://doi.org/10.3109/0886022X.2014.958953.
75. Imran M, Bhat R, Anijeet H. Pneumoperitoneum in peritoneal dialysis patients; one centre's experience. NDT Plus. 2011;4:120–3. https://doi.org/10.1093/ndtplus/sfq208.
76. Kawaguchi Y, Kawanishi H, Mujais S, Topley N, Oreopoulos DG. Encapsulating peritoneal sclerosis: definition, etiology, diagnosis, and treatment. International Society for Peritoneal Dialysis Ad Hoc Committee on Ultrafiltration Management in Peritoneal Dialysis. Perit Dial Int. 2000;20(Suppl 4):S43–55.
77. Nakamoto H. Encapsulating peritoneal sclerosis - a clinician's approach to diagnosis and medical treatment. Perit Dial Int. 2005;25(Suppl 4):S30–8.
78. Kawaguchi Y, Saito A, Kawanishi H, Nakayama M, Miyazaki M, Nakamoto H, Tranaeus A. Recommendations on the management of encapsulating peritoneal sclerosis in Japan, 2005: diagnosis, predictive markers, treatment, and preventive measures. Perit Dial Int. 2005;25(Suppl 4):S83–95.
79. Holland P. Sclerosing encapsulating peritonitis in chronic ambulatory peritoneal dialysis. Clin Radiol. 1990;41:19–23.
80. Hollman AS, McMillan MA, Briggs JD, Junor BJ, Morley P. Ultrasound changes in sclerosing peritonitis following continuous ambulatory peritoneal dialysis. Clin Radiol. 1991;43:176–9.
81. Campbell S, Clarke P, Hawley C, Wigan M, Kerlin P, Butler J, Wall D. Sclerosing peritonitis: identification of diagnostic, clinical, and radiological features. Am J Kidney Dis. 1994;24:819–25.
82. Krestin GP, Kacl G, Hauser M, Keusch G, Burger HR, Hoffmann R. Imaging diagnosis of sclerosing peritonitis and relation of radiologic signs to the extent of the disease. Abdom Imaging. 1995;20:414–20.
83. Tarzi RM, Lim A, Moser S, Ahmad S, George A, Balasubramaniam G, Clutterbuck EJ, Gedroyc W, Brown EA. Assessing the validity of an abdominal CT scoring system in the diagnosis of encapsulating peritoneal sclerosis. Clin J Am Soc Nephrol. 2008;3:1702–10. https://doi.org/10.2215/CJN.01820408.
84. Vlijm A, Stoker J, Bipat S, Spijkerboer AM, Phoa SS, Maes R, Struijk DG, Krediet RT. Computer tomographic findings characteristic for encapsulating peritoneal sclerosis: a case-control study. Perit Dial Int. 2009;29:517–22.
85. Térébus Look M, Lubrano J, Courivaud C, Bresson Vautrin C, Kastler B, Delabrousse E. CT in predicting abdominal cocoon in patients on peritoneal dialysis. Clin Radiol. 2010;65:924–9. https://doi.org/10.1016/j.crad.2010.06.014.
86. Ti JP, Al-Aradi A, Conlon PJ, Lee MJ, Morrin MM. Imaging features of encapsulating peritoneal sclerosis in continuous ambulatory peritoneal dialysis patients. Am J Roentgenol. 2010;195:W50–4. https://doi.org/10.2214/AJR.09.3175.
87. Vlijm A, van Schuppen J, Lamers AB, Struijk DG, Krediet RT. Imaging in encapsulating peritoneal sclerosis. NDT Plus. 2011;4:281–4. https://doi.org/10.1093/ndtplus/sfr068.
88. Goodlad C, Tarzi R, Gedroyc W, Lim A, Moser S, Brown EA. Screening for encapsulating peritoneal sclerosis in patients on peritoneal dialysis: role of CT scanning. Nephrol Dial Transplant. 2011;26:1374–9. https://doi.org/10.1093/ndt/gfq533.
89. Upponi S, Butler AJ, Watson CJ, Shaw AS. Encapsulating peritoneal sclerosis--correlation of radiological findings at CT with underlying pathogenesis. Clin Radiol. 2014;69:103–9. https://doi.org/10.1016/j.crad.2013.09.004.
90. Stuart S, Stott D, Goode A, Cash CJ, Davenport A. Can radiological assessment of abdominal computerized scans diagnose encapsulating peritoneal sclerosis in long-term peritoneal dialysis patients. Nephrology (Carlton). 2017;22:19–24. https://doi.org/10.1111/nep.12718.
91. Hüser N, Stangl M, Lutz J, Fend F, Kreymann B, Gaa J. Sclerosing encapsulating peritonitis: MRI diagnosis. Eur Radiol. 2006;16:238–9. https://doi.org/10.1007/s00330-005-2746-5.
92. Wright B, Summers A, Fenner J, Gillott R, Hutchinson CE, Spencer PA, Wilkie M, Hurst H, Herrick S, Brenchley P, Augustine T, Bardhan KD. Initial observations using a novel "cine" magnetic resonance imaging technique to detect changes in abdominal motion caused by encapsulating peritoneal sclerosis. Perit Dial Int. 2011;31:287–90. https://doi.org/10.3747/pdi.2010.00078.

22 Ultrasound-Guided Central Venous Catheter Placement for Hemodialysis

Antonio Granata, Morale Walter, Ricciardi Carlo Alberto, Fiorini Fulvio, Forneris Giacomo, and Gallieni Maurizio

22.1 Introduction

Central venous catheter placement is a common procedure, which has been introduced in the clinical setting over the past 50 years. It is performed in 8% of hospitalized patients and more than 5 million central venous catheters are placed every year in the United States [1, 2]. A central venous access is usually necessary for specific intravenous therapies, such as chemotherapy, parenteral nutrition, central venous and arterial pressure monitoring, heart pacemaker positioning, and extracorporeal therapies, such as plasma exchange and hemodialysis.

Since the introduction of Seldinger technique in 1953, central venous catheter insertion has become an easier and safer procedure [3, 4]. The addition of ultrasound (US) has been shown to decrease complications even further [3, 4]. Ultrasounds, indeed, allow clinicians to visualize vein target and its anatomical features, as well as needle path. Moreover, US-guided central venous catheter placement is characterized by a lower incidence of unsuccessful attempts and requires less time to be performed [5–8]. For these reasons international guidelines recommend the use of ultrasounds in case of central venous catheter positioning [9–13].

In the following paragraphs, we will describe internal jugular vein catheterization, but this technique can be used in case of central vein catheter placement in other sites (i.e., femoral vein) as well.

22.2 Type of Ultrasound Scanner

Ultrasound scanner technical features vary depending on the manufacturing companies and the type of monitors, utilizing B-mode, color Doppler, and pulsed Doppler function to perform

A. Granata (✉)
Department of Nephrology and Dialysis, "Cannizzaro" Emergency Hospital, Catania, Italy

M. Walter
Nephrology and Dialysis Unit, P.O. "Maggiore", Modica, ASP Ragusa, Italy

R. C. Alberto
Faculty of Life of Cardiovascular Medicine & Sciences, Section Vascular Biology and Inflammation, British Heart Foundation Centre for Research Excellence, King's College of London, London, UK

F. Fulvio
Nephrology and Dialysis Unit, AULSS 5 Polesana, Ospedale SM della Misericordia, Scuola Nazionale SIUMB di Ecografia Nefrologica, Rovigo, Italy

F. Giacomo
SC Universitaria di Nefrologia e Dialisi, Centro di Ricerche di Immunopatologia e Documentazione Malattia Rare, "Giovanni Bosco" Hospital e University of Torino, Torino, Italy

G. Maurizio
Nephrology and Dialysis Unit, ASST Fatebenefratelli "Sacco", Milano, Italy

Department of Biomedical and Clinical Sciences "Luigi Sacco", School of Medicine, Università degli Studi di Milano, Milan, Italy

A. Granata, M. Bertolotto (eds.), *Imaging in Nephrology*, https://doi.org/10.1007/978-3-030-60794-4_22

US-guided central venous catheter placement. In particular, B-mode (brightness mode) provides bidimensional images of tissues in a gray scale, whereas color Doppler and pulsed Doppler provide information about both direction and speed of blood flow. To optimize ergonomy of the procedure ultrasound scanner should be placed in front of the operator, allowing an effortless control of needle advancement and reducing the risk of complications.

22.2.1 Type and Position of Ultrasound Probe

Central veins used for venous catheter placement are located few millimeters under skin surface; the use of linear probes (high-frequency probes of 5–12 mHz) provides high-resolution images of deep tissues. The probe should be kept between the inch and the other fingers of the hand, which should lay on patient's body, in order to reach a stable position of the transducer and, subsequently, a stable image of the vein target. It is important that the probe is properly oriented and to maintain side correspondence of probe marker and lead on the monitor (Fig. 22.1). Wrong position of the transducer may lead to an incorrect visualization of the needle progression with respect to the anatomical structures near the vein. In fact probe marker (a bright LED located on a side of the transducer) is usually positioned at the left of the operator and the scanner, so that the left of the patient is visualized on the left of the scanner and the needle movements through the patient's tissues correspond to those of ultrasound images.

22.2.2 Ultrasound Setting

Ultrasound setting is fundamental to perform any US-guided procedure. Each type of setting has specific parameters, such as probe frequency, total gain, focus position, and number, which allow to obtain the best quality of ultrasonography images with respect to the anatomical region of interest. Usually, vascular setting is the ideal modality for central venous catheter placement [14, 15]. After setting adjust and vein visualization, total gain (image brightness in B-mode), depth (number of tissue centimeters under the probe), and focus position (depth corresponding to one of the veins to be cannulated) might be modified in order to improve the quality of the ultrasonographic image even further [14, 15].

22.3 Ultrasound Scan and Anatomy

Central vein to be cannulated may be visualized in a longitudinal axis (*in-plane*—long axis) with probe positioned parallelly to the longitudinal axis of the vein or in a transversal scan (*out-of-plane*—short axis), perpendicularly to the longitudinal axis of the vein (Fig. 22.2a, b) [14–16]. By transversal approach, both the artery and vein appear as round anechoic images. Usually, the vein presents thinner walls than the artery, collapses with a slight probe pressure in the absence of thrombosis, and dilates in case of increased venous blood pressure (Valsalva maneuver, Trendelenburg position) [14–16]. Conversely, the artery does not collapse due to endovascular pressure and thick wall. In the longitudinal scan, both the vein and the artery appear as ribbon images with an anechoic lumen delimited by parallel and echogenic walls [14–16]. The use of color Doppler and pulsed Doppler may help clinicians in distinguishing the artery from the vein. It is important to remember that red and blue colors indicate only blood flow direction with respect to the probe (the red color indicates that flow is towards the probe, while the blue color indicates that flow is leaving). Pulsed Doppler provides graphic and acoustic images of both arterial and venous flow. In particular, arterial flow is characterized by a Doppler wave with a typical systolic peak and an acute sound which are expression of the cardiac systolic activity. Venous flow is rather characterized by a Doppler wave which changes according to respiratory and cardiac activity and hydration state.

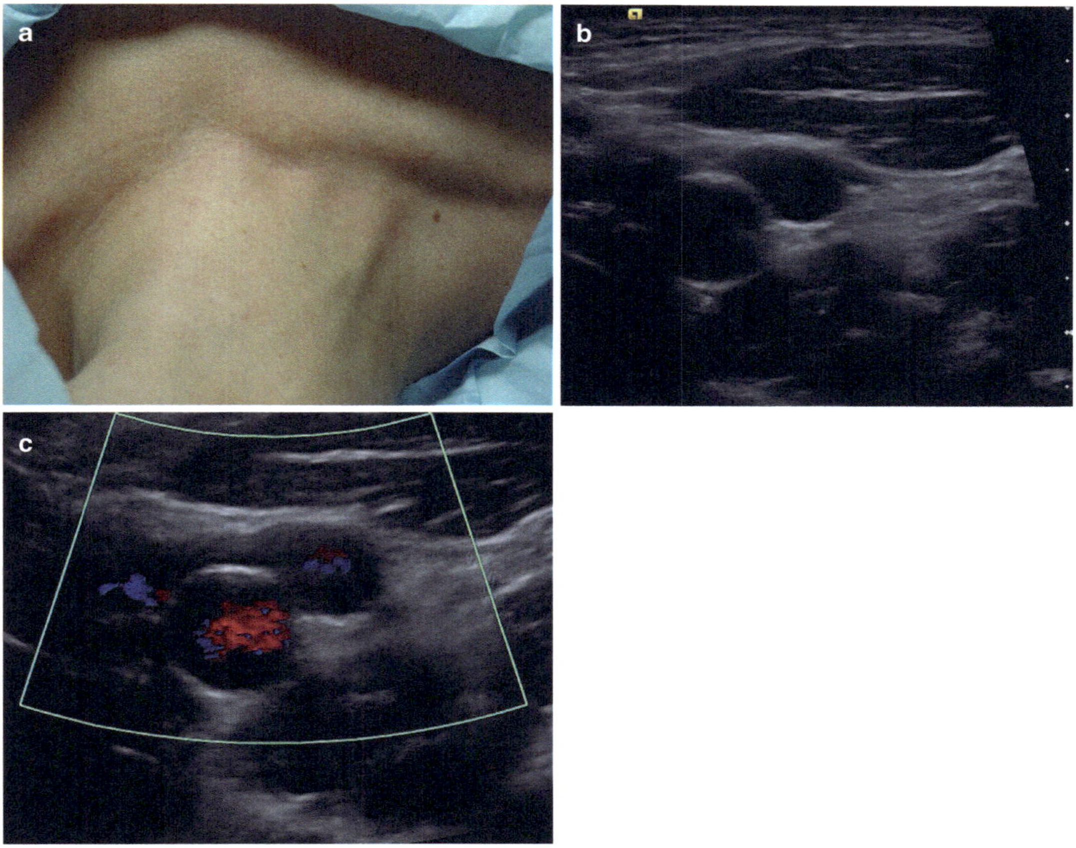

Fig. 22.1 Anatomical landmarks. (**a**)The localization of the internal jugular vein is based on its relationships with the sternocleidomastoid muscle (SCM). It is considered as a landmark of the apex of the triangle formed by the two ends, sternal and clavicular, of the sternocleidomastoid muscle at its insertion. The needle comes inserted at the apex of the triangle and advanced to the ipsilateral nipple. To the emergency point from the chest, the VGI is lateral and slightly anterior to the carotid artery. The B-mode (**b**) and the color Doppler (**c**) allow to visualize the vessels of the neck easily, and in particular to establish the anatomical relationships with the adjacent structures (common carotid artery and thyroid lobe, tracheal axis)

22.4 Preoperative Evaluation of the Patient

Before central venous catheter placement, meticulous prescan should be performed. Echo-color Doppler allows clinicians to rule out the presence of thrombosis and possible vascular injury due to previous catheter placement, as well as to evaluate anatomical characteristics of the vein (Fig. 22.3a–c). In some cases before the procedure, it may be useful to check the presence of "pleural sliding" (Fig. 22.4a–b). Indeed, after central venous catheter placement, it will be possible to rule out the presence of pneumothorax, a possible complication of the technique which is characterized by "pleural sliding" loss in real-time ultrasonography [17]. Optimal prescan is fundamental to confirm the indication for precise site of needle insertion and best technique to use (out-of-plane or in-plane approach).

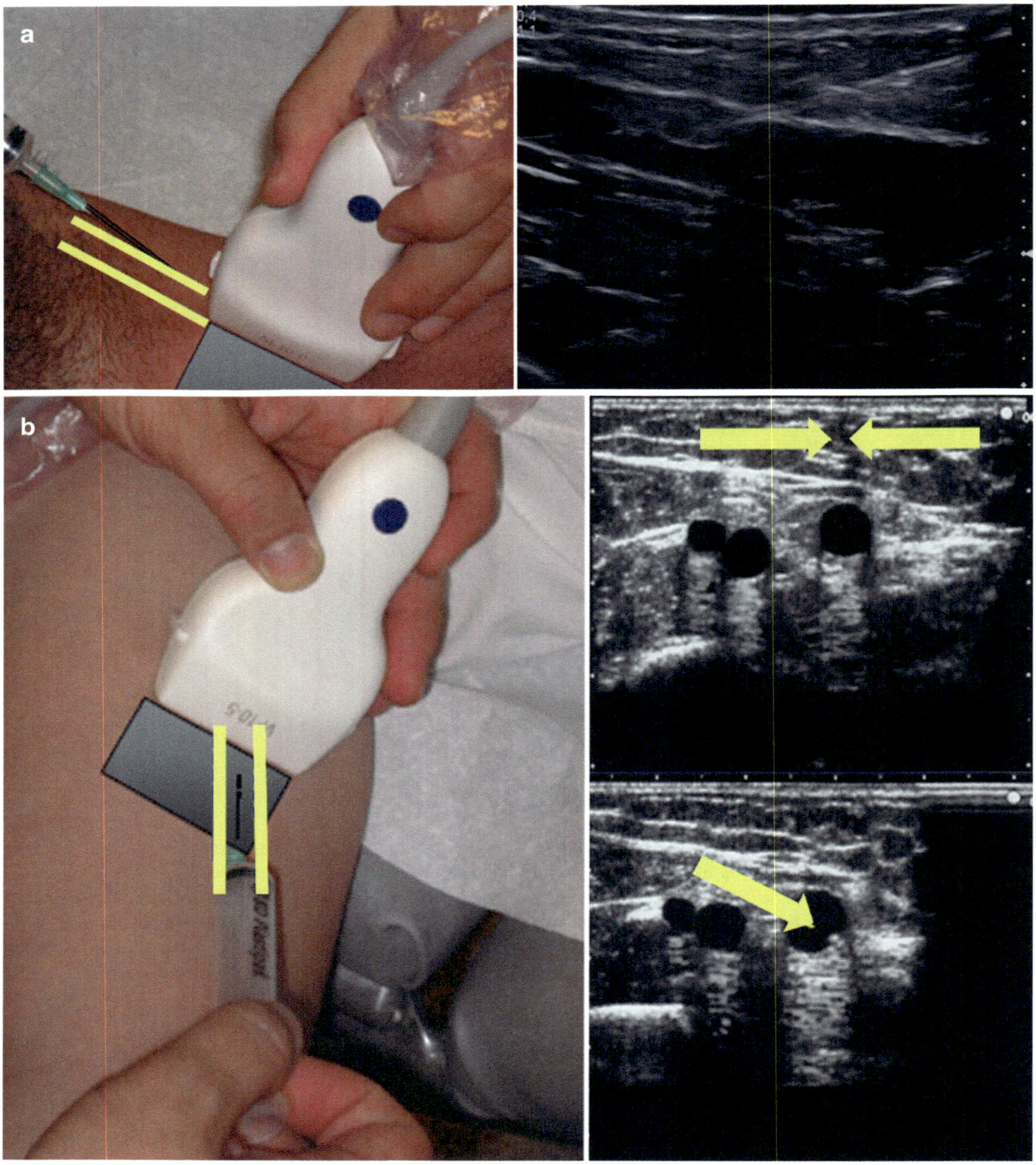

Fig. 22.2 Ultrasound scan. (**a**) Longitudinal scan. The probe is positioned parallel to the longitudinal axis of the vein. (**b**) Transverse scan. The probe is positioned parallel to the short axis (arrows indicate the route of the needle)

22.5 Ultrasonography Techniques

There are two different techniques of ultrasound-guided central venous catheter placement [14–16]:

1. "Static" ultrasound-guided technique
2. "Dynamic" or "real-time" ultrasound-guided technique

In the first one, ultrasonography is used only to identify the vein to be cannulated and confirm

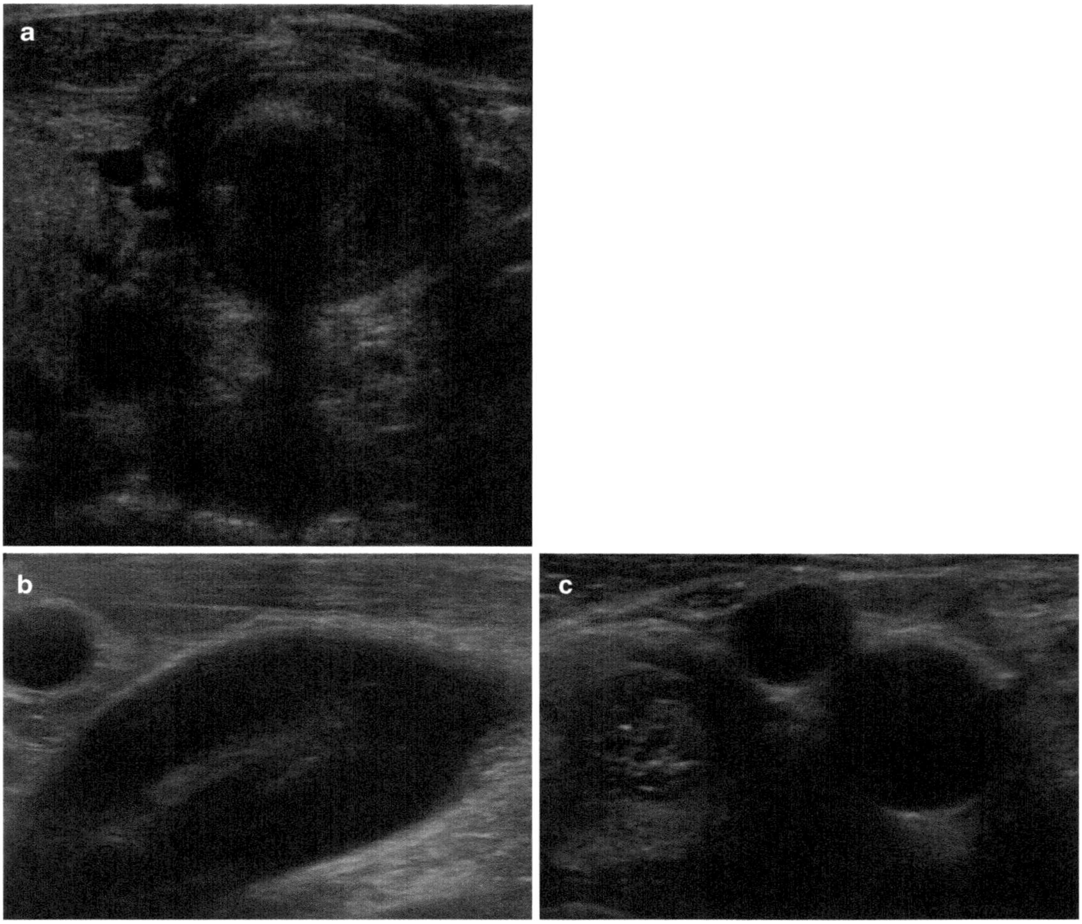

Fig. 22.3 Preoperative evaluation of the patient. Presence of thrombus in the lumen of the jugular vein visible on both the transverse (**a**) and longitudinal (**b**) scans. (**c**) Abnormal position of the jugular vein (posterior to the common carotid artery); besides right thyroid nodule is visible

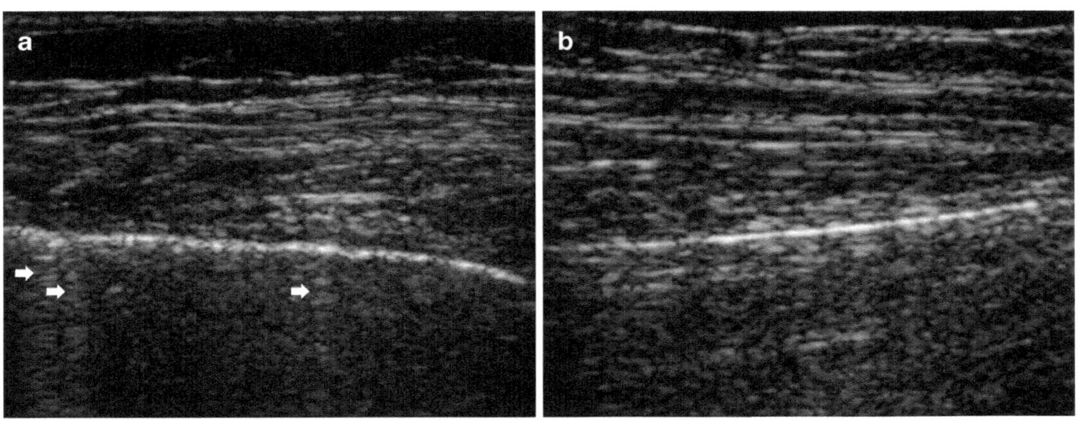

Fig. 22.4 Pneumothorax during the procedure. The absence of movement of the pleura is recognizable to B-mode (no sliding); moreover the lines B (comet-tail artifacts, arrows) are no longer recognizable (**a–b**)

the absence of thrombosis. The exact region should be marked with an indelible pen and the procedure is performed without ultrasounds [14–16].

In the "dynamic" ultrasound-guided technique, the probe is used during all the procedures in order to follow the needle trajectory in real time. This technique has been shown to be superior to the first one [18] that should be abandoned. In the "dynamic" ultrasound-guided technique, it is possible to keep the needle free (ultrasound-assisted procedure) or to allocate the needle in a system which does not allow to change direction or angulation (ultrasound-guided procedure) [14–16]. According to our experience, the ultrasound-assisted procedure should be preferred because it lets clinicians free to correct needle direction and inclination, required in particular anatomic situation.

In the transversal scan of the "dynamic" ultrasound-guided technique, the needle appears as a hyperechoic image and its trajectory may be followed in real time with minimal probe movements. In the longitudinal scan the entire shaft of the needle is advanced and visualized within the electronic beam (Fig. 22.5). Nevertheless, according to our experience longitudinal scan is not the scan of choice in case of central venous catheter placement in the neck for several reasons.

In fact when using linear probes, needle insertion point results to be too far from the clavicle in

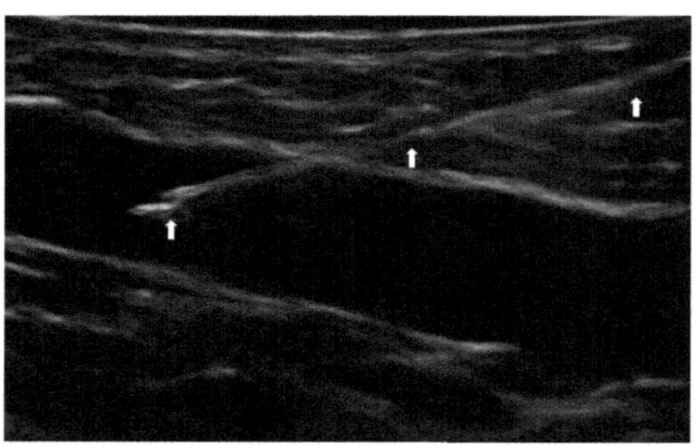

Fig. 22.5 Ultrasonography techniques. Longitudinal scan of the entire shaft of the needle is advanced and visualized within the electronic beam (arrows indicate the route of the needle)

the longitudinal scan, thus promoting subsequent kinking and malfunctioning of permanent catheters when performing subcutaneous tunneling. Secondly, during vein cannulation it may be more difficult to distinguish the vein from the artery in the longitudinal scan; moreover transversal scan allows changing needle trajectory more easily. Dynamic technique requires more experience since a precise coordination between eyes and hands is necessary.

22.6 Materials

Materials and instruments for ultrasound-guided central venous catheter placement should include:

1. Kit for central venous catheter placement (catheter of different dimensions and lengths depending on the clinical characteristic of the patient, guide wire, venous dilator, 18-gauge needle, syringe to perform venipuncture)
2. 10–20 mL syringes to administer anesthetic and to check catheter function and flushing
3. Antiseptic towels, sterile gloves and labs
4. Mask, glasses, and headset
5. Disinfectant (chlorhexidine 2% is preferred)
6. Antiseptic gauzes
7. Needle holder, surgical tweezer, and sutures
8. Local anesthetic (lidocaine 1–2%), optionally with vasoconstrictor (i.e., adrenaline 1:200,000)
9. Scalpel
10. Ultrasound scanner with a high-resolution linear probe (7–10 mHz)
11. Antiseptic gel for US
12. Sterile probe and US cover
13. Elastics to fix probe and cover
14. Monitor with ECG and oximeter
15. Stable peripheral iv access

22.7 Procedure

1. The patient should lay in a supine position. Trendelenburg position should be kept if internal jugular vein has to be cannulated in

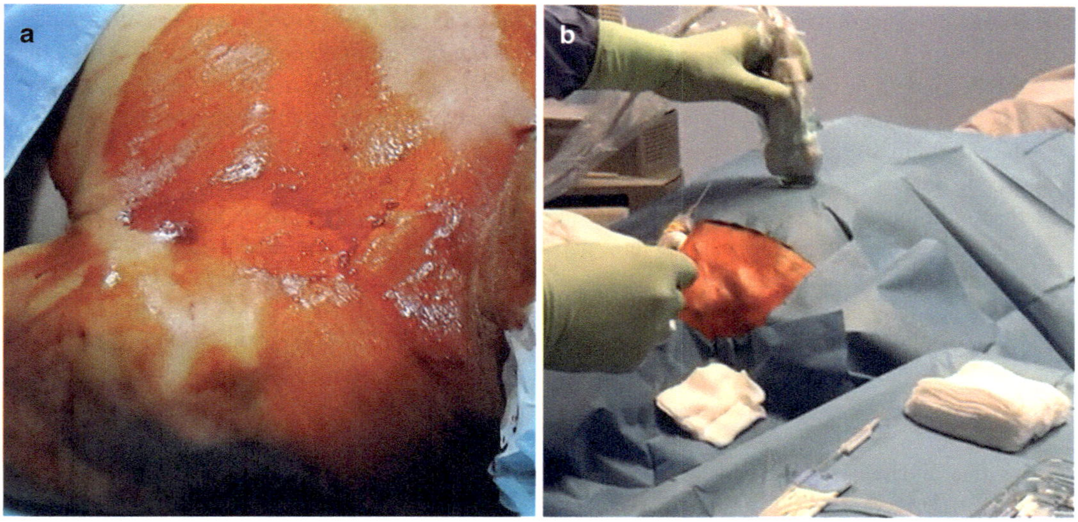

Fig. 22.6 Ultrasonography techniques. Create a sterile field before the procedure (**a**) and use a probe cover and antiseptic gel during the procedure (**b**)

order to increase venous return and to reduce air embolism risk.

2. Evaluation of the anatomical referral points of the region where the catheter should be inserted is fundamental—prescan.
3. Site for cannulation is disinfected and antiseptic towels are positioned (Fig. 22.6).
4. Ultrasound probe with antiseptic gel and cover should be positioned in order to obtain a clear image of the vein near anatomical structures; some gel or disinfectant solutions (chlorhexidine or iodopovidone) or saline solution can be used as a means of ultrasound conducting (Fig. 22.7).
5. Administer local anesthetic under ultrasound guidance in order to avoid stinging the vein or the artery, and to deliver an excessive amount of the drug.
6. The needle should be positioned under the probe and the syringe should be kept in aspiration, until blood is drawn.
7. The probe is then laid down, and the syringe is detached from the needle, and firmly kept still.
8. It is important to verify that the blood comes out from the needle continuously and not in a pulsatile way.

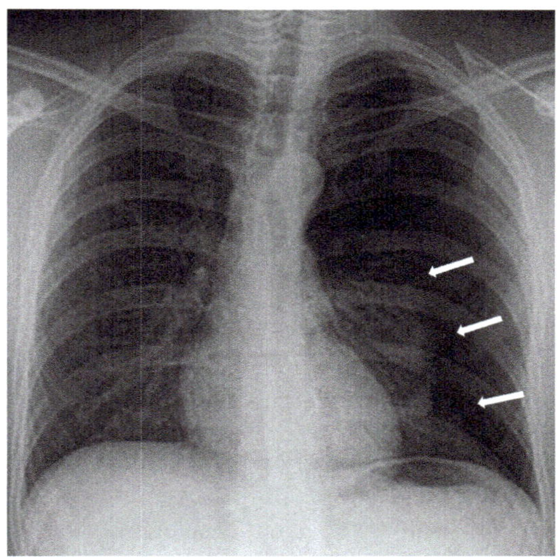

Fig. 22.7 Pneumothorax. A chest X-ray shows the right lung collapse due to the presence of an important pneumothorax

9. Insert the guide into the needle and advance in the vein forward without tissue resistance; check for cardiac rhythm disturbance: in this eventuality it may be useful to pull back the guide a few centimeters until cardiac rhythm returns to normal.

10. Remove the needle, leaving the guide in situ; perform a short skin incision near the vein entry site with a scalpel.
11. Check for correct position of guide wire into the vein and store it in US machine before proceeding.
12. Insert dilator over the guide in order to dilate skin-vessel tract for a few centimeters, performing the pull-and-through maneuver of guide just to exclude guide entrapment.
13. Remove the dilator and insert the catheter (with stylet) over the guide into the vein.
14. Remove the guide (and the stylet), verify the correct functioning of the catheter with syringe, and then flush the catheter with saline.
15. Verify correct position of the tip by chest X-ray or an endocavitary ECG.
16. In case of long-term catheter, tunneling (anterograde or retrograde) should be performed by anesthetic infiltration before or after catheter insertion into the vein.
17. Fix the catheter with surgical sutures and perform an antiseptic medication.
18. Perform chest X-ray (in case of internal jugular vein and subclavian vein) in order to confirm the right catheter tip placement and identify possible complication of the procedure.

22.8 Indications: Anatomical Sites Compared

Although several studies have demonstrated a greater global and cardiovascular mortality in patients with CVC rather than native arteriovenous fistula [19–20], central venous catheters are increasingly used in nephrology and dialysis units for starting hemodialysis even in young and nondiabetic patients [21]. The development of new biocompatible materials, the recent innovations in bioengineering, and the widespread use of ultrasound guidance for CVC placement have certainly contributed to increased number of CVC placement procedures. The placement of a CVC can be required in two possible scenarios:

1. Urgency: CVC can be required for patients needing hemodialysis for acute pulmonary edema not responsive to diuretics, severe acute hyperkalemia, or severe metabolic acidosis. Moreover, CVC can be helpful for performing dialysis sessions in patients with AVF complications (stenosis, thrombosis). In these scenarios, venous access is usually obtained through the cannulation of the femoral vein at bedside, in emergency room, in intensive care unit, or in dialysis room.
2. Scheduled procedure: It can be performed in patients waiting a complete AVF maturation or patients about to start peritoneal dialysis. Moreover, CVC placement can be scheduled to allow dialysis as a "bridge" to renal transplant or when no other vascular accesses are available. In these cases, the internal jugular vein or another venous vessel can be cannulated using either temporary or tunneled catheter, with respect to the same rules of asepsis and safety of any other surgical intervention.

The right internal jugular vein is universally considered the best site for both temporary and tunneled CVC placement. Its superficial position and straight course with drainage directly into the superior vena cava reduce the traumatism of the vascular walls, increase the success rate, and lower the risk of pneumothorax. The right internal jugular vein is also preferred for bedridden patients with BMI >28 or patients who have undergone major abdominal surgery. The possible disadvantages consist of the accidental puncture of the carotid artery (with consequent hematoma of the neck, hemothorax, hemopericardium, and/or mediastinal hemorrhage) or of the nervous structures (vagus and inferior laryngeal nerves, brachial plexus).

CVC placement in both right and left femoral vein is considered a fast and technically noncomplex procedure with a high success rate. Moreover, it does not interfere with any cardiopulmonary resuscitation maneuvers and avoids the risk of pneumothorax. It must however be remembered that the femoral site is at major risk of thrombotic and infectious complications [22]. Therefore, it should be avoided (when possible) in patients who are candidates for renal transplant because the eventual steno-thrombosis of the iliac vein would compromise the vascular anastomosis of the graft [23].

The left internal jugular vein and subclavian vein cannulations are both intricate because their angulated course increases the risk of procedural complications and of CVC malfunction due to venous stenosis or catheter tip malposition. The subclavian site has a further potential disadvantage consisting of the impossibility to create an arteriovenous fistula in the ipsilateral upper limb in the case of steno-thrombosis of the subclavian axis.

In summary, all the principal international guidelines [9, 24, 25] agree in indicating the right internal jugular vein as the first choice and the subclavian vein as the last option for CVC placement. The question if the femoral vein must be preferred or not to the left internal jugular vein remains controversial. The optimal site for a CVC placement must be chosen taking into consideration the clinical setting (acute vs. chronic) and planning the possible future perspectives for the patient.

22.9 Early Complications

Early complications can occur in conjunction with CVC insertion or within 24–48 h. The most common are arterial puncture, hematoma, hemorrhage, pneumothorax, hemothorax, air embolism, cardiac arrhythmias, and CVC malposition.

22.9.1 Arterial Puncture, Hematoma, Hemorrhage

Arterial puncture occurs in 3–15% of the CVC placement procedures. In patients with normal blood pressure and partial pressure of oxygen, it can be easily recognized for the appearance of a bright red blood into the syringe with pulsatile flow. In these cases, the needle should be removed immediately and a direct and continuous compression should be applied at the site of needle insertion. If necessary, antihypertensive drugs can be administered in order to prevent hematomas and/or hemorrhage. A simple method to determine whether or not the artery was really cannulated consists of taking blood samples from CVC and a periphery artery and performing a blood gas analysis in order to compare the partial pressures of oxygen. If the values are similar, the CVC is really inside the artery and must be therefore removed [26].

22.9.2 Pneumothorax

The incidence of pneumothorax is greater for the subclavian vein than for the internal jugular vein (1.5–3.1% vs. 0.1–0.2%) due to the anatomical proximity to the pleura. When the operator notices the presence of air inside the syringe, the correct connection between the needle and the syringe must be verified before suspecting a pneumothorax. Typical clinical signs are cough, dyspnea, sweating, tachycardia, and thoracic pain, but it can be asymptomatic. A chest X-ray is usually helpful in recognizing a large pneumothorax (Fig. 22.7). Conversely, lung ultrasound is more sensitive in detecting small amounts of air trapped in the pleural space (occult pneumothorax), showing the disappearance of the *pleural sliding* at the site of pneumothorax. If the clinical conditions make it necessary to place a CVC, it is advisable to avoid a new attempt in the contralateral supradiaphragmatic site and to move into the femoral vein as a bilateral pneumothorax could be lethal [1].

22.9.3 Hemothorax

Hemothorax is the passage of blood inside the pleural cavity and follows the lesion of the vascular structures during the CVC-positioning procedure. Similarly to pneumothorax, it can manifest with thoracic pain and dyspnea. When the blood loss is conspicuous, hypotension and tachycardia may appear up to hemorrhagic shock and death [6]. Hemothorax requires an immediate therapeutic intervention, including blood drainage from the pleural cavity, blood transfusions to correct anemia, procoagulant drug administration, and use of inotropes and vasopressors to improve circulation.

22.9.4 Air Embolism

Air embolism is due to the passage of air through the catheter into the bloodstream. The negative intrathoracic pressure generated by patient's inspiration during CVC placement facilitates the entry of air in the venous system. Some precautions such as maintaining the patient in the Trendelenburg position, Valsalva maneuver, and correct closure of the CVC-line clumps reduce the risk of air embolism. Tachycardia, thoracic pain, cough, and dyspnea are classical symptoms, but when the volume of air is >20 mL cardiovascular collapse can occur [6]. In these cases, the patients should be placed in the Trendelenburg position with left lateral decubitus in order to trap the air in the apex of the right ventricle. 100% oxygen administration can speed air reabsorption.

22.9.5 Cardiac Arrhythmias

Premature ventricular contractions, ventricular tachycardia, and right or left bundle branch blocks can occur during CVC placement and are due to guide-wire progression along the superior vena cava. They can be prevented by advancing the guide wire not more than 16 cm. Failure to recognize cardiac arrhythmias significantly increases the risk of cardiac arrest [5, 27, 28]. Therefore, ECG monitoring during the CVC placement procedure is mandatory.

22.9.6 CVC Malposition

CVC malposition occurs when the tip is not in the correct position. The ideal position of the tip differs between temporary and tunneled catheters. The former are rigid and have a pointed end; therefore the tip should be positioned into the superior vena cava 2–3 cm above the atriocaval junction in order to avoid the perforation of the venous and/or cardiac wall [29]. The latter are not rigid and have blunt ends, so the tips can be placed into the right atrium with no risk of cardiac perforation, higher blood flow rates, and lower incidence of steno-thrombosis and malfunction compared to superior vena cava [1]. CVC malposition is much more likely when the left internal jugular vein is cannulated, because the presence of multiple collateral veins increases the risk that the CVC enters alternative routes or encounters difficulties in progressing along the vein [30]. The most critical points are the union between left jugular vein and left anonymous vein and the union between left anonymous vein and superior vena cava. International guidelines recommend checking the correct positioning of the tip before using CVC. For temporary CVC, a chest X-ray in both anteroposterior and latero-lateral projection is recommended, whereas fluoroscopy is mandatory for tunneled catheters. Fluoroscopy is the gold standard for evaluating the correct tip position, allowing a real-time visualization of the guide wire and the catheter and an early recognition of procedural complications. A valid alternative to imaging techniques is endocavitary ECG, which is able to indicate the position of the tip through the recognition of typical P wave patterns [31]. The only limit is the absence of P waves at the basal ECG (for example in patients with atrial fibrillation, supraventricular arrhythmias, and/or pacemaker carriers).

22.10 Conclusion

The use of ultrasounds for central venous catheter placement reduces the incidence of complications related to the technique and allows the clinician to perform a correct procedure. Nevertheless, the use of US in central venous catheterism does not exclude complication and operator's training and experience are essential to execute a successful and safe procedure.

References

1. Ruesch S, Walder B, Tramar MR. Complications of central venous catheters: internal jugular versus subclavian access - a systematic review. Crit Care Med. 2002;30(2):454–60.
2. McGee DC, Gould MK. Preventing complications of central venous catheterization. N Engl J Med. 2003;348(12):1123–33.
3. Seldinger SI. Catheter replacement of the needle in percutaneous arteriography; a new technique. Acta Radiol. 1953;39:368–76.
4. Higgs ZC, Macafee DA, Braithwaite BD, Maxwell-Armstrong CA. The Seldinger technique: 50 years on. Lancet. 2005;366(9494):1407–9.
5. Rabindranath KS, Kumar E, Shail R, et al. Use of real-time ultrasound guidance for the placement of hemodialysis catheters: a systematic review and meta-analysis of randomized controlled trials. Am J Kidney Dis. 2011;58(6):964–70.
6. Hind D, Calvert N, McWilliams R, et al. Ultrasonic locating devices for central venous cannulation: meta-analysis. BMJ. 2003;327:361.
7. Rabindranath KS, Kumar E, Shail R, Vaux EC. Ultrasound use for the placement of haemodialysis catheters. Cochrane Database Syst Rev. 2011:CD005279.
8. Londrino F, Floccari F, Granata A, et al. Internal jugular vein cannulation: why ultrasound guidance should be expanded as much as possible. J Vasc Access. 2013;14(4):400–1.
9. NKF-K/DOQI Vascular Access Work Group. Clinical practice guidelines for vascular access. Am J Kidney Dis. 2006;48:S176–273.
10. Dariushnia SR, Wallace MJ, Siddiqi NH, et al. Society of Interventional Radiology Standards of Practice Committee. Quality improvement guidelines for central venous access. J Vasc Interv Radiol. 2010;21:976–81.
11. ACS Committee on Perioperative Care. Revised statement on recommendations for use of real-time ultrasound guidance for placement of central venous catheters. Bull Am Coll Surg. 2011;96:36–7.
12. Lamperti M, Bodenham AR, Pittiruti M, et al. International evidence-based recommendations on ultrasound-guided vascular access. Intensive Care Med. 2012;38:1105–17.
13. Rupp SM, Apfelbaum JL, Bitt C, et al. American Society of Anesthesiologists Task Force on central venous access: a report by the American Society of Anesthesiologists Task Force on central venous access. Anesthesiology. 2012;116:539–73.
14. Siverberg MJ, Kory P. Intensive care ultrasound: II. Central vascular access and venous diagnostic ultrasound. Ann Am Thorac Soc. 2013;10(5):549–56.
15. Mitchell E and Averill LW. Principles of ultrasound-guided venous access. www.uptodate.com - last access 11 July 2014.
16. Troianos CA, Hartman GS, Glas KE, et al. Guidelines for performing ultrasound guided vascular cannulation: recommendations of the American Society of Echocardiography and the Society of Cardiovascular Anesthesiologists. J Am Soc Echocardiogr. 2011;24:1291–318.
17. Fiorini F, Zanforlin A, D'Amelio A, et al. L'ecografia polmonare in nefrologia. G Ital Nefrol. 2014;31(3):1–11.
18. Milling TJ, Rose J, Briggs WM, et al. Randomized, controlled clinical trial of point-of-care limited ultrasonography assistance of central venous cannulation: the third sonography outcomes assessment program (SOAP-3) trial. Crit Care Med. 2005;33:1764–9.
19. Bray BD, Boyd J, Daly C, et al. Vascular access type and risk of mortality in a national prospective cohort of haemodialysis patients. QJM. 2012;105(11):1097–103. https://doi.org/10.1093/qjmed/hcs143.
20. Ocak G, Halbesma N, Le Cessie S, et al. Haemodialysis catheters increase mortality as compared to arteriovenous accesses especially in elderly patients. Nephrol Dial Transplant. 2011;26(8):2611–7. https://doi.org/10.1093/ndt/gfq775.
21. Chaudhry M, Bhola C, Joarder M, et al. Seeing eye to eye: the key to reducing catheter use. J Vasc Access. 2011;12(2):120–6.
22. Merrer J, De Jonghe B, Golliot F, et al. Complications of femoral and subclavian venous catheterization in critically ill patients: a randomized controlled trial. JAMA. 2001;286(6):700–7.
23. Clark EG, Barsuk JH. Temporary hemodialysis catheters: recent advances. Kidney Int. 2014;86(5):888–95. https://doi.org/10.1038/ki.2014.162.
24. KDIGO Clinical practice guidelines for acute kidney injury section 5: dialysis interventions for treatment of AKI. "Kidney inter", Suppl. 2012;2:89–115.
25. Practice guidelines for central venous access: a report by the American Society of Anesthesiologists Task Force on Central Venous Access. Anesthesiology. 2012;116(3):539–73. doi: https://doi.org/10.1097/ALN.0b013e31823c9569.
26. Work J. Chronic catheter placement. Semin Dial. 2001;14(6):436–40.
27. Graham AS, Ozment C, Tegtmeyer K, et al. Videos in clinical medicine. Central venous catheterization. N Engl J Med. 2007;356(21):e21.
28. Wirsing M, Schummer C, Neumann R, et al. Is traditional reading of the bedside chest radiograph appropriate to detect intra-atrial central venous catheter position? Chest. 2008 Sep;134(3):527–33. https://doi.org/10.1378/chest.07-2687.
29. Young MP. Complication of central venous catheter and their prevention. www.uptodate.com
30. Granata A, Figuera M, Basile A. Right internal thoracic cannulation by CVC for hemodialysis therapy. Am J Kidney Dis. 2008;51(5):A42–4. https://doi.org/10.1053/j.ajkd.2007.12.025.
31. Calabria M, Zamboli P, D'Amelio A, et al. Use of ECG-EC in the positioning of central venous catheters. G Ital Nefrol. 2012;29(1):49–57.

Part V

Non-renal Imaging in Nephrologic Patients

23 Parathyroid

Antonio Granata, Mancuso Salvatore, and Stefano Spiezie

23.1 Introduction

Secondary hyperparathyroidism (sHPT) is a common complication of chronic kidney disease (CKD). The humoral changes related to uremia impair the enteric calcium absorption and promote phosphate retention and 1,25-hydroxycholecalciferol deficiency. Serum parathyroid hormone (PTH) and fibroblast growth factor-23 (FGF-23) levels increase in order to maintain calcium homeostasis, causing changes in parathyroid cell biology and leading to a diffuse hyperplasia of the parathyroid glands. As the disease progresses, cell clones with reduced calcium receptor (CaR) and vitamin D receptor (VDR) density are selected. The histological pattern varies from polyclonal and widespread to monoclonal and nodular glandular hyperplasia, making the parathyroid glands less responsive to hormonal stimuli and more resistant to medical treatments, such as vitamin D pulse therapy [1]. In CKD patients with long-standing sHPT, parathyroid tissue loses the normal feedback inhibition by calcium. The resultant autonomous parathyroid hormone secretion and hypercalcemia lead to tertiary hyperparathyroidism (tHPT). sHPT and tHPT are responsible for the so-called *chronic kidney disease-mineral bone disease (CKD-MBD)*, which correlates with higher cardiovascular risk, fracture rates, and morbidity and mortality than the general population [2]. Nowadays, sHPT diagnosis is based on biochemical parameters of mineral metabolism because the identification of normal parathyroid glands is difficult with all imaging techniques. Radionuclide localization of the parathyroid glands with ^{99m}Tc sestamibi is efficacious for primary hyperparathyroidism, whereas its role in sHPT and tHPT is poorly defined. High-resolution ultrasound with color Doppler (US/CD) is helpful in localizing parathyroid glands. Moreover, US/CD is able to detect volumetric variations of parathyroid glands and to provide semi-quantitative parameters for glandular perfusion during the progression of sHPT [3]. A broad spectrum of therapy options is available. Vitamin D analogs and phosphate binders are widely used in order to lower serum PTH levels; however some studies have demonstrated that they do not stop the course of the disease. Calcimimetics could reduce the occurrence of severe sHPT, although randomized clinical trials demonstrating the long-term efficacy of these drugs are still lacking [4]. A parathyroidectomy is necessary in approximately 5–10% of patients with sHPT or tHPT [5] if a large amount of parathyroid tissue is present.

A. Granata (✉)
Department of Nephrology and Dialysis, "Cannizzaro" Emergency Hospital, Catania, Italy

M. Salvatore
Advanced School of Nephrology, A.O. per l'Emergenza "Cannizzaro", Catania, Italy

S. Spiezie
Endocrine Surgery Unit, "Ospedale del Mare" ASL Napoli1 Centro, Naples, Italy

A. Granata, M. Bertolotto (eds.), *Imaging in Nephrology*,
https://doi.org/10.1007/978-3-030-60794-4_23

23.2 Anatomical Characteristics of Parathyroid Glands

The parathyroid glands are located on the posterior aspect of the lateral lobes of the thyroid gland. They are flattened and oval in shape, situated external to the gland itself, but within its sheath. The majority of people have four parathyroid glands (two superior, two inferior), although variation in number is common: the absence of one parathyroid gland is found in 3% of cases, accessory or supernumerary glands in 13% of cases, and ectopic glands in 15–29% of cases (Fig. 23.1). The embryological origin of the superior parathyroid glands is the fourth pharyngeal pouch. They are located approximately 1 cm superior to the entry of the inferior thyroid arteries into the thyroid gland and the recurrent laryngeal nerve (at the level of the inferior border of the cricoid cartilage). The embryological origin of the inferior parathyroid glands is the third pharyngeal pouch. The inferior parathyroid glands are usually found near the inferior poles of the thyroid gland. In a small percentage of people, the glands can be found as far inferiorly as the superior mediastinum. Parathyroid glands are supplied by the branches of the inferior thyroid arteries. The parathyroid veins drain into the thyroid plexus of veins. The lymphatic vessels drain into the deep cervical lymph nodes and paratracheal lymph nodes, along with those of the thyroid gland. Nerves are made up of vasomotor fibers deriving from the thyroid branches of the cervical sympathetic ganglia [6].

23.3 Echographic Evaluation of the Cervical Region

The examination of the cervical region should be performed supine with a pillow placed beneath the shoulders to slightly extend the neck. The

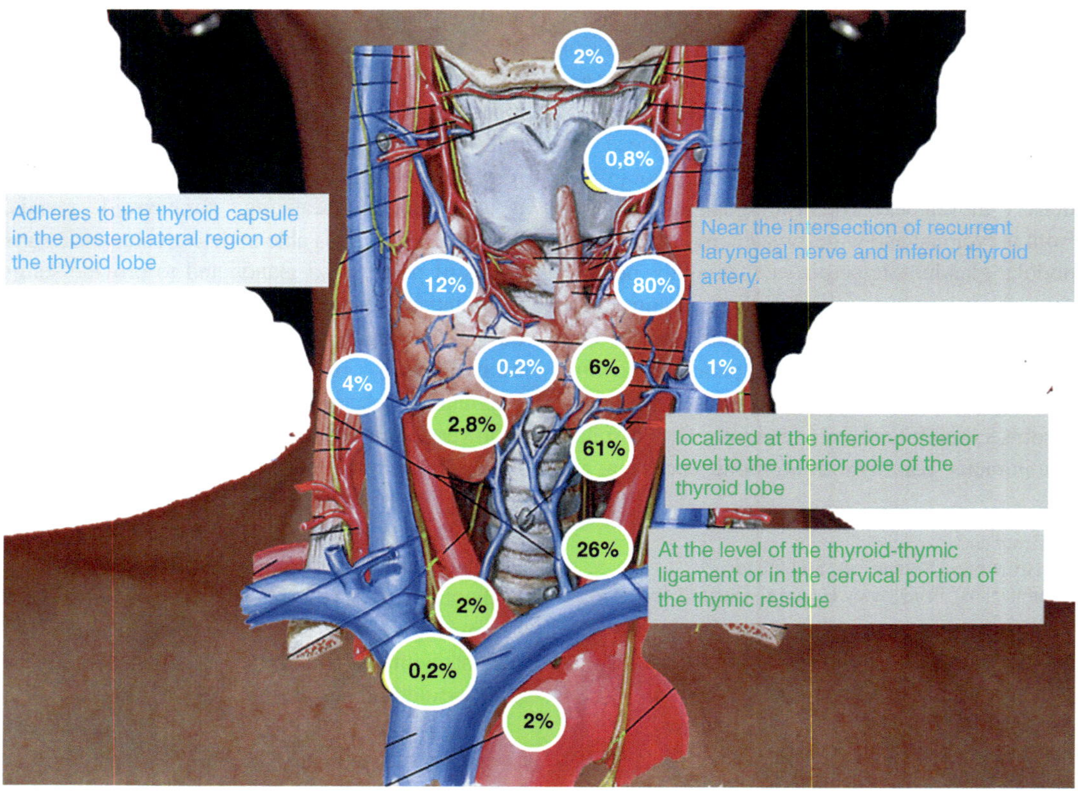

Fig. 23.1 The possible positions of the parathyroid glands, with their respective percentages

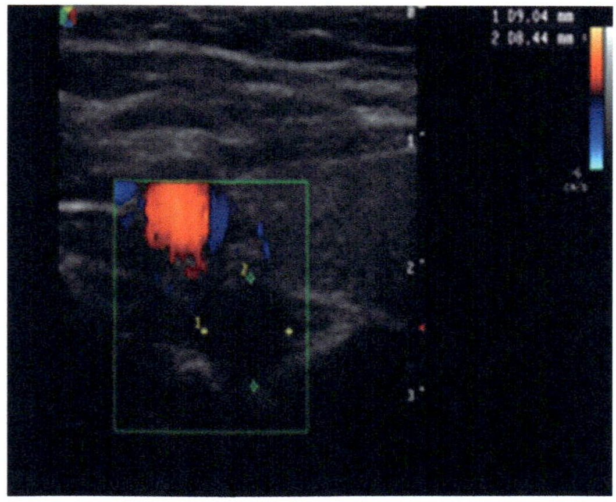

Fig. 23.2 Evaluation of the parathyroid gland: echogenicity (typically hypoechoic), morphology (oval shaped or roundish), and two diameters in the axial scan

neck must be deviated, first to the right and then to the left, in order to allow the exploration of the laterocervical region from the corner of the jaw to the superior mediastinum. Ultrasound examination should be performed with high-resolution linear probes (7.5–14 MHz). Initial scanning should be performed with real-time grayscale imaging in the transverse plane, beginning at the level of the superior pole of the thyroid and continuing inferiorly to the sternal notch. Just above the clavicle, the probe should be angled inferiorly to visualize the neck to the level of the subclavian vein. Scans then should be performed in the longitudinal plane before moving to the contralateral side [7]. As parathyroid glands may be hidden below the clavicles in the lower neck and upper mediastinum, it may be helpful to have the patient swallow during the examination with constant real-time observation.

The presence of numerous adipose cells makes parathyroid glands structurally similar to the thyroid parenchyma, so that they are difficult to distinguish even using high-resolution probes. Primary or secondary cellular hyperplasia, however, makes the glands diffusely hypoechoic compared with thyroid tissue and well outlined by a thin hyperechoic edge. Once visualized, the location, size, and number of the enlarged parathyroid glands should be documented, and measurements should be made in three dimensions (Fig. 23.2). If no lesions are identified on real-time grayscale imaging, longitudinal scans of the thyroid should be repeated using color and power Doppler imaging to look specifically for asymmetry of the thyroid vasculature. In sHPT the increase in volume of parathyroid glands is associated with the evidence of an enlarged feeding artery at the hilum and a widespread increase in vascularity characterized by the presence of a peripheral arc and/or raylike endonodular vessels (Fig. 23.3).

Although US/CD is an operator-dependent procedure, diagnostic ultrasound of the neck is very useful in evaluating parathyroid gland abnormalities, with a reported sensitivity of 90% in detecting cervical glands and a better resolution than computed tomography and magnetic resonance. Sensitivity is reduced for the identification of ectopic glands, with a reported value of 44% for glands localized below the sternal notch [8]. As mentioned above, the trend over time of serum PTH levels and other mineral metabolism parameters is pivotal for sHPT diagnosis and for therapeutic decisions. In this setting, US/CD can act as a surrogate marker of sHPT by identifying the number and the volume of hyperplastic glands. Although a size limit to define a pathological parathyroid gland has not been identified, the presence of at least a hypoechoic gland with at least two diameters >5 mm and a volume >500 mm^3 are strongly associated with hyperplasia [9]. Some authors have proposed US scores in order to simplify the diagnosis of nodular hyperplasia. Onoda et al. [10] elaborated a US score in which the power Doppler signals at periphery (P-signal) and at the center of parathyroid glands (C-signal) were classified in ordinal scale. Vulpio et al. [11] combined the power Doppler P- and C-signals with the echostructural pattern of the glands (EP score). Both the authors concluded that the findings of abundant power Doppler signal inside the glands with a highly heterogeneous or an evident nodular ultrasound pattern are associated with nodular hyperplasia, as demonstrated by a post-parathyroidectomy histological comparison.

It must be emphasized that the presence of high serum PTH levels is not always associated

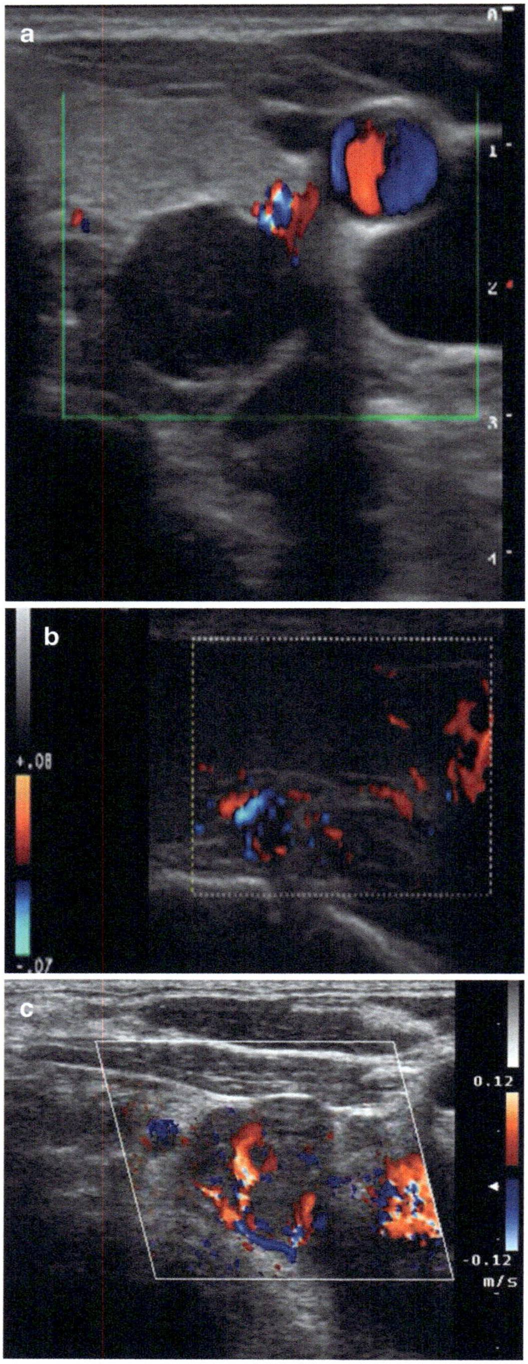

Fig. 23.3 Echo-color Doppler of the parathyroid gland: (**a**, **b**) In many cases it is possible to recognize the hilum (57% of cases). (**c**) Rich and uniformly distributed vascularization (25% of cases)

with ultrasound evidence of enlarged parathyroid glands at the time of diagnosis of sHPT. Similarly, the trend of serum PTH levels is not indicative of the functional state of the parathyroid glands during the course of the disease. Based on actual evidence, morpho-functional parameters such as a reduction of glandular diameter and volume, hyperechogenicity (due to a reversed ratio between cellularity and stromal adipose tissue), and presence of calcifications and/or involutive anechoic cysts without vascularization seems to be more indicative of the response to medical therapy [12].

The availability of calcimimetics has revolutionized the therapeutic approach to sHPT. Some studies have investigated the role of cinacalcet in promoting a reversal in the progression of sHPT, demonstrating a progressive serum PTH level reduction, stabilization of mineral metabolism, and reduction of glandular volume and vascularization [13, 14]. However, data regarding the superiority of calcimimetics over vitamin D analogs and phosphate binders are conflicting due to the lack of randomized clinical trials [4]. Therefore, parathyroidectomy is still the last therapeutic option in nonresponder patients. The presurgical ultrasound evaluation of parathyroid glands in sHPT is not diriment as for primary hyperparathyroidism because hyperplasia does not involve equally all the glands and an exploratory cervicotomy is mandatory for a complete excision. The role of US/CD is therefore to establish the surgical timing. In fact, according to international guidelines [15], parathyroidectomy is indicated when US/CD shows at least one hyperplastic gland with a volume $\geq$500 mm^3.

Finally, US/CD is useful as a guidance for percutaneous ethanol injection therapy (PEIT), which consists of a selective chemical ablation of the parathyroid glands [16]. Although the procedure is safe and the short-term results are promising, the long-term outcomes are still unknown. Actually, the only indication for PEIT is recurrent sHPT untreatable with parathyroidectomy [17].

23.4 Parathyroid Scintigraphy

Parathyroid glands can be localized using a radionuclide thanks to the capacity to concentrate a variety of chemical substances in their parenchyma. ^{99m}Tc sestamibi is the radiotracer of choice because it ensures a superior image quality and an improved accuracy compared to other molecules. After intravenous administration, this cationic and lipophilic radiopharmaceutical is rapidly cleared from circulation and passively accumulates within the mitochondria of metabolically active cells. In patients with sHPT the intensity of the focal uptake of ^{99m}Tc sestamibi in the parathyroid glands is considered to be directly related to the phase of the cell cycle. Higher uptake levels correlate with the active phase of cell growth, indicating that ^{99m}Tc sestamibi scintigraphy reflects the functional state of the gland [18]. Because it washes out more rapidly from the thyroid than from the abnormal parathyroid tissue, ^{99m}Tc sestamibi (sometimes used with ^{123}I, a tracer specific to the thyroid) reduces the number of false positive due to the simultaneous presence of thyroid nodules and/or lymph nodes. Conventional scintigraphic evaluation of parathyroid glands was performed with planar imaging. Modern techniques, such as single-photon emission computed tomography (SPECT) and SPECT with CT scanning (SPECT-TC), allow a three-dimensional visualization of the parathyroid lesions, distinguishing them from a thyroid lesion and thus increasing the sensitivity of the technique [19]. Although the role of scintigraphy in the management of sHPT and tHPT is not well defined, SPECT and SPECT-TC are both helpful in detecting ectopic or supernumerary glands, especially in the mediastinum where they have shown a greater capacity than planar imaging to distinguish anterior from posterior mediastinum lesions. The imaged field should span from the angle of the mandible to the heart because ectopic glands may be widely distributed along the parathyroid cell migration routes. A correct identification of ectopic or supernumerary glands is very important especially before parathyroidectomy, because it avoids surgical failure and reduces the extent of dissection. Another useful information is the identification of the parathyroid gland with the lowest ^{99m}Tc-MIBI uptake intensity, which can be partially autografted or maintained in situ in order to maintain a correct mineral balance and avoid adynamic bone disease [20]. Positron-emission tomography (PET) using ^{11}C-methionine can be a useful method in patients with secondary hyperparathyroidism when the results of echography and gammagraphy have proved negative or inconclusive. Furthermore, ectopic glands are identified with greater precision by PET than by conventional scintigraphy, as it enables three-dimensional images to be obtained [21].

23.5 Computed Tomography (CT) and Nuclear Magnetic Resonance (NMR)

CT has a marginal role in the management of sHPT because the enhancement patterns of parathyroid glands are extremely variable and the presence of lymph nodes and/or thyroid nodules can all cause false-positive results. Moreover, it must be considered that the use of contrast media in patients with sHPT due to chronic kidney disease should be avoided. Nevertheless, CT can locate parathyroid glands with less than 4 mm in size, as well as peri-thyroid, substernal, or retroclavicular soft-tissue masses. Some series have reported that its sensitivity is similar to that of scintigraphy and echography in the diagnosis of multiglandular parathyroid disease, but the cost is greater and the detection of parathyroid tissue which is adjacent to the thyroid gland may be difficult [22]. Nuclear magnetic resonance (NMR) seems to be more sensitive and offers the possibility of improving images by the use of contrast agent and 3-D reconstruction. Several studies refer to NMR as an imaging test which is more sensitive than CT [23, 24] although it is more difficult to differentiate parathyroid adenomas from thyroid lesions. Currently, the only indication to CT and NMR is the localization of parathyroid hyperplasia when the above tests (echography and scintigraphy) have proved negative [21].

References

1. Drüeke TB. Cell biology of parathyroid gland hyperplasia in chronic renal failure. J Am Soc Nephrol. 2000;11(6):1141–52.
2. Block GA, Klassen PS, Lazarus JM, et al. Mineral metabolism, mortality, and morbidity in maintenance hemodialysis. J Am Soc Nephrol. 2004;15(8):2208–18. https://doi.org/10.1097/01.ASN.0000133041.27682.A2.
3. Katoh N, Nakayama M, Shigematsu T, et al. Presence of sonographically detectable parathyroid glands can predict resistance to oral pulsed-dose calcitriol treatment of secondary hyperparathyroidism. Am J Kidney Dis. 2000;35(3):465–8.
4. Vulpio C, Bossola M, De Gaetano A, et al. Parathyroid gland ultrasound patterns and biochemical findings after one-year cinacalcet treatment for advanced secondary hyperparathyroidism. Ther Apher Dial. 2010;14(2):178–85. https://doi.org/10.1111/j.1744-9987.2009.00781.x.
5. Dumasius V, Angelos P. Parathyroid surgery in renal failure patients. Otolaryngol Clin N Am. 2010;43(2):433–40, x-xi. https://doi.org/10.1016/j.otc.2010.01.010.
6. Steward DL, Hainston JA. Development and surgical anatomy of the thyroid compartment. In: Terris DJ, Goirin CG, editors. Thyroid and parathyroid disease. New York: Thieme; 2009. p. 11–7.
7. Alkhalili E, Tasci Y, Aksoy E, et al. The utility of neck ultrasound and sestamibi scans in patients with secondary and tertiary hyperparathyroidism. World J Surg. 2015;39(3):701–5. https://doi.org/10.1007/s00268-014-2878-3.
8. Meola M, Petrucci I, Cupisti A. Ultrasound in clinical setting of secondary hyperparathyroidism. J Nephrol. 2013;26(5):848–55. https://doi.org/10.5301/jn.5000219.
9. Pavlović D, Brzac HT. Prevention and treatment of secondary hyperparathyroidism: still a challenge for the nephrologist? Nephrol Dial Transplant. 2003;18(Suppl 5):v45–6.
10. Onoda N, Kurihara S, Sakurai Y, et al. Evaluation of blood supply to the parathyroid glands in secondary hyperparathyroidism compared with histopathology. Nephrol Dial Transplant. 2003;18(Suppl 3):iii34–7.
11. Vulpio C, Bossola M, De Gaetano A, et al. Ultrasound patterns of parathyroid glands in chronic hemodialysis patients with secondary hyperparathyroidism. Am J Nephrol. 2008;28(4):589–97. https://doi.org/10.1159/000116875.
12. Matsuoka S, Tominaga Y, Sato T, et al. Relationship between the dimension of parathyroid glands estimated by ultrasonography and the hyperplastic pattern in patients with renal hyperparathyroidism. Ther Apher Dial. 2008;12(5):391–5. https://doi.org/10.1111/j.1744-9987.2008.00615.x.
13. Komaba H, Nakanishi S, Fujimori A, et al. Cinacalcet effectively reduces parathyroid hormone secretion and gland volume regardless of pretreatment gland size in patients with secondary hyperparathyroidism. Clin J Am Soc Nephrol. 2010;5(12):2305–14. https://doi.org/10.2215/CJN.02110310.
14. Meola M, Petrucci I, Barsotti G. Long-term treatment with cinacalcet and conventional therapy reduces parathyroid hyperplasia in severe secondary hyperparathyroidism. Nephrol Dial Transplant. 2009 Mar;24(3):982–9. https://doi.org/10.1093/ndt/gfn654.
15. Kidney Disease: Improving Global Outcomes (KDIGO) CKD-MBD Work Group. KDIGO clinical practice guideline for the diagnosis, evaluation, prevention, and treatment of Chronic Kidney Disease-Mineral and Bone Disorder (CKD-MBD). Kidney Int Suppl. 2009;113:S1–130. https://doi.org/10.1038/ki.2009.188.
16. Fukagawa M, Kitaoka M, Tominaga Y, et al. Selective percutaneous ethanol injection therapy (PEIT) of the parathyroid in chronic dialysis patients--the Japanese strategy. Japanese Working Group on PEIT of Parathyroid, Tokyo, Japan. Nephrol Dial Transplant. 1999;14(11):2574–7.
17. Hindié E, Ugur O, Fuster D, et al. 2009 EANM parathyroid guidelines. Eur J Nucl Med Mol Imaging. 2009;36(7):1201–16. https://doi.org/10.1007/s00259-009-1131-z.
18. Torregrosa JV, Fernández-Cruz L, Canalejo A, Vidal S, Astudillo E, Almadén Y, et al. 99mTc-sestamibi scintigraphy and cell cycle in parathyroid glands of secondary hyperparathyroidism. World J Surg. 2000;24:1386–90.
19. Sharma J, Halkar R, Weber CJ. Imaging of parathyroid glands in end stage renal disease. Semin Dial. 2017;30(4):369–72. https://doi.org/10.1111/sdi.12608.
20. Taïeb D, Ureña-Torres P, Zanotti-Fregonara P, et al. Parathyroid scintigraphy in renal hyperparathyroidism. The added diagnostic value of SPECT and SPECT/CT. Clin Nucl Med. 2013;38(8):630–5. https://doi.org/10.1097/RLU.0b013e31829af5bf.
21. Torregrosa JV, Félez I, Fuster D. Usefulness of imaging techniques in secondary hyperparathyroidism. Nefrologia. 2010;30(2):158–67. https://doi.org/10.3265/Nefrologia.pre2010.Jan.10231.
22. Weber AL, Randolph G, Aksoy FG. The thyroid and parathyroid glands-CT and imaging and correlation with pathology and clinical findings. Radio Clin North Am. 2000;38:1105.
23. McDermott VG, Fernández RJM, Meakem TJ, et al. Preoperative MR imaging in hyperparathyroidism: results and factors affecting parathyroid detection. Am J Roentgenol. 1996;166:705–10.
24. Stevens SK, Chang JM, Clark OH, et al. Detection of abnormal parathyroid glands in postoperative patients with recurrent hyperparathyroidism sensitivity of MR imaging. Am J Roentgenol. 1993;160:607–12.

24 The Role of Doppler Ultrasound in Preoperative Vascular Mapping and Postoperative Follow-Up of Arteriovenous Fistula for Hemodialysis

Antonio Granata, Irene Campo, Rosario Maccarrone, Slave Boicef, Fiorini Fulvio, and Pasquale Zamboli

24.1 Introduction

Arterio-venous fistulas (AVFs) created with native vessels are the vascular access of choice for hemodialysis: compared with grafts and central venous catheters, AVFs have longer survival and fewer complications and are associated with better clinical outcomes (mortality, infection, hospitalization, and cardiovascular events) [1, 2]. However, nephrologists and vascular surgeons find it increasingly difficult to locate native vessels suitable for creation of a well-functioning, persistently patent AVF because of increasing prevalence among patients requiring dialysis of advanced age and comorbidities, such as diabetes mellitus and vascular disease [3]. The use of Doppler ultrasound (DUS) by physicians performing vascular access surgery has increased the number of cases in which AVFs can be created with native vessels by allowing preoperative mapping and identification of suitable vessels. Indeed DUS, providing more information about arm vascularization, reduces the unsuccessful surgical exploration rate and identifies the most appropriate target vessels; in a recent meta-analysis DUS mapping significantly reduced the risk of immediate AVF failure [4, 5]. DUS can also extend native AVF survival by improving early diagnosis and rapid correction of fistula's complications (postoperative surveillance) [6].

This review examines the numerous roles played by DUS in the construction and postoperative follow-up of AVFs with particular attention to preoperative vascular mapping, maturation, and surveillance of AVF.

24.2 The Doppler Ultrasound in the Presurgical Phase: "Preoperative Vascular Mapping"

For decades, the selection of vessels to be used for constructing an AVF was based exclusively on physical examination of the upper limbs,

A. Granata (✉)
Department of Nephrology and Dialysis, "Cannizzaro" Emergency Hospital, Catania, Italy

R. Maccarrone
Nephrology and Dialysis Unit, "San Giovanni Di Dio" Hospital, Agrigento, Italy

I. Campo
Department of Radiology, Civile Hospital, Conegliano, Italy

S. Boicef
Vascular Surgery Unit, Maggiore Hospital, Cremona, Italy

F. Fulvio
Nepherology and Dialysis Unit, Santa Maria della Misericordia Hospital, Rovigo, Italy

P. Zamboli
Vascular Access Department, Second University of Naples, Naples, Italy

A. Granata, M. Bertolotto (eds.), *Imaging in Nephrology*, https://doi.org/10.1007/978-3-030-60794-4_24

which is a low-cost, bedside procedure that requires no additional equipment. Although this approach can provide acceptable information on the superficial venous circulation (vessel palpability, caliber, patency, and course), it furnishes much more limited data on the arterial vessels (pulse palpability and patency of the arterial circulation of the hand based on the results of the Allen test) [7, 8]. In addition, physical examination alone is insufficient in a considerable percentage of patients (~25–50%) [8].

DUS provides more information on the superficial and deep veins of the arm and a wealth of additional data on the arterial circulation in comparison to physical examination. In addition, DUS is noninvasive, safe, and repeatable; it is the only diagnostic imaging technique that allows simultaneous visualization of the anatomy of an area (B-mode) and its blood supply (color Doppler); and it can be performed directly by the physician who will create the vascular access. Routine preoperative mapping results in a marked increase in placement of AVFs, in the success rate of fistula creation, and in an improvement in the adequacy of forearm fistulas for dialysis as well as in a reduction of primary failure and of fistula abandonment. Ultrasound examination improves moreover times to functional fistula maturation and secondary patency [4, 5, 9–11]. Therefore, although some authors maintain (suggest) that DUS should not be part of the routine preoperative assessment but should be used only in the presence of anomalies during the physical examination (because it is time consuming, and requires an experienced examiner and special equipment) [9], preoperative vascular mapping is recommended by main international guidelines for all patient candidates for an AVF, as a natural complement to the physical examination [12, 13]. In our opinion DUS is mandatory prior to vascular access surgery because the goal of the preoperative evaluation is not only to establish the next vascular access but also to design a sequence of surgical options for the individual patient [14, 15].

24.2.1 Technical Requirements and Examination Technique

The ultrasound scanner used to map the upper extremity vasculature must be equipped with a linear probe with minimum frequencies of 7 MHz for the B-mode examination and 5 MHz for the Doppler study [16]. The patient should be examined in the supine position with the trunk moderately elevated to avoid flexion of the elbow. Alternatively, he/she may be seated in front of the operator with the forearm resting on a stand. Most examiners prefer the supine position because it simplifies the assessment of the vascular structures of the arm (subclavicular axillary region) and is more comfortable for the patient [16, 17]. The examination should be carried out in a comfortably warm room, and the gel should also be warmed to avoid triggering vasoconstriction of the structures being examined [16, 17]. Ideally, the arterial and venous districts should be evaluated consecutively, with transverse and/or longitudinal scans of the arteries (from the root of the arm towards the hand) and veins (from the periphery towards the thorax). The examination can begin with the arterial or the venous district, depending on operator preferences and characteristics of the individual patient. A thorough examination of the circulation of the arm must include B-mode assessment of morphological aspects as well as color Doppler evaluation of arterial and venous blood flow.

24.2.2 Preoperative Arterial Mapping: Morphological Parameters

The arterial evaluation tries to identify an artery able of delivering adequate inflow to the AVF while preserving flow to the hand. DUS allows thorough assessment of the arterial circulation of the arm based on a series of morphological and functional parameters [8]. The morphological aspects include vessel diameter, wall thickness, wall alterations, vessel course, and any steno-obstructive lesions that may be present. The functional evaluation involves the assessment of blood flow and the artery's ability to dilate.

Preoperative arterial DUS should include evaluation of subclavian, axillary, brachial, radial, and ulnar arteries [18]. In clinical practice, however, most arterial evaluations begin with the distal subclavian artery or even the brachial artery [7, 19]: only when anomalies are found at these levels is the investigation extended to the proximal portion of the subclavian artery.

The internal diameter of an artery can be measured on either longitudinal or transverse scans [17], but the former allows visualization of the intimal layers of the superficial and deep vessel walls, thereby facilitating more precise measurement of the intima–intima distance (i.e., the internal diameter of the vessel) [7]. The internal diameter is measured at the site of the expected anastomosis. To verify the precision of these measurements, sonographically measured vessel diameters have been compared with measurements obtained directly during surgery, and the correlation between the two proved to be good [20]. The relationship between arterial diameters and AVF outcomes has been studied in radial-cephalic fistulas. In the first major publication on this subject, Silva et al. proposed a minimal arterial diameter of 2 mm, which in their experience was associated with an early failure rate of 8% and a 1-year primary patency rate of 83% [21]. Although this threshold has been questioned by other investigators, this 2 mm recommendation for the minimum arterial diameter threshold is the one that is more commonly accepted in adults. However, the disparities in the studies available on this topic do not allow to make a recommendation on the minimum diameter of the artery used for AVF creation. Therefore, indicating an ideal threshold for the diameter of the artery is inappropriate; this also reflects the fact that the arterial diameter is only one of the factors that affect the probability of successful AVF creation. It has to be evaluated in conjunction with other clinical and ultrasound parameters which provide indications on the anatomic and functional status of the artery. In other words, the functional quality of the artery is an important determinant of AVF success, and it is not necessarily related to the internal diameter of the vessel (as shown, for example, by experience with AVFs created in pediatric patients).

The presence of arteriopathy that can jeopardize the success of the AVF can be easily detected with a high-resolution B-mode examination of the thickness and alterations of the vessel walls. Arterial wall changes are, in fact, common in patients with chronic renal insufficiency, diabetes, and atherosclerosis [8]. The intima-media thickness is estimated in a longitudinal scan of the distal wall of the artery. The ultrasonographic measurement shows good correlation with histologic measurement, and increased thickness seems to be closely correlated with fistula failure [22]. Calcifications are sonographically depicted as areas of hyperechogenicity (with or without posterior shadowing) within the arterial wall and irregularities of the intimal lamina. Although these alterations are easy to identify, they are difficult to quantify. In addition, they do not represent contraindications to the creation of a fistula although they can influence its outcome and/or render surgery more difficult [17].

DUS is also a very accurate method for identifying stenotic arterial lesions (sensitivity and specificity: 91% and 100%, respectively, for the subclavian artery; 93% and 100% for the arteries of the arm; 89% and 99% for those of the forearm), obstructive arterial lesions (sensitivity and specificity of 90% and 99%) [23], and vascular abnormalities such as brachial artery bifurcation in the most proximal portion of the arm.

24.2.3 Preoperative Arterial Mapping: Functional Parameters

Likely more important than the diameter of the artery is its functional capacity (its ability to dilate and accommodate the increased blood flow demands of an AV fistula). As noted earlier, the functional study involves the assessment of blood flow and the artery's ability to dilate. Blood flow can be evaluated by measuring the vessel diameter and mean flow velocity (cm/s) on longitudinal scans (see below for calculation of flow volume). However, the value of these measurements in predicting AVF outcome has been assessed in relatively few studies on this subject [8, 24]. Malovrh et al. [8] found that successful radial-cephalic AVF construction was associated with radial artery flow exceeding 50 mL/min while in the study by Sato et al. [24] a preoperative radial artery flow <20 mL/min was associated with an increased risk of "primary AVF failure" within 8 months of surgery. The peak systolic velocity of the inflow artery has also been evaluated as a predictor of a successful AVF. Sedlacek suggests a threshold of at least 50 cm/s for successful creation [25].

After surgery, adequate fistula maturation is associated with dilation of the artery that feeds the AVF. As a result, blood flow within the vascular access increases and the previously triphasic (high resistance) arterial spectrum becomes biphasic (low resistance). The artery's ability to increase its caliber (distensibility) can be estimated preoperatively on the basis of variations in the radial artery Doppler spectrum during the reactive hyperemia test (Fig. 24.1) [8]. The term "reactive hyperemia" refers to the physiological increment in blood flow through an artery that occurs after a period of ischemia. In this test, ischemia is induced by having the patient make a fist for 2 min (others have used 3 min), and the increase in arterial flow (reactive hyperemia) is observed immediately after the hand is reopened [8]. During the phase of ischemia, the Doppler spectrum of the artery is normally triphasic, reflecting high resistance. If the vessel is capable of dilatation, the arterial spectrum becomes biphasic during the phase of reactive hyperemia (Fig. 24.1) [8]. This effect is mediated by nitric oxide released from the endothelium. This spectral variation can be quantified by calculating the resistance index (RI) [RI = (peak systolic velocity − end diastolic velocity)/peak systolic velocity]); in particular, the greater the intensity of the reactive hyperemia, the lower the RI [8]. Malovrh et al. demonstrated that the absence of reactive hyperemia (reflected by an RI >0.7 after the fist is opened) indicates an insufficient increase in

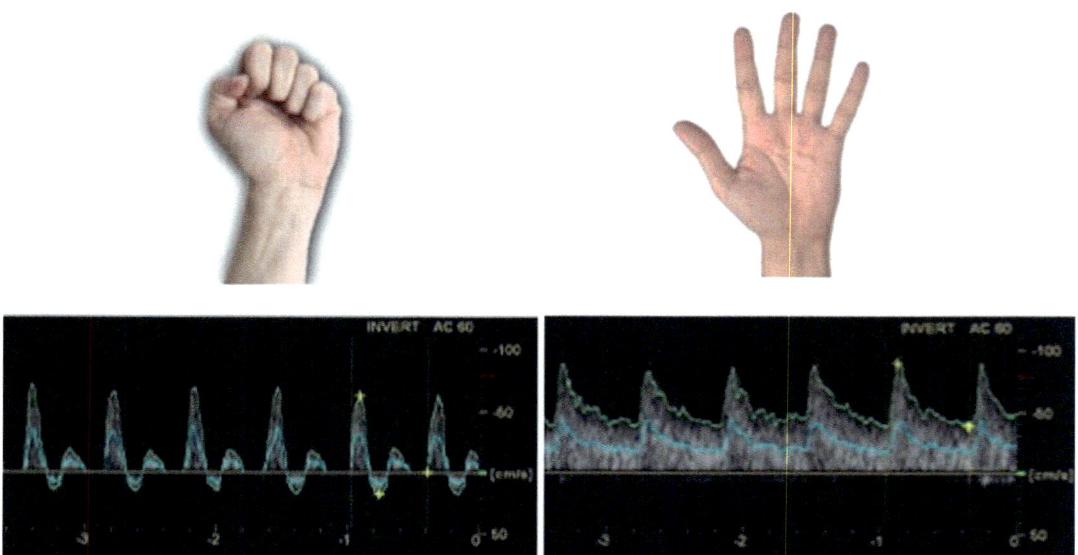

Fig. 24.1 Reactive hyperemia test. *Left:* Ischemic phase with fist closed and corresponding Doppler spectrum. *Right:* Doppler spectrum during the reactive hyperemia phase with the hand opened

arterial flow during the test, which is predictive of immediate postoperative AVF failure [8]. In another report, the hyperemic response was elicited by inflating a blood pressure cuff placed on the upper arm to 20 mmHg above the systolic pressure for 3 min [26]. The response in the artery being evaluated was measured by subtracting the peak systolic velocity (PSV) at rest from the PSV obtained after the period of ischemia. The hyperemic response was recorded for both brachial and radial arteries. They concluded that an AV fistula created using an artery with a hyperemic response that is less than a 5 cm/s increase in PSV was twice as likely to fail as was the one created with a response greater than that level. In addition, an AV fistula constructed using a radial artery with a hyperemic response that is less than a 5 cm/s increase in PSV was 4.5 times as likely to fail as was the one created using a brachial artery with a response >5 cm/s increase in PSV.

These findings show that the reactive hyperemia test provides an excellent index of the functional status of the artery, and it is particularly useful for selecting the artery and the surgical site (wrist, forearm, elbow) for AVF construction.

As we stated before, the arterial evaluation tries to identify an adequate artery for AVF construction but also preserving of flow to the hand. Regarding this latter purpose, the Allen test is used to evaluate the blood supply of the hand. The presence of an optimally functioning dual circulation to the hand, as represented by the radial and ulnar arteries communicating distally through the superficial and deep palmar arches, is an important safeguard against hand ischemia. When the radial artery is used for the AV access, a normal and patent ulnar artery can usually support the perfusion of the hand. In those cases in which the Allen test is clinically difficult to assess, the test can be performed using ultrasound. The radial artery is manually occluded near the wrist and the ultrasound probe is placed distal to the occlusion. Retrograde flow indicates a patent palmar arch and a negative Allen test.

24.2.4 Preoperative Venous Mapping: Morphological Parameters

Preoperative venous DUS involves evaluation of the superficial and deep venous systems of the upper limb from the wrist up to the central veins. With ultrasound, the latter veins can be easily examined up to the distal segment of the subclavian vein, but direct visualization of the proximal portions of the subclavian vein and the innominate vein is not always possible [16]. The superior vena cava cannot be evaluated with DUS because it lies inside the rib cage.

A tourniquet is placed around the root of the arm, and the superficial venous circulation is examined with transverse scans, beginning with the cephalic vein, from the wrist to the point where it drains into the deep venous system [7]. The full course of the basilic vein should also be examined, but this is often done only if the cephalic vein is not suitable for AVF creation [7]. With this assessment a map of the superficial venous circulation can be drawn.

Several ultrasound parameters can be helpful in deciding whether a superficial vein can be used to create an AVF. They include the appearance of the vein wall, the course of the vessel, its patency, caliber, and the presence of collateral circuits [7, 16].

A normal vein is characterized by thin, regular walls and a completely anechoic lumen. The course of the vein must be sufficiently linear (for a distance of at least 8–10 cm), and it should lie less than 6 mm below the skin surface to facilitate venipuncture [12]. Vein patency is assessed by exerting intermittent pressure with the transducer which causes complete collapse of the vessel walls [7]. The non-compressibility of the vein under the transducer's pressure is a sign of obstruction and is often associated with the presence of echogenic material in the lumen. If doubts arise, the patency of the vein can be confirmed using the color Doppler module with a low pulse repetition frequency or by verifying the presence of the Doppler trace in a longitudinal scan. A normal venous Doppler spectrum is characterized by continuous, low-velocity flow, which becomes increasingly phasic as the examination proceeds towards the central veins; the absence of such flow confirms the presence of an obstruction. Doppler spectral analysis can also provide an accurate indirect index of the patency of the innominate veins and the superior vena cava. In fact, the presence at the level of the subclavian and internal jugular veins of flow that varies in velocity with the respiratory and cardiac activity is an indirect index of the patency of the ipsilateral innominate vein and the superior vena cava, whereas a monophasic curve is indicative of steno-occlusion [8, 16, 17]. The suspicion of steno-thrombotic lesions involving a central vein should in any case be confirmed with phlebography [12].

The diameter of the vein should be measured at several points in the arm. This can be done on longitudinal or transverse scans [17]. To reduce the risk of underestimation, gel should be applied copiously to prevent the exertion of excessive pressure with the transducer. As with arterial size, a generally recognized standard for vein size does not exist. It is widely agreed that fistulas created with small-caliber veins (<1.6 mm) are at high risk for early failure [27], but there is no consensus on the minimum cephalic vein diameter that will ensure good maturation of a radial-cephalic AVF. Based on their findings, Silva et al. [21] suggest a minimum diameter of ≥2.5 mm when a tourniquet has been applied; in the absence of a tourniquet, Mendes et al. [28] propose a diameter of >2 mm. Well-documented indications on the minimum diameter for the veins of the arm are also lacking, but a value of at least 3 mm is recommended [17].

Some authors have suggested that the likelihood of nonmaturation is related to the presence and diameter of accessory veins. Wong et al. found that the presence of accessory veins less than 5 cm from the site chosen for the anastomosis can alter the functionality of the fistula [27], while Beathard et al. stressed the importance of the dimensions of these veins and reported higher frequencies of nonmaturation when the AVF was near large collateral veins [29].

24.2.5 Preoperative Venous Mapping: Functional Parameters

Several reports have stressed the importance of evaluating vein distensibility when performing vascular mapping. Indeed, after the AVF has been created, the vein tends to dilate as a result of the increased blood flow and the vein's ability to dilate (venous distensibility) can be evaluated during preoperative mapping. The diameter of the vessel is measured before and at least 2 min after placement of a tourniquet (or a sphygmomanometer cuff inflated to a pressure of 50–60 mmHg), and the increase of diameter is evaluated [17, 30] (Fig. 24.2). The impact of venous distensibility on AVF outcomes has been evaluated in some studies. Malovrh et al. con-

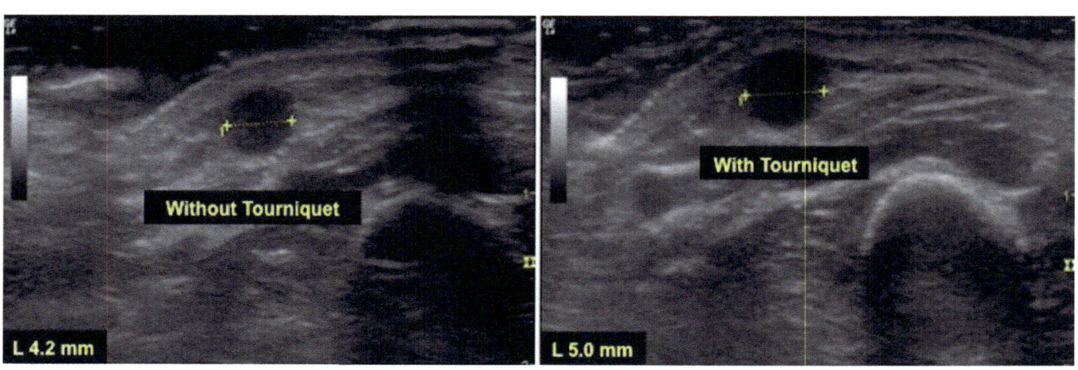

Fig. 24.2 Venous distensibility test using a tourniquet at the root of the limb for 2 min

cluded that venous distensibility is a predictor of outcome since venous diameter increased by an average of 48% in patients with successful fistulas compared with only 11% in failed fistulas [8]. In another study of 50 cases, procedural success was significantly improved for cephalic veins which diameters increased more than 0.35 mm after inflating a blood pressure cuff on the upper arm to a level sufficient to stop superficial venous return for 1 min [31]. In a larger observational study involving 122 patients, the venous distensibility threshold separating successful from unsuccessful cases was >0.4 mm, the difference in vein diameter before and after application of a tourniquet for 2 min [32].

24.3 The Doppler Ultrasound in the Postsurgical Phase: "Maturation and Surveillance of AVF"

24.3.1 Role of DUS in the Assessment of AVF Maturation

The term *maturation* refers to the development of those physical characteristics that render an AVF suitable for venipuncture with large-gauge needles [12]. In many cases, nonmaturation is the reason an AVF cannot be used for dialysis. In fact, despite the obvious long-term advantages in terms of morbidity and mortality that make AVFs the vascular access of choice for hemodialysis patients [12], arterio-venous anastomoses with native vessels have been associated with a high incidence of early occlusion and failure to mature (FTM) during the postoperative period. In different case series, the incidence of FTM for radiocephalic AVFs ranged from 30 to 60% [18, 33].

But how does one assess AVF maturation? Generally, the physical examination conducted by an experienced dialysis nurse is sufficiently reliable for determining whether the fistula is mature and therefore ready for puncture [18]. The problem arises when the fistula does not appear clearly mature based on inspection alone, a situation that occurs with obese patients and with slow-maturing AVFs. In these cases, the ultrasound examination and assessment of hemodynamic parameters (AVF blood flow, RI) can help determine whether the AVF is suitable for cannulation or it has failed to mature and is therefore likely to undergo thrombosis or have a low flow volume.

In obese subjects, for example, even veins that are well developed can be difficult to visualize or palpate because of their depth; in these cases, DUS can reveal whether the fistula is mature, and US mapping of the outflow veins can facilitate the first cannulation and simplify subsequent punctures [18]. In this regard, it is important to recall the proposal of Rayner et al. [34], which was incorporated in the K-DOQI Guidelines [12] as "the Rule of 6." It identifies the ultrasound characteristics that confirm that a fistula is mature and, therefore, ready for use: a flow volume of >600 mL/min, an outflow vein diameter of ≥6 mm, and an outflow vein depth of ≤6 mm below the skin surface.

For slowly maturing AVFs, it is fundamental to determine whether the fistula is actually maturing—albeit slowly—or not (i.e., FTM). In these cases, the diagnosis can be made with DUS assessment and periodic calculation of the vascular access flow volume at the level of the brachial artery. Normally, the Doppler spectrum of brachial artery is classically triphasic (high resistance), with flow rates that vary from 80 to 150 mL/min [35, 36]. As soon as the arterio-venous anastomosis has been completed, a *locus minoris resistentiae* is created, and the velocity/time curve of the brachial artery becomes biphasic (low resistance). Blood flow increases dramatically in the first 24 h after surgery and more gradually thereafter, until after varying periods of time the vascular access reaches full maturity [14]. Lomonte and coworkers evaluated 17 radiocephalic AVFs, measuring brachial artery flow volumes preoperatively and 1, 7, 28, and 258 days after construction of the arterio-venous anastomosis. They confirmed that the most dramatic percentage increase in AVF flow occurs on postoperative day 1, and it accounts for approximately 50% of the flow volume measured on postoperative day 28. Subsequent increases were more gradual [37]. The authors concluded that serial measurement of AVF flow volumes during the first month after surgery can help distinguish fistulas that will mature correctly from those destined to fail. Based on the data they collected, it appears that maturation is likely if blood flow through the fistula is 250–500 mL/min on postoperative day 1 and 500–900 mL/min 1 month after construction of the anastomosis [37]. If lower flow rates are encountered or—worse yet—if the brachial artery flow volume tends to decline over time, proper maturation is unlikely, and the fistula will probably become unsuitable for use in dialysis owing to problems of thrombosis or low flow. Therefore, assessments of AVF maturation should always include a physical examination as well as DUS measurements of the flow volume. The latter allows one to predict the probable outcome of the vascular access, and if FTM is observed, it can be helpful in identifying and in some cases correcting the cause.

In conclusion, in response to our initial question regarding the role played by DUS in assessing AVF maturation, the data discussed above clearly show that maturation should be sonographically monitored until the fistula is used, especially when maturation seems to be proceeding slowly and in patients whose veins cannot be easily assessed with physical examination alone (e.g., due to obesity). DUS measurement of AVF flow volumes is perhaps the only imaging tool that can be used to monitor the fistula even during its maturation. Even so, DUS should always be done before an AVF is first used. This examination provides baseline data on the vascular access, which can be useful in subsequent examinations performed to evaluate functional problems [18].

24.3.2 Calculation of AVF Flow Volume

When performed correctly, calculation of the AVF flow volume by DUS is a simple procedure that can be completed in a few minutes and is highly reproducible.

The formula used to calculate flow volumes is (area x mean velocity x 60), where *area* is the cross-sectional area of the vessel in square centimeters (since the vessel is cylindrical, its section is a circle whose area is calculated as the square of the radius × 3.14) (Fig. 24.3), *mean velocity* (in cm/sec) is that of the red blood cells measured from the Doppler trace recorded at the site used to measure *area*, and *60* is the number of seconds in a minute (since flow volumes are expressed in milliliters per minute) [14, 16]. The vessel diameter and mean flow velocity necessary for calculating flow volume according to this formula can be measured on a single longitudinal scan of the vessel. First, the vessel diameter is measured on the appropriately enlarged B-mode image. The pulsed Doppler module is then activated, the PRF is adjusted to eliminate artifacts, and the mean flow velocity is calculated from the time/velocity curve (using the time-averaged velocity option available on most scanners) (Fig. 24.3). Measuring both variables on the same scan ensures that both have been made at the same site in the vessel. In fact, once the two measurements have been made, further calculations are really not necessary: modern ultrasound scanners are equipped with computing algorithms for automatic calculation of the AVF flow volume (Fig. 24.3).

As for the sampling site, the arterialized vein is punctured during hemodialysis, so the outflow vein of the AVF should be an ideal site for measuring the vascular access flow volume. However, measurements made at this level are actually fairly imprecise because this vein can be easily compressed with the probe. In addition, its diameter varies widely due to its tortuous course and the presence of collateral circuits, and these variations make it difficult to calculate the cross-sectional area of the vessel with any degree of precision. Moreover, calculation of the mean velocity is complicated by the turbulent flow that characterizes the venous side of the AVF. For these reasons, measuring the flow volume at the level of the inflow artery improves accuracy and reproducibility. However, measuring the flow volume of a distal AVF at the level of the radial artery can lead to underestimation because a variable portion of the fistula flow (approximately 25–30%) may come from the ulnar artery, via the palmar arch. This "reverse flow" occurs if the

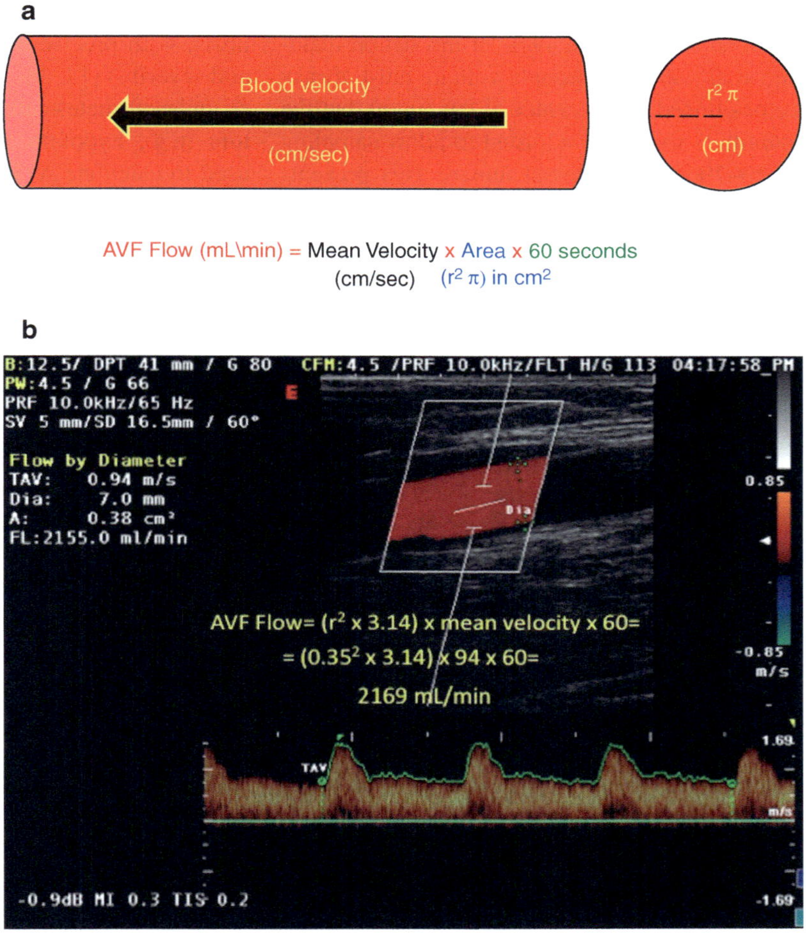

Fig. 24.3 Calculation of the AVF blood flow volume. *Left:* Theoretical basis of the formula used to calculate blood flow volume of a blood vessel. *Right:* Example of AVF flow volume calculated at the level of the brachial artery, manually with the proposed formula ("AVF flow") and with the scanner software ("Flow by Diameter")

diameter of the anastomotic chamber is larger than that of the artery that supplies arterial blood to the fistula. Therefore, in clinical practice, the brachial artery is the preferred site for measuring the flow volume of distal and proximal/proximalized AVFs [12, 14, 16, 37], for several reasons. It is easy to sample and does not collapse under normal transducer pressures. In addition, just above the elbow crease, there is an oblique segment of the brachial artery, where the sample volume can be easily positioned at an appropriate insonation angle. And finally, its laminar flow allows one to record suitable tracings for precise calculation of the mean velocity. In patients with proximal or prosthetic fistulas, the brachial artery flow downstream from the AV anastomosis should be subtracted from the value obtained to improve the accuracy of the flow volume measurement. Alternatively, in prosthetic grafts the flow volume can be measured directly in the prosthetic conduit, which is more regular in caliber than a native outflow vein and more resistant to pressure exerted with the transducer.

To reduce the risk of over- or underestimating the AVF flow volume, several things should be kept in mind. In the first place, use of the zoom function: measurement of the vessel diameter must be as precise as possible because minimal variations in diameter translate into major variations in flow volume (indeed, the formula used to calculate flow volume entails squaring the vessel radius, which thus becomes an important determinant of flow). Second, when data for the Doppler curve is being acquired, the sample volume should be oriented parallel to the direction of blood flow and the angle of insonation maintained at <60°. The sample volume must always be positioned at the center of the vessel, but the amplitude should be adjusted to allow sampling of 50–70% of the vessel lumen. This prevents measurement from being restricted to the red blood cells that pass through the central part of the vessel, which move faster than those flowing close to the vessel walls. Acquisition of velocity data must be as precise as possible; this can be achieved by careful regulation of the PRF to eliminate all types of artifacts.

24.3.3 Role of DUS in the Surveillance of AVF (Follow-Up and Detection of Complications)

For a well-functioning AVF, the nephrologist's job is to maximize its survival by prevention, early detection, and prompt treatment of complications. To this end, the international guidelines recommend a specific protocol for vascular access monitoring (physical examination of the AVF before each dialysis session) and surveillance (assessment of recirculation, venous/arterial pressures, calculation of flow volume, and other parameters, which provide information on AVF function and should be evaluated on a monthly basis) [12]. Measurement of blood flow is now considered the best means of surveillance for a vascular access [12]: reduced flow volumes or values that decrease over time are predictive of thrombosis for both native and prosthetic AVFs [14, 38, 39]. There are several methods for calculating AVF flow (DUS, MR angiography, ultrasound dilution technique, the Crit-Line monitor, glucose infusion, differential conductivity, ionic dialysance), and none is considered unequivocally superior to the others in the main international guidelines [12, 40]. One of the drawbacks of DUS with respect to the other methods is that it cannot be used during hemodialysis, but it also offers a major advantage, i.e., it can be used to document the presence of a low AVF flow volumes and simultaneously explore possible causes (e.g., by providing direct visualization of an area of stenosis, with precise information on its location and severity) [14, 16, 18]. To minimize the risk of underestimates caused by hemodynamic factors (e.g., hypotension), DUS should not be used to calculate AVF flow volumes during the immediate post-dialysis period: measurements made between one session and the next or immediately before a dialysis session are preferable.

Data in the literature on DUS flow volume assessment indicate that a well-functioning AVF will be characterized by a flow rate of 700–1300 mL/min [14, 37]. Values of <500 mL/min [12, 16] and <300 mL/min [14, 16] are considered predictive of access dysfunction and imminent thrombosis, respectively. Aside from these absolute values, subsequent studies have shown that, in a vascular access that has previously been stable with flow volumes of >1000 mL/min, further investigation is warranted when consecutive monthly measurements reveal a decrease in flow volume of >25% over a relatively short period of time (1–4 months) since these findings are predictive of stenosis and vascular access thrombosis [12, 18, 38, 39].

DUS calculation of AVF flow volume can also be useful for assessing the effectiveness of a therapeutic intervention carried out to resolve a complication. The absence of an increase in flow of at least 20% after such an intervention (e.g., percutaneous transluminal angioplasty to eliminate stenosis) indicates that the treatment has failed and an alternative solution is needed [12].

As mentioned, in AVF surveillance DUS can also be used to explore the possible causes of vascular access malfunction. However, while flow volume calculation is fairly simple and takes very little time, systematic assessment of an AVF with DUS is a challenging and more time-consuming procedure that should be done only by experienced operators. Therefore, this examination should be used only when monitoring/surveillance methods have revealed anomalies or when problems arise that prevent regular dialysis (difficult venipuncture, insufficient blood flow, high venous pressure, prolonged bleeding after removal of fistula needles).

The minimal technical requirements and the position of the patient are those used for preoperative mapping. Given the relatively superficial position of the vessels used to create an AVF, high-frequency (7.5–13 MHz) linear probes are fundamental for obtaining maximum anatomical details on the vessel walls and for accurate assessment of the superficial wall of the outflow vein, where puncture damage is more likely (approximately 300 punctures/year with 15–16 gauge needle) [35]. The wall of the outflow vein is only a few millimeters below the skin surface. If a lower frequency transducer is used, this area will inevitably be out of focus, and it will be very difficult to identify wall lesions [35]. The vessels of an AVF almost always run parallel to the skin surface. Therefore, the Doppler examination should always be performed with a beam-steering transducer that will allow the operator to maintain the correct angle of incidence (30–60°) relative to the direction of flow [35].

The examination should include the following steps:

1. Study of arterial inflow side of the fistula (including AVF flow volume)
2. Study of anastomotic chamber
3. Study of venous outflow side of the fistula

A thorough evaluation of the AVF includes exploration of each of these three areas with both transverse and longitudinal scans and assessment of morphological (B-mode) as well as hemodynamic aspects (with color Doppler and Doppler analysis).

B-mode, color Doppler, and Doppler analysis findings that are typical of a well-functioning AVF are described separately below (for purely educational purposes, as in clinical settings the three studies are generally carried out concomitantly). Descriptions of the ultrasound findings associated with the main complications of AVFs would render this review excessively long, and the reader is therefore referred to specialist publications on this subject [35, 41].

24.4 Morphological Assessment (B-Mode)

The study typically begins proximally, with an examination of the brachial artery. On a longitudinal view, a normal artery appears as a completely anechoic band delimitated by two three-layered walls. On real-time images, the arteries can be easily distinguished from the veins by their walls, which move in synchrony with cardiac systole, and by their non-compressibility under probe pressure.

The brachial artery is followed down to the antecubital crease, where it divides into radial and ulnar arteries, which run along the lateral and medial sides of the forearm, respectively. The AVF inflow artery, generally the radial artery, is characterized by a constant, regular increase in caliber and modest tortuosity, which are more marked in high-flow AVFs. Another common finding is pulsatility, which is much stronger than that of the same vessel in the contralateral arm (especially in the area near the anastomosis) [14, 35].

Exploration of the arterial side of the fistula proceeds distally to the surgical anastomosis, which frequently has a winding course. Vessel pulsatility at the anastomotic region is so marked that it produces a "thrill" caused by the turbulence of the flow. It is characterized by fine, rapid, palpable, and sonographically documented vibrations involving the tissues surrounding the vessel [14, 35]. The sonographic image of the anastomotic region can help us to define the AVF type: end-to-end (E-E), side-to-end (S-E), or side-to-side (S-S) (Fig. 24.4).

If the nonlinearity of the anastomotic chamber precludes acquisition of such images, the presence or absence of the arterial and distal venous segment with respect to the site of the anastomosis can be used to identify the type of anastomosis.

The outflow vein is characterized by tortuosity, ectasia, and segmental variations in caliber that are generally due to wall damage caused by repeated venipuncture. The vessel walls gener-

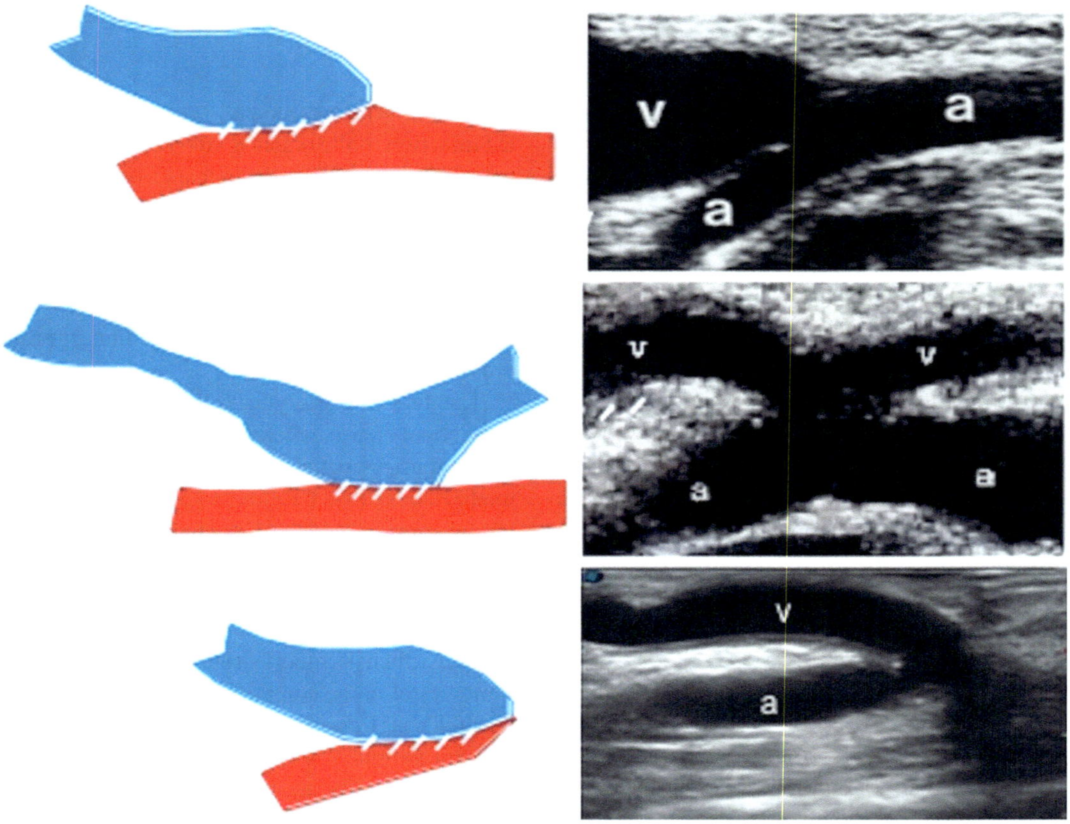

Fig. 24.4 Longitudinal ultrasound scans of the anastomotic region of various AVF types. *Top:* Side-to-end AVF. *Center:* Side-to-side AVF. *Bottom:* End-to-end AVF

ally appear to be mildly thickened as a result of intimal hyperplasia, a phenomenon that renders the vessel capable of withstanding repeated venipuncture with large-caliber needles [14, 35].

24.5 Color Doppler Examination

The appearance of color confirms the patency of the vessels being examined. As a general rule, the scanner is usually set to "map" arterial flow in red (flow moving towards the transducer) and venous flow in blue (moving away from the transducer).

The pulse repetition frequency (PRF) is one of the most important settings that need to be adjusted for a proper flowmetric analysis. The PRF selected for AVFs is usually higher (1000–6000 Hz) than that commonly used to study the upper limbs, because of the higher flow velocities in AVFs [14, 35]. It is important to recall that this is a "dynamic" setting, which has to be readjusted several times during the examination to eliminate aliasing (especially near the anastomosis, where the flow is faster) and to avoid noncoding of the venous flow, which can occur, for example, during exploration of the outflow vein after assessment of the AVF with a high PRF [14, 35]. Lower PRFs (less than 1000 Hz) can be used when a vessel seems to be patent on the basis of morphological findings and responses to compression maneuvers, but intraluminal flow signals are lacking. This can occur, for example, at the level of large venous aneurysms, where flow slows considerably as a result of the large caliber of the lumen. Low PRFs are also recommended—although not absolutely necessary—during exploration of collateral vessels near a thrombosed or complex AVF [14, 35].

On color Doppler imaging, the inflow artery of the AVF is characterized by relatively homogeneous, laminar flow (with maximum velocity at the center of the lumen and the lowest values near the vessel walls). Near the anastomosis, there is an increase in flow velocity (reflected by lighter colors, even white) and turbulence (reflected by a disorderly alternation of reds and blues within the same luminal segment). Because of the high flow volumes and caliber irregularities that characterize the outflow vein, areas of vortex flow are often observed at this level, especially near the anastomosis. They are reflected by alternating intraluminal color signals with a typical spiroidal configuration [14, 35]. Moving away from the AVF, the caliber of the vessel tends to decrease, vortexing diminishes, and the venous flow gradually becomes more homogeneous and regular [14, 35].

24.6 Doppler Ultrasound Assessment

On Doppler ultrasound imaging, the inflow side of a normal AVF is characterized by an appreciable reduction in peripheral resistance relative to the contralateral limb, with copious anterograde flow during the entire diastolic phase [14, 35]. As the transducer moves closer to the anastomosis, flow through the afferent artery undergoes a progressive and constant increase in velocity that involves both the systolic and diastolic phases, and spectral broadening is observed, which is maximal in the vicinity of anastomosis, where it reaches the baseline with the disappearance of the acoustic window [14, 35]. At the level of anastomosis, purely turbulent flow profiles are observed, with loss of arterial phasicity, a broad spectrum extending above and below the baseline, and high peak systolic velocities that are extremely variable in subsequent moments [14, 35]. On the venous side, near the anastomosis, flow is "arterialized" with obvious systolic-diastolic phasicity and a particularly broad spectrum. As the distance from the AVF increases, arterial phasicity is progressively lost, the mean flow velocity diminishes, and the spectrum takes on the characteristics of regular venous flow [14, 35].

24.7 Diagnosis of Stenosis

The development of a stenosis at any point of the access conduit is the most frequent cause of fistula dysfunction and is the main predisposing factor for AVF thrombosis (80–85% of cases) [42]. Stenosis is a narrowing of the vessel lumen ≥50% compared to the adjacent normal vessel. In native AVFs, stenosis rarely affects the arterial side of AVF and in this case is mainly linked to degenerative phenomena on an atherosclerotic basis; such situations should be recognized with preoperative vascular mapping before the creation of AVF and eventually resolved. Stenosis of the anastomosis generally results from technical errors during the surgical intervention. Therefore, the most frequent site of stenosis in native AVFs is the venous side (outflow vein), less resistant to wall stress (due to high velocities and turbulence of the flow) and subjected to the traumatism associated with repeated punctures [42].

Venous stenoses generally develop in areas of surgical vein mobilization (swing points), vein bifurcations, venipuncture sites, and areas where valves are present [42]. Moreover, in native forearm AVFs, venous stenoses are mainly localized in the peri-anastomotic area (~50% of cases), generating problems in aspiration during hemodialysis [42]. In AVFs of the arm, instead, the venous narrowings are mainly localized far from the anastomosis (50–55% of the cases) generating problems of increased venous pressure during restitution of blood [42]. In prosthetic AVFs, stenoses usually develop in the venous outflow tract at the site of anastomosis between the graft and the vein (~85% of cases) generating, even in this case, problems of increased venous pressure [42].

During DUS examination of an AVF, a stenosis is identified by three main findings [16]:

1. Vessel lumen reduction >50% (B-mode)
2. "Aliasing" phenomenon (color Doppler)
3. Peak systolic velocity (PSV) >400 cm/s at the site of stenosis or twofold increase of PSV at the site of stenosis compared to the VPS measured on a healthy vein segment (PSV ratio >2)

For sonographic assessment of stenosis, the AVF is examined with a transverse B-mode scan from the feeding artery across the anastomosis and the arterialized draining vein as far into the central venous system as possible; this approach allows to easily identify the tract of vessel characterized by important reduction of size [14, 43]. Once identified the stenosis in this way, a longitudinal scan must be obtained to evaluate the stenotic area together with the pre- and post-stenotic tract in order to determine the severity of the stenosis itself [14, 43]; indeed, to calculate the percentage of stenosis, the residual vessel diameter at the site of stenosis is compared with the diameter of a nearby normal segment using the formula [16]

(Normal lumen − residual lumen)/normal lumen × 100 = percent stenosis (Fig. 24.5)

The calculation of the percentage of a venous stenosis is not as simple as it might seem because often it is difficult to identify a normal segment of vein; in fact, the caliber of the efferent vein of an AVF is generally very irregular and the pre-stenotic tract is frequently characterized by an aneurysmal dilatation. These problems can easily lead to under- or overestimation of the degree of stenosis; therefore, for the calculation of the percentage of stenosis it is considered most appropriate to refer to the post-stenotic vein tract [14, 16, 43].

At the color Doppler evaluation, the stenotic area is characterized by the appearance of "aliasing" (i.e., a mosaic of colors) due to the particular turbulence of the blood flow at the level of the stenosis site; this artifact is not present in the pre-stenotic and in the post-stenotic area where the blood flow remains laminar [14, 16, 43].

The pulsed Doppler analysis shows an increase in PSV in the area of stenosis and a demodulation of the spectral curve due to the high velocities and the turbulence of blood flow in the stenotic segment. To diagnose a stenosis, we have to find a PSV >400 cm/s at the site of stenosis or a two-fold increase of PSV at the site of stenosis zone in comparison to PSV in a non-stenotic segment (PSV ratio >2) [14, 16, 43].

In the presence of a stenosis, however, the importance of DUS examination is not only due to the possibility of diagnosing such complications; in fact, DUS allows to evaluate a series of parameters (site of the stenosis, extension of the stenosis, residual lumen, presence of parietal thrombosis, vascular access blood flow, resistive index of the feeding artery) that can suggest us whether to treat the stenosis or not [44]. In the past, it was sufficient that a stenosis was >50% to direct the patient to the endovascular treatment; therefore, such a treatment was often too precocious and counterproductive because traumatizing the vessel wall accelerated the appearance of restenosis and reduced the survival of the vascular access itself. In order to avoid this negative effect of a too early treatment of stenosis, alongside the three "classical" criteria of stenosis, "additional" DUS criteria have been established; such additional criteria allow us to define a stenosis as "significant", i.e., a stenosis that requires treatment [45]. Additional criteria are shown in Table 24.1. In particular, the presence of three main criteria without any additional criterion

Fig. 24.5 Calculation of the percentage of stenosis in the presence of a venous stenosis

% Stenosis =
[(A-B)/A x 100] =
[(4.9-2.0)/4.9 x 100]= 59%

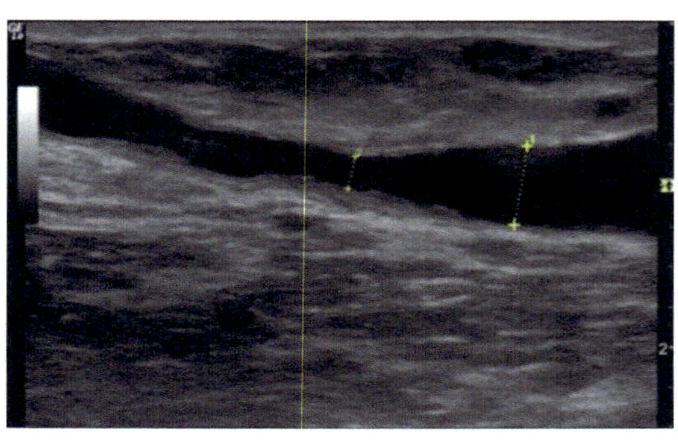

Table 24.1 DUS criteria for stenosis and definition of borderline and significant stenosis

Main criteria	Additional criteria
Luminal diameter reduction >50%	Blood flow volume <600 mL/min
Aliasing phenomenon	>25% decrease of flow volume between 2 controls
PSV >400 cm/s or >2-fold increase of PSV	Residual diameter <2 mm
	RI increase of the brachial artery (>0.70)
	Presence of parietal thrombosis

PSV = Peak systolic velocity; RI = resistive index
Only 3 main criteria = "Borderline" stenosis
3 main criteria + ≥1 additional criteria = "Significant" stenosis

allows us to diagnose a "borderline" stenosis, that is, a stenosis that does not need to be treated but needs an ultrasound follow-up (within 6–8 weeks). On the contrary, the stenosis is "significant" if there is a combination of the three main criteria with at least one of the "additional" criteria: residual lumen <2 mm, AVF low blood flow (<600 mL/min) or blood flow reduction of >25% since the previous examination, increase of resistive index of the feeding artery, and presence of parietal thrombosis. In case of the significant stenosis early endovascular treatment is suggested.

24.8 Conclusions

The native AVF is the vascular access of choice for patients who require hemodialysis: it lasts longer and is associated with fewer complications than other types of vascular access; for hemodialysis patients, these benefits translate into better quality of life and longer survival. Physicians involved in the construction and maintenance of vascular accesses for hemodialysis know that DUS is fundamental for identifying vessels that are suitable for creating an AVF (preoperative mapping) and for early detection of complications (surveillance) and is perhaps the only imaging tool that can be used to monitor the fistula even during its maturation process. Indeed, DUS is the only method that allows to monitor AVF blood flow and simultaneously explore possible causes of vascular access malfunction. This facilitates timely, targeted salvage interventions that can prolong the survival of the vascular access and consequently that of the patient as well.

References

1. Ravani P, Palmer SC, Oliver MJ, et al. Associations between hemodialysis access type and clinical outcomes: a systematic review. J Am Soc Nephrol. 2013;24:465–73.
2. Gibson KD, Gillen DL, Caps MT, et al. Vascular access survival and incidence of revisions: a comparison of prosthetic grafts, simple autogenous fistulas, and venous transposition fistulas from the United States renal data system dialysis morbidity and mortality study. J Vasc Surg. 2001;34:694–700.
3. Konner K, Hulbert-Shearon TE, Roys EC, et al. Tailoring the initial vascular access for dialysis patients. Kidney Int. 2002;62:329–38.
4. Georgiadis GS, Charalampidis DG, Argyriou C, et al. The necessity for routine pre-operative ultrasound mapping before arteriovenous fistula creation: a meta-analysis. Eur J Vasc Endovasc Surg. 2015;49:600–5.
5. Ilhan G, Esi E, Bozok S, et al. The clinical utility of vascular mapping with Doppler ultrasound prior to arteriovenous fistula construction for hemodialysis access. J Vasc Access. 2013;14(1):83–8.
6. Shenoy S, Darcy M. Ultrasound as a tool for pre-operative planning, monitoring and interventions in dialysis arteriovenous access. AJR Am J Roentgenol. 2013;201(4):W539–43.
7. Ferring M, Henderson J, Wilmink A, et al. Vascular ultrasound for the pre-operative evaluation prior to arteriovenous fistula formation for haemodialysis: review of the evidence. Nephrol Dial Transplant. 2008;23:1809–15.
8. Malovrh M. Native arteriovenous fistula: preoperative evaluation. Am J Kidney Dis. 2002;39:1218–25.
9. Allon M, Lockhart ME, Lilly RZ, et al. Effect of preoperative sonographic mapping on vascular access outcomes in hemodialysis patients. Kidney Int. 2001;60:2013–20.
10. Wong CS, McNicholas N, Healy D, et al. A systematic review of preoperative duplex ultrasonography and arteriovenous fistula formation. J Vasc Surg. 2013;57:1129–33.
11. Hossain S, Sharma A, Dubois L, et al. Preoperative point-of-care ultrasound and its impact on arteriovenous fistula maturation outcomes. J Vasc Surg. 2018;68(4):1157–65.
12. NKF-K/DOQI. Clinical practice guidelines for vascular access update 2006. Am J Kidney Dis. 2006;48(Suppl 1):s176–322.

13. Ibeas J, Roca-Tey R, Vallespin J, et al. Spanish clinical guidelines on vascular access for hemodialysis. Nefrologia. 2017;37(Suppl 1):1–177.
14. Zamboli P, Fiorini F, D'Amelio A, et al. Color Doppler ultrasound and arteriovenous fistulas for hemodialysis. J Ultrasound. 2014;17(4):253–63.
15. Clausen LL. Ultrasound mapping. In vascular accesses for hemodialysis. Castelli P and Setacci P. Edizioni. Minerva Med. 2018;
16. Wiese P, Nonnast-Daniel B. Colour Doppler ultrasound in dialysis access. Nephrol Dial Transplant. 2004;19:1956–63.
17. Malovrh M. The role of sonography in the planning of arteriovenous fistulas for hemodialysis. Semin Dial. 2003;16:299–303.
18. Davidson I, Chan D, Dolmatch B, et al. Duplex ultrasound evaluation for dialysis access selection and maintenance: a practical guide. J Vasc Access. 2008;9:1–9.
19. Ferring M, Claridge M, Smith SA, et al. Routine preoperative vascular ultrasound improves patency and use of arteriovenous fistulas for hemodialysis: a randomized trial. Clin J Am Soc Nephrol. 2010;5(12):2236–44.
20. Malovrh M. Non-invasive evaluation of vessels by duplex sonography prior to construction of arteriovenous fistulas for haemodialysis. Nephrol Dial Transplant. 1998;13:125–9.
21. Silva MB Jr, Hobson RW 2nd, Pappas PJ, et al. A strategy for increasing use of autogenous hemodialysis access procedures: impact of pre-operative noninvasive evaluation. J Vasc Surg. 1998;27:302–7.
22. Ku YM, Kim YO, Kim JI, et al. Ultrasonographic measurement of intima-media thickness of radial artery in pre-dialysis uremic patients: comparison with histological examination. Nephrol Dial Transplant. 2006;21:715–20.
23. Wittenberg G, Schindler T, Tschammler A, et al. Value of color coded duplex ultrasound in evaluating arm blood vessels-arteries and haemodialysis shunts. Ultraschall Med. 1998;19:22–7.
24. Sato M, Io H, Tanimoto M, et al. Relationship between preoperative radial artery and postoperative arteriovenous fistula blood flow in hemodialysis patients. J Nephrol. 2012;25(5):726–31.
25. Sedlacek M, Teodorescu V, Falk A, et al. Hemodialysis access placement with preoperative noninvasive vascular mapping: comparison between patients with and without diabetes. Am J Kidney Dis. 2001;38:560–4.
26. Wall LP, Gasparis A, Callahan S, et al. Impaired hyperemic response is predictive of early access failure. Ann Vasc Surg. 2004;18:167–71.
27. Wong V, Ward R, Taylor J, et al. Factors associated with early failure of arteriovenous fistulae for haemodialysis accesses. Eur J Vasc Endovasc Surg. 1996;12:207–13.
28. Mendes RR, Farber MA, Marston WA, et al. Prediction of wrist arteriovenous fistula maturation with preoperative vein mapping with ultrasonography. J Vasc Surg. 2002;36:460–3.
29. Beathard GA, Arnold P, Jackson J, et al. Physician Operators Forum of RMS Lifeline. Aggressive treatment of early fistula failure. Kidney Int. 2003;64:1487–94.
30. Planken RN, Keuter XH, Hoeks AP, et al. Diameter measurement of the forearm cephalic vein prior to vascular access creation in end-stage renal disease patients: graduated pressure cuff versus tourniquet vessel dilatation. Nephrol Dial Transplant. 2006;21:802–6.
31. Kim JT, Chang WH, Oh TY, et al. Venous distensibility as a key factor in the success of arteriovenous fistulas at the wrist. Ann Vasc Surg. 2011;25:1094–8.
32. Jemcov TK. Morphologic and functional vessels characteristics assessed by ultrasonography for prediction of radiocephalic fistula maturation. J Vasc Access. 2013;14:356–63.
33. Dember LM, Beck GJ, Allon M, et al. Effect of clopidogrel on early failure of arteriovenous fistula for hemodialysis: a randomized controlled trial. JAMA. 2008;299(18):2164–71.
34. Rayner HC, Pisoni RL, Gillespie BW, et al. Creation, cannulation and survival of arteriovenous fistulae: data from the dialysis outcomes and practice patterns study. Kidney Int. 2003;63:323–30.
35. Rabbia C, Matricardi L. Eco-Color-Doppler Vascolare. III Edizione: Minerva Medica; 2006.
36. Zamboli P, Calabria M, Camocardi A, et al. Color-Doppler imaging and arteriovenous fistula: preoperative evaluation and surveillance. G Ital Nefrol. 2012;29(Suppl 57):S36–46.
37. Lomonte C, Casucci F, Antonelli M, et al. Is there a place for duplex screening of the brachial artery in the maturation of arteriovenous fistulas? Semin Dial. 2005;18(3):243–6.
38. Smits JH, van der Linden J, Hagen EC, et al. Graft surveillance: venous pressure, access flow or the combination? Kidney Int. 2001;59:1551–8.
39. Kim YO, Yang CW, Yoon SA, et al. Access blood flow as a predictor of early failures of native arteriovenous fistulas in hemodialysis patients. Am J Nephrol. 2001;21:221–5.
40. Tordoir J, Canaud B, Haage P, et al. EBPG on Vascular Access. Nephrol Dial Transplant. 2007;22(Suppl 2):ii88–ii117.
41. Napoli M. Echo color Doppler & vascular access for hemodialysis. Wichtig Editor. 2011;
42. Quencer KB, Arici M. Arteriovenous fistulas and their characteristics sites of stenosis. Am J Roentgenol. 2015;205:726–34.
43. Granata A, Zamboli P, Fatuzzo P, et al. US and arteriovenous fistulas for hemodialysis. In: Atlas of ultra-

sonography in urology, andrology and nephrology: Springer Editor; 2017.
44. Malik J, Kudlicka J, Novakova L, et al. Surveillance of arteriovenous accesses with the use of duplex Doppler ultrasonography. J Vasc Access. 2014;15(Suppl 7):S28–32.
45. Schmidli J, Widmer MK, Basile C, et al. Vascular access: 2018 clinical practice guidelines of the European Society for Vascular Surgery (ESVS). Eur J Vasc Endovasc Surg. 2018;55:757–818.

Carotid Artery Evaluation

25

Ilaria Fiorina, Annalisa Nanni, Shaun Muzic, Filippo Richelmi, Maria Vittoria Raciti, Fabrizio Calliada, and Chandra Bortolotto

25.1 Carotid Arteries: Normal Anatomy

All the major arteries of the neck take origin from the aortic arch through three main vessels: the brachiocephalic trunk, the left common carotid, and the left subclavian artery.

The common carotid arteries (CCA), right and left, are the main arterial vessels that supply the vascularization of the head and neck.

The right CCA usually originates from the brachiocephalic trunk, at the base of the neck, just behind the right sternoclavicular joint. The left CCA, instead, originates directly from the arch of the aorta, at thoracic level. So, while the right CCA is exclusively cervical, the left one has a thoracic and a cervical tract and for this reason the left CCA is about 20–25 mm longer than the right one.

In the neck tract the two common carotids follow the same path: they course superiorly in the neck, anteromedial to the jugular vein and the vagus nerve, and they divide into internal (ICA) and external (ECA) carotid arteries [1, 2]. They typically divide at the level of C3 or C4 vertebral body, as the height of the carotid bifurcation (HCB) is classically defined in relation with vertebral levels. This anatomical level is highly variable across literature; thus C3–C4 and C4–C5 are the most common levels of bifurcation, as we can see later in this paragraph [3, 4].

The ECA distributes itself over the external surface of the skull, to the face and to the upper part of the neck, while the internal carotid artery supplies the organs contained in the cranial cavity and in the orbital cavities. The carotid arteries, together with the internal jugular vein and the vagus nerve (tenth cranial nerve), are wrapped in the carotid sheath, a connective structure that covers them and continues with the middle cervical fascia: all these structures together constitute the neurovascular bundle of the neck [1, 2].

At its upper end, near the bifurcation, the CCA has an expansion that is named carotid sinus or carotid bulb and which usually extends also to the initial tract of the internal carotid artery. The common carotid artery usually has no collateral branches, except for small branches for its own sheath and directed to the carotid glomus. As anatomical variants it can rarely provide some collateral branches such as the vertebral artery, the upper thyroid artery, the ascending pharyngeal artery, the lingual artery, the lower thyroid artery, and the occipital artery [1].

Bouthillier classification system, firstly described in 1996 and the most widely used,

I. Fiorina (✉)
Radiology and Neuroradiology Diagnostic and Interventional Department, Fondazione IRCSS Policlinico San Matteo, Pavia, Italy

A. Nanni · S. Muzic · F. Richelmi · M. V. Raciti
F. Calliada · C. Bortolotto
Radiology Institute, Fondazione IRCSS Policlinico San Matteo, Pavia, Italy

A. Granata, M. Bertolotto (eds.), *Imaging in Nephrology*, https://doi.org/10.1007/978-3-030-60794-4_25

divides the ICA into seven segments from the cervical tract to the intracranial course: (1) cervical segment; (2) petrous segment; (3) lacerum segment; (4) cavernous segment; (5) clinoid segment; (6) ophthalmic (supraclinoid) segment; and (7) communicating (terminal) segment.

The cervical segment of the ICA extends from the carotid bifurcation to the base of the skull, and runs up and back to the inferior orifice of the carotid canal of the temporal bone, where the artery enters the carotid canal. The ICA rises cranially, passes medially to the ECA, and is placed medially to the internal jugular vein and anteriorly to the transverse processes of the upper cervical vertebrae.

The cervical segment of the ICA usually has no branches in the neck, unless there is remnant of carotid-basilar anastomoses, such as the hypoglossal artery or proatlantal artery type I.

Following the Bouthillier classification then we have six intracranial segments starting from the petrous segment that begins when ICA crosses the carotid canal and enters the cranial cavity, where it enters into the fibrocartilage which obliterates the foramen lacerum and folds upwards, penetrating the cavernous sinus. Subsequently, in correspondence of the anterior clinoid process, the artery turns superiorly, with vertical course, and perforates the dura mater. Finally, it terminates below the anterior substance of the brain, dividing into anterior and middle cerebral arteries, posterior communicating artery, and anterior choroidal artery [1, 2, 5, 6].

The cervical segment of the ECA heads up to divide into its terminal branches about 4 cm above the corner of the jaw, and runs anteromedial to ICA. It gives six collateral branches in the neck before it divides into two terminal branches entering the parotid gland. The six collateral branches are the superior thyroid artery, the ascending pharyngeal artery, the lingual artery, the facial artery, the occipital artery, and the posterior auricular artery. The terminal branches of the external carotid artery are the superficial temporal artery and internal maxillary artery [1, 2].

As anatomical variants sometimes we can observe variations in position of the carotid origins. These anatomical variants are usually related to variations of aortic arch anatomy. The most frequent one is a common origin of the brachiocephalic and left CCA, the so-called bovine arch, which occurs in 7–27% of patients. In 7.2% of patients there is a common origin of the left common carotid and subclavian arteries, leading to bilaterally symmetric brachiocephalic trunks. Rarely, in 2.5% of patients, the right CCA arises directly from the arch and is usually associated with an aberrant right subclavian artery arising distally from the arch, with the right CCA as the first branch off the arch [7, 8].

Variation in the course and position of the common carotids and carotid bifurcations are also pretty common. The position of the carotid bifurcation reflects the degree of embryologic migration of the ECA and is also very variable.

Huber reports the bifurcation at C4–C5 in 48% of 658 bifurcations, and at C3–C4 in 34%, as C3–C4 and C4–C5 are the most common levels of bifurcation.

There are extremely rare reported cases of bifurcation of the carotid in the thorax down to the T3 level, and some reported cases of a very high bifurcation, as high as C2 [7, 9, 10].

Other variations in the cervical carotids include external carotid branches off the CCA or the ICA, aplasia of the ICA, and separate origins of the internal and external carotids [11].

25.2 Imaging Techniques

25.2.1 Ultrasound

Carotid Doppler ultrasound (DUS) is the primary noninvasive imaging modality for evaluating the extracranial carotid arteries, because of its high sensitivity and specificity, and relatively low cost, avoiding ionizing radiation and the necessity of contrast medium.

The patient lies supine with the neck slightly hyperextended and turned toward the contralateral side. The US examination is usually performed with linear array transducer, through transverse and longitudinal planes, using B-mode, color Doppler, and spectral Doppler, avoiding the use of angles of insonation more than 60° to have a correct evaluation of the flow. The vessels should be examined as completely as possible, with caudal angulation of the transducer in the supraclavicular region and cephalic angulation at the level of the mandible.

The thickness of the two inner vessel layers, intima and media, in the CCA, is called intima-media thickness (IMT), which is an independent risk factor for cardiovascular disease and it is associated with the risk of myocardial infarction, sudden death, and stroke [12].

During B-mode evaluation in the longitudinal view of the CCA, the arterial walls show an internal line (the interface of the lumen-intima) and an external line (the interface of the media-adventitia); the IMT is the distance between them (see Fig. 25.1). It should be measured bilaterally, along the posterior wall of the mid CCA 1 cm below the bulb; the value varies with age, gender, and race but a measurement less than 0.7–0.8 mm should be considered normal and >1 mm pathologic.

The examiner can simply differentiate the ICA from the ECA: through the identification of branches arising from the ECA (such as lingual artery), and dimensions and location (ICA is generally larger and posterolateral to the ECA) (see Fig. 25.2).

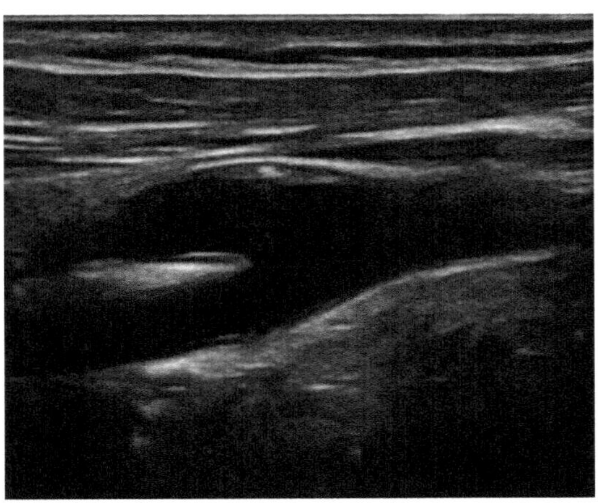

Fig. 25.1 Intima-media thickness (IMT) semiautomatic evaluation: grayscale B-mode scan performed with linear array transducer, through longitudinal plane of CCA posterior wall (about 1 cm below the bulb). The normal value varies with age, gender, and race but a measurement less than 0.7–0.8 mm should be considered normal

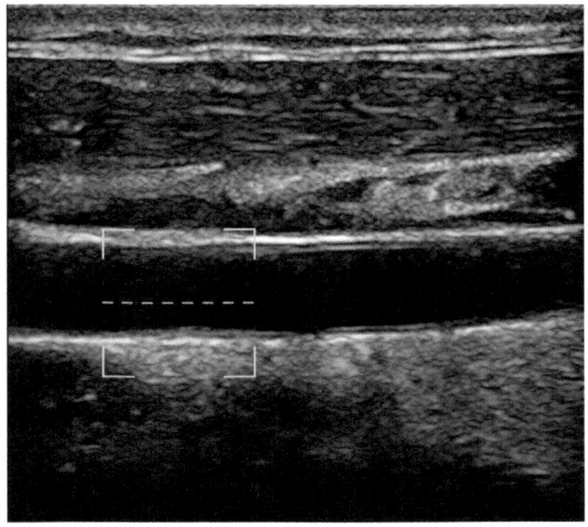

Fig. 25.2 Longitudinal color Doppler imaging of a normal carotid bifurcation. It is intuitively possible to differentiate the ICA from the ECA: ECA usually smaller than the ICA, with a branch arising from its medial wall. The focus of the probe is correctly positioned just deeper than the vessels to be examined. The insonation angle is <60°, allowing a correct flow evaluation. The flow is usually represented with caudo-cranial direction, higher speed in the center of the vessel and slower in the periphery

Carotid waveform pattern is also typical: all the carotid arteries have a sharp systolic upstroke and narrow spectral envelope; in the ICA the normal waveform is characterized by a thicker spectral envelope and continuous diastolic flow due to peripheral vascular resistance; instead the normal ECA waveform has less diastolic flow and a thinner spectral envelope, with an early diastolic notch (see Fig. 25.3a/b). Normal peak systolic velocity (PSV) in the CCA normally ranges from 60 to 100 cm/s and decreases slightly distally.

Color Doppler should be performed to detect areas of abnormal blood flow that require spectral Doppler evaluation. Spectral Doppler analysis should be performed in the mid CCA, proximal ICA, as well as proximal to, at, and immediately distal to the pathological areas.

Advantages of carotid DUS are wide availability, ease of use, and minor cost than other imaging methods. It is also a noninvasive technique, is extremely safe, and does not necessitate ionizing radiation exposure.

Main **limitations** of carotid US are operator dependence; physical characteristics of the

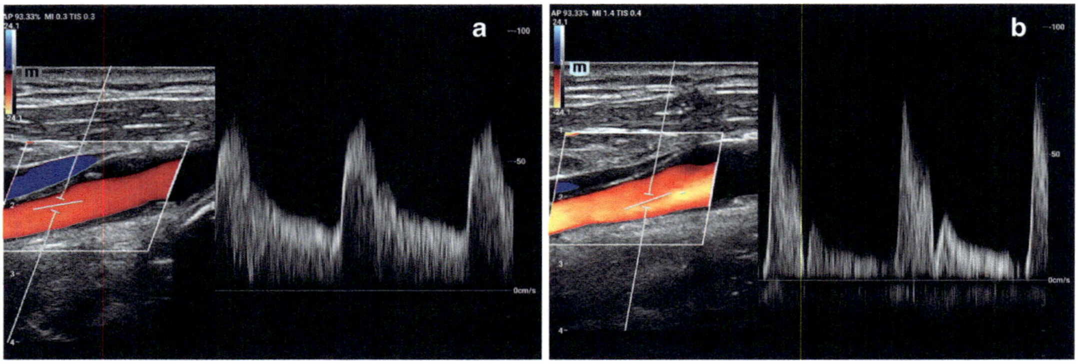

Fig. 25.3 (**a**) Normal spectral Doppler tracing of the internal carotid artery performed with linear array transducer, through longitudinal plane. The gate is positioned in the center of the vessel, with a size of about a third of the vessel diameter. Normal waveform is characterized by a thicker spectral envelope and continuous diastolic flow due to peripheral vascular resistance. There is a continuous diastolic flow, the systolic peak is slightly blunted, and the spectral envelope is slightly widened. The systolic upstroke is sharp, and velocity gradually tapers during diastole. (**b**) Normal spectral Doppler tracing of the external carotid artery, performed with linear array transducer, through longitudinal plane. The gate is positioned in the center of the vessel, with a size of about a third of the vessel diameter. The ECA has a higher resistance waveform with less diastolic flow and a thinner spectral envelope than the ICA. There is a small amount of diastolic flow; reversal of flow in early diastolic notch is a normal finding in the ECA

patient, such as a short muscular neck, the presence of a high carotid bifurcation, tortuous vessels, calcified shadowing plaques, postoperative suture, hematoma or bandages, and inability to rotate the head; and uncooperative patients.

25.2.1.1 US Technological Innovations

The multiparametric nature of US is further advanced by the introduction of new technologies including contrast-enhanced ultrasound, elastography, and vector flow.

The use of microbubble ultrasound contrast has recently obtained many emerging applications. **Contrast-enhanced ultrasound** (CEUS) is routinely employed for the differential diagnosis in focal parenchymal lesions, especially in the liver and in the kidney because the microbubbles allow to assess contrast enhancement due to malignant angiogenesis and to identify "washout" in the late phases. In the carotid arteries CEUS can be used to improve flow visualization free of artifacts and detailed plaque surface delineation [13].

Feinstein et al. reported also the use of CEUS to identify plaque neovascularity, with a better visualization of plaques with irregular surface and ulcerations than conventional Doppler [14].

Elastography is a US method which allows to evaluate in real time the elasticity and the absolute stiffness of a tissue.

In shear wave elastography (SWE) the probe produces push pulse that generates downward displacement, which can be tracked to measure shear wave propagation speed.

Carotid plaque composition, such as fibrous cap and lipid core, is related to the vulnerability of the plaque and may affect its elastic properties. SWE has shown promising results in the risk stratification of carotid plaques [15].

Vector flow imaging (VFI) is an innovative, angle-independent method, which provides a multidimensional characterization of blood flow in all directions, showing velocity vectors at any location into a vessel, streamline distribution, and vorticity distribution [16].

The multi-direction flow estimation is made possible through an acquisition with multiple incidence angles of plane wave, achieving high frame rate and a dynamic visualization of a complex flow.

Recently, several clinical studies based on VFI showed the additional information carried out from this technique analyzing different flow patterns in the human cardiocirculatory system.

The first in vivo study with vector velocity method, based on plane wave acquisition, was published in 2009 by Hansen et al., which reported the visualization of a stable vortex in the bulb of six carotid bifurcations [17].

VFI was then deployed to demonstrate the presence of a reversal blood flow from the external to the internal carotid during the systole, suggesting the possible role of retrograde embolism in case of plaques in the proximal external carotid artery [18].

Goddi et al. evaluated 60 carotid bifurcations in healthy adults, identified a complex flow in the internal carotid artery, and analyzed the location and duration of different blood flow patterns, confirming the relationship between vessel enlargement and flow disturbances [19].

VFI was also used to assess the normal values of wall shear stress in the common carotid arteries of 79 healthy volunteers, with good intraclass correlation coefficient and inter-observer reproducibility [20].

25.2.2 Computed Tomography Angiography

Computed tomography angiography (CTA) of carotid arteries is a minimally invasive, useful, and proven method for the recognition and characterization of vascular anatomy and pathologies of carotids for its high spatial resolution [21, 22].

The main **indications** for CTA of carotids include diagnosis, characterization, and/or surveillance of atherosclerotic steno-occlusive diseases, aneurysms or pseudoaneurysms, and vasculitis [21].

Furthermore, CTA is the first line of imaging in emergency department in patients with a high probability of neurovascular disease requiring immediate therapy, such as in cases of acute stroke [21, 23]. CTA can also be used to confirm the diagnosis or as preoperative evaluation of significant internal carotid stenosis or to more accurately characterize the degree of stenosis and to evaluate plaque morphology and components [23].

CTA has various **advantages** over US: it is able to evaluate in the same acquisition vessels from the aortic arch to the circle of Willis and has a better spatial resolution [21, 24]. Moreover, CTA has a significantly higher sensitivity and specificity, and it is often used routinely as a first-line examination in case of emergency for the evaluation of suspected acute vascular-nervous disease, as in cases of dissection, pseudo-occlusion, thrombosis of the ICA, pseudoaneurysms, and bleeding [23].

CTA also has various advantages over magnetic resonance angiography (MRA): a better spatial resolution, due to smaller pixels that allow to obtain a more accurate and detailed vascular anatomy and evaluation of adjacent anatomical structures; less susceptibility to artifacts, because CTA, as digital subtraction technique, relies on intraluminal contrast instead of signal changes due to alterations in blood flow and is less prone to motion artifacts because the scan is faster [23].

Main **limitations** of CTA are the exposure to ionizing radiation and the use of iodinated contrast. In pediatric patients MRA should be chosen as the first line of imaging instead of CTA, to reduce radiation exposure [21]. Due to the high doses of radiation and the potential contrast nephrotoxicity, CTA is not recommended for screening purpose [24].

The advent of multidetector (MD) CT scanners has increased spatial and temporal resolution and reduced acquisition times compared to single-layer CT. Actually, the use of MD scanners is preferred and it allows volumetric data acquisition with submillimeter isotropic voxels and complete subsecond gantry rotation that should not be greater than 1 s (preferable a gantry rotation time down to 0.33 s) [21, 25].

Gantry rotation time depends on the number of detector row. The fastest possible gantry rotation time should be used to reduce scan duration and contrast dose. The more detector rows a CT has, the smaller is the thickness of the single detector row (for example, 1–1.25 mm in a 4-detector-row CT and 0.5–0.6 mm in a 64-detector-row CT). The range of slice thickness should be 0.5–0.6 mm or at least preferably no greater than 1.5 mm. In general, in 16–64-slice CT the thinnest option is preferable [21, 25].

A reduced slice thickness allows to acquire isotropic voxels, which are mandatory to obtain high-resolution 3D reconstructions and other post-processing methods, such as the multiplanar reformation (MPR) or the maximum intensity projection (MIP).

The field of view (FOV) should include a volume from the aortic arch to the intracranial circulation, which require a scan range of approximately 200–250 mm [22, 25].

The arterial phase is often the only phase necessary for the study of the main carotid diseases. It is preferable to use a high-density iodinated nonionic contrast medium (iodine, 350 or 370 mmol/mL) to obtain a more effective opacification of the vessels. The contrast medium should be injected with a high-speed flow rate, not less than 4–5 mL/s, to obtain an appropriate arterial phase [21, 25]. The contrast volume used in adult patients (or in any patient weighing 50 or more kilograms) is about 75 mL. In pediatric patients, it is calculated based on weight (2 mL/kg). In general, however, the volume and flow of the contrast medium must be selected based on the patient's weight, age, and comorbidity [21].

The contrast medium is injected prior to venous access, with a 20-gauge or larger catheter (22 or 24 gauge for pediatric patients) possibly in the antecubital vein on the right arm, to avoid artifacts due to undiluted contrast material in the left brachiocephalic vein [21].

Furthermore, the use of a bolus of saline solution at the end of the injection may reduce the volume of contrast needed for adequate opacification of the vessels [21].

Contrast timing is mandatory to obtain a proper arterial opacification of the vessels. The time of the scan should occur during the peak contrast opacification. The main techniques used are automatic bolus tracking technique and test bolus injection [25]. The former is faster, because a single contrast medium injection is used and the scan starts when the HU preset value threshold of the region of interest (usually positioned over aortic arch) is reached. Test bolus injection, instead, relies on the peak of the curve obtained with the injection of a 10% of contrast volume to calculate the scanning time.

25.2.3 Magnetic Resonance

Magnetic resonance angiography (MRA) is a group of advanced imaging techniques based on magnetic resonance imaging (MRI) used to image blood vessels. They can be broadly divided into dark blood imaging techniques, which suppress signal from flowing blood, and bright blood imaging techniques, which can be further divided into contrast-enhanced and non-contrast MRA.

The two MRA techniques most commonly used for carotid imaging are time-of-flight imaging (TOF-MRA), which has the advantage of not requiring the use of contrast medium, and gadolinium contrast-enhanced angiography (CE-MRA), which is less dependent on blood flow compared to the former technique [23].

An important advantage of carotid MRA is the possibility of applying it in patients with important contraindications to the use of contrast agents. TOF-MRA is one such technique, based on flow-related enhancement. Radiofrequency waves continuously stimulate protons in the selected region, causing them to become magnetically saturated, so they do not generate MRI signals; protons within the blood however that are flowing into the selected region are not saturated and generate high MRI signal within the lumen. A technical distinction should be made between 2D TOF imaging where individual slices are acquired separately and 3D TOF imaging where data is acquired simultaneously from the entire tissue volume. Both 2D and 3D TOF sequences require more time to complete compared to CE-MRA, making them more susceptible to patient movement artifacts [26].

Another technique that does not rely on the use of gadolinium-based contrast agents is PC-MRA, and it has a different physical basis compared to TOF-MRA. A PC-MRA sequence modifies the precessional frequencies of protons with the application of a bipolar gradient, which makes it possible to study both blood flow and velocity. PC-MRA can also be used to study the vessel lumen, but TOF-MRA achieves similar results with a shorter scan time [27].

CE-MRA on the other hand uses the paramagnetic effect of a gadolinium-containing contrast agent in order to increase MRI signal arising from the blood. This makes CE-MRA less prone to artifacts from low velocity or turbulent blood flow. Despite recent technological developments in the field of MRA, CE-MRA seems to still be superior to TOF-MRA [28].

A more specific application of this technique is time-resolved CE-MRA, which consists of the acquisition of more temporally detailed images by repeatedly acquiring lower spatial resolution information that reflects contrast filling of vessels. This technique is especially used in the imaging of certain conditions that require imaging of the temporal dynamics of flow, such as in the case of arteriovenous fistulae [29].

MRA of the carotid arteries is frequently indicated as a follow-up exam after carotid Doppler ultrasound during screening of patients with a lower probability of neurovascular disease. These patients might present with symptoms such as amaurosis fugax, transient ischemic attacks (TIA), syncope, or episodic dizziness. MRA exams also have the advantage of being able to extend the imaging field to include an evaluation of perivascular soft tissue and brain parenchyma, providing a more precise characterization compared to a contrast-enhanced CT exam.

Both carotid DUS and MRA are capable of studying both blood flow and velocity. However, when compared with carotid DUS, MRA is less operator dependent and does produce an image of the whole artery.

MRA exams do not produce ionizing radiation, as opposed to CTA exams, making them more preferable exams in the case of pediatric patients. Some patients may not be able to undergo MRA examinations due to well-researched contraindications, such as the presence of pacemakers or foreign metallic bodies. Even in the case of MRI-compatible devices, these can still produce image-distortion artifacts that limit blood vessel evaluation if they are located in their proximity. MRI exams in general are also contraindicated in the case of claustrophobic patients, not only because of the restricted space but also because they tend to require more time, which also makes patient movement artifacts more likely. They also tend to be less readily available than CTA imaging, as well as more expensive.

25.3 Atherosclerotic Stenosis

Carotid stenosis is a narrowing of carotid arteries, which is manly a consequence of atherosclerosis and accumulation of atherosclerotic plaques in the carotid bifurcation and the initial part of the internal carotid artery.

Atherosclerosis is a chronic inflammatory disease of the arterial wall and main risk factors are hypertension, hyperlipidemia, and smoking. It is important to diagnose and determinate the degree of carotid stenosis for the prevention of stroke, the correct management, and an adequate treatment.

25.3.1 Doppler Ultrasound Evaluation for Carotid Stenosis

The operator should suspect the presence of a stenosis in the case of an endoluminal plaque, which determines a narrowing of the vessel, with a consequent turbulent flow represented with an aliasing area and a reduced flow in the post-stenotic segment.

During carotid Doppler evaluation it is highly recommended to evaluate the plaque morphology, to grade the ICA stenosis, and to analyze the waveform analysis.

25.3.1.1 Plaque Characterization

It is very important to describe the morphology and the characteristics of the parietal plaque, because the risk of distal embolization is directly related not only to the degree of stenosis but also to the plaque composition (see Fig. 25.4a/b). Unstable thrombus should be suspected in case of plaque neovascularity or hemorrhage, high lipid or necrotic content, irregular or ulcerated surface, and heterogenous echogenicity of the plaque.

Plaque echolucency on ultrasound B-mode was often associated with the presence or development of neurological events. According to

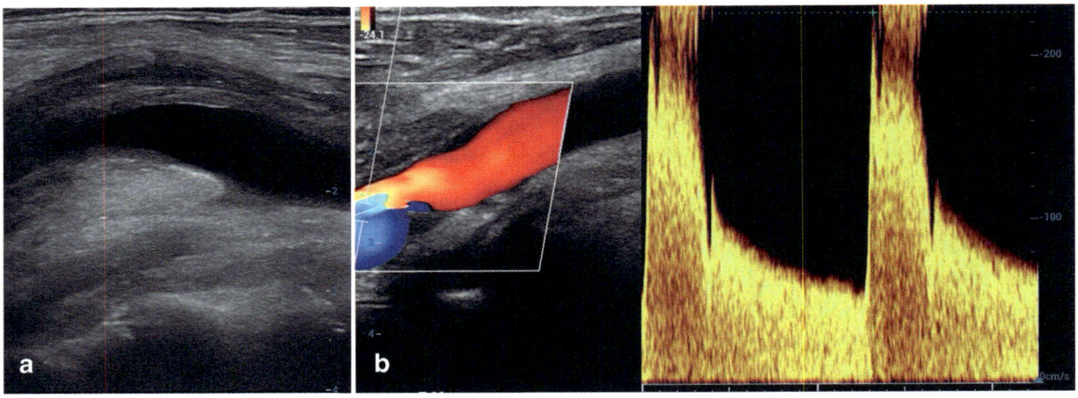

Fig. 25.4 (**a**) B-mode ultrasound of carotid bulb performed with linear array transducer, through longitudinal plane. Grayscale US image shows a plaque containing an echo-poor area, which may be due to hemorrhage or lipids. (**b**) B-mode ultrasound of carotid bulb and proximal ICA performed with linear array transducer, through longitudinal plane. The image shows an eccentric dishomogeneous type 3 plaque, predominantly hyperechoic, with an irregular surface. The plaque determines a significant stenosis of the bulb and proximal ICA

Gray-Weale classification, the plaques are distinguished into five types: type 1: uniformly hypoechoic (less than 15% of the area is occupied by hyperechoic areas); type 2: predominantly hypoechoic (hyperechoic areas from 15 to 50%); type 3: predominantly echogenic (hyper-echogenic areas from 50 to 85%); type 4: uniformly echogenic (hyperechoic areas more than 85%); and type 5: calcified surface >15% (with "shadow cone"). Types 1 and 2 are associated with a higher incidence of cerebrovascular accidents in 3 years. However, the magnitude of increased risk is not sufficient to identify patients likely to benefit from revascularization [30–32].

25.3.1.2 Grading ICA Stenosis

An atherosclerotic lesion usually determines a vessel narrowing associated with a post-stenotic dilatation. The measurement of the ICA stenosis is usually still considered the leading parameter in the choice of therapeutic options and a correct quantification of the stenosis degree is fundamental in order to plan the correct treatment. Color Doppler is based on the results of two prospective studies: the North American Symptomatic Carotid Endarterectomy Trial (NASCET) and the European Carotid Surgery Trial (ECST). They demonstrated a significant benefit of carotid endarterectomy in patients with severe carotid stenosis (≥70% for NASCET and ≥80% for ECST) to reduce the risk of stroke.

The NASCET method suggests to calculate percent ICA stenosis dividing the smallest residual ICA luminal diameter by the luminal diameter of the distal normal ICA; instead the ECST compares the diameter of the residual lumen with an estimate of the width of the ICA at the site of stenosis [33, 34].

Although NASCET method underestimates the plaque, this is the preferred technique to grade an ICA stenosis [35].

The velocity range is one of the most important ultrasound parameters. Normal velocity of blood in the ICA is typically between 60 and 100 cm/s. PSV is considered another primary Doppler criterion recommended for grading ICA stenosis, where a value >230 cm/s is indicative of a significant (>70%) stenosis [36]. But the absolute PSV should be considered unreliable in patients with increased or decreased cardiac output, in case of increased compensatory flow due to a contralateral high-grade stenosis or occlusion, in the presence of tandem lesions or a long-segment stenosis. Other Doppler criteria of a significant stenosis are a value of end-diastolic flow velocity in the stenosis >100 cm/s and a carotid ratio ICA/CCA >4.

25.3.1.3 Waveform Analysis

In the presence of a stenosis, the flow velocity increases proportionally to the degree of the stenosis with increase of both systolic and diastolic velocity.

Post-stenotic flow is characterized by a reduction in the steep systolic rise and a reduction in systolic-diastolic difference. This waveform is called "tardus parvus," which is characterized by a slow rate of systolic upstroke, rounding of the systolic peak, and decreased PSV, and it is the typical indirect sign of a more proximal stenosis even if the presence of a distal normal flow cannot rule out the presence of a proximal stenosis.

In case of complete occlusion, no flow can be identified along the carotid artery.

A "knocking waveform," which is characterized by decreased PSV, a sharp systolic upstroke, and decreased or reversed diastolic flow, is observed proximal to high-grade stenosis.

25.3.2 CTA in Carotid Stenosis

An accurate assessment of presence and degree of stenosis in the carotid artery is very important for planning therapeutic treatment. Currently, DUS remains the most used first-line method for the study of a suspected carotid stenosis. CTA, with MRA, is the method of deepening in asymptomatic patients with intermediate-grade stenosis (> or = 50%, <70%) at DUS [37, 38].

CTA and MRA can be the first-line methods in patients with a high disease probability to have a more complete assessment of intrathoracic and intracranial lesions [38]. Particularly, CTA alone, or combined with DUS, is the most convenient method in patients with a recent transient ischemic attack or a small ischemic stroke [39]. CTA may be used alone or with DUS. The choice is based on some parameters such as the patient's gender, risk profile of stroke incidence, window time between the first ischemic symptoms, and carotid endarterectomy [39].

The choice of carotid diagnostic imaging therefore depends mainly on the clinical indications and experience of individual center [38]. According to some authors (Tholen et al.), CTA should be performed in patients with transient ischemic attack (TIA) or minor stroke, if DUS is positive.

If, however, patients have a high-risk profile or a high probability of carotid stenosis, CTA should be the first-line method followed by surgical treatment for stenosis of 50–99% [39].

Unlike DUS, both CTA and MRA have the **advantage** of allowing the evaluation of carotid arteries throughout their path, from the aortic arch to the intracranial site. Moreover, the acquisition of images is faster than other methods and the evaluation is relatively less dependent on the operator [38].

Furthermore, another advantage of CTA, compared to the other two methods, is that CTA is less susceptible than MRA to overestimate the severity of carotid stenosis and the possibility to evaluate the composition of plaques [37, 38]. The ability to recognize the composition of plaques allows to evaluate the stability of the stenosis, correlating it to the risk of stroke [40]. Based on Hounsfield unit (HU) values, carotid plaques can be classified into three groups: soft plaques (attenuation values <50 HU), fatty plaques (> 50 UH and <120 HU), and calcified plaques (>120 HU) [41]. Depending on their composition, each plaque has a different ischemic risk and different imaging (see Fig. 25.5).

However, a **limitation** of CTA is to be less reliable than DUS and MRA in the evaluation of plaque morphology, especially if they have lipid component or ulcerations [37, 38]. The disadvantages of CTA, also, are related to the intravenous use of the iodinated contrast medium and radiation. Although CTA can recognize small calcifications better than DSA or MRA, extensive calcifications can reduce their accuracy. Other disadvantages of CTA are metal beam-hardening artifacts and high contrast concentrations in the brachiocephalic vein [38]. Modern multidetector CT scanners allow fast acquisitions with isotropic submillimetric voxels. This ability allows to obtain, thanks to post-processing programs, 3D reconstructions, with high spatial resolution and anatomical details that cannot be easily obtained with other methods [40]. CTA post-processing techniques include maximal intensity projection

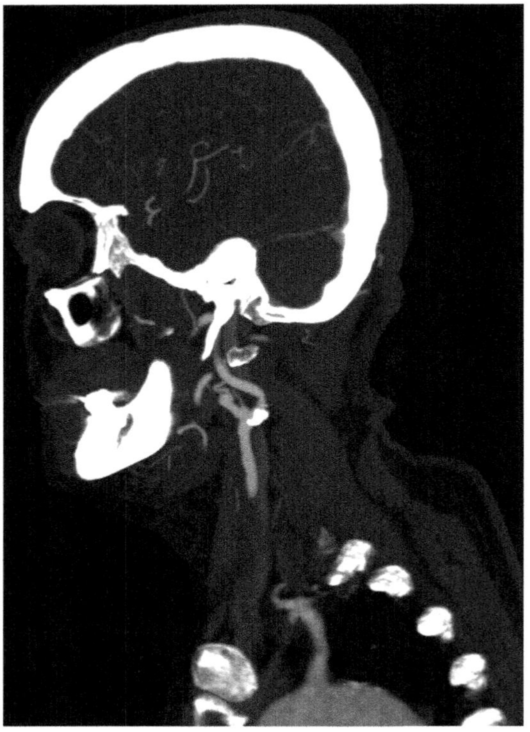

Fig. 25.5 Computed tomography angiography (CTA) of the left carotid artery bifurcation. Maximum intensity projection (MIP) reconstruction provides an overview of the target vessel, showing a calcified plaque at the origin of the internal carotid artery

(MIP), multiplanar reconstruction (MPR), and 3D volume rendering. These techniques allow to reconstruct the path of the entire carotid artery, cutting the venous structures and the bone. MIP images, on the other hand, are obtained by selecting the pixels with the highest density values, while MPR images are reconstructed by selecting the average density of all the pixels.

The volume rendering projects all the pixels and uses all data in a 3D display. It may have some limits with large calcific plaques while it works best when the vessels have small calcifications. MIP and MPR are more accurate than 3D images in the evaluation of stenosis with calcified plaques.

The only acquisition in the arterial phase is sufficient for the study of carotid stenosis [38]. In clinical practice, there are many measurement methods for quantification of internal carotid artery (ICA) stenosis. The two most used methods are North American Symptomatic Carotid Endarterectomy Trial (NASCET) and European Carotid Surgery Trial (ECST), which compare the segment of maximum stenosis with:

- The normal diameter of the post-stenotic ICA, in the North American Symptomatic Carotid Endarterectomy Trial (NASCET) [38, 42]
- The estimated width of the original artery at the point of greatest narrowing, in the European Carotid Surgery Trial (ECST) [38, 43] (see Fig. 25.6)

A third, less widespread, method is the common carotid (CC) method, which relates the diameter of the lumen remaining at the point of maximum stenosis with the diameter of the lumen of the proximal portion of the common carotid artery (CCA), because it is more reproducible [43].

All these methods have similar prognostic values but lead to different estimates of the degree of stenosis [38, 43]. However, both NASCET and ECST have shown benefits from carotid endarterectomy in cases of severe stenosis [40].

25.3.3 MRI in Carotid Stenosis and Occlusion

CTA has a slightly better performance than MRA in evaluating carotid artery stenosis [44], though to improve the accuracy of the diagnosis, the use of two imaging modalities before revascularization is suggested [38]. In the case of more urgent cases or with evidence of more severe stenosis, carotid CTA is preferred to confirm the diagnosis or more accurately determine the precise degree of stenosis, as severe ICA origin stenosis can result in complete signal dropout despite the presence of a hairline residual lumen [38].

MRA is capable of studying plaque composition with the use of additional sequences, and is more suited to studying calcified plaques compared to CTA. However, in the presence of stenting of the carotid arteries, an alternative imaging technique should be considered, as these can in some cases cause imaging acquisition artifacts that can severely hinder the study of vascular structures [45].

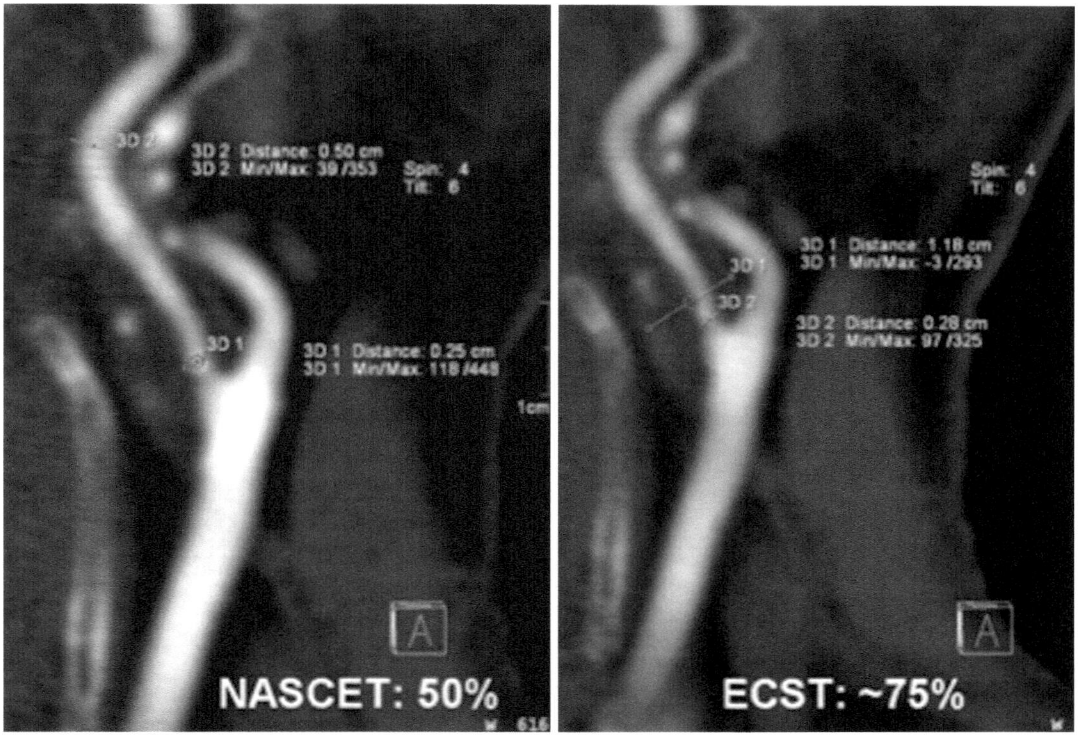

Fig. 25.6 Computed tomography angiography (CTA) of the carotid artery bifurcation. An atherosclerotic plaque in ICA determines a vessel narrowing. Stenosis grade is calculated with both NASCET (50%) and ECST (~75%) methods. The NASCET method suggests to calculate percent ICA stenosis dividing the smallest residual ICA luminal diameter by the luminal diameter of the distal normal ICA; instead the ECST compares the diameter of the residual lumen with an estimate of the width of the ICA at the site of stenosis. Although NASCET method underestimates the plaque, this is the preferred technique to grade an ICA stenosis

Though CE-MRA techniques enjoy a slightly higher sensitivity compared to TOF MRA in the case of detection of severe stenosis, 3D TOF-MRA shows a higher specificity, making it a valid option for carotid stenosis detection [46]. However, recent studies show that 3D TOF MRA at 3 T may result in significantly higher stenosis grades, and may potentially lead to inadequate therapy, which is why it should not be used as a replacement for CE-MRA [47].

25.3.4 Carotid Angiography and Stenosis Treatment

Carotid arteriography is nowadays performed just for interventional purposes, instead of diagnostic scope, because of improvements of other carotid artery imaging modalities.

Endovascular procedures are usually performed via local anesthesia. Femoral artery access is an established standard approach, but in the cases of severe kinking or untreated stenosis/occlusion of the iliac arteries or abdominal aorta, a brachial or radial access is preferred. The guidewire is then advanced into the abdominal and thoracic aorta, where the operator can perform the selective carotid artery angiography with many different kinds of catheters or a pre-shaped long sheath.

The common angiographic aspect of an atherosclerotic lesion is an eccentric narrowing, usually associated with a post-stenotic dilatation (see Fig. 25.7).

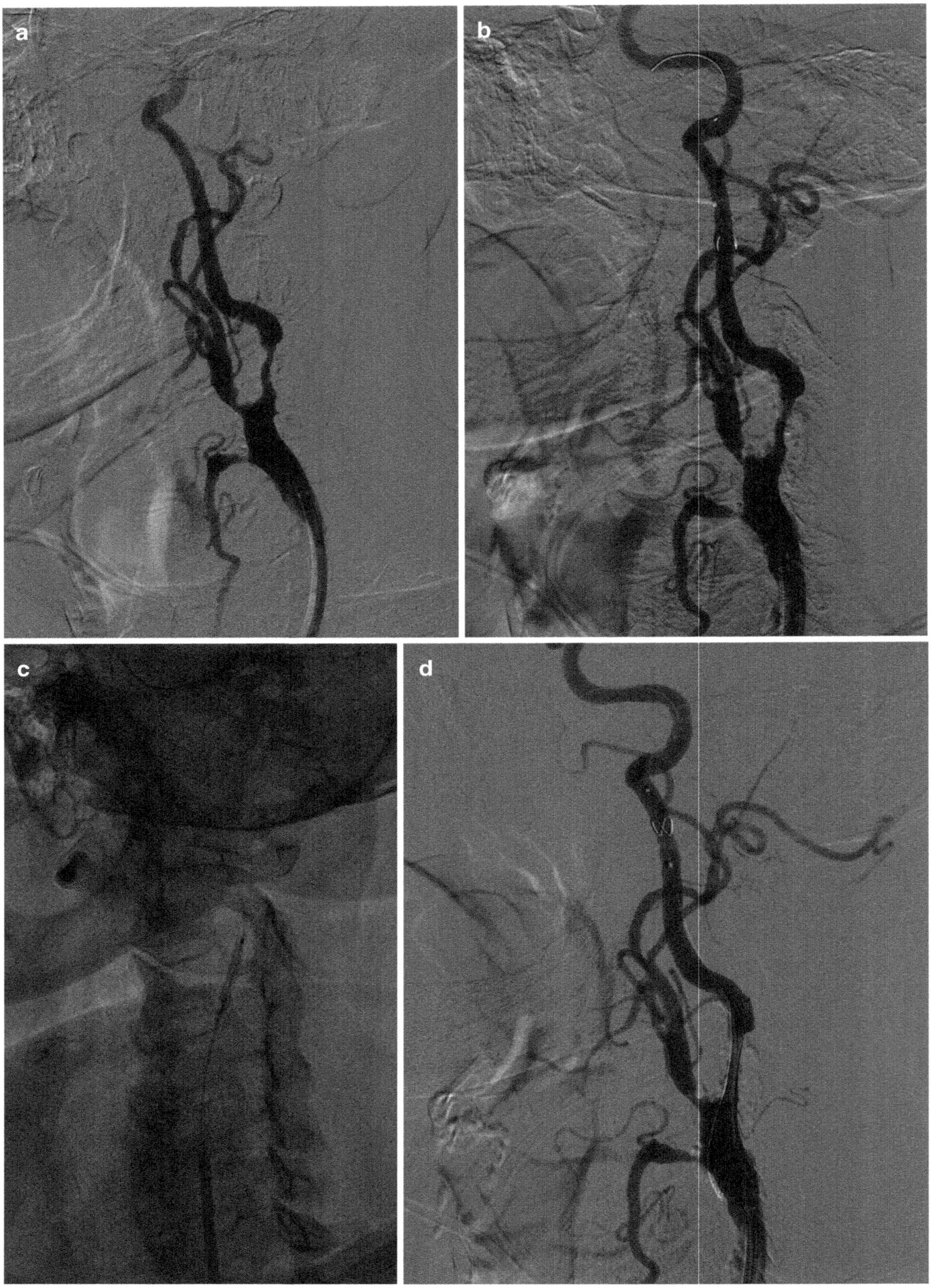

Fig. 25.7 Carotid artery stenting procedure. (**a**) Digital subtraction angiography showing the presence of a severe stenosis at the origin of the internal carotid artery. (**b**) Distal embolic filter is deployed in the internal carotid artery (**c**) inflation and deflation of a balloon catheter in correspondence of the vascular stenosis. (**d**) Deployment of the carotid stent. (**e**) Final angiographic control, with an improved caliber of the vessel after the treatment

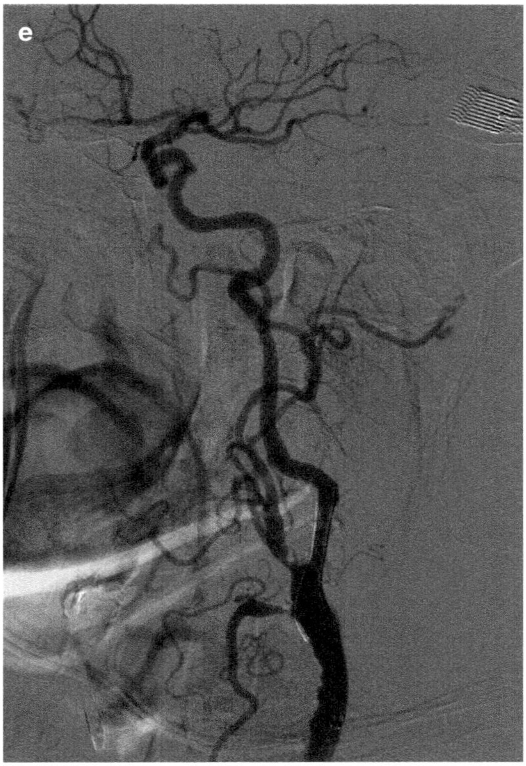

Fig. 25.7 (continued)

Distal embolic protection devices are used to reduce the peri-interventional risk of distal atheroembolism, but its usefulness is still on debate.

In cases of highly calcified tight lesions, predilatation should be performed to allow full stent expansion. Self-expandable stents are usually used with a stent-to-vessel ratio of 1.1:1 and with the minor length possible to cover the lesion.

Post-interventional angiogram, without the guidewire in place, should be performed to evaluate the treated lesion and to exclude distal embolism or other complications.

25.4 Carotid Aneurysm and Pseudoaneurysm

Extracranial carotid artery aneurysms can be divided into true and false aneurysms. True aneurysms involve all three layers of the arterial wall, and it is generally due to atherosclerosis; in the young the commonest cause is Takayasu's arteritis and less commonly the aneurysm is mycotic. The fusiform shape is more frequent in this case, though saccular aneurysms can also be seen, usually along the course of the common or internal carotid artery.

An arterial pseudoaneurysm (PSA), also known as false aneurysm, is caused by damage to the arterial wall, resulting in locally contained hematoma with turbulent blood. Unlike a true aneurysm, a pseudoaneurysm does not contain any layer of the vessel wall. Instead, there is blood containment by a wall developed with the products of the clotting cascade.

PSAs most often occur following penetrating trauma, usually iatrogenic, or as a complication of arteritis, cervical trauma, carotid dissection, and carotid neoplastic invasion.

DUS: On B-mode imaging it is possible to find an outpouching arising from the carotid artery. With color Doppler a typical Korean flag pattern (or "yin-yang" pattern) can be seen inside the sac, due to slowly swirling blood flow. By evaluating the spectral Doppler at the neck, it is probable to obtain a characteristic "to-and-fro" waveform for the presence of a flow heading toward the PSA during systole and reversed flow during diastole.

CTA is a convenient, reliable technique for detecting **aneurysms**, useful for deciding on surgical planning. Current multidetector CT scanners allow for extended diagnostic accuracy even in the detection of small intracranial aneurysms.

A limitation of CTA is that aneurysms adjacent to the skull base may not be recognizable. Some authors have described how aneurysms deriving from the intracavernous and paraclinoid tracts of the carotid artery could be hidden by bone, calcium, or venous blood. However, according to Tomandl, paraclinoid aneurysms not detected on conventional 3D CTA were optimally visualized with bone-subtraction CT angiography (BSCTA) [48].

Another limitation, highlighted by Gaughen, is that although CTA has a high sensitivity in recognizing the aneurysm blisters of the supraclinoid ICA, this sensitivity is still not 100% [49].

Pseudoaneurysms are often associated with dissection. CTA, as well as MRA, is the reference method for recognition. CTA is more precise than MRA in order to detect the aneurysm location at the skull base and their exact dimensions.

MRA techniques have an important role as a second-level imaging technique along with CTA, and can be useful in providing information regarding the size and extent of aneurysmal dilation, and the presence or absence of thrombus, as well as providing a panoramic view of the carotid arterial system along with describing the relationship with surrounding structures [38].

Though TOF-MRA can be used in these cases, it can underestimate aneurysm volume and neck size, and visualization of smaller aneurysms could be difficult when compared to CE-MRA [50]. The major disadvantage of 3D TOF-MRA is that it generally cannot be used to visualize the entire length of coverage of cervical vasculature. This makes contrast-enhanced 3D MRA the preferred method for the study of the entire cervical vasculature, while 3D TOF-MRA could be used as a supplemental study of common carotid bifurcation or degree of stenosis [38].

25.5 Carotid Artery Dissection

Carotid dissection is a major cause of cerebrovascular disease, as it represents a common cause of stroke in young patients. Dissections commonly occur in the presence of bifurcations and in places where vessels transition from flexible to fixed. In general, extracranial carotid dissection is more common compared to intracranial ICA dissection.

ICA dissection in the extracranial tract involves the cervical portion of the artery distal to the carotid bulb and tends not to extend beyond its entrance into the petrous sinus [51]. The dissection therefore tends to spare the carotid bifurcation as well as the intracranial portion of the ICA [51].

DUS: On B-mode imaging it is possible to visualize an intraluminal hematoma or an echogenic intraluminal flap. The true lumen typically has a normal Doppler waveform or an increased PSV may be demonstrated in case of secondary compression by the false lumen. The most common US finding is a high-resistance waveform pattern in the proximal ICA.

CTA: The dissection appears as an eccentric narrowing of the vessel lumen, with an increase of the external diameter of the artery [51].

In addition to the arterial contrastographic phase, a basal acquisition could be useful. The basal acquisition allows the finding of a crescent-shape hyperdense area, corresponding to the wall hematoma, which occurs in acute dissections usually at the level of the upper portion of the cervical ICA, which otherwise would not be recognized in arterial acquisition because it is isodense compared to the surrounding muscle tissue [51].

The typical findings of an acute dissection are the eccentric narrowing of the lumen surrounded by a crescent-shape wall thickening and a thin and annular contrastographic enhancement or a presence of an intimal flap. These features are very specific but less sensitive [51, 52].

MRI: In addition to showing luminal abnormalities, such as intimal flaps, focal stenosis, long-segment stenosis, "flame-shaped" occlusion, or a pseudoaneurysm, both MRA and CTA images are able to show mural findings. An advantage of MRA imaging is the possibility of detection of intramural hematomas as a bright signal material on unenhanced images, particularly with dark blood techniques, as well as detection of blood products through axial flow-suppressed MRI images which increase the specificity for dissection [53]. Time-resolved MRA imaging can provide further information on the dissection by watching the temporal filling patterns [54].

25.6 Carotid Vasculitis

In vasculitis inflammatory leukocytes are present in vessel walls; this leads to swelling and damage of mural structures. The lumen is narrowed or occluded leading to ischemia and necrosis.

The carotid arteries are affected by the vasculitis of the large vessels like giant-cell arteritis

(GCS) and Takayasu's arteritis (TA). These pathologies have affinity to affect the branches of the carotid artery, but subclinical involvement of the other cranial arteries and the wider arterial tree is not uncommon. Takayasu's arteritis is less common than giant-cell arteritis. The annual incidence of TA is 0.4–2/million/year [55].

The pattern of artery involvement may be similar for GCA and Takayasu's arteritis; however, Takayasu's arteritis may occur less symmetrically.

DUS: In large-vessel vasculitis the artery wall is thickened, usually to more than 1 mm, and a homogeneous wall swelling, preferably circumferential, of 1.5 mm or more is often associated. In acute flares the wall is hypoechoic because of wall edema, whereas in most cases it tends to be hyperechoic. Furthermore, arteriosclerosis in large-vessel arteritis is possible. For the causes mentioned above, vasculitis may lead to stenosis. In few cases it may be difficult to differentiate hypoechoic plaques from vasculitic lesions. However, usually it is easy to differentiate arteriosclerosis from vasculitis with ultrasound [56].

Some authors have suggested a possible role for carotid CEUS in the assessment of disease activity in patients with large-vessel vasculitis. Carotid CEUS can improve the visualization of the lumen border and allows the assessment of carotid wall vascularization. The visualization of contrast microbubbles through the thickened artery wall was construed as a potential sign of inflammation and consequently a marker of disease activity [57].

CTA: In general, CT angiography allows to detect the presence and the extent of stenosis, occlusion, aneurysm, and wall thickening, which could be related to vasculitis disease. In particular, CT angiography can detect the modification of vessel walls (see Fig. 25.8), before a significant stenosis could be found by conventional catheter angiography [58, 59].

The role of computed tomography is quite limited in the detection of cerebral vasculitis. In particular, CT is less sensitive than MRI and it has less resolution than US. However, it could be useful in case of hemorrhage [58]. The use of contrast medium allows to detect enhancement and a hypovascular halo in mural thickening wall in active vasculitis. In inactive diseases, mural calcifications could be found with mild thickening and enhancement [60].

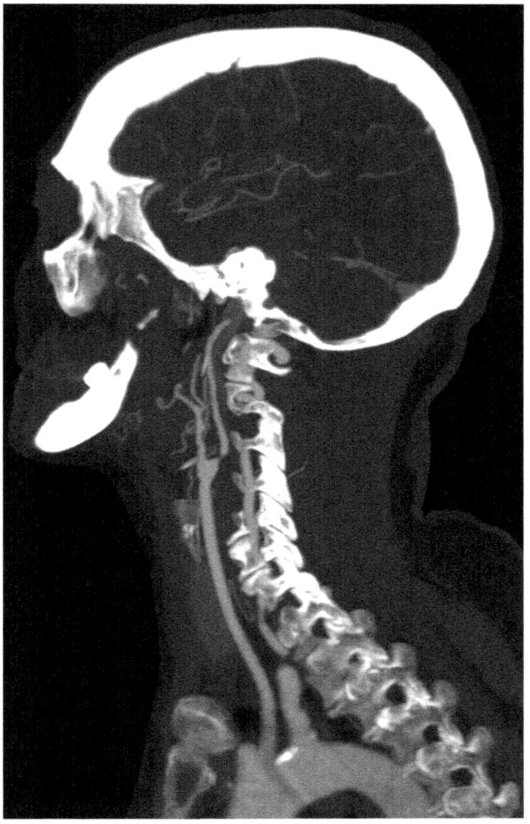

Fig. 25.8 Computed tomography angiography (CTA) of the left carotid artery bifurcation. Maximum intensity projection (MIP) reconstruction provides an overview of the target vessel, showing the irregularities of the vessel walls due to vasculitis

In order to evaluate carotid arteries, CT has shown a sensitivity and specificity of 93% and 98% to detect carotid stenosis in patients with Takayasu's arteritis [61].

The main advantages of CT are an excellent high spatial resolution, the use of multiple planes and three-dimensional view, and an accurate cross-sectional imaging in demonstrating vessel wall change [59]. The disadvantages are exposure to ionizing radiation and contraindication to contrast media [59].

MRI: In large vessels such as the carotid arteries, vasculitides commonly manifest as vessel wall irregularity, multifocal stenosis, or aneurysm formation. While these changes can be detected both by MRA and CTA, MRI has the added benefit of being able to use additional sequences such as short T1 inversion recovery (STIR) images to detect vessel wall edema [60]. Dark blood imaging techniques do not require the use of IV contrast, and can be used to evaluate the vessel wall for signs of thickening and inflammation [62]. However, the use of gadolinium-containing contrast medium in these cases provides an indispensable contribution to the diagnosis by highlighting vessel wall enhancement and perivascular edema as signs of active inflammation, as opposed to vessel wall thickening which can persist chronically beyond the active periods of inflammation [63].

25.7 Fibromuscular Dysplasia

Fibromuscular dysplasia (FMD) is a non-atheromatous, non-inflammatory arteriopathy of unknown etiology with segmental manifestation on medium-sized arteries in various regions of the body. The disease can occur at any age but is usually diagnosed in middle-aged, predominately female individuals. The TSAs, especially the internal carotid artery, are involved, often bilaterally. The proximal section of the ICA is generally not affected, except in a rare FMD subtype characterized by proximal involvement with a web-like membrane.

DUS: B-mode can show typical string-of-beads pattern with alternating regions of lumen narrowing and vessel dilatation, over a length of 3–5 cm. Color Doppler imaging also reveals the segmental string-of-beads pattern distally to a completely normal segment of the vessel. Dependent on the degree of stenosis, direct or indirect hemodynamic criteria may be recognized. In comparison to other imaging techniques, the sensitivity of US is low; the vascular lesion can only be visualized with ultrasound when it is located not too far cranially on the ICA [64].

References

1. Anastasi G, Capitani S, Carnazza ML, et al. Trattato di Anatomia Umana. Volume Primo – Edi.Ermes. 2010:341–57.
2. Saba L, Raz E. Neurovascular imaging: from basics to advanced concepts. Springer Ref. 2016:87–92.
3. Michalinos A, Chatzimarkos M, et al. Anatomical considerations on surgical anatomy of the carotid bifurcation. Anatomy Research International. 2016;2016:1.
4. Schulz UGR, Rothwell PM. Major variation in carotid bifurcation anatomy: a possible risk factor for plaque development? Stroke. 2001;32(11):2522–9.
5. Bouthillier A, Van Loveren HR, Keller JT. Segments of the internal carotid artery: A new classification. Neurosurgery. 1996;38(3):425–33.
6. Lasjaunias P, Santoyo-Vazquez A. Segmental agenesis of the internal carotid artery: angiographic:133–41.
7. Dungan DH, Heiserman JE. The carotid artery: embryology. Normal Anat Physiol. 1996:1052–51.49.
8. Newton TH, Potts DG. Radiology of the skull and brain. CV Mosby: St Louis; 1974.
9. Huber P. Cerebral angiography, ed 2: Thieme Medical Publishers; 1982.
10. Vitek JJ, Reaves P. Thoracic bifurcation of the common carotid artery. Neuroradiology. 1973;5:133–9.
11. Lie TA. Congenital anomalies of the carotid arteries: an angiographic study and a review of the literature. Amsterdam: Excerpta Medica; 1968.
12. O'Leary DH, Polak JF, Kronmal RA, et al. Carotid-artery intima and media thickness as a risk factor for myocardial infarction and stroke in older adults. Cardiovascular Health Study. N Engl J Med. 1999;340:14–22.
13. Rafailidis V, Charitanti A, Tegos T, et al. Contrast-enhanced ultrasound of the carotid system: a review of the current literature. J Ultrasound. 2017;20:97–109.
14. Feinstein SB. Contrast ultrasound imaging of the carotid artery vasa vasorum and atherosclerotic plaque neovascularization. J Am Coll Cardiol. 2006;48:236–43.
15. Rafailidis V, Sidhu PS. Vascular ultrasound, the potential of integration of multiparametric ultrasound into routine clinical practice. Ultrasound. 2018;26:136–44.
16. Goddi A, Bortolotto C, Fiorina I, et al. High-frame rate vector flow imaging of the carotid bifurcation. Insights Imaging. 2017;8:319.
17. Hansen KL, Udesen J, Gran F, Jensen JA, Bachmann NM. In-vivo examples of flow patterns with the fast vector velocity ultrasound method. Ultraschall Med. 2009;30:471–7.
18. Meyer P, Pelz JO. Blood flow reversal from the external into the internal carotid artery-New insights into the hemodynamics at the carotid bifurcation. Brain Behav. 2018;8(11)
19. Goddi A, Fanizza M, Bortolotto C, et al. Vector flow imaging techniques: a new way to study vessel flow with ultrasound. J Clin Ultrasound. 2017;45:582–8.

20. Qiu Y, Yang D, Zhang Q et al. V Flow technology in measurement of wall shear stress of common carotid arteries in healthy adults: Feasibility and normal values. Clin Hemorheol Microcirc 2019
21. ACR-ASNR-SPR Practice Parameter for the Performance and Interpretation of Cervico-cerebral Computed Tomography Angiography (CTA) Res.19–2015.
22. Varga A, Di Leo G, et al. Multidetector CT angiography of the circle of Willis: association of its variants with carotid artery disease and brain ischemia. Eur Radiol. 2019;29:46–56. https://doi.org/10.1007/s00330-018-5577-x.
23. Jaff MR, Goldmakher GV, et al. Imaging of the carotid arteries: the role of duplex ultrasonography, magnetic resonance arteriography, and computerized tomographic arteriography. Vascular Medicine. 2008;13(4):281–92. https://doi.org/10.1177/1358863X08091971.
24. Aboyans V, Ricco JB, et al. 2017 ESC guidelines on the diagnosis and treatment of peripheral arterial diseases, in collaboration with the European Society for Vascular Surgery (ESVS): document covering atherosclerotic disease of extracranial carotid and vertebral, mesenteric, renal, upper and lower extremity arteries. Heart Journal. 2018;39(9):763–816. https://doi.org/10.1093/eurheartj/ehx095.
25. Lell MM, Anders K, et al. New Techniques in CT Angiography. Radiographics. 2006;26(Suppl 1):S45–62.
26. Morelli JN, et al. Technical considerations in MR angiography: an image-based guide. J Magn Reson Imaging. 2013;37(6):1326–41. https://doi.org/10.1002/jmri.24174.
27. Yucel EK, et al. Magnetic resonance angiography. Circulation. 1999;100(22):2284–301. https://doi.org/10.1161/01.CIR.100.22.2284.
28. Boujan T, et al. Value of contrast-enhanced MRA versus time-of-flight MRA in acute ischemic stroke MRI. AJNR. 2018;39(9):1710–6. https://doi.org/10.3174/ajnr.A5771.
29. Binek A, et al. Detection and grading of DAVF: prospects and limitations of 3T MRI. Eur Radiol. 2012;22(2):429–38. https://doi.org/10.1007/s00330-011-2268-2.
30. Mathiesen EB, Bønaa KH, et al. Echolucent plaques are associated with high risk of ischemic cerebrovascular events in carotid stenosis: the tromsø study. Circulation. 2001;103(17):2171–5.
31. Grønholdt ML, Nordestgaard BG, et al. Ultrasonic echolucent carotid plaques predict future stroke. Circulation. 2001;104(1):68–73.
32. Gupta A, Kesavabhotla K, et al. Plaque echolucency and stroke risk in asymptomatic carotid stenosis: a systematic review and meta-analysis. Stroke. 2015;46(1):91–7.
33. Barnett HJM, Taylor DW, Eliasziw M, et al. Benefit of carotid endarterectomy in patients with symptomatic moderate or severe stenosis. North American Symptomatic Carotid Endarterectomy Trial Collaborators. N Engl J Med. 1998;339(20):1415–25.
34. European Carotid Surgery Trialists' Collaborative Group. Randomized trial of endarterectomy for recently symptomatic carotid stenosis: final results of the MRC European Carotid Surgery Trial (ECST). Lancet. 1998;351(9113):1379–87.
35. Brott TG, Halperin JL, Abbara S, et al. 2011 ASA/ACCF/AHA/AANN/AANS/ACR/ASNR/CNS/SAIP/ SCAI/SIR/SNIS/SVM/SVS guideline on the management of patients with extracranial carotid and vertebral artery disease. J Am Coll Cardiol. 2011;57(8):1002–44.
36. Grant EG, Benson CB, Moneta GL, et al. Carotid artery stenosis: gray-scale and Doppler US diagnosis–Society of Radiologists in Ultrasound Consensus Conference. Radiology. 2003;229(2):340–6.
37. Ricotta JJ, AbuRahma A, et al. Updated Society for Vascular Surgery guidelines for management of extracranial carotid disease. J Vasc Surg. 2011;54:e1.
38. Adla T, Adlova R. Multimodality imaging of carotid stenosis. Int J Angiol. 2015;24:179–84.
39. Tholen A, De Monye C, et al. Suspected carotid artery stenosis: cost-effectiveness of CT angiography in work-up of patients with recent TIA or minor ischemic stroke. Radiology. 2010;256(2):585–97. https://doi.org/10.1148/radiol.10091157.
40. Bartlett ES, Walters TD, et al. Quantification of carotid stenosis on CT angiography. Am J Neuroradiol. 2006;27:13–9.
41. Saba L, Mallarini G. Window setting for the study of calcified carotid plaques with multidetector CT angiography. AJNR Am J Neuroradiol. 2009;30:1445–50.
42. Samarzija K, Milosevic P, et al. Grading of carotid artery stenosis with computed tomography angiography: whether to use the narrowest diameter or the cross-sectional area. Insight into Imaging. 2018;9:527–34.
43. U-King-Im JM, Trivedi RA, et al. Measuring carotid stenosis on contrast-enhanced magnetic resonance angiography. Diagnostic performance and reproducibility of 3 different methods. Stroke. 2004;35(9):2083–8.
44. Anzidei M, et al. Diagnostic accuracy of colour Doppler ultrasonography, CT angiography and blood-pool-enhanced MR angiography in assessing carotid stenosis: A comparative study with DSA in 170 patients. Radiol Med. 2012;117(1):54–71. https://doi.org/10.1007/s11547-011-0651-3.
45. Frölich AMJ, et al. Comparing different MR angiography strategies of carotid stents in a vascular flow model: toward stent-specific recommendations in MR follow-up. Neuroradiology. 2011;53(5):359–65. https://doi.org/10.1007/s00234-010-0753-y.
46. Debrey SM, et al. Diagnostic accuracy of magnetic resonance angiography for internal carotid artery disease. Stroke. 2008;39(8):2237–48. https://doi.org/10.1161/STROKEAHA.107.509877.
47. Platzek I, et al. Carotid artery stenosis: comparison of 3D time-of-flight MR angiography and contrast-enhanced MR angiography at 3T. Radiol Res Pract. 2014;2014:508–715. https://doi.org/10.1155/2014/508715.

48. Tomandl BF, Hammen T. Bone-subtraction CT angiography for the evaluation of intracranial aneurysms. AJNR Am J Neuroradiol. 2006;27:55–9.
49. Gaughen JR, Raghavan P, Jensen ME, et al. Utility of CT angiography in the identification and characterization of supraclinoid internal carotid artery blister aneurysms. AJNR Am J Neuroradiol. 2010;31(4):640–4. https://doi.org/10.3174/ajnr.A1893.
50. Deutschmann HA, et al. Diagnostic accuracy of 3D time-of-flight MR angiography compared with digital subtraction angiography for follow-up of coiled intracranial aneurysms: influence of aneurysm size. Am J Neuroradiol. 2007;28(4):628–34. http://www.ajnr.org/content/28/4/628.
51. Rodallec MH, Marteau V, et al. Craniocervical arterial dissection: Spectrum of imaging findings and differential diagnosis. Radiographics. 2008;28:1711–28.
52. Leclerc X, Godefroy O, Salhi A, Lucas C, Leys D, Pruvo JP. Helical CT for the diagnosis of extracranial internal carotid artery dissection. Stroke. 1996;27(3):461–6.
53. Mehdi E, et al. Craniocervical dissections: radiologic findings, pitfalls, mimicking diseases: A pictorial review. Curr Med Imag Reviews. 2018;14(2):207–22. https://doi.org/10.2174/157340561366617040310223 5.
54. Schneider G, et al. Magnetic resonance angiography: Springer-Verlag; 2005. https://doi.org/10.1007/b138651.
55. Mukhtyar C, Guillevin L, et al. EULAR recommendations for the management of large vessel vasculitis. Ann Rheum Dis. 2009;68(3):318–23.
56. Schmidt WA. Role of ultrasound in the understanding and management of vasculitis. Ther Adv Musculoskel Dis. 2014;6(2):39–47.
57. Germano G, Macchioni P, et al. Contrast-enhanced ultrasound of the carotid artery in patients with large vessel vasculitis: correlation with positron emission tomography findings. Arthritis Care Res. 2017;69(1):143–9.
58. Razek AAKA, Alvarez H, Bagg S, et al. Imaging spectrum of CNS vasculitis. Radiographics. 2014;34(4):873–94.
59. Hur JH, Chun EJ, et al. CT features of vasculitides based on the 2012 International Chapel Hill Consensus Conference Revised Classification. Korean J Radiol. 2017;18(5):786–98.
60. Broncano J, Vargas D, et al. CT and MR imaging of cardio-thoracic vasculitis. Radiographics. 2018;38(4):997–1021. https://doi.org/10.1148/rg.2018170136.
61. Pipitone N, Versari A, Salvarani C. Role of imaging studies in the diagnosis and follow-up of large-vessel vasculitis: an update. Rheumatology (Oxford). 2008;47(4):403–8.
62. Saam T, et al. High-resolution black-blood contrast-enhanced T1 weighted images for the diagnosis and follow-up of intracranial arteritis. Br J Radiol. 2010;83(993):e182–4. https://doi.org/10.1259/bjr/74101656.
63. Adler S, et al. Diagnostic value of contrast-enhanced magnetic resonance angiography in large-vessel vasculitis. Swiss Med Wkly. 2017;147:0708. https://doi.org/10.4414/smw.2017.14397.
64. Arning C, Grzyska U. Color Doppler imaging of cervicocephalic fibromuscular dysplasia. Cardiovasc Ultrasound. 2004;2:7.

Echocardiography in Nephrology 26

Luca Di Lullo, Antonio Granata, Vincenzo Barbera, and Antonio Bellasi

26.1 Introduction

Renal function impairment, indicated by reduced estimated glomerular filtration rate (eGFR), is a powerful prognostic predictor of mortality, cardiovascular events, and hospitalization [1, 2]. In addition, despite advances in dialysis therapy and patient care, end-stage renal disease (ESRD) is still notorious for high mortality [1–4]. There are several possible explanations for poor prognosis of CKD patients, including traditional cardiovascular risk factors (i.e., hypertension, diabetes mellitus, and dyslipidemia), nontraditional factors (e.g., malnutrition, inflammation, and oxidative stress), and CKD-related risk factors (e.g., atherosclerosis, anemia, altered calcium-phosphate metabolism) [5, 6]. These factors may contribute to the development and deterioration of the coronary artery disease (CAD), microvasculopathy, valvulopathy, cardiomyopathy, and arrhythmias [7, 8]. Cardiac abnormalities, especially abnormal left ventricular (LV) geometry and functions, are frequently detected in CKD patients and have been proven to be correlated with high cardiovascular mortality/morbidity and all-cause mortality [9, 10]. Early identification of such high-risk patients should thus allow physicians to optimize the therapeutic interventions, which may lower morbidity and mortality [4].

26.2 Role of Echocardiography

Cardiac magnetic resonance imaging (cMRI) is the widely accepted reference standard of noninvasive imaging modalities to evaluate cardiac morphology (e.g., LV volume and mass) and function [e.g., ejection fraction (EF) and cardiac output] [11]. However, there are several major limitations of cMRI in daily practice, such as its high costs, nonportability, and having little or no prognostic evidence of several CVDs [12]. These factors limit its clinical application. In addition, although the risk of gadolinium toxicity in advanced CKD patients is rare, the serious complication of nephrogenic systemic fibrosis is still the major concern [13]. Echocardiography is another option to evaluate cardiac geometry and functions. Although echocardiography is operator dependent, over the past several years the accuracy of echocardiographic measurements had been proven to be closely correlated with histologic findings and had also been well validated in epidemiologic studies. Therefore, echocardiographic study may play a critical role in evaluating

L. Di Lullo (✉) · V. Barbera
Department of Nephrology and Dialysis,
"L. Parodi – Delfino Hospital", Colleferro, Italy

A. Granata
Department of Nephrology and Dialysis,
"Cannizzaro" Emergency Hospital, Catania, Italy

A. Bellasi
Research, Innovation and Brand Reputation, ASST
Papa Giovanni XXIII, Bergamo, Italy

A. Granata, M. Bertolotto (eds.), *Imaging in Nephrology*,
https://doi.org/10.1007/978-3-030-60794-4_26

cardiac functions, stratifying prognostic risk factors, and assessing the effect of therapeutic interventions. Traditionally, two-dimensional echocardiography (2DE) and M-mode imaging have been viewed as capable of assessing LV geometry and quantifying LV mass, end-diastolic and end-systolic volumes, and systolic function [14]. Furthermore, the Doppler modality can provide indirect information about LV relaxation, which indicates the LV diastolic function [15].

26.3 Echocardiography: Principles of Cardiac Ultrasonography

Echocardiography is a group of interrelated applications of ultrasound including two-dimensional imaging, M-mode echocardiography, Doppler techniques, and contrast echocardiography, all relying on sound waves in a frequency range of 2–10 MHz [16].

This section will mainly focus on M-mode ultrasound investigation which represents a peculiar aspect of cardiovascular ultrasound with respect to other tissues' investigation in kidney disease patients [16].

In the M-mode echocardiography, the image is acquired by interrogating returning ultrasound signals from a single line of interrogation. Each returning packet is analyzed for its round-trip transit time, which is then converted to a distance from a transducer face, and it is then displayed as a discrete point which intensity is directly related to the amplitude of the returning signal. This process is usually repeated at a frequency of 1000–3000 per second and then recorded [16].

The M-mode interrogation line can be "swept" over an area of cardiac anatomy and the image is then displayed as a series of side-by-side M-mode interrogation lines (Fig. 26.1) [16].

Standard M-mode examination can be integrated by color M-mode that integrates routine M-mode scanning with superimposed color Doppler information. As with standard M-mode echocardiography, the x-axis represents time and y-axis the distance from the transducer. Along the M-mode single line of interrogation, Doppler information is then color encoded and superimposed on the M-mode display. Color M-mode echocardiography, providing high temporal resolution for timing of intracardiac flow, holds value in determining the timing of potential regurgitant volume into left ventricle [16].

26.4 Echocardiography Views

Heart can be examined by four approaches: parasternal, apical, subcostal, and suprasternal according to patient's accommodation and referral's lines of examination.

26.4.1 Parasternal Long- and Short-Axis View

In this view (Fig. 26.2) the infero-posterior wall and intraventricular septum are visualized, each concave toward the other. The normal ascending aorta is also visualized, including annulus, sinuses of Valsalva, and proximal portion of ascending aorta. Mitral valves' leaflets are also visualized with the anterior leaflet appearing more elongated. Anterior to the aorta, a portion of right ventricle could be evaluated [16]. From the long-axis view, a series of short-axis views can be obtained by rotating the transducer 90°. At the base of the heart, circular aorta and aortic valve with three (or two, if it is a bicuspid aortic valve) leaflets are also visualized. With further angulation, circular cavity of left ventricle can also be studied. The normal left ventricle holds circular geometry, whether it is visualized at the level of mitral valve, papillary muscles, or apex [16].

26.4.2 Apical Views

Apical views are obtained by transducer at heart's apex. From this transducer position, normal left ventricle has a bullet-shaped geometry and the anterior and posterior mitral valve leaflets can be visualized. Left atrium and pulmonary veins are also visualized (Fig. 26.3). In the four-chamber apical view, right ventricle appears as a triangle,

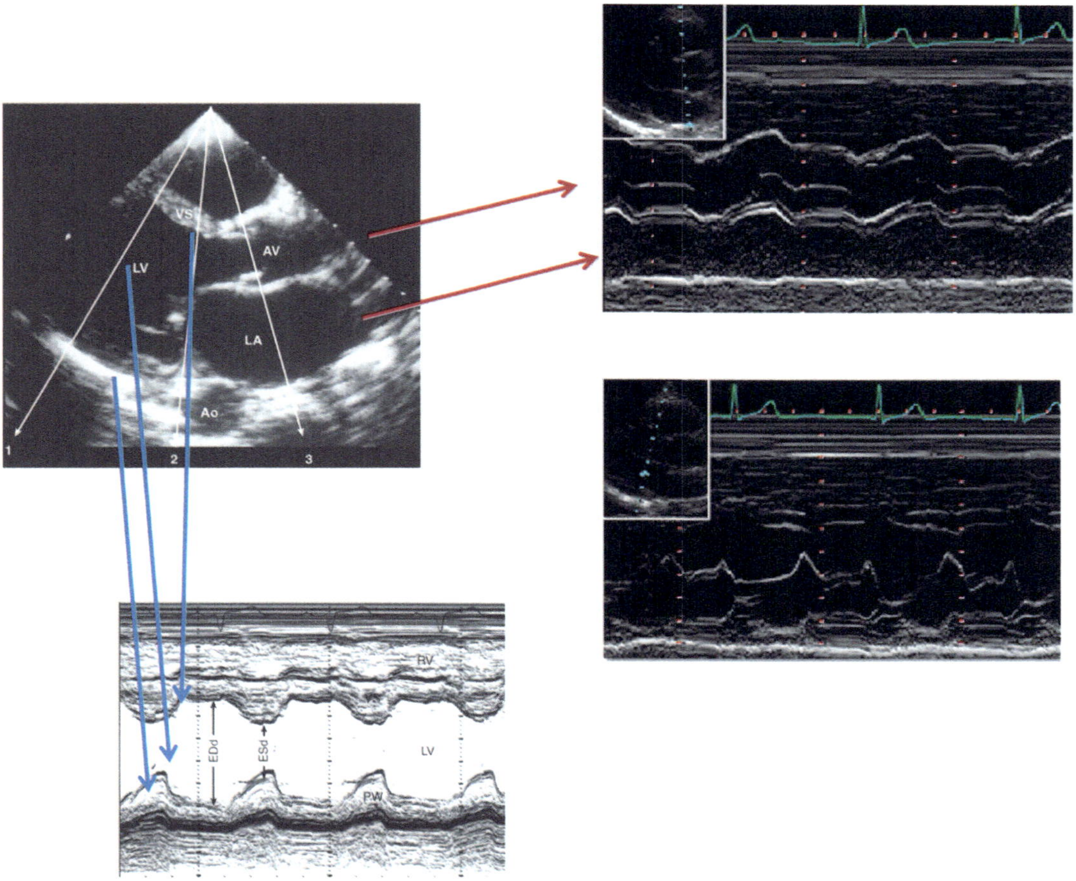

Fig. 26.1 M-mode echocardiography showing side-by-side M-mode interrogation lines. Abbreviations: *LV* left ventricle, *LA* left atrium, *AV* left ventricular outflow tract

while tricuspid valve gets inserted into the annulus of the right ventricle slightly more apical than mitral valve [16].

By rotating the transducer 90° from the four-chamber view, a two-chamber view of the left ventricle and left atrium can be obtained. At the same time, by picking up transducer 40–45°, a five-chamber apical view can be visualized with aortic root (Fig. 26.4) [16].

26.4.3 Subcostal and Suprasternal Views

In addition to parasternal and apical transducer positions, subcostal and suprasternal views can be more effective in patients with chronic lung disease in whom previous views are obscured by interfering lung tissue. For subcostal imaging, patients are usually placed in supine position and transducer is placed in subxiphoid position. Subcostal views provide excellent visualization of atrial septum and connection between inferior vena cava (IVC) and right atrium [16].

26.5 Principles of the Doppler Echocardiography

All four cardiac valves can be interrogated using either pulsed, continuous-wave, or color-flow Doppler. In normal heart, maximum velocity encountered is less than 1.5 m/s. Color-flow Doppler provides the ability to track mitral and

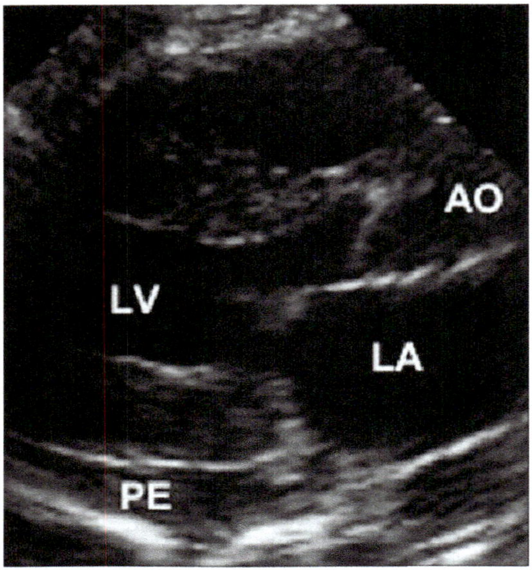

Fig. 26.2 Parasternal long-axis view. Abbreviations: *LV* left ventricle, *LA* left atrium, *AO* aorta, *PE* pericardium

tricuspid inflow patterns and left and right ventricular outflow as well as to detect abnormal flow. Normal mitral inflow appears as a red signal moving from the mitral orifice along the lateral wall to the left ventricular apex, where it reverses

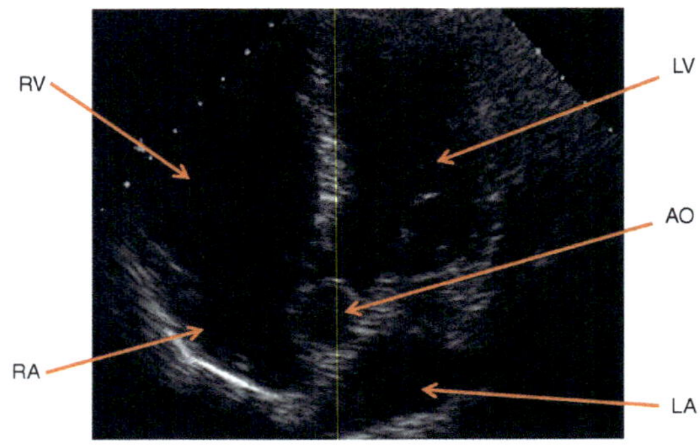

Fig. 26.4 Five-chamber apical view. Abbreviations: *LV* left ventricle, *LA* left atrium, *RV* right ventricle, *RA* right atrium, *AO* aorta

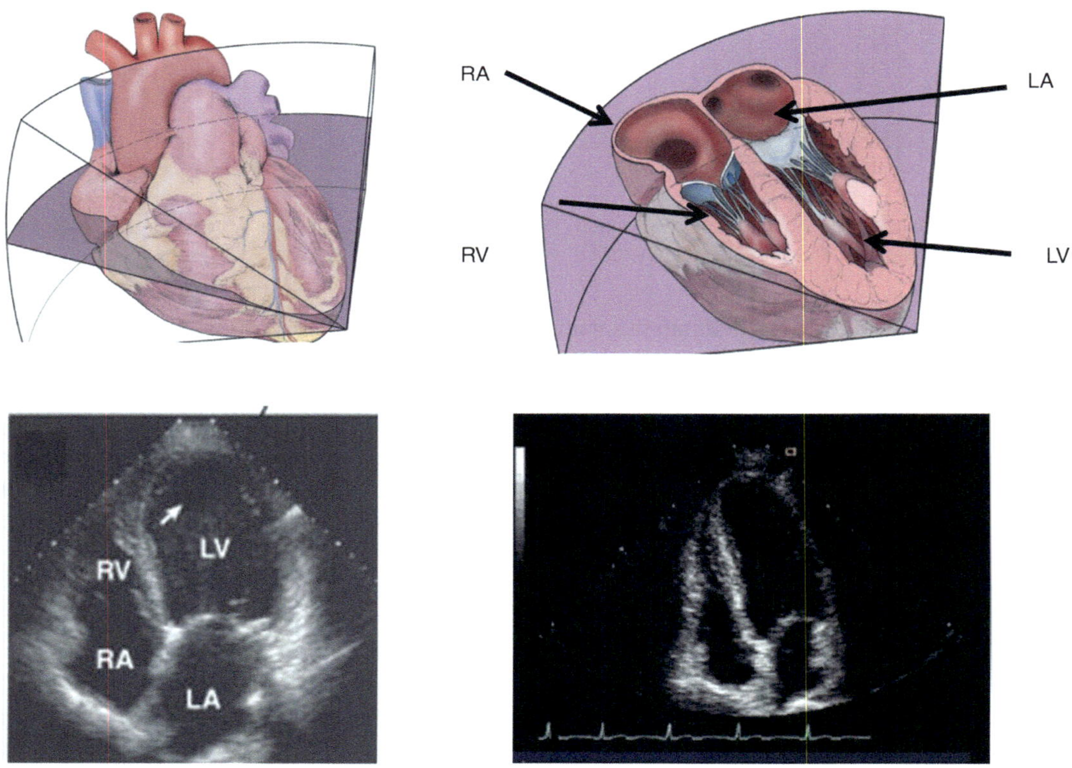

Fig. 26.3 Four-chamber apical view. Abbreviations: *LV* left ventricle, *LA* left atrium, *RV* right ventricle, *RA* right atrium

course and appears as blue signal along the septum. Pathologic flow will be detected either as a turbulence due to restricted orifice, such as flow through a stenotic valve, or as a regurgitant flow signal in a downstream chamber. With Doppler evaluation, a calculation of pressure gradients (according to Bernoulli equation) and regurgitant volume (by calculating the area of regurgitant volume) can also be performed. In fact, because the Doppler spectral profile provides an accurate measure of the velocity of the moving blood, this value, combined with a measured or calculated area, can provide data regarding the actual volumetric flow [16].

26.6 Contrast Echocardiography

Contrast echocardiography represents an evolving field especially used in the evaluation of myocardial perfusion [17]. All forms of contrast echocardiography are based on microbubbles that are intense echo reflectors. Reflectivity of a microbubble is greater than that of tissue, and as such in low concentrations creating a highly reflective target. Depending on the power of insonating beam, the interaction may be simple reflection back at the fundamental frequency, generation and reflection back of harmonic frequencies, or stimulated acoustic omission [17].

First and simplest interaction is reflection, characterized by reflection back of an intensive echo target from each individual microbubble. Microbubbles can be detected in blood or tissue using direct reflection in either the fundamental or the harmonic domains [17].

In clinical practice, contrast echocardiography is used on a daily basis for detection of shunts and characterization of suspect cardiac masses [17].

The commercially developed perfluorocarbon agents contain populations of smaller (4–6 ųm) microbubbles of uniform size [18]. Because perfluorocarbon has low diffusibility, microbubbles have persistence after injection and they can cross pulmonary capillary bed opacifying left ventricular structures and enhancing left heart borders [18].

26.7 Echocardiography in CKD

26.7.1 CKD-Related Cardiomyopathy

Cardiomyopathy in hemodialysis (HD) patients is due to a critical obstruction of coronary vessels, reduction of coronary reserve, and/or microvascular alterations. In CKD and ESRD patients, pressure and volume overload lead to left ventricular remodeling [16]; if no intervention will be provided, cell death and myocardial sclerosis and fibrosis can occur, leading to diastolic dysfunction, disturbances in intraventricular conduction, dilatation, and more compensatory hypertrophy [16]. Consequent electric instability could be accountable of greater incidence of sudden cardiac death in those patients [19]. Doppler echocardiography allows to evaluate ventricular mass and volume also holding great sensibility and specificity in assessing left ventricular hypertrophy (eccentric or concentric) and systolic function [16]. Left ventricular hypertrophy (LVH) is a major issue in CKD and ESRD patients and it is associated with poor cardiovascular outcome. LVH's incidence increases together with renal function decline with a prevalence between 16 and 31% increasing to 60–75% in patients starting renal replacement therapy. LV mass is proportional to body size and traditionally indexing body surface was utilized for correction in classic studies. Concerning cutoff values, Silberberg et al. used a reference value of 125 g/m^2, while Parfrey et al. used the values employed in the Framingham study (132 g/m^2 for males and 100 g/m^2 for females) [16]. It is quite important to stress that the geometry of LV in CKD patients can be related to the moment at which the echocardiogram was performed; timing is crucial in performing an echocardiographic exam in hemodialysis patients. Shortly after the dialysis session, it is common to see a reduction in diastolic diameter of the LV and an increase in the thickness of the LV wall as a pure consequence of volume depletion by ultrafiltration. At the same time, the exam performed shortly before beginning the session can present a diagnosis of LV dilatation with eccentric hypertrophy becoming concentric at the end of the dialysis session.

This incorrect evaluation could be minimized by performing the echocardiogram during the interdialytic period. Evaluation of cardiac mass represents a key feature in CKD patients because progression of LVH in individuals with CKD is predictive of cardiovascular events. An increase in mass of 1 g/m$^{2.7}$/month was associated with a 62% increase in the incident risk of fatal and nonfatal cardiovascular events in a study with dialysis patients [16].

26.7.2 Left Ventricular Systolic and Diastolic Dysfunction

Left ventricular systolic dysfunction's prevalence ranges from 15 to 28% in patients on dialysis and it represents a strong predictor of unfavorable prognosis in patients on HD as well as those in the post-renal transplant phase [20]. Systolic dysfunction is performed by evaluating ejection fraction (EF) and fractional shortening both based on measures taken in the endocardium that could overestimate systolic function in patients with LVH. Alternatively, a method based on the measure of the myocardial midwall can be employed diagnosing lower systolic performance in patients with normal ejection fraction [21]. Anyway, LV systolic dysfunction is independently associated with fatal and nonfatal cardiovascular events, and, although the adverse effect of systolic dysfunction is independent of LV mass, these alterations interact in the prediction of cardiovascular outcome [22]. EF is currently evaluated by employing Simpson's rule (Fig. 26.5). On the other side, diastolic dysfunction is characterized by alterations in ventricular relaxation and compliance, frequently followed by a compensatory increase in filling pressure in more advanced stages. Prevalence of LV diastolic dysfunction in CKD patients varies from 50 to 65%, including pre-dialysis, dialysis, and posttransplant populations [23]. Doppler parameters derived from mitral inflow are highly load dependent, while tissue Doppler imaging (TDI) of mitral annulus or myocardial walls represents

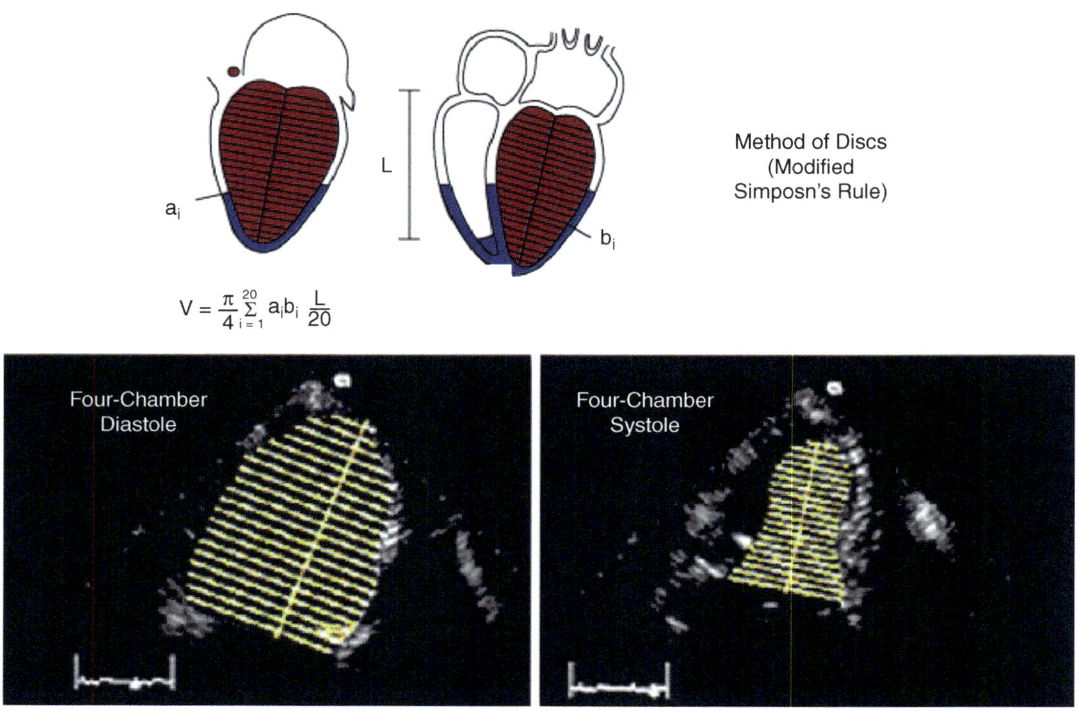

Fig. 26.5 Left ventricular systolic function evaluation by Simpson's method

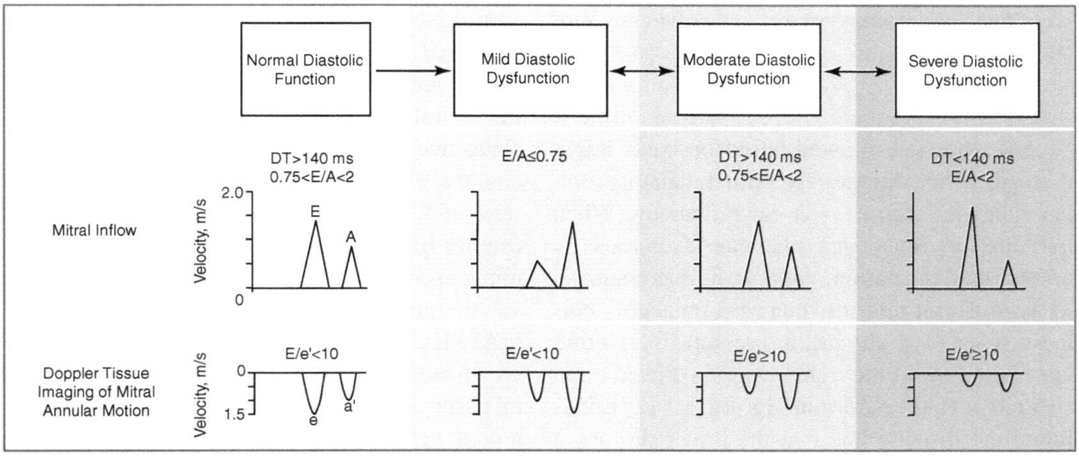

Fig. 26.6 Left ventricular diastolic dysfunction's classification

an important method of evaluation of segmental and global diastolic function. TDI-derived diastolic velocities (early E' and late A') are "relatively" preload independent, without significant variation after one HD session [24]. As a consequence, E' (an index of relaxation) and E/E' can be particularly helpful for HD patients in differentiating pseudonormalization from the true normal profile of diastolic function [24] (Fig. 26.6). Diastolic function can also be studied by investigating left atrial (LA) volume. In contrast to Doppler-derived indices, LA volume acts as a chronic marker of diastolic function, reflecting the long-term effect of increased filling pressure. Recent data reported that this index was an independent predictor of mortality in patients on renal replacement therapy. An indexed LA volume >32 mL/m^2 provides information complementary to ejection fraction, E/E' ratio, and LV ventricular mass [20].

26.7.3 Right Heart Dysfunction and Pulmonary Hypertension

Right heart failure is a major issue in ESRD patients since it is closely linked to presence of vascular access for hemodialysis. Evaluation of systolic pulmonary pressure is easily performed by standard transthoracic echocardiography. AHA (American Heart Association) and SIEC (Italian Society of Cardiovascular Echography) guidelines list it among the essential parameters to investigate in basic echocardiography [25]. Preliminary B-mode echocardiography, however, allows the detection of some ultrasound aspects that could suggest pulmonary hypertension:

1. Right heart chamber dilation
2. "D" shape of the right ventricle by flattening of the interventricular septum
3. Absence of inferior vena cava inhalatory collapse

The M-mode view will show small or absent "a" (atrial) wave. The diagnostic accuracy of these echocardiographic findings is quite poor, both with respect to specificity and sensibility. Therefore, they are all qualitative features and they do not allow the evaluation of the degree of right ventricular impairment and of the response to pharmacological therapy [25]. It is crucial to complete the echocardiographic test with a Doppler evaluation; assessment of pulmonary arterial pressure is performed by tricuspid and pulmonary regurgitation speed assay. Tricuspid regurgitation speed (V TR) is evaluated by four-chamber echocardiographic apical view with ultrasound probe following transvalvular flow to collect regurgitation volume [26]. V TR reveals the systolic pressure gradient between the two right heart sections. If right atrial pressure (RAP) is added, pulmonary artery systolic pressure (PASP) is obtained:

$$PASP = 4(V\ TR)\ 2 + RAP$$

RAP can be estimated based on basic transthoracic echocardiography with inhalatory collapse in the inferior vena cava diameter. When the inferior vena cava diameter decreases by >50% with inhalation, right atrium pressure is <10 mm Hg; if inferior vena cava inhalatory collapse is <50%, right atrium pressure is >10 mm Hg. Therefore, if the right atrium is dilated (area >15 cm^2), RAP is 15 mm Hg at least [27]. It is important to underline that the issues discussed above are not validated for the presence of pulmonary valve stenosis or any other mechanical obstruction to right ventricle outflow.

Pulmonary hypertension is characterized by a V TR ≥2 m/s (the normal value is <1 m/s). Telediastolic pulmonary regurgitation speed (V PR) represents a telediastolic pressure gradient between the pulmonary artery and the right ventricle. At the end of diastole, right ventricular pressure should be the same as RAP:

$$PAEDP = 4 \times V\ PR\ 2 + RAP$$

where PAEDP is telediastolic pulmonary arterial pressure [26].

Pulmonary arterial pressure is usually increased in patients with high left ventricle inflow pressures; pulsed-wave Doppler study of the mitral valve allows the identification of a restrictive pattern of transmitral flow (increase of E wave, decrease of A wave, and deceleration time of E wave, E/A ratio >2) [28]. Right ventricular function is often assessed by measuring upper caudal excursion capability of the tricuspid valve annulus during ventricular systole (TAPSE). TAPSE index can be easily evaluated on M-mode echocardiography without referring to tissue Doppler and has good reproducibility among echocardiographic physicians (Fig. 26.7) [29]. A compliant right ventricle allows wide excursion of the tricuspid annulus, while this is prevented or strongly restricted in progressive right heart impairment and failure. TAPSE is well related with diastolic function of the right ventricle and blood inflow towards the right atrium. TAPSE also represents a good prognostic marker to stratify cardiovascular risk and it is not affected by heart rate and rhythm. Thus, TAPSE can also be performed in patients with tachycardia or atrial fibrillation in which evaluation of diastolic function is prevented by only one atrial wave on transmitral Doppler. TAPSE scoring also represents a cardiovascular prognostic index together

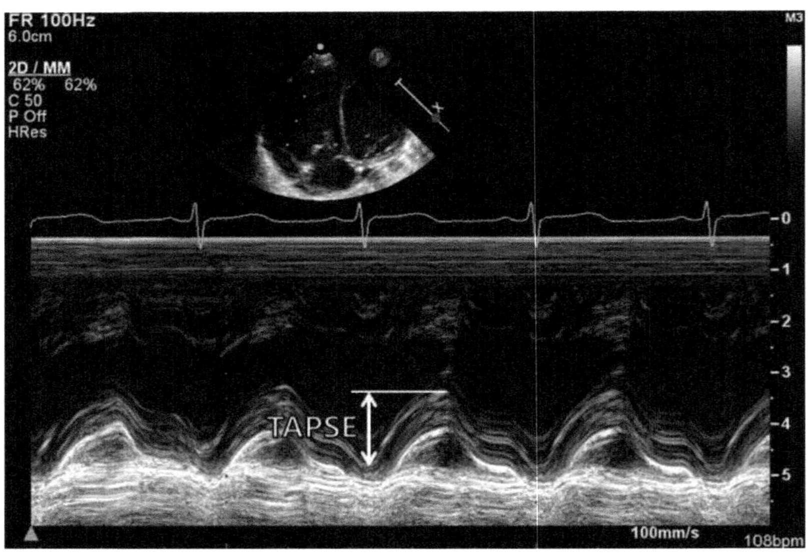

Fig. 26.7 M-mode echocardiography showing TAPSE evaluation

with the NYHA (New York Heart Association) classification [29]. According to our experience, single hemodialysis treatment does not affect PAP values, while it significantly affects TAPSE values as a consequence of volume overload reduction following ultrafiltration, which is not related to the myocardial stunning hypothesis because ejection fraction improves after the hemodialysis session [30]. Our results seem to confirm those of Beigi et al. [31] both concerning long-term effects of arteriovenous fistulae on cardiac output and pulmonary circulation and epidemiological data on the prevalence of pathological PAP values [30].

26.7.4 Pericardial Disease

Later stage CKD patients (especially those on renal replacement's therapies) often present pericardial involvement due to fluid overload and/or specific diseases (e.g., pericarditis) [16, 29]. A variety of disease processes can result in a pericardial effusion with a differential diagnosis similar to that for pericarditis (infections, malignancies, inflammatory diseases, and post-cardiac surgery complications). Physiologic consequences of fluid's presence in the pericardial space depend on both the amount and the rate of fluid accumulation. A slowly expanding pericardial effusion can become quite large (>1000 mL) with little increase in pericardial pressures, whereas rapid accumulation of even a small volume of fluid (50–100 mL) can lead to a marked increase in pericardial pressure [16, 29]. This process could even lead to a cardiac tamponade when pressure in the pericardium exceeds pressure in cardiac chambers, resulting in impaired cardiac filling. As pericardial pressure increases, filling of each cardiac chamber is sequentially impaired, with lower pressure chambers (atria) affected before higher pressure chambers (ventricles). Compressive effect of the pericardial fluid is seen most clearly in the phase of cardiac cycle when pressure is lowest in that chamber systole for the atrium and diastole for the ventricles. Filling pressures become elevated as a compensatory mechanism to maintain cardiac output. In fully developed tamponade, diastolic pressures in all four cardiac chambers are equal (and elevated) due to exposure of the whole heart to the elevated pericardial pressure [16, 29]. A pericardial effusion is recognized on 2D echocardiography as an echolucent space adjacent to the cardiac shape. In the absence of prior pericardial disease or surgery, pericardial effusions are usually diffuse and symmetric with clear separation between visceral and parietal pericardium (Fig. 26.8) [29]. M-mode views are helpful especially with small effusion, showing the flat posterior pericardial echo reflection and the moving epicardial echo with separation between the two in both systole and diastole [16]. In patients with recurrent or long-standing pericardial disease, fibrinous stranding within the fluid and on the epicardial surface of the heart may be seen. The size of the pericardial effusion is considered to be small when the separation between parietal and visceral pericardium is less than 0.5 cm, moderate when it is 0.5–2 cm, and large when it is greater than 2 cm [16, 29]. Sometimes, as it occurs in the postoperative patients, pericardial effusion can be a loculated one. In this occasion, effusion is localized by adhesions to a small area of the pericardial space and it consists of several separate areas of pericardial effusion, separated by adhesions [16, 29]. Recognition of such kind of pericardial effusion is particularly important because hemodynamic compromise can occur with even a small, strategically located fluid collection. Therefore, drainage of a loculated effusion may be difficult (and even impossible) from a percutaneous approach [29].

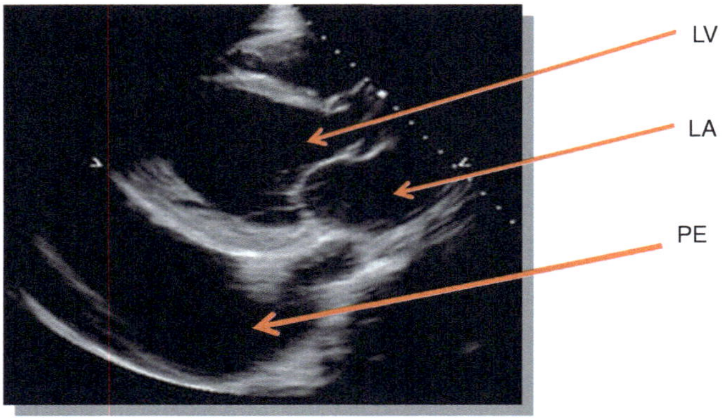

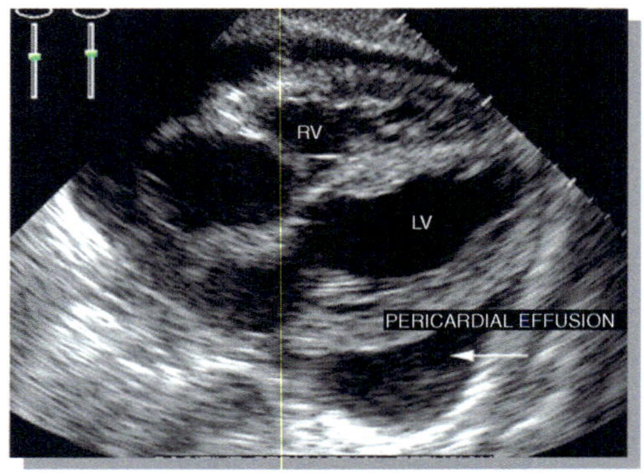

Fig. 26.8 Examples of pericardial effusions in parasternal long-axis views. Abbreviations: *LV* left ventricle, *LA* left atrium, *RV* right ventricle, *PE* pericardial effusion

References

1. Heimdal A, Støylen A, Torp H, Skjaerpe T. Real-time strain rate imaging of the left ventricle by ultrasound. J Am Soc Echocardiogr. 1998;11:1013e9.
2. Go AS, Chertow GM, Fan D, McCulloch CE, Hsu CY. Chronic kidney disease and the risks of death, cardiovascular events, and hospitalization. N Engl J Med. 2004;351:1296e305.
3. Wen CP, Cheng TY, Tsai MK, Chang YC, Chan HT, Tsai SP, et al. All-cause mortality attributable to chronic kidney disease: a prospective cohort study based on 462,293 adults in Taiwan. Lancet. 2008;371:2173e82.
4. deFilippi C, Wasserman S, Rosanio S, Tiblier E, Sperger H, Tocchi M, et al. Cardiac troponin T and C-reactive protein for predicting prognosis, coronary atherosclerosis, and cardiomyopathy in patients undergoing long-term hemodialysis. JAMA. 2003;290:353.
5. Akdag I, Yilmaz Y, Kahvecioglu S, Bolca N, Ercan I, Ersoy A, et al. Clinical value of the malnutrition-inflammation atherosclerosis syndrome for long-term prediction of cardiovascular mortality in patients with end-stage renal disease: a 5-year prospective study. Nephron Clin Pract. 2008;108:c99e105.
6. Liu YW, Su CT, Chang YT, Tsai WC, Su YR, Wang SP, et al. Elevated serum interleukin-18 level is associated with all-cause mortality in stable hemodialysis patients independently of cardiac dysfunction. PLoS One. 2014;9:e89457.
7. McCullough PA. Cardiovascular disease in chronic kidney disease from a cardiologist's perspective. Curr Opin Nephrol Hypertens. 2004;13:591e600.
8. Best PJ, Reddan DN, Berger PB, Szczech LA, McCullough PA, Califf RM. Cardiovascular disease and chronic kidney disease: insights and an update. Am Heart J. 2004;148:230e42.
9. Foley RN, Parfrey PS, Harnett JD, Kent GM, Martin CJ, Murray DC, et al. Clinical and echocardiographic disease in patients starting end-stage renal disease therapy. Kidney Int. 1995;47:186e92.
10. Wang AY, Lam CW, Yu CM, Wang M, Chan IH, Lui SF, et al. Troponin T, left ventricular mass, and function are excellent predictors of cardiovascular congestion in peritoneal dialysis. Kidney Int. 2006;70:444e52.
11. Pennell DJ, Sechtem UP, Higgins CB, Manning WJ, Pohost GM, Rademakers FE, et al. Clinical indications for cardiovascular magnetic resonance (CMR): consensus panel report. Eur Heart J. 2004;25:1940e65.

12. Flett AS, Westwood MA, Davies LC, Mathur A, Moon JC. The prognostic implications of cardiovascular magnetic resonance. Circ Cardiovasc Imaging. 2009;2:243e50.
13. Perazella MA. Current status of gadolinium toxicity in patients with kidney disease. Clin J Am Soc Nephrol. 2009;4:461e9.
14. Lang RM, Bierig M, Devereux RB, Flachskampf FA, Foster E, Pellikka PA, et al. Recommendations for chamber quantification: a report from the American Society of Echocardiography's Guidelines and Standards Committee and the Chamber Quantification Writing Group, developed in conjunction with the European Association of Echocardiography, a branch of the European Society of Cardiology. J Am Soc Echocardiogr. 2005;18:1440e63.
15. Nagueh SF, Appleton CP, Gillebert TC, Marino PN, Oh JK, Smiseth OA, et al. Recommendations for the evaluation of left ventricular diastolic function by echocardiography. J Am Soc Echocardiogr. 2009;22:107e33.
16. Di Lullo L, Floccari F, Granata A, D'Amelio A, Rivera R, Fiorini F, Malaguti M, Timio M. Ultrasonography: Ariadne's thread in the diagnosis of the cardiorenal syndrome. Cardiorenal Med. 2012;2(1):11–7.
17. Mulvagh ST, DeMaria AN, Feinstein SB, et al. Contrast echocardiography: current and future applications. J Am Soc Echocardiogr. 2000;13:331.
18. Gldberg BB, Liu JB, Forsberg P. Ultrasound contrast agents: a review. Ultrasound Med Biol. 1994;20:319.
19. Di Lullo L, Rivera R, Barbera V, Bellasi A, Cozzolino M, Russo D, De Pascalis A, Banerjee D, Floccari F, Ronco C. Sudden cardiac death and chronic kidney disease: from pathophysiology to treatment strategies. Int J Cardiol. 2016;217:16–27.
20. Barberato SH, Pecoits Filho R. Prognostic value of left atrial volume index in hemodialysis patients. Arq Bras Cardiol. 2007;88:643–50.
21. Shimizu G, Hirota Y, Kita Y, Kawamura K, Saito T, Gaasch WH. Left ventricular midwall mechanics in systemic arterial hypertension. Myocardial function is depressed in pressure-overload hypertrophy. Circulation. 1991;83:1676–84.
22. Zoccali C, Benedetto FA, Mallamaci F, Tripepi G, Giacone G, Cataliotti A, Seminara G, Stancanelli B, Malatino LS. Prognostic value of echocardiographic indicators of left ventricular systolic function in asymptomatic dialysis patients. J Am Soc Nephrol. 2004;15:1029–37.
23. Kunz K, Dimitrov Y, Muller S, Chantrel F, Hannedouche T. Uraemic cardiomyopathy. Nephrol Dial Transplant. 1998;13(suppl 4):39–43.
24. Barberato SH, Mantilla DE, Misocami MA, Goncalves SM, Bignelli AT, Riella MC, et al. Effect of preload reduction by hemodialysis on left atrial volume and echocardiographic Doppler parameters in patients with end-stage renal disease. Am J Cardiol. 2004;94:1208–10.
25. Hammerstingl C, Schueler R, Bors L, Momcilovic D, Pabst S, Nickenig G, Skowasch D. Diagnostic value of echocardiography in the diagnosis of pulmonary hypertension. PLoS One. 2012;7:e38519.
26. Otto CM. Pulmonary heart disease: echocardiographic approach. Textbook of Clinical Echocardiography, ed 2. Elsevier Saunders. 2004:250–2.
27. Brennan JM, Blair JE, Goonewardena S, Ronan A, Shah D, Vasaiwala S, Kirkpatrick JN, Spencer KT. Reappraisal of the use of inferior vena cava for estimating right atrial pressure. J Am Soc Echocardiogr. 2007;20:857–61.
28. Wong SP, Otto CM. Echocardiographic findings in acute and chronic pulmonary disease. In: Otto CM, editor. The Practice of Clinical Echocardiography. 3rd ed: WB Saunders; 2002. p. 739–60.
29. Di Lullo L, Floccari F, Rivera R, Granata A, D'Amelio A, Logias F, Otranto G, Villani A, Santoboni A, Malaguti M, Timio M, Fiorini F. The nephrologist and the role of ultrasound imaging in the diagnosis of cardiorenal syndrome. G Ital Nefrol. 2012;29:321–7.
30. Di Lullo L, Floccari F, Polito P. Right ventricular diastolic function in dialysis patients could be affected by vascular access. Nephron Clin Pract. 2011;118:c258–62.
31. Beigi AA, Sadeghi AM, Khosravi AR, Karami M, Masoudpour H. Effects of the arteriovenous fistula on pulmonary artery pressure and cardiac output in patients with chronic renal failure. J Vasc Access. 2009;10:160–6.

Basic Lung Ultrasonography for the Nephrologist

27

Luna Gargani, Giovanni Volpicelli, and Luciano Cardinale

27.1 Introduction

Quite recently, lung ultrasound (LUS) opened new perspectives in the bedside evaluation of pulmonary congestion. Many authors produced a growing number of papers showing the power of LUS in diagnosing pulmonary diseases. Rather than from technologic progress, development of modern LUS is mainly based on discovering the significance of sonographic artifacts. Particularly, some vertical echogenic linear artifacts, known as B-lines, are simple, noninvasive signs of increased extravascular lung water (EVLW) that can be easily evaluated at bedside [1]. B-lines likely originate from multiple small subpleural air/fluid acoustic interfaces, which are generated when the lung loses air and fluids increase. This phenomenon is based on the physical properties of air and water, which are characterized by opposite values of acoustic impedance. The contrast between air-filled and water-rich structures generates multiple reverberations of the ultrasound beam that are visualized on the screen as linear vertical artifacts, the B-lines. In the normally aerated lung, only a very few B-lines can be detected by sonography. When the water content increases and air decreases due to disease, the fluid into the interstitial and alveolar spaces causes the appearance of multiple and diffuse B-lines.

Any condition of the lung where pulmonary air is partially lost and fluids or cellularity is diffusely increased, causes the appearance of B-lines at LUS examination. In critically ill patients and in emergency situations, B-lines depict the so-called interstitial syndrome with high accuracy in terms of sensitivity and specificity, thus demonstrating a valid support in orientating the diagnostic process of acute respiratory failure. However, this technique has two main limitations. First, in the diagnostic process for the interstitial syndrome, the sonographic examination of the lung can only be limited to the pulmonary surface. Thus, it is only indicative in diseases and conditions involving the whole organ and not in those situations where the lung periphery is spared. Second, B-lines are highly specific to diagnose the generic interstitial syndrome but cannot differentiate the etiology of the disease, as the origin of these artifacts can be related to pulmonary edema of any cause, including noncardiogenic edema (acute lung injury/acute respiratory distress syndrome, ALI/ARDS), cardiogenic edema, fluid overload, and also fibrosis

L. Gargani (✉)
Institute of Clinical Physiology, National Research Council, Pisa, Italy

G. Volpicelli
Department of Emergency Medicine, San Luigi Gonzaga University Hospital, Orbassano, Torino, Italy

L. Cardinale
Department of Radiology, San Luigi Gonzaga University Hospital, Orbassano, Torino, Italy

A. Granata, M. Bertolotto (eds.), *Imaging in Nephrology*, https://doi.org/10.1007/978-3-030-60794-4_27

and interstitial infections. As a consequence, the power of LUS is strictly related to the clinical interpretation at bedside, taking into account also other LUS signs and the ultrasound evaluation of other organs, when available. Indeed, in more specific settings where the diagnosis is already established, as it may happen for patients on dialysis, LUS examination has a great potential as the interpretation of B-lines is already oriented, and these ultrasound signs can be used for the noninvasive estimation and monitoring of EVLW.

27.2 Lung Ultrasound in Kidney Disease: Current Knowledge and Future Perspectives

27.2.1 Detection of Volume Overload

Volume overload is a main determinant of prognosis in end-stage renal disease (ESRD) patients [2]. It is common especially in patients with combined kidney and heart dysfunction, and is a determinant of further cardiovascular deterioration [3, 4]. The clinical evaluation of volume overload is not accurate; therefore any technique that may enable to easily assess and monitor fluid status is extremely useful in this population. There are a few methods for estimating the patient's hydration status: isotope dilution and neutron activation analysis are considered the gold standard for body fluid compartment assessment, but their use is limited to research settings; bioelectrical impedance analysis (BIA), ultrasound estimation of the inferior vena cava (IVC) diameter and collapsibility index, and natriuretic peptides are indirect methods that are quite used in the clinical arena, although all of them carry significant limitations [4]. In particular, BIA is a quite widespread method to noninvasively assess the patient's hydration status bedside, but its measurements are largely based on mathematical assumptions validated mainly on European subjects with normal renal function; moreover, it is significantly affected by fluid intake, and cannot evaluate hydration changes during hemodialysis.

Lung ultrasound has been firstly proposed in patients with kidney disease in 2009. Noble et al. evaluated 40 patients undergoing hemodialysis before, at the midpoint, and after dialysis. 34 of 40 patients had a statistically significant reduction in the number of B-lines from predialysis to the midpoint scan, and from predialysis to postdialysis; 6 patients had no B-line predialysis, and none of them gained B-lines during dialysis. Interestingly, there was no association between subjective dyspnea scores and number of B-lines removed. These results highlighted for the first time that B-line resolution could occur real time as the fluid was drained from the body, supporting LUS as a useful method for evaluating real-time changes in extravascular lung water [5]. These data were further confirmed by Mallamaci et al., who also established B-line correlations with different echocardiography parameters including left atrial volume, pulmonary artery systolic pressure, E/e' ratio as index of diastolic function, and ejection fraction. They also found that, although B-lines were more numerous in patients with NYHA functional classes III and IV, the vast majority of asymptomatic patients had moderate-to-severe B-lines [6]. Another study showed that whereas the number of B-lines was significantly related to fluid overload both before and after dialysis, inferior vena cava evaluation was related to weight gain and to the number of B-lines only before and not after dialysis, suggesting that vena cava measurements are useful for detecting fluid overload, but they seem less informative than B-lines to estimate rapid volume status variation [7].

Pulmonary congestion measured by B-lines is common not only in hemodialysis [5–10], but also in peritoneal dialysis, where it is even more often asymptomatic [11–13]. The correlation between B-lines and crackles detected by lung auscultation is also poor, as demonstrated by a subproject of a large multicentric randomized trial testing whether the use of LUS in high-risk hemodialysis patients may improve clinical outcomes ("Lung water by Ultra-Sound guided Treatment to prevent death and cardiovascular complications in high-risk ESRD patients with cardiomyopathy—LUST"). Although lung auscultation to detect crackles at the lung bases is a cornerstone for the diagnosis and monitoring of congestion in patients with heart failure and chronic kidney disease, its reliability to detect interstitial edema is known to be low, and not surprisingly, congestion evaluated by crackles and/or edema poorly reflected the severity of congestion as detected by B-lines [14]. A linear correlation between B-lines and fluid overload has been demonstrated also in children with acute kidney injury and ESRD [15]. Also in the pediatric population, dynamic changes in B-lines were observed real time with fluid removal during individual hemodialysis sessions. The non-ionizing nature of the technique makes LUS even more suitable to assess pulmonary congestion in the pediatric population. In patients with active nephrotic syndrome, although asymptomatic, the number of B-lines has been shown to correlate with serum albumin ($r = -0.45$, $P = 0.005$) and with the severity of peripheral edema 60 min of supine position. This study evaluated also the postural changes of B-lines in comparison with stage 5 ESRD patients on chronic hemodialysis and healthy individuals, showing wider postural variations of B-lines compared to ESRD patients with a similar degree of baseline lung congestion [16].

27.2.2 Prognosis

Interesting data have been published also on the role of B-lines in prognosis. In a multicenter study with 392 hemodialysis patients, Zoccali et al. showed that patients with very severe congestion immediately before dialysis had a 4.2-fold risk of death compared to patients having mild or no congestion, and a 3.2-fold risk of cardiac events, adjusted for NYHA class and other risk factors. Including the degree of pulmonary congestion evaluated by LUS significantly improved the risk reclassification for cardiac events by 10%. In this study population, patients with more B-lines were significantly older, with higher C-reactive protein and lower serum albumin; they were more frequently affected by cardiovascular comorbidities and worse dyspnea (NYHA classes III–IV), compared with patients with less B-lines [17].

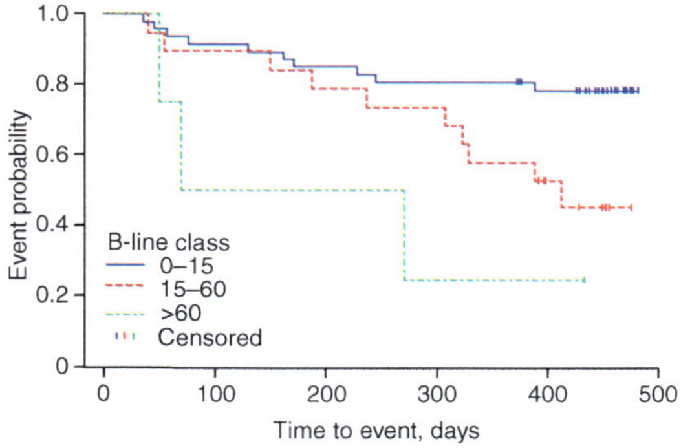

0–15	47	45	43	42	40	38	38	38	31	21
15–60	19	18	17	17	15	14	14	11	7	5
> 60	4	4	2	2	2	2	1	1	1	0

Fig. 27.1 Kaplan-Meier curves showing survival probability according to the number of B-lines (ref. [18])

Very similar results were obtained also in patients evaluated immediately after dialysis, when they had achieved their target weight. Seventy-one subjects were followed for a mean duration of 1.2 years with a total of 9 deaths and 20 incident cardiac events: survival analysis demonstrated an interval decrease in survival times in all-cause mortality and cardiac events with increased B-lines (Fig. 27.1). Thus, the number of B-lines was an independent predictor of hospitalizations, cardiovascular events, and death also at dry weight [18].

B-lines in hemodialysis patients were found to be associated with survival, even after adjustments for echocardiographic or bioimpedance-derived parameters [19], although in one study the relative fluid overload, defined as the absolute fluid overload-to-extracellular water ratio, was superior to B-lines in improving risk prediction for death, beyond classical and echocardiographic based risk prediction scores [20].

27.2.3 Methodology

LUS has demonstrated high intra- and interobserver reproducibility in ESRD patients, as well as in heart failure patients [6, 21–23]. With LUS being a relatively easy application of ultrasound, a good reproducibility can be reached also after a brief online training, as shown. This was applied within the framework of the LUST trial (LUng water by Ultra-Sound guided Treatment to prevent death and cardiovascular events in high-risk end-stage renal disease patients), where a group of 30 nephrologists and 14 cardiologists completed an online training consisting of a demonstrating video. At the end of the training, a set of 47 LUS videos were provided to trainees who were asked to estimate the number of B-lines in each video; the intraclass correlation coefficient for the whole series of 47 videos between trainees and the expert trainer was high (average 0.81 ± 0.21) [24].

The scanning scheme most frequently used in the different studies has been the previously described 28-scanning site technique [25–27], which is a bit more time consuming than the standard 8-zone technique [27], but more precise to detect dynamic changes in B-lines. However, a simplified scheme limited to the lateral chest regions has demonstrated a similar performance with reduced scanning time [9]. A cardiac or a convex or microconvex probe can be used to detect B-lines in hemodialysis patients. When a specific "pulmonary" setting is not available, a cardiac or abdominal setting can be selected. Gain and depth should be adjusted in order to clearly visualize the pleural line, the reference point for all LUS examinations [27, 28]. The probe should be placed in the intercostal space, avoiding the ribs, in order to visualize the pleural line all over the upper part of the screen (Fig. 27.2). B-lines should be recorded in each site, and then the sum of all scanning sites should be taken into account as an overall score of pulmonary congestion: the more B-lines, the less the air in the lung due to interstitial pulmonary edema. B-lines move with respiration and it can be difficult to count the artifacts separately, especially when they are more numerous and tend to be confluent. There is however a quite simple rule to quantify them, taking into account the percentage of the scanning site occupied by B-lines (i.e., the percentage of white screen compared to black screen below the pleural line) and then dividing it by ten (i.e., 30% corresponds to about 3 B-lines, 70% corresponds to about 7 B-lines). Overall, the more the white of B-lines we see, the less the air in the lung because of the presence of extravascular lung water [28].

Lung ultrasound allows also the visualization not only of B-lines, as a sign of pulmonary interstitial edema, but also of pleural effusion, which can be present in decompensated patients (Fig. 27.3), and lung consolidations. In the presence of a radio-opacity on chest X-ray, LUS can easily reveal whether the radio-opacity is related to an effusion or consolidation. Moreover, it can show a complex pleural effusion (Fig. 27.4), which can help to better characterize the patient. The highest value of LUS is gained when imaging data and their changes are strongly linked to the clinical picture. In this view, LUS should be interpreted as an extension—not a substitute—of the pulmonary auscultation. In the following years, point-of-care sonography is expected to become the fifth pillar of the physical examination [29].

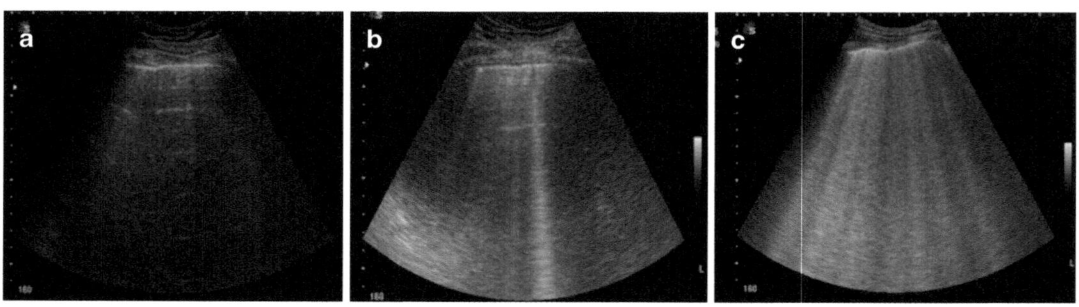

Fig. 27.2 Panel A: no B-lines; panel B: a few separated B-lines; panel C: many coalescent B-lines

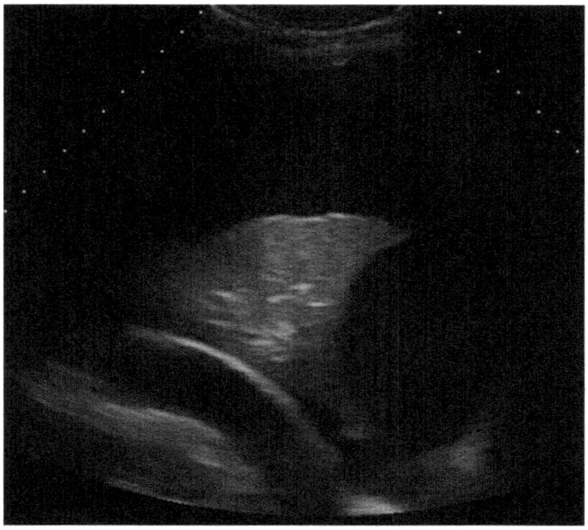

Fig. 27.3 Pleural effusion with compression atelectasis of the lung

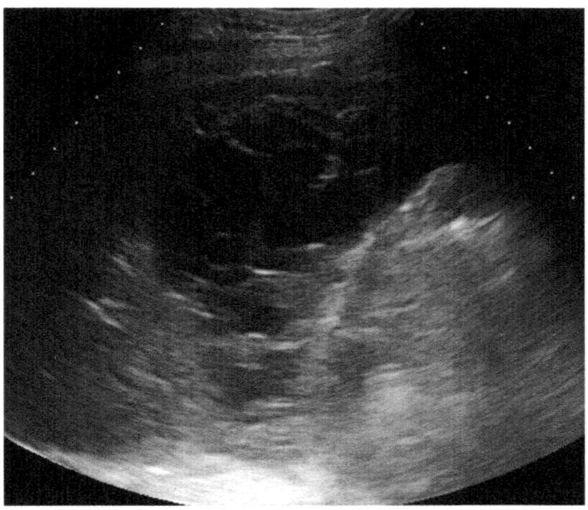

Fig. 27.4 Complex pleural effusion

27.3 Conclusions

The application of LUS in patients with ESRD has relevant clinical implications and a high potentiality [30–32]. The technique is easy to be performed and interpreted, low cost, and nonionizing, which makes it very appealing in patients with a chronic disease. It can be done bedside with virtually any ultrasound machine, including hand-held device [28, 33].

However, the real cost efficacy of adding LUS to standard management in this subset of patients needs to be tested in randomized trials, to confirm that assessing pulmonary congestion by ultrasound B-lines not only is reliable, feasible, and user friendly, but also clearly improves the prognosis of these vulnerable patients.

References

1. Volpicelli G. Lung sonography. J Ultrasound Med. 2013;32:165–71.
2. Agarwal R. Hypervolemia is associated with increased mortality among hemodialysis patients. Hypertension. 2010;56(3):512–7.
3. Onofriescu MS, Voroneanu L, Hogas S, et al. Overhydration, cardiac function and survival in hemodialysis patients. PLoS One. 2015;10(8):e0135691.
4. Covic A, Siriopol D, Voroneanu L. Use of lung ultrasound for the assessment of volume status in CKD. Am J Kidney Dis. 2018;71(3):412–22.
5. Noble VE, Murray AF, Capp R, Sylvia-Reardon MH, Steele DJR, Liteplo A. Ultrasound assessment for extravascular lung water in patients undergoing hemodialysis. Time course for resolution. Chest. 2009;135(6):1433–9.
6. Mallamaci F, Benedetto FA, Tripepi R, Rastelli S, Castellino P, Tripepi G, et al. Detection of pulmonary congestion by chest ultrasound in dialysis patients. JACC Cardiovasc Imaging. 2010;3(6):586–94.
7. Trezzi M, Torzillo D, Ceriani E, Costantino G, Caruso S, Damavandi PT, et al. Lung ultrasonography for the assessment of rapid extravascular water variation: evidence from hemodialysis patients. Intern Emerg Med. 2013;8(5):409–15.
8. Vitturi N, Dugo M, Soattin M, Simoni F, Maresca L, Zagatti R, et al. Lung ultrasound during hemodialysis: the role in the assessment of volume status. Int Urol Nephrol. 2014;46(1):169.
9. Donadio C, Bozzoli L, Colombini E, Pisanu G, Ricchiuti G, Picano E, et al. Effective and timely evaluation of pulmonary congestion: qualitative comparison between lung ultrasound and thoracic bioelectrical impedance in maintenance hemodialysis patients. Medicine (Baltimore). 2015;94(6):e473.
10. Enia G, Torino C, Panuccio V, Tripepi R, Postorino M, Aliotta R, et al. Asymptomatic pulmonary congestion and physical functioning in hemodialysis patients. Clin J Am Soc Nephrol. 2013;8(8):1343–8.
11. Panuccio V, Enia G, Tripepi R, Torino C, Garozzo M, Battaglia GG, et al. Chest ultrasound and hidden lung congestion in peritoneal dialysis patients. Nephrol Dial Transplant. 2012;27(9):3601–5.
12. Enia G, Tripepi R, Panuccio V, Torino C, Garozzo M, Battaglia GG, et al. Pulmonary congestion and physical functioning in peritoneal dialysis patients. Perit Dial Int. 2012;32(5):531–6.
13. Paudel K, Kausik T, Visser A, Ramballi C, Fan SL. Comparing lung ultrasound with bioimpedance spectroscopy for evaluating hydration in peritoneal dialysis patients. Nephrology. 2015;20(1):1–5.

14. Torino C, Gargani L, Sicari R, Letachowicz K, Ekart R, Fliser D, et al. The agreement between auscultation and lung ultrasound in hemodialysis patients: the LUST study. Clin J Am Soc Nephrol. 2016;11(10):2005–11.
15. Allinovi M, Saleem M, Romagnani P, Nazerian P, Hayes W. Lung ultrasound: a novel technique for detecting fluid overload in children on dialysis. Nephrol Dial Transpl. 2016:1–6.
16. Marino F, Martorano C, Tripepi R, Bellantoni M, Tripepi G, Mallamaci F, Zoccali C. Subclinical pulmonary congestion is prevalent in nephrotic syndrome. Kidney Int. 2016;89(2):421–8.
17. Zoccali C, Torino C, Tripepi R, Tripepi G, D'Arrigo G, Postorino M, et al. Pulmonary congestion predicts cardiac events and mortality in ESRD. J Am Soc Nephrol. 2013;24(4):639–46.
18. Saad MM, Kamal J, Moussaly E, Karam B, Mansour W, Gobran E, Abbasi SH, Mahgoub A, Singh P, Hardy R, Das D, Brown C, Kapoor M, Demissie S, Kleiner MJ, El Charabaty E, El Sayegh SE. Relevance of B-lines on lung ultrasound in volume overload and pulmonary congestion: clinical correlations and outcomes in patients on hemodialysis. Cardiorenal Med. 2018;8(2):83–91.
19. Siriopol D, Hogas S, Voroneanu L, Onofriescu M, Apetrii M, Oleniuc M, et al. Predicting mortality in haemodialysis patients: a comparison between lung ultrasonography, bioimpedance data and echocardiography parameters. Nephrol Dial Transplant. 2013;28(July):2851–9.
20. Siriopol D, Voroneanu L, Hogas S, Apetrii M, Gramaticu A, Dumea R, et al. Bioimpedance analysis versus lung ultrasonography for optimal risk prediction in hemodialysis patients. Int J Cardiovasc Imaging. 2016;32(2):263–70.
21. Basso F, Milan Manani S, Cruz DN, Teixeira C, Brendolan A, Nalesso F, et al. Comparison and reproducibility of techniques for fluid status assessment in chronic hemodialysis patients. Cardiorenal Med. 2013;3(2):104–12.
22. Bedetti G, Gargani L, Corbisiero A, Frassi F, Poggianti E, Mottola G. Evaluation of ultrasound lung comets by hand-held echocardiography. Cardiovasc Ultrasound. 2006;4:34.
23. Noble VE, Lamhaut L, Capp R, Bosson N, Liteplo A, Marx J-S, et al. Evaluation of a thoracic ultrasound training module for the detection of pneumothorax and pulmonary edema by prehospital physician care providers. BMC Med Educ. 2009 Jan;9:3.
24. Gargani L, Sicari R, Raciti M, Serasini L, Passera M, Torino C, et al. Efficacy of a remote web-based lung ultrasound training for nephrologists and cardiologists: a LUST trial sub-project. Nephrol Dial Transplant. 2016:gfw329.
25. Jambrik Z, Monti S, Coppola V, Agricola E, Mottola G, Miniati M, et al. Usefulness of ultrasound lung comets as a nonradiologic sign of extravascular lung water. Am J Cardiol. 2004;93(10):1265–70.
26. Gargani L. Lung ultrasound: a new tool for the cardiologist. Cardiovasc Ultrasound. 2011;9:6.
27. Volpicelli G, Elbarbary M, Blaivas M, Lichtenstein DA, Mathis G, Kirkpatrick AW, et al. International evidence-based recommendations for point-of-care lung ultrasound. Intensive Care Med. 2012;38(4):577–91.
28. Gargani L, Volpicelli G. How I do it: lung ultrasound. Cardiovasc Ultrasound. 2014;12(1):1–10.
29. Narula J, Chandrashekhar Y, Braunwald E. Time to add a fifth pillar to bedside physical examination: inspection, palpation, percussion, auscultation, and insonation. JAMA Cardiol. 2018;3(4):346–50.
30. Di Nicolò P, Magnoni G, Granata A. In-depth review lung ultrasound in hemodialysis: a card to be played? Blood Purif. 2017;44:1–7.
31. Zoccali C. Lung ultrasound in the management of fluid volume in dialysis patients: potential usefulness. Semin Dial. 2017;30(1):6–9.
32. Sherman RA. Crackles and comets: lung ultrasound to detect pulmonary congestion in patients on dialysis is coming of age. Clin J Am Soc Nephrol. 2016:1–3.
33. Sicari R, Galderisi M, Voigt J-U, Habib G, Zamorano JL, Lancellotti P, et al. The use of pocket-size imaging devices: a position statement of the European Association of Echocardiography. Eur J Echocardiogr. 2011 Feb;12(2):85–7.

GPSR Compliance

The European Union's (EU) General Product Safety Regulation (GPSR) is a set of rules that requires consumer products to be safe and our obligations to ensure this.

If you have any concerns about our products, you can contact us on ProductSafety@springernature.com

In case Publisher is established outside the EU, the EU authorized representative is:

Springer Nature Customer Service Center GmbH
Europaplatz 3
69115 Heidelberg, Germany

Batch number: 10732801

Printed by Printforce, the Netherlands